Professor D. v. Zerssen,
mit herzlichsten Grüßen!

von

Andreas Marneros

Bonn 6. 1. 92

A. Marneros · N. C. Andreasen · M. T. Tsuang (Eds.)

Negative Versus Positive Schizophrenia

Contributors
N. C. Andreasen, G. E. Berrios, B. Bogerts, H. D. Brenner
W. T. Carpenter, T. J. Crow, A. Deister, C. Eggers, H. Häfner
A. Klimke, R. R. J. Lewine, J. A. Lieberman, A. Marneros
K. Maurer, P. McGuffin, C. S. Mellor, H. Y. Meltzer, H.-J. Möller
Ch. Mundt, H. Remschmidt, A. Rohde, R.-D. Stieglitz, M. T. Tsuang
D. P. van Kammen, and others

Springer-Verlag
Berlin Heidelberg New York
London Paris Tokyo Hong Kong
Barcelona Budapest

Professor Dr. med. ANDREAS MARNEROS
Psychiatrische Universitätsklinik
Sigmund-Freud-Straße 25, W-5300 Bonn, FRG

NANCY C. ANDREASEN, MD., Ph. D.
University of Iowa
Department of Psychiatry
500 Newton Road, Iowa City, IO 52242, USA

MING T. TSUANG, MD., Ph. D., D. Sc.
Harvard Departments of Psychiatry and Epidemiology
Brockton/West Roxbury VA Medical Center
940 Belmont Street, Brockton, MA 02401, USA

With 84 Figures and 111 Tables

ISBN 3-540-54388-0 Springer-Verlag Berlin Heidelberg New York
ISBN 0-387-54388-0 Springer-Verlag New York Berlin Heidelberg

Typesetting: Fotosatz-Service Köhler, W-8700 Würzburg, FRG
25/3130-543210 – Printed on acid-free paper

Preface

The positive versus negative distinction of schizophrenic disorders has promoted ongoing research. Phenomenology, psychopathology, biology, genetics, pharmacological and nonpharmacological treatment, psychosocial and longitudinal research: all have found a new focus of interest. This volume attempts to provide an unbiased picture of the status of American and European knowledge regarding the positive/negative distinction. Researchers from North America and Europe describe the relation of modern concepts of positive and negative symptomatology to the original models of Reynolds and Jackson. Integrating phenomenological, genetic, and biological factors, the authors depict current methods of assessing positive and negative symptomatology, differentiating between primary and secondary symptomatology, and using pharmacological and nonpharmacological treatment. The stability of positive and negative symptoms over time and evidence for the occurrence of separate positive and negative episodes over a long-term course of schizophrenia are extensively discussed in terms of their implications on the positive/negative construct. The relevance of the positive/negative dichotomy to child and adolescent schizophrenia is also debated.

The main aim of this book is not to advocate a single concept and present only arguments supporting it, but to discuss important controversies. Problems concerning a concept cannot be solved by ignoring them. However, unanswered questions may be resolved through discussion, debate, and constructive compromise.

A concept cannot be useful and fruitful if it is monolithic, rigid, and unamenable to change and development. A psychiatric concept can be beneficial for the patients and useful for scientific research only if it is able to integrate new developments, adapt to criticism, and address open questions.

This approach was our motivation and our goal in bringing international experts on the topic together around the table. Our intent in editing this book is to present and foster constructive scientific dialogue.

Autumn, 1991

A. Marneros, Bonn, FRG
N. C. Andreasen, Iowa City, USA
M. T. Tsuang, Boston, USA

Contents

List of Contributors

You will find the address at the beginning of the respective contribution

Dichotomies and Other Distinctions in Schizophrenia

A. MARNEROS[1] and M. T. TSUANG[2]

Introduction

Homogeneity in psychiatric disorders is a rare phenomenon. The richness of variation in phenomenology, patterns in the course, the quality and quantity of persisting aberrations, treatment response, possible etiopathological agents, etc. creates a very complex picture of mental disorders. Even when some variables are sufficient to mark and distinguish some relatively distinct groups of disorders, such as schizophrenic disorders, affective disorders, or organic mental disorders, some degree of heterogeneity always remains.

This state of affairs was one of the reasons why the early psychiatrists preferred either asceticism in classification, like Griesinger (1817–1868), in Germany, who distinguished only between mental exaltation and mental depression; or "poly pragmatism in classification", like Kahlbaum (1828–1899), also in Germany, who described a plethora of types in mental diseases. The heterogeneity of mental disorders was one of the more serious difficulties faced by Kraepelin (1856–1926) during his lifelong efforts in the classification of mental diseases. In Kraepelin's formulation, dementia praecox and manic-depressive insanity are groups of phenomenologically diverse disorders. In the same fashion, Bleuler (1911, 1950) did not describe "schizophrenia," but "the group of schizophrenias."

Within the heterogeneous construct of schizophrenia, Kraepelin distinguished between four subtypes: paranoid-hallucinatory, catatonic, hebephrenic, and the simplex type. These subtypes are similar to those postulated by Bleuler and the distinctions between them have been accepted for many decades.

Regarding affective disorders – apart from various other distinctions – the dichotomy between bipolar and unipolar types differing on several levels is well established (Angst 1980, 1986; Angst et al. 1973, 1978, 1980; Goodwin and Jamison 1990; Marneros et al. 1990a, b, c, 1991a).

A bipolar and unipolar distinction is also accepted for schizoaffective disorders, perhaps in addition to a schizo-dominant and affect-dominant distinction (Marneros et al. 1989a, b, c; overviews in Marneros and Tsuang 1986, 1990). Aside from their phenomenological validity, these two dimensions

[1] Psychiatrische Universitätsklinik, Sigmund-Freud-Straße 25, W-5300 Bonn 1, FRG
[2] Harvard Depts. of Psychiatry and Epidemiology, Brockton/West Roxbury VA Medical Center, 940 Belmont Street, Brockton, MA 02401, USA

A. Marneros / N. C. Andreasen / M. T. Tsuang (Eds.)
Negative Versus Positive Schizophrenia

in schizoaffective disorders are associated with external validators, such as patterns in the course, outcome, premorbid and social variables, treatment response, etc. Clear-cut distinctions in the group of schizophrenias, however, remain much more elusive.

Distinctions Within the Group of Schizophrenic Disorders

The classical distinction between paranoid-hallucinatory, catatonic, hebephrenic, and simplex forms remained for many decades the primary approach to subgroup schizophrenia. However, the correctness of the classical distinctions was, from the very beginning, associated with some doubts which continued to increase over the years: for example, the hebephrenic type is not always manifested in very young people; the paranoid-hallucinatory form frequently shifts into another type; the catatonic type has become increasingly infrequent, especially after the introduction of pharmacological treatment and long-term out-patient treatment; and the simplex form did not always prove to be identifiable, or at least proved only with difficulty to be distinguishable from personality disorders, organic mental disorders, or other types of mental illness. In addition, the Kraepelinian distinction did not have any place for the so-called mixed states, i.e., what we would today call schizoaffective disorders. The same concerns apply to Bleuler's classification system (1911, 1950). The inclusion of the mixed psychoses (i.e., the schizoaffective disorders) in the category of schizophrenia eventually proved to be incorrect (see overview in Marneros 1989; Marneros and Tsuang 1986, 1990). Nevertheless, the classical distinction continued in modern classification systems, such as the ICD-9 and in modified form in DSM-III. In DSM-III and in DSM-III-R, the hebephrenic type was identified as the "disorganized type," and the mixed type as "undifferentiated."

Huber (1957) added another type of schizophrenia to the classical distinctions, the so-called "coenaesthetic schizophrenia", which is mainly characterized by abnormal body sensations which are not due to any physical disease. A residual type was also added (DSM-III, DSM-III-R). Independently of phenomenology, other distinctions – mainly dichotomies – described other aspects, such as prognostic aspects: good-/poor-prognosis schizophrenia (Fowler et al. 1972; Taylor and Abrams 1975), process/non-process schizophrenia (Stephens 1970), benign/non-benign schizophrenia (Blau 1957), and reactive or psychogenic versus non-reactive schizophrenia (Strömgren 1986; Retterstoel 1978). A pseudoneurotic or a pseudopsychopathic type of schizophrenia was also described (Hoch 1912).

One of the most fruitful divisions in schizophrenia, which has stimulated research on clinical strategies, is the positive/negative dichotomy introduced recently by Andreasen (1982, 1983, 1990a, b).

Positive/Negative Distinction

Andreasen identified two highly reliable and internally consistent groups of symptoms, namely the negative and the positive group (Andreasen 1990a, b; Andreasen et al., 1991). The terms "negative" and "positive" refer, respectively, to a loss in function and "more than normal" functions. Andreasen's formulation marks the beginning of modern research in the subject, although the origin of the positive/negative distinction in psychiatry is an old one (Berrios 1985, 1991). Apart from the conceptualization of consistent symptomatology in schizophrenia, the positive/negative dichotomy formed the foundation of research in etiopathogenesis, in course and outcome variables, in treatment strategies, and in biology and genetics. The question of whether positive and negative symptomatology represented distinct syndromes or even distinct diseases became the subject of debate (Andreasen 1990b). The most comprehensive formulation was that of Crow (1980), who distinguished between type I (positive) and type II (negative) schizophrenia. Type I was characterized by good premorbid functioning, relatively favorable outcome, acute onset, good response to treatment, and hyperdopaminergic activity in a structurally normal brain. Type II was characterized by poor premorbid functioning, impaired cognition and poor response to treatment, as well as structural brain abnormalities. In a similar fashion, Farmer et al. (1983, 1984) developed a formulation of H-type and P-type schizophrenia, corresponding to the traditional distinction between hebephrenic and paranoid schizophrenia. Researchers are still working towards identifying the most relevant biological, genetic, and pharmacological correlates to a negative or positive phenomenology (Andreasen et al., 1991; Bogerts et al., 1991; McGuffin et al., 1991; Meltzer, 1991; Möller, 1991; Tsuang et al., 1991; van Kammen et al. 1991).

Unanswered Questions and Perspectives

Criticisms of the negative/positive dichotomy have come mainly from psychopathologists and investigators of the long-term course of schizophrenia: phenomenologically similar symptoms identified as negative symptoms are assumed to be secondary to positive symptoms or to other psychological and social disturbances caused by the illness (Carpenter et al., 1991; Mundt, this volume; Brenner et al., 1991). It could be a source of error if "symptoms" having protective functioning are assumed to be a result of a deficit or loss of functions (Carpenter et al., 1991; Mundt, 1985; Mundt, 1991; Lewine, 1991). Studies of negative symptoms in schizophrenia should attend to their primary or secondary nature. Another essential criticism of the negative/positive dichotomy concerns the nature of the positive symptoms: positive symptoms are assumed to be developmental stages of so-called basic symptoms (most of them are negative symptoms) (Huber 1983). In fact, positive and negative symptoms are interdependent, and they exist in parallel (Häfner and Maurer 1991, Maurer and Häfner, 1991).

Certainly the most important questions regarding the value of the negative/positive distinction have come from longitudinal investigations. The classical longitudinal studies of schizophrenia, with an observation time of more than 20 years, found that the classical subtypes of schizophrenia changed during the long-term course (Bleuler 1972; Ciompi and Müller 1976; Huber et al. 1979; Marneros et al. 1991; Tsuang et al. 1979; Winokur et al. 1985).

The research of the Mannheim group of Häfner and of Marneros and co-workers, using modern scales of assessment of negative and positive symptoms, confirmed the findings of the above-mentioned clinical studies. The long-term course of schizophrenia seems to be bimorphous regarding positive and negative symptomatology in general (Marneros et al. 1991a, b).

An essential question which has to be answered is: how can distinct phenomenological subtypes be correlated with biological, genetic, or outcome parameters if they are not longitudinally stable, but often change from one to the other? Assuming that the long-term course of schizophrenia is bimorphous or polymorphous, then the positive/negative approach has to be incorporated in a manner other than a simple dichotomy between pure "positive" and pure "negative" subtypes. Examples of such an approach would include assessing the relevance of predominance of groups of symptoms over the course of illness, or the relevance of the type of initial episode.

References

Andreasen NC (1982) Negative syndromes in schizophrenia: definition and reliability. Arch Gen Psychiatry 39:784–788

Andreasen NC (1983) The scale for assessment of negative symptoms. University of Iowa: Iowa City

Andreasen NC (1990a) Positive and negative symptoms: historical and conceptual aspects. In: Andreasen NC (ed) Schizophrenia: Positive and negative symptoms and syndromes. Karger, Basel

Andreasen NC (1990b) Methods for assessing positive and negative symptoms. In: Andreasen NC (ed) Schizophrenia: Positive and negative symptoms and syndromes. Karger, Basel

Andreasen NC, Flaum M, Arndt S, Alliger R, Swayze VW (1991) Positive and negative symptomes: assessment and validity. In: Marneros A, Andreasen NC, Tsuang MT (eds) Negative vs. positive schizophrenia. Springer, Berlin Heidelberg New York

Angst J (1980) Verlauf unipolarer depressiver, bipolar manisch-depressiver und schizoaffektiver Erkrankungen und Psychosen. Fortschr Neurol Psychiatr 48:3–30

Angst J (1986) The course of affective disorders. Psychopathology 119 (Suppl 2):47–52

Angst J, Baastrup P, Grof P, Hippius H, Pöldinger W, Weis P (1973) The course of monopolar depression and bipolar psychoses. Psychiatr Neurol Neurochir 76:489–500

Angst J, Felder W, Frey R, Stassen HH (1978) The course of affective disorders. I. Change of diagnosis of monopolar, unipolar, and bipolar illness. Arch Psychiatr Nervenkr 226:57–64

Angst J, Frey R, Lohmeyer B, Zerbin-Rüdin E (1980) Bipolar manic-depressive psychoses: results of a genetic investigation. Hum Genet 55:237–254

Berrios GE (1985) Positive and negative symptoms and Jackson. Arch Gen Psychiatry 42:95–97

Berrios GE (1991) Positive and negative signals: a conceptual history. In: Marneros A, Andreasen NC, Tsuang MT (eds) Negative vs. positive schizophrenia. Springer, Berlin Heidelberg New York
Blau A (1957) Benign schizophrenia. Arch Neurol Psychiatry 78:605–611
Bleuler E (1911) Dementia praecox oder Gruppe der Schizophrenien. In: Aschaffenburg G (ed) Handbuch der Psychiatrie. Spezieller Teil, Vol. 4. Deuticke, Leipzig
Bleuler E (1950) Dementia praecox or the group of schizophrenias. International University Press, New York
Bleuler M (1972) Die schizophrenen Geistesstörungen im Lichte langjähriger Kranken- und Familiengeschichten. Springer, Berlin Heidelberg New York
Bogerts B, Falkai P, Degreef G, Lieberman J (1991) Neuropathological and brain imaging studies in positive and negative schizophrenia. In: Marneros A, Andreasen NC, Tsuang MT (eds) Negative vs. positive schizophrenia. Springer, Berlin Heidelberg New York
Brenner HD, Hodel B, Merlo MCG (1991) Nonpharmacological treatment concepts of negative symptomatology. In: Marneros A, Andreasen NC, Tsuang MT (eds) Negative vs. positive schizophrenia. Springer, Berlin Heidelberg New York
Carpenter WT, Buchanan RW, Kirkpatrick B, Thaker G, Tamminga C (1991) Negative Symptoms: A critique of current approaches. In: Marneros A, Andreasen NC, Tsuang MT (eds) Negative vs. positive schizophrenia. Springer, Berlin Heidelberg New York
Ciompi L, Müller C (1976) Lebensweg und Alter der Schizophrenen. Eine katamnestische Langzeitstudie bis ins Senium. Springer, Berlin Heidelberg New York
Crow TJ (1980) Molecular pathology of schizophrenia: More than one disease process? Br Med J (Clin Res) 280:66–68
Farmer AE, McGuffin P, Spitznagel E (1983) Heterogeneity in schizophrenia. A cluster analytic approach. Psychiatry Res 8:1–12
Farmer AE, McGuffin P, Gottesman II (1984) Searching for the split in schizophrenia: A twin study perspective. Psychiatry Res 13:109–118
Fowler RC, McCabe MS, Cadoret RJ, Winokur G (1972) The validity of good prognosis schizophrenia. Arch Gen Psychiatry 26:182–185
Goodwin FK, Jamison KR (1990) Manic-depressive illness. Oxford University Press, New York
Häfner H, Maurer K (1991) Are there two types of schizophrenia? – True onset and sequence of positive and negative syndromes prior to first admission – In: Marneros A, Andreasen NC, Tsuang MT (eds) Negative vs. positive schizophrenia. Springer, Berlin Heidelberg New York
Hoch A (1912) Die Bedeutung der Symptomkomplexe in der Psychiatrie. Zentralbl Gesamte Neurol Psychiatr 12:540–551
Huber G (1957) Pneumencephalographische und psychopathologische Bilder bei endogenen Psychosen. Springer, Berlin Heidelberg New York
Huber G (1983) Das Konzept substratnaher Basissymptome und seine Bedeutung für Theorie und Therapie schizophrener Erkrankungen. Nervenarzt 54:23–32
Huber G, Gross G, Schüttler R (1979) Schizophrenie. Eine verlaufs- und sozialpsychiatrische Langzeitstudie. Springer, Berlin Heidelberg New York
Lewine RJ (1991) Anhedonia and the amotivational state of schizophrenia. In: Marneros A, Andreasen NC, Tsuang MT (eds) Negative vs. positive schizophrenia. Springer, Berlin Heidelberg New York
Lieberman JA, Jody D, Alvir JMJ, Borenstein M, Mayerhoff DI (1991) Negative symptoms in schizophrenia: relationship to positive symptoms and outcome. In: Marneros A, Andreasen NC, Tsuang MT (eds) Negative vs. positive schizophrenia. Springer: Berlin Heidelberg New York
Marneros A (1989) Schizoaffektive Psychosen. Diagnose, Therapie und Prophylaxe. Springer, Berlin Heidelberg New York
Marneros A, Tsuang MT (1986) Schizoaffective psychoses. Springer, Berlin Heidelberg New York

Marneros A, Tsuang MT (eds) (1990) Affective and schizoaffective disorders. Similarities and differences. Springer, Berlin Heidelberg New York
Marneros A, Deister A, Rohde A (1989a) Unipolar and bipolar schizoaffective disorders: a comparative study. I. Premorbid and sociodemographic features. Eur Arch Psychiatry Neurol Sci 239:158–163
Marneros A, Rohde A, Deister A (1989b) Unipolar and bipolar schizoaffective disorders: a comparative study. II. Long-term course. Eur Arch Psychiatry Neurol Sci 239:158–163
Marneros A, Deister A, Rohde A, Jünemann (1989c) Unipolar and bipolar schizoaffective disorders: a comparative study. III. Long-term outcome. Eur Arch Psychiatry Neurol Sci 239:171–176
Marneros A, Deister A, Rohde A (1990a) The concept of distinct but voluminous bipolar and unipolar diseases. I: The bipolar diseases. Eur Arch Psychiatry Clin Neurosci 240:77–84
Marneros A, Rohde A, Deister A (1990b) The concept of distinct but voluminous bipolar and unipolar diseases. II: The unipolar diseases. Eur Arch Psychiatry Clin Neurosci 240:85–89
Maerneros A, Deister A, Rohde A (1990c) The concept of distinct but voluminous bipolar and unipolar diseases. III: Unipolar and bipolar comparison. Eur Arch Psychiatry Clin Neurosci 240:90–95
Marneros A, Deister A, Rohde A (1991a) Affektive, schizoaffektive und schizophrene Psychosen. Eine vergleichende Langzeitstudie. Springer, Berlin Heidelberg New York
Marneros A, Deister A, Rohde A (1991b) Long-term investigations in stability of negative/positive distinction. In: Marneros A, Andreasen NC, Tsuang NC (eds) Negative versus positive schizophrenia. Springer, Berlin Heidelberg New York
Maurer K, Häfner H (1991) Dependence, independence or interdependence of positive and negative symptoms. In: Marneros A, Andreasen NC, Tsuang MT (eds) Negative vs. positive schizophrenia. Springer, Berlin Heidelberg New York
McGuffin P, Harvey I, Williams M (1991) The negative/positive dichotomy: Does it make sense from the perspective of the genetic researcher? In: Marneros A, Andreasen NC, Tsuang MT (eds) Negative vs. positive schizophrenia. Springer, Berlin Heidelberg New York
Meltzer HY (1991) The Effect of Clozapine and other atypical antipsychotic drugs on negative symptoms. In: Marneros A, Andreasen NC, Tsuang MT (eds) Negative vs. positive schizophrenia. Springer: Berlin Heidelberg New York
Möller HJ (1991) Typical neuroleptics in the treatment of positive and negative symptoms. In: Marneros A, Andreasen NC, Tsuang NC (eds) Negative versus positive schizophrenia. Springer, Berlin Heidelberg New York
Mundt C (1985) Das Apathiesyndrom der Schizophrenen. Eine psychopathologische und computertomographische Untersuchung. Springer, Berlin Heidelberg New York
Mundt C (1991) Constituting reality – its decline and repair in the long-term course of schizophrenic psychoses. In: Marneros A, Andreasen NC, Tsuang MT (eds) Negative vs. positive schizophrenia. Springer, Berlin Heidelberg New York
Retterstoel N (1978) The scandinavian concept of reactive psychosis, schizophreniform psychosis and schizophrenia. Psychiatr Clin 11:180–187
Stephens JH (1970) Long-term course and prognosis in schizophrenia. Sem Psychiatry 2:464–485
Strömgren E (1986) Reactive (psychogenic) psychoses and their relations to schizoaffective psychoses. In: Marneros A, Tsuang MT (eds) Schizoaffective psychoses. Springer, Berlin Heidelberg New York
Taylor MA, Abrams R (1975) Manic-dpressive illness and good prognosis schizophrenia. Am J Psychiatry 132:741–742
Tsuang MT, Woolson RF, Fleming JA (1979) Long-term outcome of major psychoses. Arch Gen Psychiatry 36:1295
Tsuang MT, Gilbertson NW, Faraone SV (1991) Genetic transmission of negative and positive symptoms in the biological relatives of schizophrenics. In: Marneros A, Andreasen NC, Tsuang MT (eds) Negative vs. positive schizophrenia. Springer, Berlin Heidelberg New York

van Kammen DP, Peters JL, Yao J, van Kammen WB, Neylan T, Shaw D (1991) Noradrenergic mechanisms, state dependency, and negative symptoms in schizophrenia. In: Greden JF, Tandon R (eds) Negative schizophrenic symptoms: pathophysiology and clinical implications. American Psychiatric Press, Washington DC

Winokur G, Scharfetter C, Angst J (1985) Stability of psychotic symptomatology (delusions, hallucinations), affective syndromes, and schizophrenic symptoms (thought disorders, incongruent affect) over episodes in remitting psychoses. Eur Arch Psychiatry Neurol Sci 234:303–307

Positive and Negative Signals: A Conceptual History

G. E. Berrios [1]

The terms "positive" and "negative", used to categorize the symptoms of schizophrenia, have "burst in the horizon as a recurrent comet" (Zubin 1985). More popular, perhaps, amongst researchers than clinicians, they have thrived almost beyond the reach of evaluation. Unimpressed by fashion, the conceptual historian must ask:

1. What do these terms contribute (that others do not) to the understanding of the symptoms of schizophrenia? In the past, it must be remembered, other (less successful) pairs of words have been used for the same purpose: primary versus secondary, first rank versus second rank, florid versus deficit, active versus passive. etc.
2. What would be *lost* if the terms "positive" and "negative" were replaced, say, by some meaningless initials?
3. Are the categories "positive" and "negative" symptom-specific to schizophrenia? Would understanding of *other* mental disorders be improved by their use? If so, could this extra-understanding be specified? and
4. Is their popularity due only to scientific reasons? In this regard, scientific or "internal" reasons (i.e. those pertaining to the facts of observation), must be distinguished from "external factors" (extra-scientific, non-cognitive, social, etc.) which reflect the power structures controlling fashion in the psychiatric community. Terms may become fashionable not because they add anything to *knowledge*, but because they are favoured by forceful individuals or by "invisible Colleges" controlling funds, research and publications (Blashfield 1982; Latour 1988).

Sponsors of the "positive and negative" distinction may feel that these questions are naive or that they have already been answered. Perusal of the recent literature, however, indicates that this is not, in fact, the case. So, what is the uncommitted scholar to do? Answers should be sought in three evidential fields: historico-conceptual, clinical and statistical. This chapter deals only with the first of these areas of inquiry.

Unpacking the conceptual furniture of the "positive/negative" distinction reveals three semantically sequential layers: the oldest, constituted by original meanings; the intermediate, by historical readjustments; and the top-most, by

[1] Department of Psychiatry, University of Cambridge, Addenbrooke's Hospital (Level 4), Hills Road, Cambridge CB2 2QQ, United Kingdom

A. Marneros / N. C. Andreasen / M. T. Tsuang (Eds.)
Negative Versus Positive Schizophrenia

the shining definitions deposited by current sponsors. This palimpsest should be studied from three points of view: meanings and usages of the words "positive" and "negative"; their referents (i.e. what do these terms "positivise" or "negativise"); and the nature of their relationship (whether, for example, they can only work in tandem).

Meaning and Usage of the Words Positive and Negative

According to current clinical lore, the term "positive" describes a symptom whose content is an exaggeration of a function or is a behaviour "that normal people do not have". Hence its contents can be said to be active, florid, describable and measurable. A "negative" symptom, on the other hand, describes a deficit or an absence of a function or signal, a vacuum, a state of "not having a behaviour that normal people have".

Both terms were first used by Sir John Russell Reynolds (1828–1896) to refer to two *independent* forms of physical sign.Reynolds, a grandson of Henry Revell Reynolds FRS (Goulstonian Lecturer and Harveian Orator) was born in Romsey, Hampshire in 1828. In 1846 he started his medical career at University College, London, where he became a medallist in Physiology, Anatomy and Medicine. He was a disciple of Marshall Hall, and in 1862 became professor of Medicine at his old medical school. In addition to his classical work on epilepsy, after 1866 he also published a "*System of Medicine*". He was awarded his FRS in 1869 having had the support of Sharpey, Carpenter and Fergusson. Reynolds was appointed to the National Hospital in 1862 and resigned in 1869, so he and Jackson overlapped for about 5 years (personal communication from Dr MacDonald Critchley CBE). Reynolds first mentioned the terms "positive" and "negative" in 1857 in a lecture he gave to the North London Medical Society (Berrios 1985). Reynolds died in 1896 (Reynolds 1896).

The categories positive and negative were brought together by J. H. Jackson (1835–1911), who linked them both logically and ontologically (Berrios 1985). Jackson formulated this association in evolutionary terms (López Piñero 1973; Dewhurst 1982; Smith 1982). Non-evolutionary forms of hierarchical organisation of mental functions, however, had been in circulation at least since the time of Maine de Biran and Jouffroy (both of whom held a creationist view of such hierarchies) (Delay 1942; Paulus 1941). *Evolutionism* refers here to a "family of ideas which affirms that the universe and some or all of its parts have undergone irreversible, cumulative changes such that the number, variety, and complexity of the parts have increased" (Goudge 1973, p. 174).

Hierarchical models of mental function (i.e. the view that mental faculties are stratified, with the higher ones controlling or inhibiting the lower ones) may be couched in both evolutionary and non-evolutionary terms. According to the former, the order in which the mental faculties have been deposited is controlled by a natural mechanism called *evolution*; this model predates

Darwin's and has many variants. For example, French spiritualist philosophers such as Théodore Simon Jouffroy (1796–1842) sponsored a "creationist" view, i.e. that mental faculties and the manner of their organization had been fixed by God at the time of the creation (for further details on these philosophers, some of them important to the history of psychiatry, see Benrubi 1933; Ravaisson 1984; Taine 1901).

Jackson, on the other hand, believed that consciousness (a human function) was diffusely represented on the cortex (Riese 1943) and that the older layers or faculties belonged to our animal ancestors. Jackson's conception of positive and negative symptoms and of how they relate to each other was based upon (a) an hierarchical view of the functions of the brain, (b) a dismissal of the notion of "mental" functions (based on the assumption that all functions were organic), (c) an evolutionary view of the formation of the functional hierarchy, (d) an anti-localisationistic view of the anatomy of the brain, and (e) a strong conception of "dissolution" as a mechanism parallel to evolution (López Piñero 1973; Dewhurst 1982). Each component Jackson (acknowledgedly) borrowed from a different writer. Surprisingly, however, not all his attributions can be confirmed by historical analysis. Jackson's model was influential, particularly in French psychiatry, and some of these developments will be discussed presently.

Ribot. In his "*Diseases of memory*" (1882), Théodule Armand Ribot (1839–1916) used the word "negative" in a Jacksonian sense:

"Hypermnesia would then only be the result of conditions entirely negative; regression would result, not from a normal return to consciousness, but from the suppression of more activity and more intense states, like a weak voice that could only make itself heard when more powerful organs of speech had relapsed into silence" (pp 183–184).

Ribot was a "Normalien" who became professor of Experimental Psychology at the Sorbonne in 1885, and at the Collège de France in 1889 (Cleparède 1916). A disciple of H. A. Taine (1828–1893) and J. E. Renan (1823–1892), he entertained a positivist, physiological, anti-faculty psychology view of mental functions (Benrubi 1933). He was influenced by Herbert Spencer (1820–1903) and translated the latter's "*Principles of Psychology*" into French (Delay 1953). The influence of Spencer and, particularly, of Jackson shows in books written during the second period of his life, characterized by a strong interest in psychopathology (Delay 1953). Jackson quoted with approval Ribot's hierarchical view of nervous function and his views on the cerebral cortex (Jackson 1931, vol 2, p. 82).

Ribot's so-called law of regression (describing the chronological order in which information dissipates in retrograde amnesia) is based on his evolutionary views. Indeed, in "*Diseases of memory*", he attempted to show that memory was not a simple mental function [as leading philosophers in France, like Victor Cousin (1792–1867), had postulated] but a complex phenomenon, as attested by the various clinical modes in which it broke down. Following W. B. Carpenter (1813–1885) and E. Hering (1834–1918), Ribot developed a biologistic notion of memory (Walser 1974; Gasser 1988).

De Clérambault. Another French writer to use the positive/negative terminology was Gaëtan Gatian de Clérambault. This great alienist, born in Bourges, France, in 1871, trained first as a decorator and lawyer and then as a physician (Anguera 1984). From 1905 on, he worked at the Infirmerie Spéciale de la Préfecture de Police (Anguera 1989), a section of the famous Dépôt or Central Police Station which E. C. Lasègue (1816–1883) had started in 1872 (Pichot 1984, p. 27; Soubrier and Gourevitch 1984). His views on acute mental disorders, organicity, psychoses and mental automatism reflect, however, the type of patients which he saw at the "Infirmerie". He is known in Anglo-Saxon psychiatry for his views on erotomania (e.g. Segal 1989) which, in fact, constitute an aside to his work (Brousseau 1934; Ey 1952). Towards the end of his life, De Clérambault suffered from a right eye cataract, and after unhelpful surgery (which he described in vivid detail; Clérambault 1987, pp. 821–838) he killed himself in 1934.

At the 1927 Congress of French alienists in Blois, Clérambault was asked to comment on a paper by Paul Nayrac summarising French views on "mental automatism" (see Clérambault 1987; Nayrac 1974). Nayrac had concluded that:

"The human mind has its own rules which normally allow it to carry out certain actions automatically... in the pathological state normal automatism shows variations... the pathological causes are often unknown but it is likely that they are always organic... it seems that the concept of automatism may be particularly useful for the understanding of certain phenomena which occur in dementia praecox and obsessional illness" (pp 428–429).

The words "positive" and "negative" occurred once in Nayrac's presentation: "frequently motor automatism does not have a *positive* character. It may be *negative* or rather inhibitory. Patients often complain that they are being prevented from making this or that movement or from acting in a certain way..." (p. 416; may underlining). This paragraph is important on two accounts: firstly, because it highlights the view that negative symptoms may follow a temporary *inhibition* of function (on this concept see section below); and secondly, because it shows that subjective elements (i.e. what the patients actually experience) entered into the decision as to whether a particular symptom was to be called positive or negative. In this case, the subject's *feeling of passivity* induced Nayrac to consider his symptom as "negative".

This metaphorical usage re-appeared in Strauss et al. (1974), who used "the terms primarily descriptively without necessarily implying Jackson's theoretical conceptions..." (p. 65). In a later paper, Strauss (1985) suggested that even classing certain symptoms as "negative" may not add much to their understanding as they are likely to have "various etiologies, biological relationships, treatment response characteristics..." (p. 458). Strauss also made the penetrating observation that although "integration" might be desirable once "the pieces are on the table, they will never fit neatly together again" (p. 458).

De Clérambault (1987) started his comments by saying:

"To avoid the confusion generated by the terms normal or pathological automatism, I shall simply refer to Syndrome S (pp. 580–581)...Syndrome S includes a series of *positive, negative and mixed phenomena*, it can be found in a number of psychoses, both transient and chronic, and the 'phenomena' in question will vary accordingly" (p. 581; my italics).

In fact, de Clérambault had first used the positive/negative terminology in 1924 in a presentation to the Société Clinique de Maladies Mentales when he classified the symptoms of psychoses into (a) continuous or episodic *positive* processes, (b) *negative* processes and (c) *mixed* processes. The clinical states included under each heading cannot readily be fitted into any current classification. The point, however, is that neither in 1924 nor in 1927 did Clérambault presume an evolutionary or hierarchical link between the functions underlying his negative and positive symptoms. In fact, it is even unclear whether he believed that the said symptoms were related to specific mental functions at all. This explains why he had no difficulty in combining positive and negative processes in his mixed group (e.g. "substitutions of thinking" and "forgetting"). Negative phenomena, according to de Clérambault, resulted from "deficits" or "inhibitions". His descriptive technique consisted in naming groups of symptoms by a general characteristic without specifying the mental functions or modules that might be involved in each case. This is, indeed, redolent of current Anglo-Saxon usage. De Clérambault was an idiosyncratic, often Delphic writer, who rarely gave his sources and, as far as I am aware, never quoted Jackson.

The Concept of Inhibition. An important concept to the Jacksonian model, the concept of inhibition, was introduced into medicine by Brown-Séquard (Herrick 1901). He defined it thus:

"inhibition is an act in virtue of which a property or activity ... disappears, totally or partially, slowly or rapidly, temporarily or permanently, and in one or in many organs of the body, due to the influence of an irritation of the nervous system ..." (Brown-Séquard 1889, p. 1).

The mechanism of inhibition was first used in psychiatry to account for stupor (Berrios 1981, pp. 472–473).

Jackson considered it as a fundamental physiological mechanism:

"I have nothing to say on the nature of the inhibitory process. I would urge, however, that here, as in other cases we should distinguish between the psychical and the physical; we cannot legitimately speak of any mental processes as inhibitory of any physical processes, any more than we can speak of them as producing movements ..." (Jackson 1931, vol 2, p. 481).

The mechanisms of inhibition and repression have also been compared (Grinker 1939).

Von Monakow and Mourgue. Yet another interesting usage of the positive/negative distinction is provided by the work of Von Monakow and Mourgue. Constantin Von Monakow was born in Bobretzovo, north of Moscow, in 1853, and brought up in Switzerland (Mourgue 1931; Yakolev 1970). An eminent neuropathologist (his most important book is entitled "*Gehirnpathologie*"), after the First World War he became deeply interested in the conceptual aspects of neuropsychiatry. He died in 1930.

In 1918, Raoul Mourgue (by then already a distinguished neuropsychiatrist and historian of neurobiology) "by chance" discovered Von Monakow's monograph on "*Brain localization*" in the Bibliothèque National, and after corresponding for a while the two men decided to write a book on the conceptual aspects of neuropsychiatry. This monumental and much neglected volume appeared in 1928. The influence of their views can be found in Goldstein, Schilder and the great holistic neurologists of the inter-bellum period.

Von Monakow and Mourgue criticized and improved upon Jackson's view, and this contributed to the acceptance of Jacksonism in France. Their criticisms were that Jackson had (a) applied to higher mental functions principles obtained from the analysis of disturbances of lower functions (i.e. motor and sensory), and (b) had not developed a concept of cerebral centre, as required by the deep semantics of his positive/negative distinction. They also claimed that Jackson's approach was (c) cross-sectional and neglected longitudinal modes of disintegration, characteristic of the nervous system, (d) that his concept of lesion was an exogenous one, and "instinct" did not play a function in his model, and (e) that Jackson's conception of "dissolution" was too mechanical, and did not take into account the fact that the organism is also endowed with internal drives and mechanisms for self-repairing and the maintenance of homoeostasis (Von Monakow and Mourgue 1928, pp. 172–173).

There is little doubt that the first three points are correct. Von Monakow and Mourgue (1928) themselves were not very keen on the terms positive and negative although their model remained Jacksonian in structure. They went on to develop important views, whose wider diffusion was marred by the coining of complex neologisms and by the introduction of latter day vitalist principles such as "hormé". In their seminal 1928 book, they even tried to apply their model to the analysis of schizophrenia (pp. 282–322).

Ey. The fourth twentieth century writer to have used the positive/negative distinction is Henri Ey (1900–1977). A disciple of H. Claude, he converted the mental hospital of Bonneval, where he worked for 37 years, into one of the psychiatric shrines of France. He was a prolific writer, and his conceptual and historical work somewhat outweighs his clinical contribution (Albernhe and Roux 1990). His more important books include the three volumes of "*Études Psychiatriques*" (1948–1954), a monograph on "*Consciousness*" (1963), and the magnificent "*Treatise on Hallucinations*" (1974). He attempted (unsuccessfully) to link the concepts of traditional French psychiatry (which he both loved and hated) with the Jacksonian paradigm and psychoanalysis. Few of his writings have been published in English (Ey 1962; Evans 1972). The main problem with Ey's "organ-dynamic" model is that it has not generated many testable hypotheses.

Ey (1975) took up the views put forward by Von Monakow and Mourgue and went on to criticise Jackson for assuming that anatomical "dissolution" necessarily led to or meant psychological dissolution. He believed that

Jackson's much praised "principle of concomitance" was not sufficient to explain this extrapolation. Ey himself emphasized a "dialectic interaction" between positive and negative symptoms and, according to whether the disorganization occurred in a cross-sectional or a longitudinal frame, he classified negative symptoms into "synchronic and diachronic". These two terms, not very well known in Anglo-Saxon psychiatry, originated at the beginning of this century in the linguistic theory of Ferdinand de Saussure (1916) and have had some influence in the historiography and philosophy of the social sciences. In the Saussurian definition, "synchrony" refers to the system formed by the simultaneous relationship that linguistic facts hold with one other; "diachrony" to the "happenings" or "changes" occurring in a linguistic system, and to their operative factors. De Saussure conceived of synchrony and diachrony as two different forms of explanation (structural and historical, respectively) and emphasised the former as a counterbalance to nineteenth century historicism (Koerner 1982; Malberg 1986).

The unbalanced application of this model has generated much theoretical debate, but it is likely that the two approaches are complementary (Coseriu 1978; Ducrot and Todorov 1972). A modified version of this model has served well the understanding of the history of descriptive psychopathology considered as a system of descriptions (Lanteri-Laura 1966; Berrios 1984). Ey believed that positive symptoms could result from either type of disorganization. For example, a toxic psychosis resulted from *synchronic* (i.e. cross-sectional) disorganization of the structure of consciousness; in this situation the commonest positive symptom were *visual hallucinations*. In schizophrenia, on the other hand, there was a longitudinal (*diachronic*) disintegration of the self, leading to the development of *delusions* as the core positive symptom.

Ey was influenced by Julien Rouart, a psychoanalyst with whom he coauthored an important book on Jackson (Ey and Rouart 1938). Rouart (1950) himself was to publish an important paper on Janet and Jackson. The evolution of his thought, however, led him away from the Jacksonian emphasis on "negative" symptoms to concentrate on the analysis of "unconscious intentionality", which he considered as more related to positive symptoms (Ey 1975, pp. 200–205).

Ey eventually was to reach the view that positive symptoms were psychodynamic in nature and suggested that they constituted a convergence point for the Jacksonian and Freudian models. He remained deeply Jacksonian to the end of his life and upheld the belief that negative symptoms were organic and the real manifestations of the disease, whilst positive symptoms were restitutive, a healthy reaction of the "psychological structures", and hence not a manifestation of disease.

The Referent of the Terms "Positive and Negative"

The term "referent" is used here to mean "the real or imaginary object to which a word refers" (Greimas and Courts 1979); and mental "functions" will be considered as real, albeit abstract, objects. Both in the Reynoldian and Jacksonian usages, "positive" and "negative" *refer* to the activity status of some abstract or hypothetical brain functions. Negative symptoms consist in an absence of such activity, positive symptoms in an increase which on occasions may take the form of *a new form of behaviour*. Jackson hypothesized that in the normal individual the latter were "inhibited" by higher strata: so, positive symptoms were not a direct manifestation of brain pathology. They are an expression of "evolution", i.e. of the remaining level of organization. In all cases, therefore, the referent was a brain function.

Brain Functions and Brain Centres

During the second half of the nineteenth century, the term "function" had a variety of meanings (Carlet 1878; Dallenbach 1915). It was, for example, defined as the term for "the action of an organ" or as the "power or faculty by the exercise of which the vital phenomena are produced" (Mayne 1860). The phrase "functional disease" arose during this period to refer to a symptom cluster in which no "anatomical or structural change [could] be detected" (Quain 1894, vol 1, p. 710; Trimble 1982). By the turn of the century a distinction between physical and mental function had become well established, the latter being defined as "any conscious process considered as taking part in a larger system of processes" (Baldwin 1901, vol 1, p 397; Ruckmich 1913).

In general, the concept of function was related to a discrete operation by an organ, and hence it was possible conceptually to separate it from its supporting anatomical structure. This explains why the concept of functional disease became possible. But Jackson rejected this separation:

> "I do not use the term 'function' in the sense often given to it in clinical accounts of nervous maladies, as for example, when it is said of a patient that his case is entirely functional... I do not believe that there is such a thing as loss or defect of function of any nervous elements *without* a proportionate material alteration of their structure and nutrition... I think a better term for my present purpose than 'loss of function' would be negative lesion" (Jackson 1931, vol 2, p. 411; my italics).

Jackson's views on function were both anti-localisationistic, and anti-phrenological. In this he followed Spencer who, nonetheless, had had an early dalliance with phrenology (Denton 1921). This latter term refers here to a scientific and social movement, influential in the Western world during the first half of the nineteenth century, which included original views on the nature and classification of mental functions and on their brain representation (Young 1970; Cooter 1984).

Marshall (1984) has suggested that the notion of mental function as conceived by Gall and Spurzheim (the creators of the phrenological movement) has little to do with the Kantian and Scottish view of mental faculties as "abstract functions". This is an important point. Faculty psychology, common to both phrenology and the Scottish Schools, was one of the two most important psychological theories during the nineteenth century (Berrios 1988). It postulated that the mind was divided into more or less autonomous functions or faculties. One of the offshoots of this view, the tripartite classification of the faculties into intellectual (cognitive), affective (orectic) and volitional (conative), has been crucial to the formation of psychiatric nosology (Berrios 1987). Current "modular" models of mental function also see themselves as a modern version of Faculty psychology (Fodor 1983). Marshall's claim that phrenologists

"individuated [faculties] solely in terms of the *specific content domains* with which they respectively deal... the mental organs that Gall locates in the cerebral substance are therefore *incommensurate* with the traditional faculties ..." (p. 215; my italics) is therefore important.

Marshall's interpretation may lead to a review of opinions on the influence of phrenology on Jackson. Interestingly enough, Jackson often seems to be suggesting that what is represented in the brain is not something like memory or attention, but complete psychomotor routines needed for certain actions. More to the point, he suggested that these routines have multiple representation at various levels of the hierarchy (with increasing complexity from bottom to top). Jackson used his model to explain, for example, functional recovery from brain injury. He believed that this did not occur on account of new brain areas "taking over" or "learning" the lost function, but simply because lower levels *already contained* simpler engrammes of the same plan.

Most, if not all, neurobiologists during Jackson's time were brain localisers in the conventional sense (Hecaen and Lanteri-Laura 1978). Jackson's views were in this regard so absolutely different that it is likely that few really understood what he was trying to say. Indeed, he was more admired for his clinical observations than for his theorising. In this regard, some politely called him a "Bedlamite theorist" (Taylor 1925, p. 10; on Jackson's contribution to the philosophy of neurology and psychiatry see Savage 1917, Mercier 1925, Stengel 1963, Dewhurst 1982, and the rich contribution of Riese 1942, 1943, 1944, 1954, 1955, 1965).

Links Between Positive and Negative Symptoms

In Jackson's usage, positive symptoms must follow negative symptoms, their meanings are interdependent and they cannot exist independently from each other; in Reynolds's usage, however, this is not the case (Berrios 1985). This latter view can already be found in the work of Monro (1817–1889), who had strong phrenological and vitalist sympathies and in 1851 published an important theoretical book on insanity which both Jackson (Jackson 1931, vol 1, p. 123; vol 2, p. 8) and Tuke (Tuke 1882, pp. 470–473) mentioned with approval. Monro had "long ago stated his opinion that there is in insanity a negative and a positive condition" (Jackson 1931, vol 2, p. 8). This claim is, however, not correct. In fact, Monro did not actually use the words positive and negative, nor did he assume any cerebral hierarchical organization (i.e. both types of symptoms could be produced independently and "coincidentally" by brain centres as a result of either destruction or irritation; Monro 1851, pp. 12–15). Monro's notion of mental function was (as he put it) "partially phrenological" (p. 145). Furthermore, he was clear about the fact that he had not created a "new doctrine" for the view was already popular that "nervous excitement [accounted] for impetuosity and violence, and nervous torpor and decay for mental imbecility" (p. vii). In spite of claims to the contrary, there is more of Monro and of Reynolds than of Jackson in current American usage. An interesting variant of the latter is the suggestion by Zubin (1985) that positive symptoms may, in fact, occur first, and negative symptoms follow (caused by institutionalization or drugs).

The historical analysis so far carried out in this paper suggests that, sooner or later, current sponsors of the positive/negative distinction will have to make up their minds in regards to the *nature of the link* between the symptoms named by these words. The clinical usefulness of these terms is likely to be in direct proportion to the amount of theoretical furniture one is prepared to accept. If none is allowed, the terms become little more than empty names; on the other hand, to accept that positive and negative symptoms are related to increases or decreases in the activity of putative brain functions commits one to specifying them and, if possible, their brain representation in modular terms.

A modular view conceives of functions as sited in different loci which may or may not be hierarchically organized. Modularity models have been back in fashion since the work of the late David Marr, who based them on the view that "any large computation should be split up and implemented as a collection of small subparts that are as nearly independent of one another as the overall task allows" (Marr 1976, quoted in Shallice 1988; see also Fodor 1983; Marshall 1984). A "modular" view might just make the positive/negative symptoms distinction intelligible, and favour a more empirical approach.

Dissolution

The concept of "dissolution" had not been in use in medicine before Jackson. He borrowed it from Spencer around 1876 (Jackson 1931, vol 1, p. 147) to mean:

"a reverse of evolution" (Jackson, 1931, vol 2, p 6)... a process of underdevelopment... a taking to pieces in the order from the least organized towards the most organized" (Jackson 1931, vol 2, p. 46).

Jackson also believed that the phenomena that Baillarger (1809–1890) had described in relation to aphasia (Jackson 1931, vol 2, p. 3, p. 171), and Anstie in association with alcohol intoxication could be better understood as forms of dissolution. Baillarger himself sponsored a hierarchical, creationist view of the organization of the mental faculties (which he borrowed from Jouffroy; Baruk 1967). His work ranged from neuroanatomy to clinical descriptions and his views on insanity were shaped by his strong religious beliefs (Fournet 1867). Anstie's (1833–1874) pharmacological work is mentioned by Jackson as evidence for the principle of "over-action of the lower centres by mere removal of the influence of the higher centres" (Jackson, vol 2, p. 6).

Jackson saw "dissolution" as a counterpart of the process of evolution. Darwin had only been concerned with evolution which he considered as a law of nature; in fact, he used the process of natural selection (and not dissolution) to explain why some species did not survive (Mayr 1982; Richards 1987). In Jackson's usage, dissolution applied not to species, but to individuals. Moreover, in his work as in Spencer's, "dissolution" fulfils an "eschatological" role, i.e. it represents a metaphysical force of destruction. Spencer wrote that:

"In 1858 (or else the latter part of 1857) [he] had the added perception that increasing heterogeneity cannot go on without limit, but must end with the arrival at a state of equilibrium; and then, or soon after, came the further perception that since the state of equilibrium eventually reached cannot last for ever, *there must afterwards come a process of dissolution;* and that thus dissolution is everywhere complementary to evolution" (Spencer 1904, vol 2, p 168). And "this rhythm of evolution and dissolution... is so far as we can see *universal and eternal* ..." (Spencer 1904, vol 1, p. 554; my italics).

Spencer linked dissolution to the essence of nature: "evolution under its most general aspect is the integration of matter and concomitant dissipation of motion; while dissolution is the absorption of motion and concomitant disintegration of matter" (Spencer 1904a, p. 228). Jackson followed this notion closely.

According to Jackson, dissolution acted at a clinical level in a *general* and a *partial* way. Intoxication with alcohol, which (as Anstie had suggested) diffusely affected the higher centres, was an example of the former; the insanities an example of the latter. Diseases were the cause of dissolution of the higher centres and hence of negative symptoms. On one occasion, at least, however, Jackson seems to have countenanced that evolution and dissolution might go on in *normal* humans; his use of these two words also suggests that he meant by them organization and disorganization, respectively:

"Of course, there is in *normal states* a rhythm of evolution and dissolution – a going in and a going out of function. There is a big rhythm of evolution and dissolution in healthy people..." (Jackson 1931, vol 2, p. 415).

In the case of insanity, the intensity of the positive symptoms depended upon the rate and magnitude of the dissolution. Rapid dissolutions might even release "superpositive" symptoms (what Jackson meant by superpositive is unclear; the term appears in brackets twice in "*Factors of Insanities*"; Jackson 1931, vol 2, p. 414). Positive symptoms were the expression of healthy tissue, of the activity of "evolution" (so, Jackson's views on this are different from Monro's), and so it was wrong to talk about positive mental symptoms being "caused" by disease. Positive symptoms could not occur without negative ones, although the latter might be mild or difficult to identify. For example, an insane patient may look normal apart from, say, a few delusions (positive symptoms), but the negative symptoms were present nonetheless. For, in order for the patient to have a wrong belief (i.e. a delusion) he *must have ceased believing in the truth* (this constituted the negative symptom). Jackson reported the case of a man who believed that his nurse was his wife:

"It is not enough to dwell only on the positive element, that he supposes the person attending on him is his wife, for this delusion of *necessity implies the coexisting negative element* that he does not know her to be his nurse" (Jackson 1931, vol 2, p. 415; my italics).

It should be noted that this analysis is no longer based on empirical observation: it is definitional or "analytical" in a Kantian sense.

McPherson (1889), one of the very few alienists who followed Jackson during his lifetime, suggested that the insanities might be classified according to the principle of dissolution into three groups: dissolutions of the emotions or feelings (e.g. melancholia and mania), of intelligence (e.g. delusional insanity), and of volition (dipsomania, kleptomania, etc.). Five years later, Jackson attacked these efforts:

"I have never put forward the opinion that nervous maladies should be classified on the principle of dissolution for clinical purposes... it would be absurd to attempt to arrange patients in an asylum on the principle of dissolution as it would be to arrange plants in a kitchen garden on the 'natural system' of botanists" (Jackson 1931, vol 2, p. 411).

In spite of Jackson's repeated claims that he was a full "disciple" of Spencer, the question of the real sources for his evolutionary philosophy remain unclear (Riese 1943; Garcia 1987). His work was transfixed by a rigid metaphysical evolutionism, particularly his hierarchical ideas: in this the not-too-disguised influence of Fiske can be detected. John Fiske (1842–1901) was an American philosopher (Oldenquist 1967) who followed Spencer's views and came to England to complete his "*Outlines of Cosmic Philosophy*", a book that included an extreme form of evolutionary theory that, nonetheless, Jackson quoted with approval (Jackson 1931, vol 2, p. 6). (A recent book edited by Kennard and Swash (1989) has totally missed the opportunity of throwing some light on these important issues.) Finally, there is the question of the sources of Jackson's notion of concomitance. On this W. K. Clifford (1845–1879) played an important role. The untimely death of this promising Cambridge philosopher and mathematician deprived England of a major thinker (Smokler 1967). Clifford's philosophy of mind included a "doctrine of concomitance" which Jackson quoted in support of his own (e.g. Jackson 1931, vol 2, p. 72, p. 84).

Mental Automatism and Positive Signals

"Mental automatism" describes a mechanism according to which the symptoms of mental disease result from the release of mental representations deposited in the lower layers of the mind or brain. Outside France, this interesting psychopathological mechanism has been little explored. Its conceptual history can be traced back to Descartes's "automate", La Mettrie's "l'homme machine" and Pinel's demented patients leading an "existence automatique".

In the middle of the nineteenth century, mental automatism became combined with three other notions to provide alienists with a powerful explanatory mechanism. It was combined, firstly, with a non-evolutionary hierarchical model of the mind; for example, Baillarger suggested that the soul controlled the organs of the body "as a teacher his pupils" and that madness occurred when, due to an organic disease, the "pupils became incoherent". Madness was "external to the soul", that is, it was never due to problems affecting the "teacher" (Fournet 1867). Secondly, mental automatism was also combined with "oniric activity", i.e. with dreaming during wakefulness; for Baillarger (1848), Moreau de Tours and Delasiauve (Ey 1952a), dreaming was a form of automatic behaviour, an expression of activity normally inhibited. Finally, mental automatism was also linked to dissociation and somnambulism. It could be objective and subjective: objective automatism giving rise to insanity (Bailey 1927), subjective automatism to the neuroses. Janet (1889) developed this third association in "*L'Automatisme Psychologique*", where he put forward a purely "psychological" account, that is, automatism is no longer dependent (as it is in Jackson) upon the dismantling of physiological function. Nor did Janet believe (as did Jackson) that the lower psychological levels were lacking in "consciousness" (Ellenberger 1970, pp. 358–364). French views influenced the English forensic notions of "sane and insane automatism" (Walker 1968; Fenwick 1990).

Mental automatism was thus used in a descriptive and an explanatory manner, and its definition depended upon the validity of various conceptual dichotomies: voluntary versus involuntary, inhibition versus release, higher versus lower, more advanced versus less advanced, and psychological versus organic. As these pairs of terms have changed meaning since the late nineteenth century so has the semantic field of mental automatism.

Pre-evolutionary versions of mental automatism appeared in European philosophy of mind at the beginning of the nineteenth century in the work of Maine de Biran (1766–1824) and Jouffroy (1796–1842), Baillarger and Moreau de Tours (Porot 1975; Paulus 1941). Something needs to be said *in passim* about the role played by J. J. Moreau de Tours (1804–1884) in this historical process. Moreau had trained under Esquirol and his contribution to psychiatry ranges from descriptive psychopathology to pharmacology. After a 3-year visit to the near East where he learned about "hachisch" and other drugs, he returned to France with new views concerning the nature and management of insanity. With Aubert-Roche and Gautier, he became involved in the "club de hachischins", where he is supposed to have observed behavioural changes caused by drugs (Brau 1974). In 1845, he published his classic "*Du hachisch et de l'aliénation mental*". He believed that drugs caused a form of experimental insanity by exciting the lower centres (thus generating forms of mental automatism), and also that insanity was a form of dreaming during wakefulness.

Mental automatism was imported into neurology by Jackson, who linked it to evolutionary theory. His views included: (a) a belief in brain representation, (b) a stratified or hierarchical organization (deposited by evolution) of the brain according to which lower layers are under the control of higher ones, and (c) the assumption that lower strata were able to "escape" the control of higher ones. "Control" was exercised by means of the mechanism of *physiological inhibition*. The psychological consequences of automatism are, in fact, positive symptoms. Jackson suggested that mental automatism could explain the presentation of a number of mental disorders. To this day, little evidence has been presented in favour of this view (Balan 1989), whose sterility in earlier times bedevilled the work of Nayrac, de Clérambault and Ey himself.

Discussion

This paper has explored the history of the terms positive and negative before, during and after Jackson. This it has done in regards to question concerning their meaning, referent and the nature of their conceptual link. Jackson's final model was but a collection of borrowed ideas: metaphysical evolutionism and the concept of dissolution he took from Spencer; hierarchical organization of the brain from Maine de Biran and Jouffroy (via Baillarger and Moreau de Tours); the "functional" account of symptoms from Anstie and Monro; the positive/negative terminology from Reynolds; and the doctrine of "concomitance" from Clifford.

Jackson drew his neuropsychiatric model of disease from the observation of conditions such as aphasia and epilepsy and felt able to apply it to some idealised forms of insanity. In all cases, he divided symptoms into positive and negative, assumed a conceptual hierarchy of brain representation, and offered an algorithm for the dismantling of such hierarchies, which he called "dissolution". According to his "onion-like" model, conceptual brain layers become deposited by evolution and are dismantled by dissolution (i.e. disease). Functions, which he conceived of as content-related, were represented in each layer, with the upper layers containing the more complex (human) versions. So, destruction of the higher levels did not lead to a disappearance of a function, but to the release of earlier, albeit more primitive, versions of the same, as represented in the healthy tissue of the lower layers. This explained recovery after brain damage (Riese 1944).

To cope with the obvious restrictions of the hierarchical model Jackson postulated partial forms of "dissolution", i.e. the selective disabling of segmented functions within the hierarchy. In this apparently simple mechanism, Jackson packed complex metaphysical assumptions which concerned the evolution of man, the inhibition of animal functions, a view of insanity as resulting from loss of control and vitalist assumptions on tissue function.

This model has been attractive to some for it is general, diffuse, holistic and deals with the brain as a conceptual rather than a real system. Jackson rejected the notion of "mental" function as nonsense and defined function in relation to content. He also attacked the existence of specific mental functional modules or faculties such as memory or intelligence and postulated that brain representation was diffuse and widespread. Furthermore, his doctrine of "concomitance" between anatomical structures and mental events led him to believe that he could explain the pathogenesis of mental illness by simply referring to the dismantling by disease of a particular neuronal hierarchy (Prince 1891; Riese 1954; Levin 1960; Angel 1961; Engelhardt 1975; Edelheit 1976; Clark 1983).

Jackson's view that negative symptoms were the expression of the disease, and positive symptoms the expression of healthy tissue released by the functional disappearance of the higher levels denied the possibility that: (a) positive symptoms may, on occasion, be directly "pathological" (Guiraud 1950) and (b) that negative symptoms need not be a necessary accompaniment in disease. The limitations of his model, however, are understandable in terms of his narrow conception of function, hierarchy and localisation. Aware of the views expressed by many alienists that personality and exogenous factors are important in the shaping of insanity, Jackson included both factors in his model (Jackson 1931, vol 2, pp. 411–421), although he never developed them in any detail.

Jackson's usage of the distinction between positive and negative symptoms was highly theoretical, and the question in respect to current usage is whether these two terms can be emptied of all their theoretical contents without rendering them meaningless. For example, can the hierarchical model be given up (as Anglo-Saxon users have done) with impunity? The answer is that it cannot, unless it is replaced by an alternative hypothesis of brain representation; it is suggested in this paper that such replacement has (covertly) taken place. A concept of "function" as a "psychological" construct is implicit, for example, in Summers's views (1985). Cruder assumptions as to the nature of the "referent" for "negative" symptoms are found in the work of other writers (Gibbons et al. 1985; Rosen et al. 1984; Iager et al. 1985). Few current users, however, bother to specify the modules underlying the positive and negative symptoms included in their lists. This reticence is creating a current version of the old nineteenth century descriptive two-tier system which led to a pathological psychology which had little to do with normal psychology (Berrios 1984).

It is therefore essential that writers using the positive/negative terminology not only offer operational definitions for the various symptoms (as they are only too keen to do), but also list the psychological functions or modules of which their symptoms are supposed to be a pathological expression. There is, in addition, a need to explain why, the "mixed symptoms" of de Clérambault (1987), and the "disorders of personal relationships" of Strauss et al. (1974; Strauss 1985), intrinsic to their symptom taxonomies, have been allowed to disappear.

Jackson showed admirable consistency in applying his model to a number of mental disorders which included the insanities, dementia and even obsessive-compulsive disease (Berrios 1977). De Clérambault (1987) did likewise, although his main examples were taken from the psychoses, both functional and organic. Ey (1975), like Jackson, applied the "organo-dynamic" model right across the board. However, when during the 1970s the model (in its amputated form) was imported into Anglo-Saxon psychiatry (Strauss et al. 1974), it was used exclusively in relation to schizophrenia. The reasons for this selectivity are obscure and likely to be extra-scientific.

It is suggested here that if the positive/negative distinction is to have any future, it should also be applied to other clinical conditions such as major depression, mania, delirium, dementia and obsessive-compulsive disorder. There is no obvious theoretical reason why it should not work. Indeed, if the modular view of mental functioning (which now seems to underlie its usage in schizophrenia) is correct, then it is to be expected that other mental disorders will profit from its application.

Conclusions

The following conclusions can be drawn:

1. The history of the terms positive and negative symptoms starts with Reynolds in the 1850s. Since its inception, it has been used associated with a variety of models of the mind (Reynolds, Jackson, Clérambault, Ey and current users).
2. Current usage (a) almost exclusively concerns the symptomatology of schizophrenia, (b) takes an atheoretical stance and (c) bases itself on "operational-definitions". This is insufficient. The very meaning of the terms positive and negative depends on a hidden theoretical framework that includes definitions of mental function and of brain representation.
3. Analysis of the work of current users shows that Jackson's old hierarchical model has been replaced (unwittingly) by modern notions of mental function (e.g. that of "hypothetical construct") or by conventional modular models. The modules responsible for the symptoms, however, are never specified.
4. Surface mappings of abnormal behaviour are not informational enough when based on close descriptive systems. A parallel mechanism, to capture fresh signals of disease, needs to be concurrently operated.
5. The positive/negative symptom distinction should be tried in other mental disorders, as it is extremely unlikely that schizophrenia requires an entirely unique psychopathogenic model.

References

Albernhe T and Roux J (1990) La pensée de Henri Ey. Scripta, Paris

Angel RW (1961) Jackson, Freud and Sherrington on the relation of brain and mind. Am J Psychiatry 118:193–197

Anguera P (1984) Un psychiatre de légende: G G de Clérambault. Perspect Psychiatr 22:142–147

Anguera P (1989) G G de Clérambault, L'Infirmerie spéciale et al psychose hallucinatoire chronique. In: Grivois H (ed) La Psychose hallucinatoire chronique. Masson, Paris, pp. 55–58

Bailey P (1927) The syndrome of mental automatism and its role in the formation of the chronic systematized psychosis. A Review. J Nerv Ment Dis 65:345–352

Baillarger J (1848) De l'influence de l'état intermediaire a la veille et au sommeil sur la production et la marche des hallucinations. Mem Acad R Med 12:476–516

Balan B (1989) Les fondements psychologiques de la notion d'automatisme mental chez John Hughlings Jackson. Inf Psychiatr 69:609–619

Baldwin JM (1901) Dictionary of philosphy and psychology. Churchill, London
Baruk H (1967) La psychiatrie française de Pinel à nos jours. Presses Universitaires de France, Paris
Benrubi J (1933) Les sources et les courants de la philosophie contemporaine en France, vol 1. Alcan, Paris
Berrios GE (1977) Henry Ey, Jackson, et les idées obsédantes. Evol Psychiatr 42:685–699
Berrios GE (1981) Stupor revisited. Compr Psychiatry 22:466–478
Berrios GE (1984) Descriptive psychopathology: conceptual and historical aspects. Psychol Med 14:303–313
Berrios GE (1985) Positive and negative symptoms and Jackson. Arch Gen Psychiatry 42:95–97
Berrios GE (1987) Historical aspects of the psychoses: 19th century issues. Br Med Bull 43:484–498
Berrios GE (1988) Historical background to abnormal psychology. In: Miller E, Cooper PJ (eds) Adult abnormal psychology, Livingstone, Edinburgh, pp. 26–51
Blashfield R, Feighner K et al. (1982) Invisible colleges, and the Matthew effect. Schizophr Bull 8:1–12
Brau JL (1974) J Moreau (de Tours) ou le drogue qui faillit entrer a l'institut. In: Moreau de Tours (ed) Du hachisch et de l'aliénation mental. Kesselring, Paris
Brousseau A (1934) Nécrologie. G. G. de Clérambault. Encephale 29:738–739
Brown-Séquard CE (1889) Inhibition. In: Dechambre A, Lereboullet L (eds) Dictionnaire encyclopédique des sciences médicales, vol 52. Masson, Paris, pp. 1–19
Carlet G (1878) Fonction. In: Dechambre A, Lereboullet L (eds) Dictionnaire encyclopédique des sciencies médicales, vol 34. Masson, Paris, pp. 365–368
Clark MJ (1983) A plastic power ministering to organization: interpretations of the mind-body relationship in late nineteenth-century British Psychiatry. Psychol Med 13:487–497
Cleparède E (1916) Théodule Ribot. Arch Psychol 16:194–196
Cooter R (1984) The cultural meaning of popular science. Phrenology and the organization of consent in nineteenth century Britain. Cambridge University Press, Cambridge
Coseriu E (1978) Sincronía, diacronía e historia. Gredos, Madrid
Dallenbach KM (1915) The history and derivation of the word 'function' as a systematic term in psychology. Am J Psychol 26:473–484
De Clérambault GG (1987) Oeuvres psychiatriques. Frénésie, Paris
Delay J (1942) Les dissolutions de la mémoire. Presses Universitaires de France, Paris
Delay J (1953) Le Jacksonisme et l'oeuvre de Ribot. In: Delay J (ed) Études de psychologie medicale. Presses Universitaires de France, Paris, pp. 83–108
Denton GB (1921) Early psychological theories of Herbert Spencer. Am J Psychol 32:5–15
Dewhurst K (1982) Hughlings Jackson on psychiatry. Sandford, Oxford
Ducrot O, Todorov T (1972) Dictionnaire encyclopédique des sciences du langage. Seuil, Paris
Edelheit H (1976) Complementarity as a rule in psychological research. Int J Psychoanal 57:23–29
Ellenberger H (1970) The discovery of the unconscious. The history and evolution of dynamic psychiatry. Lane, London
Engelhardt HT (1975) JH Jackson and the mind-body relation. Bull Hist Med 49:137–151
Ey H (1962) Hughlings Jackson's principles and the organo-dynamic concept of psychiatry. Psychiatry 118:673–682
Ey H (1952) Une théorie mécaniciste. La doctrine de G. de Clérambault. Études Psychiatriques, vol 1. Desclée de Brouwer, Paris, pp. 83–102
Ey H (1952a) Le rêve 'fait primordial' de la psychopathologie. Etud Psychiatr 1:187–277
Ey H (1975) Des idées de Jackson à un modèle organodynamique en psychiatrie. Privately published, Paris
Ey H, Rouart J (1938) Essai d'application des principes de Jackson à une conception dynamique de la neuro-psychiatrie. Doin, Paris
Evans P (1972) Henri Ey's concepts of the organization of consciousness and its disorganization: an extension of Jacksonian theory. Brain 95:413–440

Fenwick P (1990) Automatism. In: Bluglass R, Bowden P (eds) Principles and practice of forensic psychiatry. Livingstone, Edinburgh, pp. 271–290
Fodor JA (1983) The modularity of mind. MIT Press, Cambridge
Fournet M (1867) Expose d'un doctrine organo-psychique de la folie. Ann Med Psychol (Paris) 10:296–315
Garcia C (1987) Die Schichtenregel als Grundsatz der Psychopathologie. Nervenarzt 58:589–594
Gasser J (1988) La notion de mémoire organique dans l'oeuvre de T. Ribot. Hist Philos Life Sci 10:293–313
Gibbons RD, Lewine RRJ, Davis JM, et al. (1985) An empirical test of a Kraepelinian vs Bleulerian view of negative symptoms. Schizophr Bull 11:390–395
Goudge TA (1973) Evolutionism. In Wiener PP (ed) Dictionary of the History of Ideas, vol 2, New York, Scribner's sons, pp. 174–189
Gourceix A (1989) La notion d'automatisme psychologique d'Aristote à Janet. Ann Med Psychol 147:944–945
Greimas AJ, Courts J (1979) Sémiotique. Dictionnaire raisonné de la théorie du language. Hachette, Paris
Grinker RR (1939) A comparison of psychological 'repression' and neurological 'inhibition'. J Nerv Ment Dis 89:765–781
Guiraud P (1950) Psychiatrie générale. Le François, Paris
Hecaen H, Lanteri-Laura G (1978) Evolution des connaissances et des doctrines sur les localisations cérébrales. Desclée de Brouwer, Paris
Herrick CL (1901) Inhibition. In: Baldwin JM (ed) Dictionary of philosophy and psychology, vol 1. Churchill, London, pp. 547–548
Iager AC, Kirsch DG, Wyatt RJ (1985) A negative symptom rating scale. Psychiatr Res 16:27–36
Jackson JH (1931) Selected writings of J. H. Jackson. 2 vols. Hodder and Stoughton, London
Janet P (1889) L'Automatisme psychologique. Alcan, Paris
Kennard C, Swash M (eds) (1989) Hierarchies in neurology. A reappraisal of a Jacksonian concept. Springer, Berlin Heidelberg New Yord Tokyo
Koerner EFK (1982) Ferdinand de Saussure. Génesis y evolución de su pensamiento en el marco de la linguística occidental. Gredos, Madrid
Lanteri-Laura G (1966) Les rapports de la linguistique à la psychiatrie contemporaine. Masson, Paris
Latour B (1988) The pasteurization of France. Harvard University Press, Cambridge
Levin M (1960) The mind-brain problem and Hughlings Jackson's doctrine of concomitance. Am J Psychiatr 116:718–722
López Piñero JM (1973) John Hughlings Jackson (1835–1911) Evolucionismo y neurología. Editorial Moneda y Crédito, Madrid
Malmberg B (1986) Análisis del lenguaje en el siglo XX. Gredos, Madrid
Marshall J (1984) Multiple perspectives on modularity. Cognition 17:209–242
Maurel H (1989) Approche historique de la notion d'automatisme en psychiatrie. Ann Med Psychol 147:946–950
Mayne RG (1860) An expository lexicon of the terms, ancient and modern, in medical and general science. Churchill, London
Mayr E (1982) The growth of biological thought. Harvard University Press, Cambridge
McPherson J (1889) On the dissolution of the functions of the nervous system in insanity, with a suggestion for a new basis of classification. Am J Insanity 45:387–394
Monro H (1851) Remarks on insanity: its nature and treatment. Churchill, London
Mourgue R (1931) L'oeuvre et la personnalité du Professeur Constantin Von Monakow (1835–1930). Encephale 26:417–428
Nayrac P (1974) Mental automatism. In: Hirsch SR, Shepherd M (eds) Themes and variations in European Psychiatry. Wright, Bristol, pp. 405–429
Oldenquist A (1967) John Fiske. In: Edwards P (ed) Encyclopedia of philosphy, vol 3. Macmillan, London, pp. 204–205

Paulus J (1941) Le problème de l'hallucination et l'évolution de la psychologie d'Esquirol à Pierre Janet. Les Belles Lettres, Paris
Pichot P (1984) A century of psychiatry. Dacosta, Paris
Porot A (1975) Manuel alphabétique de psychiatrie. Presses Universitaires de France, Paris
Prince M (1891) Hughlings-Jackson on the connection between the mind and the brain. Brain 14:250–269
Quain R (1894) A dictionary of medicine. 2 vols. Longmans and Green, London
Ravaisson F (1984) Rapport sur la philosophie en France au dix-neuvième siècle. Fayard, Paris
Reynolds JR (1896) Essays and addresses. Macmillan, London
Ribot T (1882) Diseases of memory. An essay in the positive psychology. Kegan Paul, Trench, London
Richards RJ (1987) Darwin and the emergence of evolutionary theories of mind and behaviour. University of Chicago Press, Chicago
Riese W (1942) The principle of integration. J Nerv Ment Dis 96:296–312
Riese W (1943) The principle of evolution of nervous function. J Nerv Ment Dis 98:255–266
Riese W (1944) The principle of compensation of nervous function. J Nerv Ment Dis 100:263–274
Riese W (1954) Hughlings Jackson's doctrine of consciousness. Sources, versions and elaborations. J Nerv Ment Dis 120:331–337
Riese W (1955) Hughlings Jackson's doctrine of aphasia and its significance today. J Nerv Ment Dis 122:1–13
Riese W (1965) The sources of Hughlings Jackson's view on aphasia. Brain 88:811–822
Rosen WG, Mohs RC, Johns CA, et al. (1984) Positive and negative symptoms in schizophrenia. Psychiatr Res 13:277–284
Rouart J, Ey E (1938) Essai d'application des principles de Jackson a une conception dynamique de la neuropsychiatrie. Doin, Paris
Rouart J (1950) Janet et Jackson. Evol Psychiatr 25:485–501
Ruckmich CA (1913) The use of the term function in English textbooks of psychology. Am J Psychol 24:99–123
Saussure F de (1945) Curso de linguística general (translation of the 1916 edition by C Bally and A Sechehaye by A Alonso). Losada, Buenos Aires
Savage G (1917) Dr Hughlings Jackson on mental disorders. J Ment Sci 63:315–328
Segal JH (1989) Erotomania revisited: from Kraepelin to DSM-III-R. Am J Psychiatr 146:1261–1266
Shallice T (1988) From neuropsychology to mental structure. Cambridge University Press, Cambridge
Smith CUM (1982) Evolution and the problem of mind: part II. John Hughlings Jackson. J Hist Biol 15:241–262
Smokler HE (1967) WK Clifford. In: Edwards P (ed) The encyclopedia of philosophy, vol 2. Macmillan, London, pp. 123–125
Sommers AA (1985) Negative symptoms: conceptual and methodological problems. Schizophr Bull 11:364–379
Soubrier JP, Gourevitch M (1984) Recherches aux archives de la préfecture de police sur les origins de l'infirmerie spéciale. Perspect Psychiatr 22:129–136
Spencer H (1904a) An autobiography. 2 vols. Williams and Norgate, London
Spencer H (1904b) First Principles. Williams and Norgate, London
Stengel E (1963) Hughlings Jackson's influence in psychiatry. Br J Psychiatr 109:348–355
Strauss JS, Carpenter WT, Bartko JJ (1974) Part III. Speculations on the processes that underlie schizophrenic symptoms and signs. Schizophr Bull 1:61–69
Strauss JS (1885) Negative symptoms: future developments of the concept. Schizophr Bull 11:457–460
Taine H (1901) Les philosophes classiques du XIXe siècle en France. Hachette, Paris
Taylor J (1925) Biographical memoir. In: Jackson JH (ed) Neurological fragments. Oxford University Press, London, pp. 1–26
Trimble M (1982) Functional diseases. Br Med J 285:1768–1770

Tuke DH (1882) Chapters in the history of the insane on the British Isles. Kegan Paul, Trench, London

Von Monakow C, Mourgue R (1928) Introduction biologique à l'étude de la neurologie et de la psychopathologie. Alcan, Paris

Walker N (1968) Crime and insanity in England. I. A historical perspective. University Press, Edinburgh

Walser HH (1974) Über Theorien des Gedächtnisses in den letzten Dezenninen des 19. Jahrhunderts und ihre Bedeutung für die Entstehung der Psychoanalyse. In: Proceedings of the 23th International Congress of the History of Medicine, vol 2. Wellcome Institute of the History of Medicine, London, pp. 1227–1232

Yakovlev PI (1970) Constantin Von Monakow. In: Haymaker W, Schiller F (eds) The founders of neurology. Thomas, Springfield, pp. 484–488

Young RM (1970) Mind, Brain and Adaptation in the nineteenth century. Clarendon, Oxford

Zubin J (1985) Negative symptoms: are they indigenous to schizophrenia? Schizophr Bull 11:461–469

Positive and Negative Symptoms: Assessment and Validity*

N. C. ANDREASEN, M. FLAUM, S. ARNDT, R. ALLIGER, and V. W. SWAYZE[1]

During the past decade, the study of the assessment and validity of negative symptoms has been restored to its rightful place in the realm of psychopathology. During the 1970s and early 1980s, negative symptoms were scarcely allowed in live in the servant's quarters. Instead, they were neglected and ignored, while positive symptoms were raised to a position of pride and popularity because of their presumed superior reliability. Positive symptoms were, therefore, made the foundation of the definition of schizophrenia in the Research Diagnostic Criteria (Spitzer et al. 1978) and Diagnostic and Statistical Manual (DSM)-III (American Psychiatric Association 1980) and DSM-III-R (American Psychiatric Association 1987), and they were also given great prominence in the Present State Examination (Wing et al. 1974) and CATEGO (Wing et al. 1974). This state of affairs was in direct contradiction to the work of the historic scholars of psychopathology, Kraepelin (1919) and Bleuler (1916), who both saw negative symptoms as the core feature of schizophrenia. During the past decade, however, clinicians and investigators have returned again to this earlier perspective. Many now agree that negative symptoms (either referred to by that name or by other terms such as the apathy syndrome, the defect state, or the residual state) are the most important and the most handicapping symptoms that patients suffering from schizophrenia experience.

The Assessment of Negative Symptoms

When Crow proposed his seminal, two-syndrome hypothesis of schizophrenia in 1980, very few resources were available to assess negative symptoms comprehensively. In fact, a standardized rating scale for positive symptoms was lacking as well. Several instruments were used initially (and continue to be used in a variety of centers) that were developed in order to provide a brief assessment of the severity of psychopathology. Perhaps the most commonly used were the Krawiecka Scale (Krawiecka et al. 1977) and the Brief Psychiatric Rating Scale (BPRS; Overall and Gorham 1962). The former is a

* This research was supported in part by NIMH grants MH 31593, MH 40856, and MHCRC 43271, The Nellie Ball Trust Fund, Iowa State Bank & Trust Company, Trustee, and a Research Scientist Award, MH 00625.

[1] The University of Iowa, Department of Psychiatry, Iowa City, IO 52242, USA

A. Marneros / N. C. Andreasen / M. T. Tsuang (Eds.)
Negative Versus Positive Schizophrenia

simple clinical rating scale that covers a limited number of symptoms and has relatively brief definitions. The BPRS was developed primarily to rate psychopathology in clinical drug trials. Its items were generated through factor analysis of a much longer list of symptoms. The terminology used (e.g., conceptual disorganization, unusual thought content, suspiciousness, etc.) does not conform directly to the classic symptoms observed in the traditional study of psychopathology because it was developed in order to compress symptoms and generate higher order factors.

Because we had a long-standing interest in negative symptoms that actually antedated the seminal Crow article (Andreasen 1979a, b, c), we decided to generate a set of rating scales in order to assess both positive and negative symptoms. The Scale for the Assessment of Negative Symptoms (SANS; Andreasen 1983) evaluates five major negative symptoms: alogia, affective blunting, anhedonia, avolition, and attentional impairment. The Scale for the Assessment of Positive Symptoms (SAPS; Andreasen 1984) evaluates five major positive symptoms: delusions, hallucinations, positive formal thought disorder, bizarre behavior, and inappropriate affect. In developing these scales, we attempted to provide a comprehensive assessment of relatively common forms of psychopathology in order to assist in description and diagnosis. In addition, we also designed them with the assumption that they should be sensitive to change rather than describe continuous and unremitting traits, so that they could be used to assess clinical exacerbations and remissions within the context of drug treatment studies or longitudinal studies.

Good clinical assessment, using scales such as the SANS and SAPS, has many aspects. We must first begin by determining the reliability of our definitions and rating scales. Good assessment also involves exploring the relative accuracy of evaluating a phenomenon using subjective approaches, such as the patient's self-report, versus objective measures. Other important aspects of assessment involve determining the relationship of a specific group of symptoms to other symptoms and evaluating their response to treatment, their evolution over time, and their specificity within diagnostic classes.

Reliability

In developing the SANS and SAPS, we placed great emphasis on determining the reliability of the symptoms that they measure. When our initial work with the scales was first published, we provided data concerning interrater reliability, which was consistently high (Andreasen 1982). In addition, interrater reliability has been evaluated in other sites throughout the world (including Italy, Spain, France, Japan, and many other places), and they have been able to establish good reliability as well (Humbert et al. 1986; Moscarelli et al. 1987; Ohta et al. 1984; Phillips 1987).

We stressed the use of objective measures in the development of the scales, because we believed this would facilitate reliability. Tables 1 and 2 show interrater and test-retest reliability measures for the various scales of the SANS

Table 1. Interrater reliability of the SANS and SAPS

	Intraclass R
Anhedonia	
Recreational interest/activity	0.78
Sexual interest and activity	0.72
Ability to feel intimacy/closeness	0.68
Relationships with friends/peers	0.89
Global rating	0.81
Affective blunting	
Unchanging facial expression	0.81
Decreased spontaneous movement	0.32
Paucity of expressive gestures	0.58
Poor eye contact	0.79
Affective nonresponsivity	0.56
Lack of vocal inflections	0.74
Global rating	0.80
Avoliton	
Grooming and hygiene	0.44
Impersistence at goal-directed activities	0.80
Physical anergia	0.91
Global rating	0.86
Alogia	
Poverty of speech	0.77
Poverty of content of speech	0.60
Blocking	0.18
Increased latency of response	0.61
Perseveration	0.54
Global rating	0.66
Attention	
Social inattentiveness	0.67
Inattentiveness during mental testing	0.65
Global rating	0.67
Hallucinations	
Auditory	1.00
Voices commenting	1.00
Voices conversing	0.82
Somatic or tactile	0.70
Olfactory	0.00
Visual	0.79
Global rating	0.93
Delusions	
Persecutory delusions	0.83
Delusions of jealousy	0.91
Delusions of guilt or sin	0.76
Grandiose delusions	0.89
Religious delusions	0.90
Somatic delusions	0.68

Table 1 (Continued)

	Intraclass R
Delusions of reference	0.84
Delusions of being controlled	0.87
Delusions of mind reading	0.93
Thought broadcasting	0.97
Thought insertion	0.89
Thought withdrawal	0.78
Global rating	0.76
Bizarre behavior	
Clothing and appearance	0.80
Social and sexual behavior	0.72
Aggressive and agitated behavior	0.73
Repetitive or stereotyped behavior	0.07
Global rating	0.62
Positive formal thought disorder	
Derailment	0.70
Tangentiality	0.83
Incoherence	0.00
Illogicality	0.00
Circumstantiality	0.72
Pressure of speech	0.40
Distractible speech	0.43
Clanging	[a]
Global rating	0.79

[a] No variability for this item.
SANS/SAPS, Scale for the Assessment of Negative/Positive Symptoms.

and SAPS, as well as the specific items that make up these scales. The data in these tables are the result of a second recent assessment of the reliability, done in the context of assessing the reliability of a large diagnostic interview that we have developed, the Comprehensive Assessment of Symptoms and History (CASH) (Andreasen 1985). As Table 1 indicates, the interrater reliability of most items on the scale as well as the global ratings remain consistently high. Occasionally, reliability is low for some items which have a low base rate (such as blocking).

These tables also indicate the way that objective phenomena have been used in order to rate the various specific negative symptoms. For example, a person is determined to have alogia (which refers to the impoverished thinking that is such an important negative symptom of schizophrenia) by assessing the amount of speech (poverty of speech), poverty of content of speech, blocking, increased latency of response, and perseveration. After the clinician makes individual ratings on each of these items, he or she then forms a global rating that summarizes his or her clinical sense of the overall severity of the symptom, based on its intensity, persistence, and interference with functioning. For example, as a clinician assesses affective blunting, he or she looks at various

Table 2. Test-retest reliability of the SANS and SAPS

	Intraclass R
Anhedonia	
Recreational interest/activities	0.44
Sexual interest and activity	0.67
Ability to feel intimacy/closeness	0.27
Relationships with friends/peers	0.64
Global rating	0.71
Affective blunting	
Unchanging facial expression	0.74
Decreased spontaneous moevement	0.61
Paucity of expressive gestures	0.57
Poor eye contact	0.74
Affective nonresponsivity	0.68
Lack of vocal inflections	0.37
Global rating	0.76
Avolition	
Grooming and hygiene	0.44
Impersistence at goal-directed activities	0.70
Physical anergia	0.76
Global rating	0.67
Alogia	
Poverty of speech	0.56
Poverty of content of speech	0.33
Blocking	0.18
Increased latency of response	0.73
Perseveration	0.32
Global rating	0.38
Attention	
Social inattentiveness	0.44
Inattentiveness during mental testing	0.37
Global rating	0.46
Hallucinations	
Auditory	0.75
Voices commenting	0.10
Voices conversing	0.70
Somatic or tactile	0.42
Olfactory	0.07
Visual	0.70
Global rating	0.65
Delusions	
Persecutory delusions	0.74
Delusions of jealousy	0.89
Delusions of guilt or sin	0.21
Grandiose delusions	0.87
Religious delusions	0.75
Somatic delusions	0.68

Table 2 (Continued)

	Intraclass R
Delusions of reference	0.37
Delusions of being controlled	0.19
Delusions of mind reading	0.41
Thought broadcasting	0.02
Thought insertion	0.20
Thought withdrawal	0.20
Global rating	0.71
Bizarre behaviour	
Clothing and appearance	0.70
Social and sexual behavior	0.47
Aggressive and agitated behavior	0.43
Repetitive or stereotyped behavior	0.00
Global rating	0.50
Positive formal thought disorder	
Derailment	0.73
Tangentiality	0.55
Incoherence	[a]
Illogicality	0.08
Circumstantiality	0.58
Pressure of speech	0.57
Distractible speech	0.66
Clanging	[a]
Global rating	0.62

[a] No variability for this item.
SANS/SAPS, Scale for the Assessment of Negative/Positive Symptoms.

objective signs such as changes in facial expression, quantity of spontaneous movements, number of expressive gestures, quality of eye contact, responsivity of affect to stimuli such as smiling or joking, and variation in vocal inflections. Similar objective and observable items are used to evaluate anhedonia, avolition, and attentional impairment. Positive symptoms, on the other hand, are evaluated more the patient's self-report. Delusions and hallucinations are evaluated almost totally by listening to the patient's description of his or her symptoms, while positive formal thought disorder and bizarre behavior rely heavily on observation.

Table 2 adds to our previous work by assessing the test-retest reliability of positive and negative symptoms. In this particular study, two different clinicians evaluated the patient, conducting the interviews on two consecutive days. We used this approach in order to ensure that the patient changed minimally over time, so that we were obtaining as pure an assessment of reliability (as opposed to stability) as possible.

As Table 2 shows, the test-retest reliability is somewhat poorer than interrater reliability, but the global ratings continue to be quite high for most of the major positive and negative symptoms. A comparison of the test-retest and interrater reliability figures illustrates some of the problems inherent in the assessment of reliability. Test-retest reliability is usually considered to be more stringent and also to approximate more accurately true sources of variance when patients are repeatedly assessed in a clinical research setting. Multiple sources of variance can enter into the assessment of reliability, however, and both rater variance and occasion variance are important components. Rater variance occurs when raters approach patients with different concepts and perceive their symptoms differently because of this variation in concepts. Occasion variance reflects changes in the patient's behavior and reporting on different occasions. If the items are observational and if the patient's behavior truly varies from one occasion to another, then interrater reliability is in some respects a truer index of agreement, since it is a pure measure of the capacity of two raters to agree with one another when they are observing precisely the same data (i.e., a pure index of rater variance). Test-retest reliability includes components of both rater variance and occasion variance and is therefore inevitably less.

In general, as one might predict, test-retest reliability tends to be substantially less on most observational items. For example, both bizarre behavior and alogia have acceptable levels of interrater reliability, but they drop to unacceptable levels when test-retest reliability is assessed. The test-retest reliability of the other observational items remains remarkably high.

Objective vs. Subjective

Our approach to quantifying positive and negative symptoms relies heavily on the thinking and descriptions of Kraepelin. Other investigators working in the FRG more recently have emphasized the importance of subjective assessment in addition to objective assessment. In a sense, this approach reflects the purest use of the concept of phenomenology, as originally presented by Jaspers. When we initially developed the SANS, we included items to evaluate the patient's subjective experience of his losses in emotional or cognitive function as well as the objective evaluations. In our own work, we found the subjective ratings to be poorly correlated with the objective ratings (Andreasen 1982). We believed that this reflected the relatively poor insight that patients have about their deficits and suggested that the objective ratings might provide a better measure. Clearly, however, more work needs to be done in this area. Clinicians all recognize that some young schizophrenics, early in their illness, experience considerable insight into the emotional and cognitive losses that they are undergoing, and they also experience substantial psychological pain as a consequence. We are continuing to explore the interrelationship between subjective and objective measures ourselves, and we believe that it is important for other investigators to do this as well.

Interrelationships Between Symptoms

When the SANS and SAPS were initially developed, the items selected for each of the scales were chosen because of apparent face validity. As has been described many times in the past, one set of symptoms was grouped together and designated as negative because they seemed to share the common property of the loss of an important cognitive or behavioral function. For example, alogia represents a loss of fluency of speech and thought, affective blunting a loss of fluency of emotional expression, and avolition/apathy a loss of the ability to pursue goal-directed behavior. Positive symptoms were grouped together because they represented an exaggeration or distortion of a normal function. For example, hallucinations involve experiencing a perception when no stimulus is present, while delusions involve making abnormal inferences from normal perceptions. General cognitive and behavioral domains were identified, such as fluency of speech, fluency of emotional expression, or perception. Then specific symptoms were identified that seemed to represent these domains. Thus, the symptoms that were selected to define alogia include poverty of speech, poverty of content of speech, blocking, and increased latency of response.

While this approach drew on both common sense and clinical experience, it required empirical evaluation as well. In our early studies of the SANS and SAPS, we therefore evaluated the interrelationship between symptoms selected for the various scales. One easy way to do this was to examine the correlation between each of the individual symptoms and the summed score for the conceptual domain (e.g., alogia), the global score for the conceptual domain, and the sum of the summed scores and the global ratings for the entire scale (e.g., the SANS). We could then use these data in order to sift through the information and make appropriate revisions in the scales, which have now been done. Table 3 illustrates an example of some early data that led to a revision in the SANS and SAPS. It shows the correlation between the various items on the original affective flattening/blunting scale. The items are reasonably closely correlated with the summed items, the global rating, the sum of sums, and the sum of globals. One notable exception is inappropriate affect, for which the correlations are consistently poor. This observation, supported by repeated factor analyses (described later in the paper), eventually led us to remove inappropriate affect from the negative symptom scale and to place it among the positive symptoms. This revision is in fact more consistent with the original

Table 3. Correlation among items evaluating affective flattening

	Summed items	Global rating	Sum of sums	Sum of globals
Facial expression	0.78429	0.79324	0.68009	0.63846
Spontaneous movements	0.71034	0.50865	0.59758	0.45773
Expressive gestures	0.84293	0.71649	0.72611	0.62932
Eye contact	0.82159	0.68250	0.75209	0.66871
Nonresponsivity	0.82605	0.67973	0.78125	0.70659
Inappropriate affect	0.28158	0.30487	0.30387	0.36616
Vocal inflections	0.74257	0.62576	0.68271	0.59857

Coefficient alpha = 0.834062.

conceptual structure of the SANS and SAPS, since inappropriate affect is an exaggeration or distortion of a normal function rather than a loss of function. It was initially grouped with the negative symptoms because it was assumed to be associated with the defect state.

Effects of Treatment

Another perspective on the assessment of positive and negative symptoms can be obtained by examining the effects of treatment. One persistent concern about the evaluation of negative symptoms is that they may be affected by neuroleptic medication, specifically worsened by the extrapyramidal side effects. Figure 1 shows some of the various confounders that can affect the assessment of negative symptoms, such as institutionalization, neuroleptic medication, depression, or positive symptoms (Andreasen and Grove 1986; Andreason 1990a, b). Any of these four factors could potentially worsen negative symptoms, obscuring our ability to see "pure negative symptoms" that are not secondary to other causes.

We attempted to evaluate the effects of medication on negative symptoms by examining a group of patients admitted to The University of Iowa Clinical Research Center for schizophrenia and who had been taken off all neuroleptic medication for a 3-week period. We wanted to look at the effects of medication on symptoms and to answer the following questions: Has the symptom improved with medication? Is the symptom worsened by medication? Is the symptom unaffected by medication?

Figures 2 and 3 show the result of our findings for the first 27 patients whom we studied. All these patients were able to successfully complete the 3-week drug wash-out period. These figures show the regression lines or the changes in positive and negative symptoms at time 1 (admission, on medication) and time 2 (the end of the 3-week drug wash-out period). A significant worsening in both positive and negative symptoms was seen when the patients were withdrawn from medication. The values on these figures are based on the sum of the global ratings. These findings might be taken to suggest that neuroleptic medications do have a therapeutic efficacy for both positive and negative symptoms. Indeed, if mean change scores for positive and negative symptoms are looked at in isolation, the change scores between time 1 and time 2 are statistically

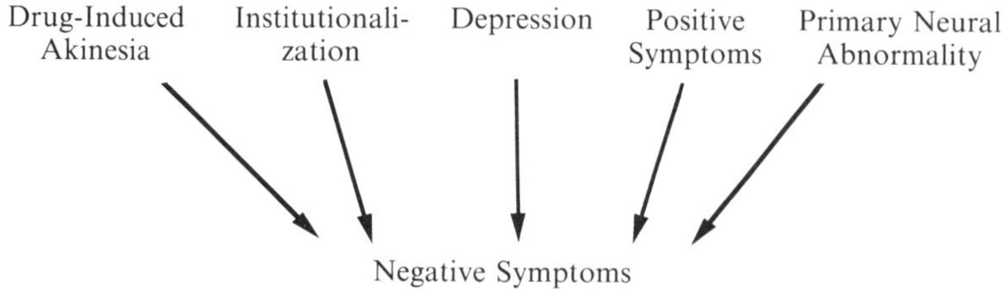

Fig. 1. Multiple paths to a final common destination

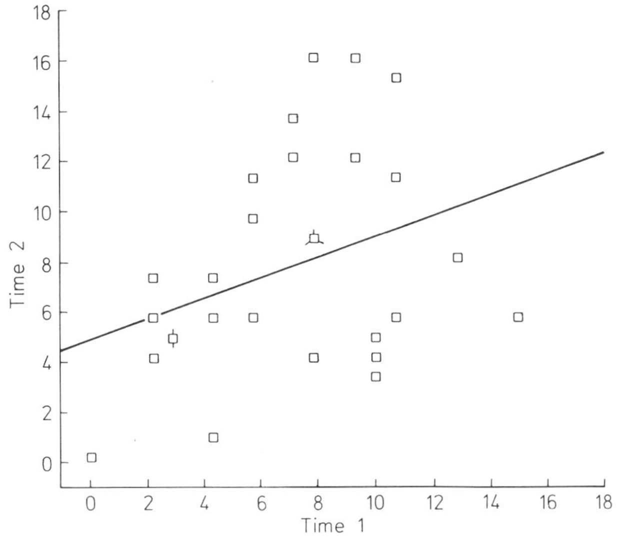

Fig. 2. Effect of medication withdrawal on total positive symptoms: $r^2 = 0.125$, $p < 0.03$ (one-tailed)

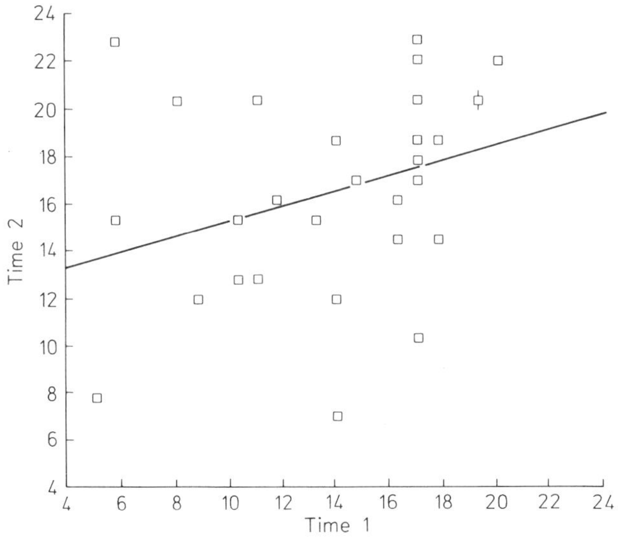

Fig. 3. Effect of medication withdrawal on total negative symptoms: $r^2 = 0.1$, $p < 0.05$ (one-tailed)

significant for negative symptoms but not for positive symptoms, suggesting that neuroleptics may have an even greater effect on negative symptoms.

As Figure 1 has indicated, however, the interrelationships between changes in positive and negative symptoms cannot be ignored. That is, negative symptoms may worsen because the direct therapeutic effect of neuroleptic drugs has been removed or secondarily to a worsening of positive symptoms: As the patient becomes increasingly suspicious and delusional, he or she may also become more withdrawn, seclusive, and reluctant to talk, thereby displaying an increase in negative symptoms that is secondary to the increase in positive symptoms. This possibility was examined by evaluating the intercorrelations between the changes in positive and negative symptoms. When this was done, the changes were found to be highly correlated with one another. That is, patients whose negative symptoms worsened tended to be those whose positive symptoms also worsened, while the patients who remained stable off-medication tended to have a minimal severity of both positive and negative symptoms. These results suggest that the worsening of negative symptoms off-medication is not due to the loss of a direct therapeutic effect of neuroleptic drugs but rather to a secondary effect.

Evolution of Symptoms Over Time

Another important question about negative symptoms is the extent to which they change over time. Some clinicians believe that they represent the "burned-out" stage of the illness, but to others it seems apparent that negative symptoms are a prominent feature of schizophrenia quite early on in the illness and that they may represent the first symptoms of schizophrenia to appear (although they may sometimes pass unrecognized).

Early studies of negative symptoms discussed this issue but did not look at it empirically. One of the first studies to attempt to evaluate the longitudinal evolution of positive and negative symptoms was done by Pfohl and Winokur (1983). They evaluated patients who had been chronically hospitalized in a long-term care facility and who were originally admitted prior to the development of neuroleptic drugs. They observed that some negative symptoms were present in these patients at index evaluation and that these symptoms tended to persist and to worsen over time, while positive symptoms diminished. This study, while a salutary initial effort, has the disadvantages that it relied on hospital records in order to document symptoms and that its patient sample may not be representative since these patients were chronically institutionalized. Several subsequent studies have employed prospective evaluations (Pogue-Geile and Harrow 1985; Johnstone et al. 1986). They show some waxing and waning of both positive and negative symptoms, but in general they suggest that positive symptoms are more prone to remit over time than are negative symptoms.

The best method for studying this question empirically is to identify a group of first episode patients and to evaluate the severity of their positive and negative symptoms. They can then be reevaluated at regular intervals, such as 6

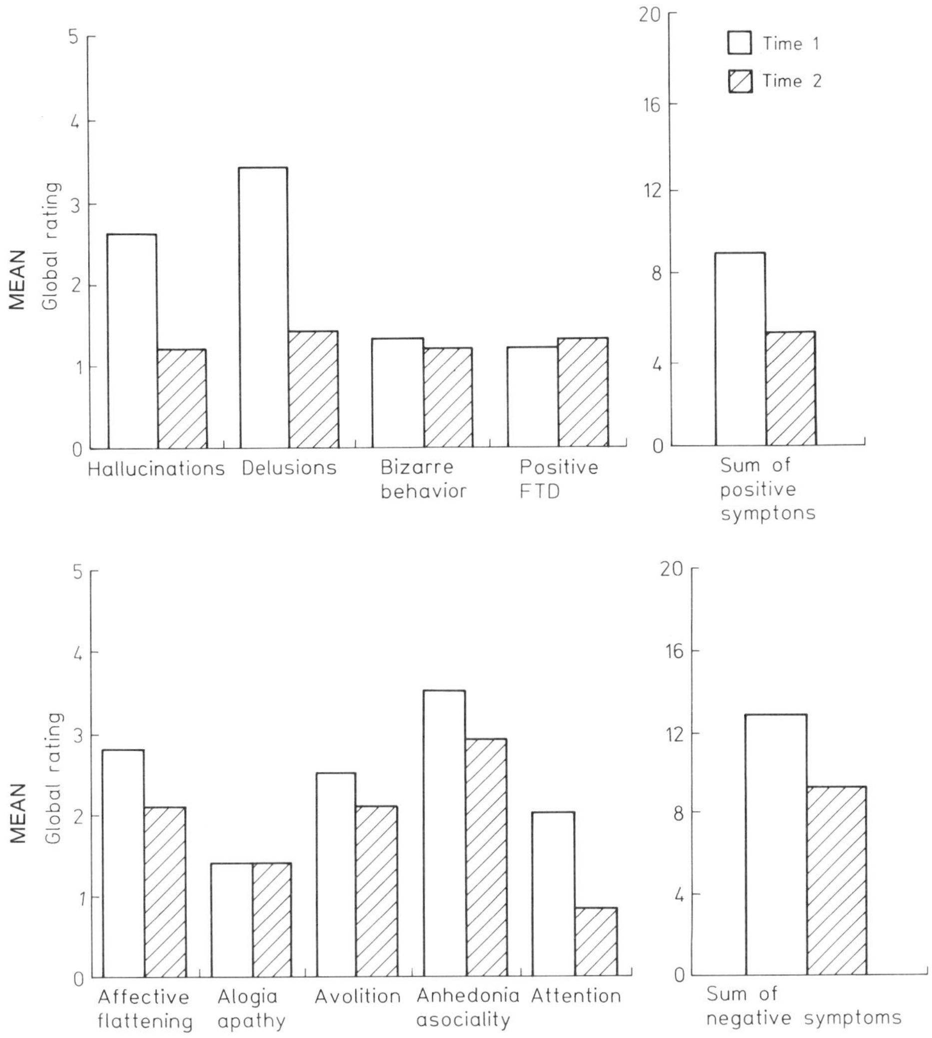

Fig. 4. Evaluation of the severity of positive (*upper diagram*) and negative (*lower diagram*) symptoms in a group of ten first episode patients. The patients' symptoms were evaluated twice (*Time 1*, *Time 2*); these two evaluations were approximately 4 years apart

months, in order to determine the extent to which these symptoms wax and wane over time.

We are currently conducting such a study at The University of Iowa. Figure 4 shows some of our preliminary data from this work. It reports on a sample of only ten first-episode patients assessed at two different times, referred to as time 1 and time 2, approximately 4 years apart. Thus, they give us some sense of how much positive and negative symptoms change over a relatively long time span after the first index assessment. As Fig. 4 shows, these young first-episode patients had a fairly high level of negative symptoms when they originally presented. These symptoms decreased slightly by time 2, but not by very much. On the other hand, their positive symptoms decreased markedly. All patients were on neuroleptic medication, which probably improved the positive symptoms and may have improved those negative symptoms that were secondary to positive symptoms. The symptoms that remain may be relatively pure negative symptoms.

In this small data set we also examined the stability and predictiveness of positive and negative symptoms. Multiple regression tended to show that negative symptoms were more stable than positive symptoms; if present initially, negative symptoms were more likely to be seen at follow-up, while there was essentially no relationship between the presence of positive symptoms at time 1 and time 2. In addition, we examined the extent to which positive and negative symptoms predicted social outcome. Again, positive symptoms had no predictive power, while the presence of negative symptoms at time 1 predicted a relatively poor social outcome at time 2, as assessed by employment, relationships with friends, and recreational functioning. Thus, the presence of negative symptoms at an initial evaluation appears to suggest a much worse prognosis.

Specificity

When an interest in negative symptoms began to reemerge in the early 1980s, some clinicians complained that they could not be important because they were not specific to, or pathognomic of, any particular illness. Such clinicians argued that negative symptoms such as avolition, apathy, asociality, or affective blunting could be observed in patients suffering from disorders such as depression. Other clinicians, who took a dimensional as opposed to a categorical approach, pointed out that there are few pathognomic symptoms in mental illnesses and argued that it is best simply to describe whatever symptoms are present.

This is a question that also lends itself to empirical exploration. We did this with a sample of 110 schizophrenic, 24 manic and 27 depressive patients admitted to The University of Iowa Hospitals and Clinics psychiatric facility. We evaluated positive symptoms, negative symptoms, and euphoric-dysphoric mood. The results are summarized in Fig. 5. As might be expected, the depressive patients score relatively low on positive symptoms, very high on dysphoria, and relatively high on many negative symptoms as well (although the ratings are considerable lower for all negative symptoms except alogia). The manic patients have a relatively high level of psychotic symptoms (although less so than for schizophrenic patients for all except positive formel thought disorder) and a high rating on euphoria. The schizophrenic patients score consistently worse on most positive symptoms and most negative symptoms and relatively low on both euphoria and dysphoria. These results indicate that both positive symptoms and negative symptoms are relatively nonspecific, with positive symptoms occurring prominently in mania and negative symptoms

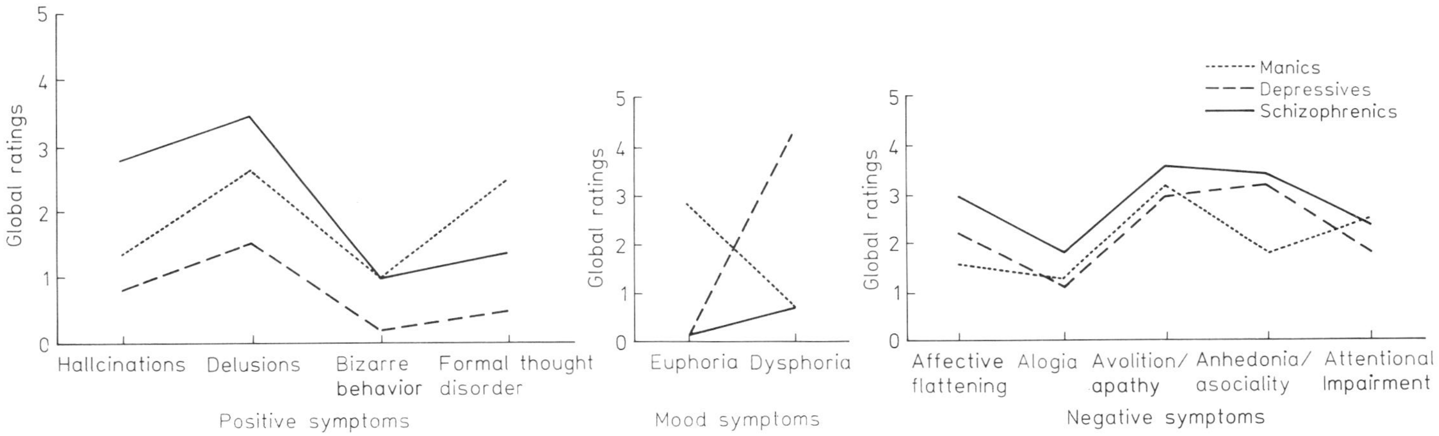

Fig. 5. Profile of positive (*left tracing*), negative (*right tracing*), and mood (*centre tracing*) in symptoms in schizophrenic (*unbroken line*), manic (*dotted line*), and depressive (*dashed line*) patients

occurring prominently in depression. What is important, however, is the overall patterning of symptoms. Schizophrenic patients tend to be relatively low on both euphoria and dysphoria, while these abnormalities of mood are distinguishing features of mania and depression. This figure illustrates graphically what each good clinican does in his or her own mind when classifying a particular patient as manic, depressive, or schizophrenic. He or she looks at the overall pattern of all types of symptoms and usually does not try to let a single symptom carry the entire diagnostic burden.

These data suggest that negative symptoms within the context of a schizophrenic syndrome can be distinguished from depressive symptoms within the context of a depressive syndrome. The issue of phenomenologic overlap between negative symptoms and depressive symptoms remains, however, and this issue is also illustrated by the data shown in Fig. 5. That is, specific symptoms of depression and the negative symptoms of schizophrenia may have similar descriptions and definitions. Alogia and avolition, as symptoms of schizophrenia, overlap closely with psychomotor retardation. The anhedonia and asociality of schizophrenia may be similar to the anhedonia of depression. This overlap can make it quite difficult to determine whether negative symptoms are secondary to depression or whether they represent primary or core negative symptoms.

A variety of studies have addressed this issue by examining correlations between negative and depressive symptoms using standard rating scales such as the Hamilton, the SANS, and the BPRS (Lewine et al. 1983; Pogue-Geile and Harrow 1984; Siris et al. 1988; Barnes et al. 1989a, b). Some of these studies find no correlation, while others find some relationship. To some extent, differences between the studies may depend on the patients sampled and the measures used to assess negative symptoms and depression. Nevertheless, the theme emerging from the bulk of these studies is that affective blunting is consistently distinguishable from depressed mood, suggesting that the presence of this symptom may be particularly powerful in investigations which attempt to separate core negative symptoms from negative symptoms that may be secondary to depression.

Validity of the Distinction Between Negative and Positive Symptoms

The assessment of the validity of a concept in psychopathology has two major components, internal and external. Internal validation refers to the internal consistency of a group of symptoms, while external validity refers to the relationship between a group of symptoms and some external correlate that is clinically useful or etiologically explanatory, such as long-term outcome or structural brain abnormalities.

Internal Consistency

From a psychometric perspective, demonstrating the internal consistency of a scale is often considered to provide a form of validation. Several approaches are available in order to evaluate internal consistence. One wide spread technique uses Cronbach's alpha, which calculates the mean of the split half-reliabilities for a scale and thereby provides an index of the extent to which the items on the scale are related to one another. A high Cronbach's alpha indicates that the scale is internally coherent.

We evaluated Cronbach's alpha when we published our first report on the SANS and demonstrated excellent internal consistency at that time (Andreasen 1982). Since that original publication, we have re-evaluated it again on several subsequent samples. By now, the results are quite consistent. Essentially, we find that the various individual negative and positive symptom scales have relatively good internal consistency (e.g., alogia, affective blunting, anhedonia). The individual negative symptom scales are also very internally consistent with one another. In our most recent calculations of Cronbach's alpha for the global ratings of all negative symptoms, it was 0.80. On the other hand, the internal consistency of positive symptoms, as assessed with Cronbach's alpha, is somewhat more spotty. In some studies, reasonably high alphas have been obtained for individual scales, but not regularly. The internal consistency of all positive symptom global ratings has been relatively poor in every analysis done. In our most recent assessment based on 100 schizophrenic patients from The University of Iowa Mental Health Clinical Research Center, we found it to be 0.49. This observation is consonant with clinical experience. That is, most patients who have one negative symptom tend to have another, but patients who have delusions do not necessarily have hallucinations or bizarre behavior or positive formal thought disorder.

An additional perspective on this problem is provided through factor analytic studies. In our original report about the SANS and SAPS published in 1982, we found a first factor that was bipolar and had strong negative weights on positive symptoms and strong positive weights on negative symptoms. In our more recent work, we have not obtained a bipolar factor. Instead, repeated factor analyses on several subsequent samples have yielded results very similar to those shown in Table 4 (Arndt et al. 1990). A first factor emerges that is essentially a negative symptom factor with strong positive weights on all five

Table 4. Varimax rotated factor loadings for global ratings of positive and negative symptoms ($n = 207$)

Symptom	Factor		
	1	2	3
Avolition	0.82	0.16	0.01
Anhedonia	0.81	−0.01	0.01
Affective flattening	0.79	0.07	0.18
Alogia	0.73	0.46	0.00
Attentional deficit	0.72	0.21	0.16
Positive formal thought disorder	0.07	0.86	0.12
Bizarre behavior	0.22	0.70	−0.01
Delusions	−0.03	0.11	0.83
Hallucinations	0.22	−0.02	0.78

negative symptoms. A second factor has strong weights on two positive symptoms: delusions and hallucinations. It appears to represent a "psychoticism" factor. A third factor has strong weights on positive formal thought disorder and bizarre behavior. It seems to represent a "disorganization factor." These results are quite similar to those reported by other investigators, such as Liddle (1984, 1987) and Bilder et al. (1985). The results of such studies are building toward a consensus that negative symptoms are relatively cohesive and intercorrelated, while positive symptoms are relatively more diverse. Positive symptoms seem to fall into at least two different broad classes that are rather independent of each another: psychoticism and disorganization.

External Validators

Traditionally, external validators of psychiatric syndromes have included family history, outcome, response to treatment, and laboratory measures (Robins and Guze 1970). More recently, greater emphasis has been placed on validators that have the potential for illuminating mechanisms and etiologies, such as cognitive function or structural and functional brain abnormalities.

Clinical Validators

The "natural history" validators of the positive/negative distinction have been recently reviewed by McGlashan (1990). In this review, McGlashan notes that there is a modest constellation of evidence indicating the validity of the positive/negative distinction. He notes that negative symptoms are more common in male patients and that there is a consistent association between negative symptoms and poor premorbid functioning, poor educational level, and compromised work capacity. The course of positive and negative symptoms has been reviewed above, and these results also support the validity of the positive/negative distinction, in that negative symptoms tend to be more stable, more persistent, and more predictive of a poor long-term outcome. The literature on response to treatment is variable and difficult to interpret, largely because of the problem of disentangling primary from secondary negative symptoms.

A modest amount of literature has accrued on the role of genetic versus environmental factors in the development of positive and negative symptoms. Theoretically, it is easy to make a case for the role of genetic/familial factors with either syndrome. Some investigators believe that schizophrenia characterized by prominent positive symptoms is more likely to be genetic, while the negative form is more likely to be environmental, positing that ventricular enlargement represents the downstream result of an environmental injury occurring early in life. Alternately, it could be argued that "negative schizophrenia" is more familial because it is a more severe and classic form of the disorder, while "positive schizophrenia" is milder and more likely to be associated with good prognosis disorders such as affective illness.

The data themselves are inconclusive. In our own work, we have looked for associations in three, large, independently collected samples of schizophrenic patients and noted none in either direction. Johnstone et al. (1981) and Pearlson et al. (1984, 1985) have also failed to find an association, while Kay et al. (1986) found a family history of psychosis to be related to negative symptoms in chronic patients but not in acute patients. Studies of twins have shown a greater concordance for negative symptoms than for positive symptoms (Dworkin and Lenzenweger 1984). If consistently supported, this finding would lend strength to the hypothesis that negative symptoms may rest at least in part on a genetic substrate.

Structural Brain Abnormalities

The early work of Crow (1980) on negative symptoms proposed a two syndrome hypothesis and argued that negative symptoms were likely to be tied to a structural brain abnormality. Since the original Crow hypothesis, numerous studies have been done using computed tomography (CT) scanning to measure ventricular size as an index of structural brain abnormality. Some studies have attempted to seek correlations between negative symptoms and ventricular enlargement, while others have examined the relationship categorically and evaluated ventricular size in patients classified as predominantly positive, negative, or mixed. The results of this work are inconclusive, but a review of the literature recently conducted did seem to indicate that the majority of studies find a relationship between ventricular size and the presence of negative symptoms. The review done by Marks and Luchins (1990) concluded that 18 investigations showed a direct relationship between neuroanatomical abnormalities and positive or negative symptoms, 5 found no relationship between structural abnormalities and positive or negative symptoms, and 3 revealed a relationship opposite to the predicted direction (i.e., normal ventricular size associated with positive symptoms and large ventricles with negative symptoms as the predicted direction).

We saw a relationship between negative symptoms and ventricular enlargement in our first CT study (Andreasen 1982) and an insignificant trend in our second CT study. The second study uncovered a relationship between ventricular enlargement and other clinical indicators of importance, such as poor premorbid adjustment, low educational achievement, or cognitive impairment.

One problem with CT studies is that they use a relatively crude measure of structural brain abnormalities and specifically of ventricular size. We have recently examined the association between ventricular size and negative symptoms with magnetic resonance imaging (MRI) using three-dimensional volumetric reconstruction. With this technique, we did find a significant relationship between negative symptoms and ventricular enlargement, as shown in Table 5 (Andreasen 1990a). The positive and mixed schizophrenic patients had relatively small ventricles, while the negative patients had extremely large ventricles. The results are highly significant. It

Table 5. Ventricular size in relation to positive, mixed, and negative subtypes of schizophrenia (subtype, mean ± SD)

Structure	Negative ($n = 5$)	Mixed ($n = 34$)	Positive ($n = 14$)	F	P
Ventricular volume (cm^3)	7.36 ± 4.17	3.84 ± 1.44	3.63 ± 1.54	8.64	0.0006
Ventricle-brain ratio[a]	7.41 ± 3.80	4.28 ± 1.64	4.19 ± 1.65	6.17	0.0041

[a] VBR = (ventricle volume/cerebral volume) × 100.

should be noted, however, that the number of negative patients is relatively small.

Functional Brain Abnormalities

Structural techniques, even relatively refined ones such as MRI, probably have less power to identify physical abnormalities or underlying mechanisms than do techniques that measure dynamic brain function, including single-photon emission computed tomography (SPECT) and positron emission tomography (PET). Such techniques have been used to explore what is perhaps the most widely held theory about the underlying mechanism producing negative symptoms, the hypofrontality hypothesis. As applied to negative symptoms, it suggests that they represent the loss of functions generally thought to reside in the frontal lobes (Andreasen 1988). The frontal lobes generate, for example, fluency of thought and speech, emotional expression, volition and drive, and the ability to form emotional attachments (Fuster 1989), and attention, alogia, affective blunting, avolition, anhedonia, and attentional impairment represent a loss of these various functions.

The hypofrontality hypothesis has been partially supported by neuroimaging studies, although not completely (Berman et al. 1986; Ingvar and Franzen 1974; Weinberger et al. 1986; Weinberger 1988; Gur et al. 1985, 1987a, b; Buchsbaum et al. 1983, 1984; Buchsbaum and Haier 1987). The failure to find consistent and replicable results with the measurement of regional blood flow with cortical probes, SPECT, or PET may be due to a variety of factors. One is the tremendous complexity of the prefrontal cortex itself. The prefrontal cortex is essentially a large association cortex that is connected to many other brain regions; it is in fact quite difficult to activate the prefrontal cortex selectively also engaging a substantial number of other brain regions that are connected to it. Another difficulty is the phenomenological complexity of schizophrenia. If one seeks a relationship between negative symptoms and hypofrontality, how does one identify a state that represents "pure negative symptoms"? Most studies are confounded by a variety of factors, such as the effects of positive symptoms or neuroleptic medication, as well as the stage of the illness. For example, if one could actually measure frontal blood flow selectively and precisely, one might find quite different patterns in a young patient presenting during the first episode with prominent negative symptoms as compared with a similar young patient who had predominantly positive symptoms. Likewise, negative symptoms seen in more chronic schizophrenic patients might result from quite different neural substrates. The patient with treatment-refractory positive symptoms could have very prominent negative symptoms which are purely secondary to the positive symptoms; when such chronic patients are mixed with those who have a more pure negative syndrome, positive findings are potentially averaged out.

In our own work with functional imaging, we have been exploring a variety of cognitive activation tasks designed to stimulate prefrontal cortical function and have used these tasks in both drug-naive and more chronic patients. These studies are still continuing and will require more extensive reporting elsewhere. At present, however, we have observed that both normal controls and patients (whether acute, drug-naive, or chronic) show a clear generalized increase in cerebral blood flow when presented with a cognitive activation task. It is extremely difficult to tease out selective prefrontal activation from the overall generalized effect, probably because the prefrontal cortex is connected with so many other brain regions.

Nevertheless, two specific findings have emerged from our data. First, drug-naive patients show evidence of hypofrontality in the left mesial frontal region, although not in other frontal regions (Table 6). The data in Table 6 reflect the performance of 13 drug-naive schizophrenic patients and 15 healthy volunteers who were performing the Tower of London, a prefrontal activation task that emphasizes planning functions, and whose blood flow was studied with a Tomomatic 64 SPECT scanner. This sample is too small to examine the relationship between positive and negative symptoms and hypofrontality. We have done this in a larger sample which pools together the drug-naive patients and the more chronic patients who have been studied using the Tower of London. We subdivided this sample of patients into two groups, those with high negative symptoms (i.e., patients who had at least two SANS global scores greater than or equal to 4) and patients with low negative symptoms (i.e., patients who did not have two SANS global scores greater than or equal to 4). The results of these analyses for the mesial and lateral frontal cortex are shown

Table 6. Frontal activation with the Tower of London task in drug-naive patients ($n = 13$) and normal controls ($n = 15$)

	Schizophrenics		Controls			
	$\bar{x}$	SD	$\bar{x}$	SD	t	P
Left mesial frontal	−3.87	8.99	5.14	6.57	3.05	0.005
Left lateral	1.23	5.98	−0.12	5.31	−0.63	0.532
Right mesial frontal	0.49	4.55	1.02	6.14	0.26	0.797
Right lateral	0.57	8.16	0.26	7.85	−0.10	0.918

The mean scores represent the mean region of interest (ROI) activation score minus the mean activation score for the brain; i.e., a positive mean activation difference score indicates greater blood flow to the ROI relative to the rest of the brain.

Table 7. Cognitive activation of the mesial and lateral frontal cortex in schizophrenia: relationship to negative symptoms

	Mesial			Lateral		
	Baseline	Activation	P	Baseline	Activation	P
Controls ($n = 16$)						
Mean	89.48	99.73	0.001	91.41	102.42	0.01
SD	15.80	15.21		14.67	16.19	
Low negative symptoms ($n = 16$)						
Mean	94.12	106.02	0.001	92.98	106.32	0.001
SD	10.86	13.44		10.79	11.84	
High negative symptoms[a] ($n = 20$)						
Mean	94.96	99.14	NS	92.57	100.03	0.05
SD	17.13	13.62		16.15	13.64	

[a] "High" patients had at least 2 SANS global scores $\geqq 4$; all patients were medication-free for at least 3 weeks.
Units are cerebral blood flow in ml/min per g of tissue.

in Table 7. Here, all three groups (controls, patients with low negative symptoms, and patients with high negative symptoms) showed significant increases in blood flow in the lateral frontal cortex when stimulated with the Tower of London, although the increase in the patients with high negative symptoms is lowest. On the other hand, the patients with high negative symptoms do not show significant activation of the mesial frontal cortex, while the controls and patients with low negative symptoms exhibit significant increases in this area.

These findings differ from those reported by the National Institute of Mental Health (NIMH) group, who found specific activation in the dorsal lateral prefrontal cortex (Berman et al. 1986; Weinberger et al. 1986). Their technique involved the use of cortical probes, however, which did not permit them to examine the mesial frontal cortex; a tomographic approach is necessary in order to evaluate activity in this region. Taken together with the findings concerning the drug-naive patients, these results suggest a potentially significant relationship between the mesial frontal cortex and the symptoms of schizophrenia and that there may be a specific relationship between this region and an increase in negative symptoms.

Future Directions

Much work needs to be done in this area in the future. As yet, the neural mechanisms that could explain positive and negative symptoms have not been determined. The initial model proposed by Crow is almost certainly too simple, since it cannot account for mixtures of positive and negative symptoms or changes in phenomenology over time. More complex models must be developed that continue to build on our growing knowledge concerning normal brain structure and function, the complex interactions of neural circuits connecting various brain regions, and the mechanism of action of neuroleptic drugs.

There are clearly some important future directions that should be explored in schizophrenia research. These include the use of in vivo imaging techniques, the careful integration of reliable clinical description and an evaluation of neural mechanisms, and recognition of the structural and neurochemical complexity of the human brain, the importance of studying patients longitudinally, and the value of examining the course of illness with dynamic rather than static models.

References

American Psychiatric Association (1987) Diagnostic and statistical manual of mental disorders (DSM-III-R). American Psychiatric Association, Washington

American Psychiatric Association and Committee on Nomenclature and Statistics (1980) Diagnostic and statistical manual of mental disorders (DSM-III). American Psychiatric Association, Washington

Andreasen NC (1979a) Thought, language, and communication disorders. I. Clinical assessment, definition of terms, and evaluation of their reliability. Arch Gen Psychiatry 36:1315–1321

Andreasen NC (1979b) Thought, language, and communication disorders. II. Diagnostic significance. Arch Gen Psychiatry 36:1325–1330

Andreasen NC (1979c) Affective flattening and the criteria for schizophrenia. Am J Psychiatry 136:944–947

Andreasen NC (1982) Negative symptoms in schizophrenia: definition and reliability. Arch Gen Psychiatry 39:784–788

Andreasen NC (1983) The scale for the assessment of negative symptoms (SANS). University of Iowa, Iowa City

Andreasen NC (1984) The scale for the assessment of positive symptoms (SAPS). University of Iowa, Iowa City

Andreasen NC (1985) Comprehensive assessment of symptoms and history (CASH). University of Iowa, Iowa City

Andreasen NC (1988) Brain imaging: applications in psychiatry. Science 239:1381–1388

Andreasen NC (1990a) Positive and negative symptoms: historical and conceptual aspects. In: Andreasen NC (ed) Modern problems of pharmacopsychiatry: positive and negative symptoms and syndromes. Karger, Basle, pp 1–42

Andreasen NC (1990b) Methods for assessing positive and negative symptoms. In: Andreasen NC (ed) Modern problems of pharmacopsychiatry: positive and negative symptoms and syndromes. Karger, Basle, pp 73–88

Andreasen NC, Grove WM (1986) Evaluation of positive and negative symptoms in schizophrenia. Psychiatr Psychobiol 1(2):108–121

Andreasen NC, Smith MR, Jacoby CG, Dennert JW, Olsen SA (1982) Ventricular enlargement in schizophrenia: definition and prevalence. Am J Psychiatry 139:292–296

Andreasen NC, Ehrhardt JC, Swayze VW, Alliger R, Yuh WTC, Cohen G, Ziebell S (1990a) Magnetic resonances imaging of the brain in schizophrenia: the pathophysiological significance of structural abnormalities. Arch General Psychiatry 47:35–44

Andreasen NC, Swayze VW, Flaum M, Alliger R, Cohen G (1990b) Ventricular abnormalities in affective disorders: clinical and demographic correlated. Am J Psychiatry 147: 893–900, 1990

Andreasen NC, Swayze VW, Flaum M, Yates WR, Arndt S, McChesney C (1990c) Ventricular enlargement in schizophrenia evaluated with computed tomographic scanning: effects of gender, age, and stage of illness. Arch Gen Psychiatry 47:1008–1015, 1990

Arndt S, Alliger RJ, Andreasen NC (1990) The distinction of positive and negative symptoms: The failure of a two-dimensional model. Br J Psychiatry 158:317–322, 1991

Barnes TRE, Curson DA, Liddle PF, Patel M (1989a) The nature and prevalence of depression in chronic schizophrenia inpatients. Br J Psychiatry 154:486–491

Barnes TRE, Liddle PF, Curson DA, Patel M (1989b) Negative symptoms, tardive dyskinesia and depression in chronic schizophrenia. Br J Psychiatry 155: (supplement 7) 99–103

Berman KF, Zec RF, Weinberger DR (1986) Physiologic dysfunction of dorsolateral prefrontal cortex in schizophrenia. II. Role of neuroleptic treatment, attention, and mental effort. Arch Gen Psychiatry 43:126–135

Bilder RM, Mukherjee S, Rieder RO, Pandurangi AK (1985) Symptomatic and neuropsychological components of defect states. Schizophr Bull 11:409–419

Bleuler E (1916) Physisch und psychisch in der Pathologie. Z Gesamte Neurol Psychiatr 30:426–475

Buchsbaum MS, Haier RJ (1987) Functional and anatomical brain imaging: impact on schizophrenia research. Schizophr Bull 13:115–132

Buchsbaum MS, Holcomb HH, Kessler R et al. (1983) Lateralized asymmetries in glucose uptake assessed by positron emission tomography in patients with schizophrenia and normal controls. In: Flor-Henry P, Gruzelier J (eds) Laterality and psychopathology. Elsevier, Amsterdam, pp 559–568

Buchsbaum MS, Capelletti J, Ball R et al. (1984) Positron emission tomographic image measurement in schizophrenia and affective disorders. Ann Neurol [Suppl] 15:S157–S165

Crow TJ (1980) Molecular pathology of schizophrenia: more than one disease process? Br Med J 280:66–68

Dworkin RH, Lenzenweger MF (1984) Symptoms and the genetics of schizophrenia: implications for diagnosis. Am J Psychiatry 141:1541–1546

Fuster J (1989) The prefrontal cortex: anatomy, physiology and neuropsychology of the frontal lobe, 2nd edn. Raven, New York

Gur RE, Gur RC, Skolnick BE et al. (1985) Brain function in psychiatric disorders. III. Regional cerebral blood flow in unmedicated schizophrenics. Arch Gen Psychiatry 42:329–334

Gur RE, Resnick SM, Alavi A et al. (1987a) Regional brain function in schizophrenia. I. A positron emission tomography study. Arch Gen Psychiatry 44:119–125

Gur RE, Resnick SM, Gur RC et al. (1987b) Regional brain function in schizophrenia. II. Repeated evaluation with positron emission tomography. Arch Gen Psychiatry 44:126–129

Humbert M, Salvador L, Segui J, Obiols J, Obiols JD (1986) Estudio interfiabilidad version espanola evaluacion de sintomas positivos y negativos. Rev Dep Psiquiatr Fac Med Univ Barcelona 13:28–36

Ingvar DH, Franzen G (1974) Abnormalities of cerebral blood flow distribution in patients with chronic schizophrenia. Acta Psychiatr Scand 50:425–462

Johnstone EC, Owens DGC, Crow TJ, Jagoe R (1981) A CT study of 188 patients with schizophrenia, affective psychosis and neurotic illness. Biol Psychiatry 9:237–240

Johnstone EC, Owens DGC, Firth CD, Crow TJ (1986) The relative stability of positive and negative features in chronic schizophrenia. Br J Psychiatry 150:60–64

Kay SR, Opler LA, Fiszbein A (1986) Significance of positive and negative symptoms in chronic schizophrenia. Br J Psychiatry 149:439–448

Kraepelin E (1919) Dementia praecox and paraphrenia. Livingstone, Edinburgh

Krawiecka M, Goldberg D, Vaughan M (1977) A standardized psychiatric assessment for rating chronic psychiatric patients. Acta Psychiatr Scand 55:299–308

Lewine RRJ, Fogg L, Meltzer HY (1983) Assessment of negative and positive symptoms in schizophrenia. Schizophr Bull 9:368–376

Liddle PF (1984) Schizophrenic symptoms, cognitive performance and neurological dysfunction. 2nd Bi-Annual Winter Workshop on Schizophrenia, Davos
Liddle PF (1987) The symptoms of chronic schizophrenia. A re-examination of the positive-negative dichotomy. Br J Psychiatr 151:145–151
Marks RC, Luchins DJ (1990) Relationship between brain imaging findings in schizophrenia and psychopathology: a review of the literature relating to positive and negative symptoms. In: Andreasen NC (ed) Modern problems of pharmacopsychiatry: positive and negative symptoms and syndromes. Karger, Basle, pp 89–123
McGlashan TH (1991) The positive/negative distinction in schizophrenia: review of natural history validators. Arch Gen Psychiatry (in press)
Moscarelli M, Maffei C, Cesana BM (1987) An international perspective on assessment of negative and positive symptoms in schizophrenia. Am J Psychiatry 144:1595–1598
Ohta T, Okazaki Y, Anzai N (1984) Reliability of the japanese version of the scale for the assessment of negative symptoms (SANS). Jpn J Psychiatry 13:999–1010
Overall J, Gorham D (1962) Brief psychiatric rating scale. Psychol Rep 10:799–812
Pearlson GD, Garbacz DJ, Breakey WR, Ahn HS, DePaulo JR (1984) Lateral ventricular enlargement associated with persistent unemployment and negative symptoms in both schizophrenia and bipolar disorder. Psychiatry Res 12:1–9
Pearlson GD, Garbacz DJ, Moberg PJ, Ahn HS, DePaulo JR (1985) Symptomatic, familial, perinatal, and social correlates of computerized axial tomography (CAT) changes in schizophrenics and bipolars. J Nerv Ment Dis 173:42–50
Pfohl B, Winokur G (1983) The micropsychopathology of hebephrenic/catatonic schizophrenia. J Nerv Ment Dis 171:296–300
Phillips M (1987) Scale for the assessment of negative symptoms and scale for the assessment of positive symptoms, Chinese version. National Center for Psychiatric Training, Shashi Psychiatric Hospital, Shashi, Hubei
Pogue-Geile MF, Harrow M (1984) Negative and positive symptoms in schizophrenia and depression: a follow-up. Schizophr Bull 10:371–387
Pogue-Geile MF, Harrow M (1985) Negative symptoms in schizophrenia: their longitudinal course and prognostic importance. Schizophr Bull 11:427–439
Robins E, Guze SB (1970) Establishment of diagnostic validity in psychiatric illness: its application to schizophrenia. Am J Psychiatry 126:983–987
Siris SG, Adan F, Cohen M, Mandeli J, Aronson A, Casey E (1988) Postpsychotic depression and negative symptoms: an investigation of syndromal overlap. Am J Psychiatry 145:1532–1537
Spitzer RL, Endicott J, Robins E (1978) Research diagnostic criteria: rationale and reliability. Arch Gen Psychiatry 35:773–782
Weinberger DR (1988) Schizophrenia and the frontal lobe. Top Neurol Sci 11:367–370
Weinberger DR, Berman KF, Zec RF (1986) Physiological dysfunction of dorsolateral prefrontal cortex in schizophrenia. I. Regional cerebral blood flow (rCBF) evidence. Arch Gen Psychiatry 43:114–124
Wing JK (1974) A standard form of psychiatric present state examinations (PSE) and a method for standardizing the classification of symptoms. In Psychiatric epidemiology. Oxford University Press, London
Wing JK, Cooper JE, Sartorius N (1974) The measurement and classification of psychiatric symptoms. Cambridge University Press, London

Assessment of Negative Symptoms: Instruments and Evaluation Criteria

R.-D. Stieglitz [1]

Introduction

Interest in negative symptoms has increased in recent years (cf. Strauss 1985; Pogue-Geile and Zubin 1988), as evidenced by a great number of theoretical as well as empirical papers dealing either with the investigation of negative symptoms or applying them as moderator variables in researching various questions.

This interest in negative symptoms and their differentiation from positive ones is connected in particular with the hope of identifying factors with different prognostic, therapeutic and pathogenetic significance (Crow 1989). Research involves prediction of the course of illness (particularly long-term; Pogue-Geile and Harrow 1985; Strauss et al. 1989: psychological and social influence of negative symptoms on the course) and the response to therapy (Andreasen 1982). Particularly fascinating are the aetiological questions (cf. also Zubin 1985) in the sense of covariation with structural brain changes, neurochemical, neurophysiological or genetic features (Crow 1985).

Origins of the concept can already be found in the nineteenth century (Berrios 1985), although no uniform theory is discernable up to the present time (Sass 1989). The definitions are broad to varying extents (Crow 1985) and are, thus, also associated in part with a number of other concepts or are even uses synonymously with them (e.g. acute vs. chronic, plus vs. minus; cf. Sass 1989). In the latter case, however, specific implications are usually additionally connected to them (e.g. residual symptoms: chronicity, course, onset and domain of function; Sommers 1985).

Many definitions of negative symptoms share the absence of or the inadequate development of normal functions (e.g. Sommers 1985; Grossman et al. 1989; Zubin 1985). According to Lenzenweger et al. (1989, p. 62), one can differentiate between positive and negative symptoms as follows:

- Positive symptoms: presence of a behaviour or function that is otherwise normally not present in an individual.
- Negative symptoms: absence of a behaviour or function that is usually present in the normal individual.

---

[1] Freie Universität Berlin, Psychiatrische Klinik, Eschenallee 3, W-1000 Berlin 19, FRG

A. Marneros / N. C. Andreasen / M. T. Tsuang (Eds.)
Negative Versus Positive Schizophrenia

Here, deficits are postulated in very different areas: cognitive, social and affective (e.g. Kay and Opler 1987; Sommers 1985).

It is generally acknowledged that when referring to negative symptoms, we are dealing with significant characteristics of the schizophrenic syndrome (Andreasen 1982). This can be concluded, for example, from the various diagnostic systems (Berner et al. 1983), although the symptoms in question are not specific to schizophrenia (Mundt et al. 1989). Other nosological groups, in particular groups of depressive patients (e.g. Stieglitz and Helmchen 1990), can also exhibit these characteristics. Thus, according to Alpert (1985), the characteristic "flat affect" can be an aspect of retardation in depressive patients, an expression of neuroleptic side-effects or a schizophrenic characteristic within the context of diagnostic systems (e.g. Diagnostic and Statistical Manual, DSM-III-R). Furthermore, negative symptoms can occur in all stages of the course of schizophrenia (Angst et al. 1989: prepsychotic, productive psychotic or post-psychotic period).

One of the basic problems includes establishing and specifying which symptoms are to be classified as negative and clearly delimiting these from the positive symptoms (Grossman et al. 1989). Moreover, there is a controversial discussion in progress regarding the extent to which a number of negative symptoms are primary or secondary (cf. e.g. Carpenter et al. 1985). Thus, for example, the frequently cited symptom of social withdrawal can be interpreted as a reaction to positive symptoms (e.g. delusions), as a consequence of the illness (Crow 1989) or as coping with the symptoms or the illness. In addition, negative symptoms are connected with a number of other characteristics of the illness, such as, for example, intellectual impairment and neurological signs (Crow 1989).

In spite of great differences in how broadly these concepts are defined (and their operationalisation by means of assessment instruments), there is a focal group of characteristics (flat affect and poverty of speech, among others), which are included in most operational definitions.

Negative symptoms range from features which are relatively easy to comprehend and define all the way to highly complex, psychopathological concepts (Rösler and Hengesch 1990).

The increasing interest in negative symptoms and their distinction from other psychopathological areas has led a number of researchers to develop assessment instruments (Grossman et al. 1989). In the more recently developed scales, one tends to find that the concept of negative symptoms is formulated more broadly.

The application of different assessment instruments is one reason for the partly discrepant results found in the literature concerning negative symptomatology (cf. e.g. Pogue-Geile 1989; Thiemann et al. 1987), for example:

- General methodological limitations (e.g. static rather than dynamic point of view; Kay and Opler 1987).
- Variously broad concepts of schizophrenia (e.g. Pogue-Geile 1989).
- Composition of the samples (e.g. different degrees of chronicity; Pogue-Geile 1989).

Moreover, the use of many – in some cases very different – instruments and the resulting limited comparability make an aggregation of data and results impossible, for example, in the context of meta-analyses.

In spite of the multiplicity of existing scales, one repeatedly hears the complaint about a shortage of reliable and valid instruments (e.g. Andreasen 1985a, b). Presently, there is no sufficiently empirical basis for preferring one scale over another (Pogue-Geile and Zubin 1988). Therefore, in the following the attempt is made to compile and define the most frequently used instruments as well as to provide evaluation criteria for assessment instruments of negative symptomatology.

Assessment Instruments

Up to now, there have been a number of very different scales developed for assessing negative symptoms. Items relating to negative symptoms are included in most of the general purpose rating scales of psychopathology (Table 1). In some scales, there are additional subscales, which exhibit a close relationship to negative symptoms. These are, for example, the "apathy syndrome" in the Association for Methodology and Documentation in Psychiatry (AMDP) system, "retardation and apathy" in the Inpatient Multidimensional Psychiatric Scale (IMPS), and the "withdrawal-retardation" (anergia) scale in the Brief Psychiatric Rating Scale (BPRS).

The item pool of these scales was often also useful in developing new scales. In this way, Gibbons et al. (1985) designed three scales based upon 11 items with a sample of 416 patients: apathy, motor retardation and loss of goal. From the BPRS, Andersen et al. (1986) developed a 10-item subscale, which is

Table 1. General purpose rating scales of psychopathology

Scale	Abbreviation	Reference	Subscale[a]
Inpatient Multidimensional Psychiatric Scale	IMPS	Lorr et al. (1966)	Retardation and apathy
Brief Psychiatric Rating Scale	BPRS	Overall and Gorham (1976)	Withdrawal-retardation (anergia)
Nurses' Observation Scale for Inpatient Evaluation	NOSIE	Honigfeld et al. (1976)	Retardation
Present State Examination	PSE	Wing et al. (1974)	–[b]
AMDP system	AMDP	AMDP (1979); Guy and Ban (1982)	Apathy syndrome
Comprehensive Psychopathological Rating Scale	CPRS	Asberg et al. (1978)	–

[a] Subscales with relation to negative symptomatology.
[b] No subscale, only negative symptoms.

Table 2. Rating scales for the assessment of negative symptomatology

Rating scale	Abbreviation	Reference	S	G	Ss	T
Activity Withdrawal Scale	AWS	Venables (1957)	10			1
Rating Scale for Chronic Schizophrenics	RSCS	Wing (1961)	4			
Manchester Rating Scale	MRS	Krawiecka et al. (1977)	4			
Rating Scale for Emotional Blunting	EBS	Abrams and Taylor (1978)	16		3	1
Scale for the Assessment of Negative Symptoms	SANS	Andreasen (1982, 1989)	19	5	5	5
Negative Symptom Rating Scale	NSRS	Iager et al. (1985)	10		4	1
Negative Symptom Behavior Rating Scale	NSBRS	Pogue-Geile and Harrow (1985)	13		3	1
Intentionalitäts-Skala	InSka	Mundt et al. (1985), Mundt (1989)	60		6	1
Positive and Negative Syndrome Scale for Schizophrenia	PANSS	Kay et al. (1987a, b, 1989)	7			1
Subjective Experience of Deficits in Schizophrenia	SEDS	Liddle and Barnes (1988)	21		5	
Schedule for the Deficit Syndrome	SDS	Kirkpatrick et al. (1989)	6		2	1
Behavioral Observation Schedule	BOS	Atakan and Cooper (1989)	82		15	5
High Royds Evaluation of Negative Scale	HEN	Mortimer et al. (1989)	18	6	6	1
WHO Psychological Impairments Rating Schedule	WHO/PIRS	Biehl et al. (1989a, b)	20			1

S, number of symptoms (not only negative symptoms); G, global rating; Ss, subscales; T, total score.

homogeneous with the unidimensional Rasch model. McGorry et al. (1988) developed a modification of the BPRS for nurses. Lewine et al. (1983) produced scales for negative symptoms from the Schedule for Affective Disorders and Schizophrenia–Change (SADS–C) as well as the Nurses' Observation Scale for Inpatient Evaluation (NOSIE), which fit the Rasch model and show sufficient stability over time.

The majority of existing scales were specially developed with regard to assessing negative symptoms and are included in Table 2. It is not possible to make a comprehensive comparison at this point. Instead, some distinguishing features and points of criticism will be dealt with here.

Rudiments of Assessment. The question arises regarding which information base should be drawn upon to assess negative symptomatology: Symptoms based on the patient's statements and/or signs based upon the observer's ratings of the patient's behaviour. All of these scales are observer rating scales (rater: physician, psychologist, in some cases nurses). Differences emerge, however, regarding what should be used as the informational base for assessment. In some scales, only observable behaviours are included (e.g. Negative Symptom Behavior Rating Scale, NSBRS, High Royds Evaluation of Negative Scale, HEN, Positive and Negative Syndrome Scale for Schizophrenia, PANSS), in others, observable and/or reported (e.g. Manchester Rating Scale, MRS, Schedule for the Deficit Syndrome, SDS, Scale for the Assessment of Negative Symptoms, SANS), and in still others, only reported characteristics (e.g. Subjective Experience of Deficits in Schizophrenia, SEDS).

Units of Assessment. The scales differ with respect to units of assessment. These include single aspects, signs or symptoms or complexes of different aspects (e.g. BPRS).

Assessment Procedure. Johnstone (1989) found that the scales can be differentiated according to how the information was assessed:

- based on general contact with the patient
- based on a non-structured interview
- based on a non-structured interview containing obligatory direct questions
- based on standardised interview.

In most of the scales, the information is assessed in a non-structured clinical interview (an exception is the MRS with obligatory direct questions).

Scaling. Graduated evaluations of severity (up to 7 graduations) are asked for in most of the scales. The graduations are unspecified (e.g. SEDS, HEN), or are at least partly operationalised, i.e. with score anchor point definitions (e.g. NSRS, PANSS, SANS).

Contents. Differences among the scales become apparent here. The majority of scales assess several areas of negative symptomatology. The most frequent are affect, speech, arousal, cognition and social functioning.

Observation Period. Very large differences between the individual scales become apparent when considering the observation period. It can be defined flexibly (e.g. NSRS), or it can refer to the interview (e.g. NSBRS). It can relate to a defined period of time (e.g. HEN), or in others, no information is given (e.g. Rating Scale for Emotional Blunting, EBS).

Development of the Scale. It is certainly problematic that the scales were often developed using very small samples (e.g. SEDS, EBS, HEN, NSRS, SDS). Test statistical analyses (e.g. item analyses) are often not available.

Reliability and Validity. Certainly the most important and complex areas are reliability and validity. For most of the scales, there are either no references to reliability or those made can be considered unsatisfactory (particularly on the symptom level). Furthermore, the available references to validity are inadequate (there is often no reference made to convergent or to divergent validity). The PANSS and SANS can be regarded as the best evaluated scales.

Aspect of Time. Besides differentiating between groups, it is important to present evidence for the applicability of the scales regarding the aspect of time. This holds true for describing both the course of illness as well as the evidence of therapeutic interventions. In addition, to prove the sensitivity of the scales for illustrating changes, one also needs to examine their temporal stability. Particularly this latter aspect has been only inadequately examined, if at all.

There are a number of other scales in addition to those presented in Table 2. For example, Rosen et al. (1984) derived a negative symptom severity score from the SANS. Otherwise, ad hoc negative symptom scales were composed based upon phenomenological considerations (e.g. Angst et al. 1989; Honigfeld and Patin 1989).

Evaluation Criteria

General

A comprehensive evaluation of the assessment instruments includes examining a number of criteria. In the following, such evaluation criteria will be introduced. Examples of their application will be presented afterwards. Most of the scales previously proposed for assessing negative symptoms are more or less explicitly oriented towards the classical test theory (CTT).

The fundamental criteria within the CTT represent objectivity, reliability and validity. They are related hierarchically and are mutually dependent. Thus, for example, a scale with high validity must necessarily exhibit high objectivity and reliability. A scale cannot be more valid than it is reliable (Lienert 1969).

By objectivity (with the elements of administrative, interpretive and scoring objectivity), Lienert (1969) means the degree to which the results of a test are independent of the examiner. In contrast to the criteria for reliability and validity, there are no numerical values here.

Essential aspects involved are:

- The (operational) definitions of the symptoms should concur with the customary terminology and be summarised in a glossary.
- An at least semi-structured interview should ensure dependable assessment of information.
- All important information relating to administration and rules for scoring as well as important data about reliability and validity should be contained in a manual.
- The scale should be simple and economic to use and allow the construction of subscales.

- Moreover, one should be able to develop an empirically supported scale. The scores obtained for the scale should also be transferable into norm scores.

The aspect of objectivity of administration can be specified even further, analogous to Hall (1980):

Description of the setting
- Purpose of the scale
- Subjects for whom the scale is intended (indication)
- Rater

Description of the procedure
- Training of raters
- Process of rating
- Information used as a basis for ratings
- Observation period
- Additional comments and quantification on the formal rating

In addition to specifying the setting in which the rating takes place, it is particularly necessary to describe the procedure in detail. The characteristics subsumed under the concept of objectivity can be regarded as necessary but not sufficient conditions for reliability and validity. They are designated as "psychometric-methodologic criteria" in the following:

Reliability
- Retest reliability
- Internal consistency
- Inter-rater reliability

Validity
- Content validity
- Concurrent or criterion-oriented validity
- Convergent validity
- Divergent validity
- Factorial validity
- Comparisons among groups
- Predictive validity
- Time invariance of the instrument

Reliability refers to the determination that the instrument is measuring a particular characteristic in a reproducible and/or consistent fashion.

Retest reliability refers to the administration of the same test twice. For scales claiming to illustrate changeable characteristics, this criterion is only important over short intervals of time.

The internal consistency of a scale (assessed by the split-half reliability or the consistency analysis) provides information about the homogeneity of a scale.

The inter-rater reliability (actually more an aspect of objectivity) gives information regarding the extent to which different raters agree in their assessments.

The parallel test reliability, a measure for the concurrence between two parallel test forms, is not listed in the table, because such parallel forms are the exception in the psychiatric field.

The decisive criteria for evaluating the scales can be subsumed under the concept of validity, i.e. the extent to which a scale measures a characteristic that it intends or purports to measure. Even less than for reliability can one say that a scale has *a* validity. There are many different aspects involved here, the most important of which are listed above. Determining the validity of a scale is an approximate or cumulative process, which in the long run is never complete.

Theoretical conceptions precede the development of a scale, and it is essential to check whether or not the scale actually is a realisation of these theoretical ideas.

By content validity, one refers to the extent to which the contents of a test instrument are representative of the characteristics or symptoms to be investigated.

The concurrent or criterion-related validity encompasses the correlations with so-called external criteria, which are or could be directly connected to the characteristic under examination.

With convergent and divergent (or discriminant) validity, one is involved in checking the relations among scales based on similar or different constructs. Both aspects are also subsumed under the term differential validity, i.e. the indication of varyingly high correlations to other scales.

A concept relevant here is factorial validity, i.e. the joint factor analysis of different scales with the expectation that scales with similar ranges of application will load on a common factor.

Comparisons among groups (e.g. comparisons of means, discriminant analyses, cluster analyses) are meant to show that the scales can differentiate, for example, between separate nosological groups.

In the area of psychiatric research, predictive validity represents the decisive criterion for validity. This includes the prediction of the therapy response as well as of the course of the illness.

One aspect frequently omitted from the discussion involves analyses of the time invariance of the instrument, because the assessment of changeable characteristics is intended by most of the scales used in the psychiatric area. In addition, there are a number of hypotheses connected with the aspect of time precisely in relation to negative symptoms (cf. Pogue-Geile and Zubin 1988: persistence of negative symptoms, prognostic value, age-related changes in the prevalence of negative symptoms). Thus, for example, it is essential to clarify first the extent to which the assessment instruments used are stable before clarifying the question of the short- or long-term stability of negative symptoms. Such investigations are scarcely ever conducted for any of the scales. Stieglitz et al. (1980) formulated pragmatic criteria for this based upon the CTT: the call for stability of the test parameters relates to the item-total correlations, distribution of the scale scores, reliability and factorial structure.

However, the fulfillment of these criteria does not solve basic problems regarding the measurement of change within classical test theory (cf. Harris 1963). Moreover, one must demand that the results attained be tested using other samples (cross validation).

The following will illustrate how to apply the criteria of evaluation presented using the examples of negative symptoms and the negative symptomatology (NS) scale "apathy symdrome" from the AMDP system. Here, references will be made to personal results as well as to the literature.

Illustration

The AMDP system (AMDP 1979; Guy and Ban 1982) is a documentation system. It consists of the following parts:

- Anamnesis 1: demographic data (e.g. education, level of employment).
- Anamnesis 2: life events (e.g. death of spouse/partner, shop/business defunct).
- Anamnesis 3: psychiatric history (e.g. birth and childhood, previous psychiatric episodes).
- Psychopathological symptoms: 100 items.
- Somatic signs: 40 items.

The formation of syndromes (e.g. apathy syndrome, paranoid-hallucinatory syndrome, depressive syndrome; Gebhardt et al. 1983; Pietzcker et al. 1983) by means of mathematic-statistical approaches can be regarded as an advantage of an economical description of the psychopathology. The "apathy syndrome" is important with respect to the assessment of negative symptoms (Table 3). The syndrome represents essential, generally accepted aspects of negative symptomatology (content validity): affect, thinking, drive, behaviour.

The ratings are based mostly upon signs or on a mixture of signs and symptoms. Only one item is based solely on a symptom.

The use of the entire AMDP system makes possible not only the assessment of NS, but also the concurrent judgement of other clinically relevant aspects of

Table 3. Items of the apathy syndrome

Items	Sign	Symptom
15 Inhibited thinking		x
16 Retarded thinking	x	
17 Circumstantial thinking	x	
18 Restricted thinking	x	
61 Blunted affect	x	
79 Affective rigidity	x	
80 Lack of drive	x	x
92 Social withdrawal	x	x

Gebhardt et al. 1983; Pietzcker et al. 1983.

Table 4. Reliability of the negative symptoms and the "apathy syndrome" of the AMDP system

Reliability	Level	Results	Reference
Inter-rater	Symptoms	$\kappa = 0.32-0.78$	Good (1989)
	Apathy syndrome	$\kappa = 0.60$	Mundt et al. (1989)
Internal consistency	Apathy syndrome	Cronbach's alpha 0.69	Gebhardt et al. (1983)
		Cronbach's alpha 0.84	Personal results

the NS (e.g. psycho-organic syndrome, depressive syndrome; assessment of neuroleptic side-effects). This is important especially in the context of therapy studies.

Evaluation Criteria for Practical Application

The evaluation criteria relevant to practical use are four. A glossary (AMDP 1979; Guy and Ban 1982) with explanations of the anamnestic sheets and definitions of the psychopathological and somatic items is available as an aid to the user. A test manual (Baumann and Stieglitz 1983, 1989) summarises the empirical studies concerning the AMDP system. An interview to obtain the information was developed by Fähndrich and Stieglitz (1989).

AMDP syndrome scales were proposed by Gebhardt et al. (1983; Pietzcker et al. 1983), with norm tables (T values) based on a heterogenous sample of psychiatric in-patients ($n = 2313$).

Psychometric Evaluation Criteria

Reliability. The inter-rater reliability for the symptoms (Table 4) of the apathy syndrome ranges from 0.32 to 0.78 (syndrome level $\kappa = 0.60$; Mundt et al. 1989). Only two symptoms fall below $\kappa = 0.40$ (blunted affect, lack of drive) as can be cited from a recent study by Good (1989).

Gebhardt et al. (1983) indicated that the internal consistency for the apathy syndrome with Cronbach's alpha was equal to 0.69. Using a sample of psychiatric patients ($n = 4114$) independent of the standardisation sample, we found an alpha equal to 0.84. This can be considered "good" to "satisfactory", particularly as the scale is relatively short, and the reliability is dependent upon the length of the scale.

Validity. 1. Comparisons Among Groups. A lot of studies exist in which comparisons among groups were made with the AMDP syndromes (cf. Baumann and Stieglitz 1983, 1989). Here, differences between groups became obvious with regard to various questions particularly in reference to the apathy syndrome:

- Various nosological groups, schizophrenic vs. neurotic and endogenous depressive at the time of admission (Pietzcker and Gebhard 1985) or in remission (Mundt and Kasper 1987)
- Various kinds of psychotherapy (e.g. Buchkremer and Fiedler 1987) or of psychopharmacotherapy (e.g. Woggon et al. 1986)

2. Concurrent Validity. The concurrent or the criterion-related validity investigates the covariation with external criteria. Here, for example, Zinner et al. (1989) found correlations between the apathy syndrome and cognitive variables, such as

- Digit cancelling ($r = -0.28$)
- Letter symbol test ($r = -0.36$)
- Substained attention test (German: Test d2); ($r = -0.39$)

in a sample of 64 chronic schizophrenic patients diagnosed according to DSM-III. Connections to additional groups of variables became apparent in two reviews (Baumann and Stieglitz 1983, 1989).

3. Convergent Validity. There is a number of papers available about convergent validity, some of which are included in Table 5. Scales were selected as criteria that also claim to assess negative symptoms or subaspects of them. The results stress that the correlations are consistently average to very high.

4. Divergent Validity. Numerous studies are also available regarding this aspect of validity (cf. survey in Baumann and Stieglitz 1983, 1989). The results of personal analyses are included in Table 6. For the entire sample of psychiatric patients ($n = 6264$) as well as for a sub-sample of schizophrenic patients (ICD-9; $n = 1490$), there appear:

- Mostly numerically low correlations (exception: depressive syndrome, which corresponds to other studies, e.g. Prosser et al. 1987).
- Low correlations with positive symptoms (e.g. paranoid-hallucinatory syndrome).

This holds true for patients with the syndromes at the time of admission as well as upon discharge.

Table 5. Convergent validity of the "apathy syndrome"

Reference	Corresponding scale(s)	*r*
Mundt (1989)	InSka	0.67–0.71
Zinner et al. (1989)	SANS	0.42–0.82
	BPRS: ANERGIA	0.79
	InSka	0.65–0.83
Straumann (1989)	SANS	0.62

For abbreviations, see Table 1, 2.

Table 6. Divergent validity (correlations of the "apathy syndrome" with the other AMDP syndromes)

	Total		ICD-9 295.3	
	A	D	A	D
Paranoid-hallucinatory syndrome	0.06	0.21	0.04	0.23
Psycho-organic syndrome	0.23	0.38	0.18	0.28
Manic syndrome	−0.27	0.03	−0.29	0.00
Depressive syndrome	0.42	0.45	0.32	0.40
Hostility syndrome	−0.03	0.28	−0.01	0.27
Autonomic syndrome	0.06	0.17	0.07	0.12
Obsessive-compulsive syndrome	0.06	0.09	0.11	0.10
n	6264		1490	

A, admission; D, discharge; ICD-9, sub-group of schizophrenic patients.

5. *Factorial Validity.* Zinner et al. (1989) performed a joint factor analysis of the apathy syndrome with other observer and self-rating scales. Along with other negative scales, the apathy syndrome was given a high factor loading ($a = 0.81$) on one factor (among others ANERGIA of the BPRS, all subscales of the SANS). It proved to be factorially independent of self-ratings and various cognitive variables.

6. *Predictive Validity.* Various studies are also available concerning predictive validity, particularly in regard to the course of the illness. Some results of Gaebel's comprehensive studies (1988) on schizophrenic patients are included in Table 7. Here in particular, significant and numerically high correlations appeared between the apathy syndrome and various course and outcome parameters (e.g. clinical global impression, social contacts), when course intervals of different lengths were involved. Fähndrich and Richter (1986) were able to discover differences between future chronic and non-chronic patients, even at the time of the first episode. Here, the apathy syndrome was more pronounced in the chronic patients. In an analysis of 12 patients presenting with their first episode of schizophrenia (ICD-9: 295.3), we found a significant correlation between the apathy syndrome at the time of release and the degree of remission (full vs. partial remission) after four relapses ($r = 0.54$, $P < 0.10$).

Table 7. Predictive validity of the "apathy syndrome" (APA) (Gebhardt et al. 1983): results of Gaebels's studies with schizophrenic patients. Significant correlations ($P < 0.05$) between:

APA	Outcome[a]	Correlation
Discharge	1 year after discharge	$r < 0.73$
Discharge	3 years after discharge	$r < 0.34$
1 year follow-up	3 years after discharge	$r < 0.44$

[a] e.g. clinical global impression, frequencies of social contacts.

Table 8. Item and test parameters (stability of time) of the "apathy syndrome"

	Admission		Discharge	
	Total ($n = 4114$)	ICD 295.3 ($n = 980$)	Total ($n = 4114$)	ICD 295.3 ($n = 980$)
Internal consistency (Cronbach's alpha)	0.84	0.80	0.89	0.78
Item-total correlation				
– Range	0.34–0.75	0.27–0.73	0.52–0.76	0.42–0.60
– Mean	0.58	0.51	0.66	0.49

7. *Time Aspect.* Test statistical analyses were performed in reference to the time aspect on a sample independent of the standardisation sample (Gebhardt et al. 1983). The results are included in Table 8. The results for the item parameters of the item-total correlation as well as for the coefficient of internal consistency for the entire scale (Cronbach's alpha) were on the whole good to satisfactory coefficients and stable over time (comparison of admission vs. discharge).

In summarising the results for the apathy syndrome, one can keep in mind that:

- The scale can be considered as sufficiently validated for assessing negative symptoms, both for the entire sample of psychiatric patients as well as for schizophrenic patients.
- This also holds true for the aspect of reliability on the scale level. One needs to strive for content revisions for two items.
- Considering the length of the scale, the apathy syndrome is an economic scale.

It is not yet definite to what extent even more items are to be assigned to the area of negative symptoms in the AMDP system. Other authors come up with more items than are included in an apathy syndrome scale (Angst et al. 1989: 14 symptoms; Rösler and Hengesch 1990: 17 symptoms). These cover the major part of the range of significance of the SANS and NSRS (Good 1989). However, it is still unclear to what extent these items can then be distinguished across several dimensions (Angst et al. 1989), i.e. to what extent negative symptoms are multi-dimensional.

The evaluation criteria investigated here using the example of the apathy syndrome should also be tested using other negative scales. Only scales assessed as satisfactory in regard to these criteria can contribute to the clarification of the construct of negative symptomatology. Naturally, this demand also applies to scales for assessing positive symptoms.

Multi-Modal Approach

Psychiatric research and practice depend upon assessing people in their entirety, i.e. on all relevant levels at the same time. Therefore, a multi-modal approach has been compulsory in psychiatry for a long time (Seidenstücker and Baumann 1987). This also applies to the study of negative symptomatology. Different data sources (e.g. self and observer ratings), data bases (e.g. somatic, psychological, social) and different constructs are to be taken into consideration. Reasons for proceeding in this way arise based upon various arguments, such as adequate description of the phenomena, i.e. mutually supplementary and complementary ways of describing the phenomena, or the ability to generate hypotheses. Furthermore, there are limits to improve the reliability and validity of individual instruments. This necessitates combining different scales to achieve a sufficiently valid measurement of the phenomenon in the centre of interest (von Zerssen and Möller 1980). The assumption involved is that each data source and each data base contribute one aspect to the respective construct under assessment.

Especially the relationship between self and observer ratings has played an important part in the discussion in recent years. Repeatedly observable discordances are considered to be a function of differing rater perspectives but can also be based upon methodological inadequacies (e.g. particular phenomena can be assessed only by self or observer ratings).

A supplementary rather than a substitutional function is granted to both groups of scales dependent upon the patient sample being investigated (Seidenstücker and Baumann 1987). Together, the two allow coverage of a broad spectrum. However, it is not only the question of varying data sources that is important. Different data bases are of central importance: very different ones are to be precisely differentiated with regard to the investigation of negative symptomatology (Wing 1989):

Somatic or biological data base (cf. survey in Crow 1985)
- Neuroanatomy
- Neuroradiology
- Neurophysiology
- Biochemistry
- Genetics

Psychological data base
- Psychopathology
- Performance (cf. survey in Pogue-Geile and Zubin 1988; Kay and Opler 1987)

Social data base (e.g. Hamilton et al. 1989)

The necessity for a multi-modal procedure is faced with the complexity of this kind of approach and the difficulties connected to it, such as the explanation of discordant findings (cross-sectional) or desynchronicity (longitudinal). Methodological studies are necessary, for example, within the approach of a multitrait/multi-method analysis (Wiggins 1973; Campbell and Fiske 1959). Here, the covariation between different parameters is systematically analysed with respect to the construct and the assessment covariation (Baumann 1986).

Appropriate systematic analyses are not available yet. They are neither carried out as separate methodological studies nor realised after the study in order to examine systematically the covariation of the individual scales (Baumann et al. 1990). References to this relation to investigating negative symptoms can be found in Sommers (1985). There, particular mention is also made to the distinction between convergent and divergent validity.

However, there are still other problems. From the statistical point of view, one must point out, for example, that an increase of the measurements included in a study increases the probability of coincidental results (Peterson 1984). This can be reduced by suitable approaches (e.g. alpha adjustment, multivariate analyses).

From the practical point of view or from the viewpoint of design, there arises the problem of the practicability of studies due, for example, to a large expenditure of time. It is essential to select those scales with satisfactory reliability and validity requiring the least expenditure of time (e.g. apathy syndrome (APA) of the AMDP system).

Regardless of these (in part solvable) problems, there are presently no alternatives to a multi-modal procedure in the area of negative symptomatology.

Perspectives

The preceding paper has shown that a large number of research efforts have been made in the past years to develop and evaluate instruments for assessing negative symptoms. In spite of much progress and the emergence of a multitude of interesting results, there are still a number of unanswered questions, particularly regarding methodology. Here are a few examples as illustrations:

- Clarification of which measurement models and test-theoretical approaches are appropriate for assessing negative symptoms, particularly when probabilistic test models are also included (e.g. Rasch model, dynamic Rasch model; Maier et al. 1990).
- Mathematical/statistical clarification of the question of the multidimensionality of negative symptomatology (cf. controversy Grau and Mueser 1986 vs. Lewine et al. 1983; Angst et al. 1989).
- Meta-analyses regarding previous studies with the same instruments.
- Multi-modal analyses with regard to construct validity, when experimental techniques (Zubin 1985) and elementary characteristics of negative symptoms are included (e.g. ratings of facial movements; Pogue-Geile and Zubin 1988).

In spite of all the existing imperfections and problems, the negative symptoms' approach provides an important contribution to understanding the heterogeneity of the phenomenology, aetiology, course and treatment of schizophrenia (Kay and Opler 1987).

References

Abrams R, Taylor MA (1978) A rating scale for emotional blunting. Am J Psychiatry 135:226–229
Alpert M (1985) The signs and symptoms of schizophrenia. Compr Psychiatry 26:103–112
AMDP (1979) Das AMDP-System. Springer, Berlin Heidelberg New York
Andersen J, Larsen JK, Schultz V, Nielsen BM, Körner A, Behnke K, Munk-Andersen E, Butler B, Allerup P, Bech P (1989) The Brief Psychiatric Rating Scale: dimension of schizophrenia – reliability and construct validity. Psychopathology 22:168–176
Andreasen NC (1982) Negative symptoms in schizophrenia. Definition and reliability. Arch Gen Psychiatry 39:784–788
Andreasen NC (1985a) Positive vs. negative schizophrenia: a critical evaluation. Schizophr Bull 11:380–389
Andreasen NC (1985b) Positive versus negative schizophrenia: criteria and validation. In: Pichot P, Berner P, Wolf R, Thau K (eds) Clinical psychopathology, nomenclature, and classification. Plenum, New York, pp 449–454 (Psychiatry. The state of the art, vol 1)
Andreasen N (1989) The Scale for the Assessment of Negative Symptoms (SANS): conceptual and theoretical foundations. Br J Psychiatry [Suppl 7] 155:49–52
Angst J, Stassen HH, Woggon B (1989) Effect of neuroleptics on positive and negative symptoms and the deficit state. Psychopharmacology 99:41–46
Asberg M, Montgomery SA, Perris C, Schalling D, Sedvall G (1978) A comprehensive psychopathological rating scale. Acta Psychiatr Scan [Suppl] 271:5–27
Atakan Z, Cooper JE (1989) Behavioural Observation Schedule (BOS), PIRS 2nd edition: a revised edition of the PIRS (WHO, Geneva, March 1978). Br J Psychiatry [Suppl 7] 155:78–80
Baumann U (1986) Angst und Depression: allgemeine methodische Überlegungen zur Begriffsbildung. In: Helmchen H, Linden M (eds) Die Differenzierung von Angst und Depression. Springer, Berlin Heidelberg New York, pp 5–13
Baumann U, Stieglitz RD (1983) Testmanual zum AMDP-System. Empirische Studien zur Psychopathologie. Springer, Berlin Heidelberg New York
Baumann U, Stieglitz RD (1989) Evaluation des AMDP-Systems anhand der neueren Literatur (1983–1987) – Überblicksarbeit. Fortschr Neurol Psychiatr 57:357–373
Baumann U, Fähndrich E, Stieglitz RD, Woggon B (1990) Probleme der Veränderungsmessung in Psychiatrie und Klinischer Psychologie. In: Baumann U, Fähndrich E, Stieglitz RD, Woggon B (eds) Veränderungsmessung in Psychiatrie und Klinischer Psychologie – Theoretische, methodische und empirische Beiträge. Profil, Munich, pp 15–45
Berner P, Gabriel E, Katschnig H, Kieffer W, Koehler K, Lenz G, Simhandl CH (1983) Diagnosekriterien für schizophrene und affektive Psychosen. Weltverband für Psychiatrie, Vienna
Berrios GE (1985) Positive and negative symptoms and Jackson – a conceptual history. Arch Gen Psychiatry 42:95–97
Biehl H, Maurer K, Jablensky A, Cooper JE, Tomov T (1989a) The WHO Psychological Impairments Rating Schedule (WHO/PIRS). I. Introducing a new instrument for rating observed behaviour and the rationale of the psychological impairment concept. Br J Psychiatry [Suppl 7] 155:68–70
Biehl H, Maurer K, Jung E, Krumm B (1989b) The WHO Psychological Impairments Rating Schedule (WHO/PIRS). II. Impairments in schizophrenics in cross-sectional and longitudinal perspective – the Mannheim experience in two independent samples. Br J Psychiatry [Suppl 7] 155:71–77
Buchkremer G, Fiedler P (1987) Kognitive versus handlungsorientierte Therapie. Nervenarzt 58:481–488
Campbell DT, Fiske DW (1959) Convergent and discriminant validation by the multitrait-multimethod matrix. Psychol Bull 56:81–105
Carpenter WT, Heinrichs DW, Alphs LD (1985) Treatment of negative symptoms. Schizophr Bull 11:440–452

Crow TJ (1985) The two-syndrome concept: origins and current status. Schizophr Bull 11:471–485
Crow TJ (1989) A current view of the type II-syndrome: age of onset, intellectual impairment, and the meaning of structural changes in the brain. Br J Psychiatry [Suppl 7] 155:15–20
Fähndrich E, Richter S (1986) Zum Verlauf schizophrener Ersterkrankungen. Eine 5-Jahres-Katamnese. Nervenarzt 57:705–711
Fähndrich E, Stieglitz RD (1989) Leitfaden zur Erfassung des psychopathologischen Befundes. Springer, Berlin Heidelberg New York
Gaebel W (1988) Indikatoren und Prädiktoren schizophrener Krankheitsstadien und Verlaufsausgänge. *Habilitationsschrift*, University of Berlin
Gebhardt R, Pietzcker A, Strauss A, Stoeckel M, Langer C, Freudenthal K (1983) Skalenbildung im AMDP-System. Arch Psychiatr Nervenkr 233:223–245
Gibbons RD, Lewine RRJ, Davis JM, Schooler NR, Cole JO (1985) An empirical test of a Kraepelinian vs. a Bleulerian view of negative symptoms. Schizophr Bull 11:390–395
Good I (1989) Minussymptomatik bei chronischer Schizophrenia. Interraterreliabilität zweier Minussymptomatik-Skalen (SANS und NSRS). Dissertation, University of Zürich
Grau BW, Mueser KT (1986) Measurement of negative symptoms. Schizophr Bull 12:7–8
Grossman LS, Luchins DJ, Harrow M (1989) Positive and negative symptoms and the neurology of schizophrenia. Curr Opin Psychiatry 2:20–25
Guy W, Ban TA (1982) The AMDP-system. Springer, Berlin Heidelberg New York
Hall JN (1980) Ward rating scales for long-stay patients: a review. Psychol Med 10:277–288
Hamilton NG, Ponzka CA, Cutler DL, Weigel RM (1989) Social networks and negative versus positive symptoms of schizophrenia. Schizophr Bull 15:625–633
Harris CW (ed) (1963) Problems in measuring change. University Wisconsin Press, Madison
Honigfeld G, Patin J (1989) Predictors of response to clozapine therapy. Psychopharmacology 99:64–67
Honigfeld G, Gillis RD, Klett CJ (1976) NOSIE. Nurses' Observation Scale for Inpatient Evaluation. In: Guy W (ed) ECDEU. Assessment manual for psychopharmacology. National Institute of Mental Health, Rockville, pp 265–273
Iager AC, Kirch DG, Wyatt RJ (1985) A negative symptom rating scale. Psychiatry Res 16:27–36
Johnstone EC (1989) The assessment of negative and positive features in schizophrenia. Br J Psychiatry [Suppl 7] 155:41–44
Kay SR, Opler LA (1987) The positive-negative dimension in schizophrenia: its validity and significance. Psychiatr Dev 2:79–103
Kay SR, Fiszbein A, Opler LA (1987a) The Positive and Negative Syndrome Scale (PANSS) for Schizophrenia. Schizophr Bull 13:261–276
Kay SR, Opler LA, Lindenmayer JP (1987b) Reliability and validity of the Positive and Negative Syndrome Scale for schizophrenics. Psychiatry Res 23:99–110
Kay SR, Opler LA, Lindenmayer JP (1989) The Positive and Negative Syndrome Scale (PANSS): rationale and standardisation. Br J Psychiatry [Suppl 7] 155:59–65
Kirkpatrick B, Buchanan RW, McKenney PD, Alphs LD, Carpenter WT (1988) The Schedule for the Deficit Syndrome: an instrument for research in schizophrenia. Psychiatry Res 30:119–123
Krawiecka M, Goldberg D, Vaughan M (1977) A standardized psychiatric assessment scale for rating chronic psychotic patients. Acta Psychiatr Scand 55:299–308
Lenzenweger MF, Dworkin RH, Wethington E (1989) Models of positive and negative symptoms in schizophrenia: an empirical evaluation of latent structures. J Abnorm Psychol 98:62–70
Lewine RRJ, Fogg L, Meltzer HY (1983) Assessment of negative and positive symptoms in schizophrenia. Schizophr Bull 9:368–376
Liddle PF, Barnes RE (1988) The subjective experience of deficits in schizophrenia. Compr Psychiatry 29:157–164
Lienert GA (1969) Testaufbau und Testanalyse. Beltz, Weinheim

Lorr M, Klett CJ, McNair DM, Lasky JJ (196) Inpatient Multidimensional Psychiatric Scale (IMPS). Consulting Psychologists, Palo Alto
Maier W, Albus M, Bech P (1990) Validitätskriterien für die Veränderungsmessung mit Ratingskalen. In: Baumann U, Fähndrich E, Stieglitz RD, Woggon U (eds) Veränderungsmessung in Psychiatrie und Klinischer Psychologie – Theoretische, methodische und empirische Beiträge. Profil, Munich, pp 286–306
McGorry PD, Goodwin RJ, Stuart GW (1988) The development, use, and reliability of the Brief Psychiatric Rating Scale (nursing modification) – an assessment procedure for the nursing team in clinical and research settings. Compr Psychiatry 29:575–587
Mortimer AM, McKenna PJ, Lund CE, Mannuzza S (1989) Rating of negative symptoms using the High Royds Evaluation of Negativity (HEN) scale. Br J Psychiatry [Suppl 7] 155:89–91
Mundt C (1989) Die psychopathologischen Grundlagen zur Psychopathometrie des schizophrenen Residualsyndroms. Fundam Psychiatr 3:2–11
Mundt C, Kasper S (1987) Zur Schizophreniespezifität von negativen und Basissymptomen. Nervenarzt 58:489–495
Mundt C, Fiedler P, Pracht B, Rettig R (1985) InSka (IntentionalitätsSkala) – ein neues psychopathometrisches Instrument zur quantitativen Erfassung der schizophrenen Residualsymptomatik. Nervenarzt 56:146–149
Mundt C, Kasper S, Huerkamp M (1989) The diagnostic specifity of negative symptoms and their psychopathological context. Br J Psychiatry [Suppl 7] 155:32–36
Overall JE, Gorham DR (1976) BPRS. Brief Psychiatric Rating Scale. In: Guy W (ed) ECDEU. Assessment manual for psychopharmacology. National Institute of Mental Health, Rockwille, pp 157–169
Peterson L (1984) A brief methodological comment on possible inaccuracies induced by multimodal measurement analysis and reporting. J Behav Med 7:307–313
Pietzcker A, Gaebel W (1987) Prospective study of course of illness in schizophrenia. I. Outcome at 1 year. Schizophr Bull 13:287–297
Pietzcker A, Gebhardt R (1985) Depressive syndromes and scales in the AMDP-system. In: Pichot P, Berner P, Wolf R, Thau K (eds) Clinical psychopathology, nomenclature, and classification. Plenum, New York, pp 655–659 (Psychiatry. The state of the art, vol 1)
Pietzcker A, Gebhardt R, Strauss A, Stöckel M, Langer C, Freundenthal K (1983) The syndrome scales in the AMDP-system. In: Bobon D, Baumann U, Angst J, Helmchen H, Hippius H (eds) The AMDP-system in pharmacopsychiatry. Karger, Basle, pp 88–89
Pogue-Geile MF (1989) The prognostic significance of negative symptoms in schizophrenia. Br J Psychiatry [Suppl 7] 155:123–127
Pogue-Geile MF, Harrow M (1984) Negative and positive symptoms in schizophrenia and depression: a follow-up. Schizophr Bull 10:371–387
Pogue-Geile MF, Zubin J (1988) Negative symptomatology and schizophrenia: a conceptual and empirical review. Int J Ment Health 16:3–45
Prosser ES, Csernansky JG, Kaplan J, Thiemann S, Becker TJ, Hollister LE (1987) Depression, Parkinsonian symptoms, and negative symptoms in schizophrenics treated with neuroleptics. J Nerv Ment Dis 175:100–105
Rosen WG, Mohs RC, Johns CA, Small NS, Kendler KS, Horvath TB, Davis KL (1984) Positive and negative symptoms in schizophrenia. Psychiatry Res 13:277–284
Rösler M, Hengesch G (1990) "Negative" Symptome im AMDP-System. In: Baumann U, Fähndrich E, Stieglitz RD, Woggon B (eds) Veränderungsmessung in Psychiatrie und Klinischer Psychologie. Theoretische, methodische und empirische Beiträge. Profil, Munich, pp 329–339
Sass H (1989) The historical evaluation of the concept of negative symptoms in schizophrenia. Br J Psychiatry [Suppl 7] 155:26–31
Seidenstücker G, Baumann U (1987) Multimodale Diagnostik als Standard in der Klinischen Psychologie. Diagnostica 33:243–258
Sommers AA (1985) "Negative symptoms": conceptual and methodological problems. Schizophr Bull 11:364–379

Stieglitz RD, Helmchen H (1990) Schizoaffective disorders in clinical routine: symptomatology, etiology, and course. In: Marneros A, Tsuang MT (eds) Affective and schizoaffective disorders: similarities and differences. Springer, Berlin Heidelberg New York
Stieglitz RD, Baumann U, Tobien H, von Zerssen D (1980) Zur Stichproben- und Zeitinvarianz von Testkennwerten einer Beschwerdenliste. Z Exp Angew Psychol 27:631–654
Straumann D (1989) Sogenannte Minussymptome bei chronischer Schizophrenie. Dissertation, University of Zurich
Strauss JS (1985) Negative symptoms: future developments of the concept. Schizophr Bull 11:457–460
Strauss JS, Rakfeldt J, Harding CM, Lieberman P (1989) Psychological and social aspects of negative symptoms. Br J Psychiatry [Suppl 7] 155:128–132
Thiemann S, Csernansky JG, Berger PA (1987) Rating scales in research: the case of negative symptoms. Psychiatry Res 20:47–55
Venables PH (1957) A short scale for rating "activity-withdrawal" in schizophrenics. J Ment Sci 103:197–199
Von Zerssen D, Möller HJ (1980) Psychometrische Verfahren in der psychiatrischen Therapieforschung. In: Biefang S (ed) Evaluationsforschung in der Psychiatrie: Fragestellungen und Methoden. Enke, Stuttgart, pp 129–166
Wiggins JS (1973) Personality and prediction. Addison-Wesley, London
Wing JK (1961) A simple and reliable subclassification of chronic schizophrenia. J Ment Sci 107:862–875
Wing JK (1989) The concept of negative symptoms. Br J Psychiatry [Suppl 7] 155:10–14
Wing JK, Cooper JE, Sartorius N (1974) Measurement and classification of psychiatric symptoms. An instruction manual for the PSE and Catego program. Cambridge University Press, Cambridge
Woggon B, Beckmann H, Heinrich K, Linden M, Krebs E, Küfferle B, Pflug B, Rüther E, Schied HW (1986) Clinical relevant differences in the therapeutic profile of fluperlapine compared to haloperidol in the treatment of schizophrenic psychosis – results of a multicentre double-blind study. Pharmacopsychiatry 19:204–205
Zinner HJ, Kraemer S, Möller HJ (1989) Empirische Untersuchungen zur Konkordanz verschiedener Minus-Symptomatik-Skalen sowie zur Korrelation mit testpsychologischen Befunden. 1st Bonner Kraepelin-Symposium, Nov 24–25, Bonn
Zubin J (1985) Negative symptoms: are they indigenous to schizophrenia? Schizophr Bull 11:461–469

Methodological Problems in Identifying and Measuring First-Rank Symptoms of Schizophrenia

C. S. MELLOR [1]

Introduction

This paper considers the question of eliciting and measuring one particular group of positive symptoms, those designated first-rank. The proposed solution to this problem is applicable to other positive symptoms that are disorders of experience. Schneider's first-rank symptoms of schizophrenia (FRS) have attracted considerable interest over the past 20 years. The literature suggests that their diagnostic use is higher than their diagnostic value. This discrepancy may originate, in some studies, from a failure to appreciate that the phenomenological method must be used to identify FRS, and, when it has been employed, its use needs to be precisely defined. The methodological difficulties that attend the clinical use of the phenomenological method and the "measurement" of the symptoms so elicited will be described, as will a solution which is based upon the concept of subjective probability.

A short review of FRS is necessary before going to the main purpose of this paper. FRS (Schneider 1959) had their origin in the difficulty of distinguishing between cyclothymia (bipolar disorder) and schizophrenia. Schneider's approach was a pragmatic one. His FRS had to distinguish between mania and schizophrenia, be reasonably easy to identify and to occur with sufficient frequency to be useful. He attached greater diagnostic value to the patient's symptoms at the time of the examination than to the course of the illness. He had a hierarchical view of diagnostic symptomatology, with organic mental disorders and their typical symptoms taking precedence over schizophrenia and FRS, which in their turn took precedence over affective disorder and typical affective symptoms. Therefore, patients with FRS had schizophrenia, but not if they had organic mental symptoms. However, the diagnosis of schizophrenia would stand even if the patients had marked affective symptoms.

Certain misunderstandings about FRS frequently appear in the literature on this subject. These arise when FRS are viewed from a theoretical standpoint, and used to define schizophrenia. Two points about FRS need emphasising. Firstly, they were arrived at empirically and, therefore, can offer no theory about the underlying nature of schizophrenia. Secondly, they do not occur in all patients with schizophrenia, and in these patients the diagnosis must be

[1] Memorial University of Newfoundland, Health Sciences Centre, St. John's, NF, A1B 3V6, Canada

A. Marneros / N. C. Andreasen / M. T. Tsuang (Eds.)
Negative Versus Positive Schizophrenia

based on other characteristic disorders of experience (second-rank symptoms) or disorders of expression. Turning to the symptoms themselves, Hoenig (1984) wrote that Schneider's own descriptions of FRS were "discursive rather than operationally precise". However, Mellor (1970) and Koehler (1979) have provided operational definitions and illustrative examples of FRS and so they will not be described here.

The use of FRS as exclusion criteria for mania was challenged by a number of investigators from 1971 onwards. Pope and Lipinski (1978) cited nine studies of mania in which the frequencies of FRS ranged from 8% to 47%. By way of explanation of some of these findings, Akiskal and Pusantian (1979) pointed out that delirium may often complicate severe bipolar disorders and could be responsible for the appearance of FRS. The diagnostic stability of FRS over time was examined by Mellor et al. (1981). During an 8-year follow-up patients who had initially presented with FRS, they did not find any who were subsequently given a diagnosis of mania.

A variety of other psychiatric disorders, in addition to mania, have been associated with the presence of FRS, including depression, neuroses and personality disorders; Hoenig (1984) cites five such studies. FRS have also been reported in normal subjects (Gharagozlou and Behin 1979). Ross et al. (1990) have reported that patients with multiple personalities had a higher frequency of FRS than those with schizophrenia. However, Tandon and Greden (1987) have reaffirmed the diagnostic specificity for schizophrenia of FRS, estimating it to be 95%. In a study of the charts from a hospital where the staff had strongly adhered to Schneiderian diagnostic orthodoxy, Marneros (1984) found that FRS differentiated schizophrenia from mania and endogenous depression. He did enter the caveat that this did not take account of the occurrence of "in-between" cases, a theme later developed in a number of publications on schizoaffective disorders (Marneros and Tsuang 1986). Another development with regard to FRS has been a series of reports from psychiatrists working with patients from a wide variety of cultures, which have demonstrated the universality of these symptoms.

In an earlier review of FRS, Mellor (1982) commented that most publications do not acknowledge the methodological problems in defining and eliciting these symptoms. Until these deficiencies are recognised and remedied, judgments about the diagnostic value of FRS should be reserved.

The Phenomenological Method and FRS

FRS are disorders of experience and Schneider (1959, p. 94) makes his approach to their identification clear: "The methods of clinical interview from the standpoint of psychopathology were established decades ago by Karl Jaspers." FRS are accessible only through the use of the phenomenological method, as described by Jaspers (1968). The application of the phenomenological method in descriptive psychopathology differs from that practised by philosophers because it involves two people, the examiner and the patient. The method, as derived from Jaspers, will be described.

1. The examiner must first empty his mind, as far as possible, of all preconceptions and biases. (It is my view that the examiner must encourage the patient to do the same. Exploring an FRS is very difficult if the patient is preoccupied with the delusional explanation rather than the experience itself.) This is similar to the "bracketing out" of the phenomenological philosophers.
2. The patient must be persuaded to reflect upon, or turn his "inner eye" upon the phenomena within his consciousness.
3. Under the guidance of the examiner, the patient explores the components of and the inter-relationships of the phenomena.
4. The patient describes the phenomena in as much detail as possible to the examiner.
5. The next step, that of "actualising" the patient's experience, is a departure from philosophical practice. The examiner uses the experiential data derived from the patient's descriptions, and any other expressive data that are relevant, to recreate within his own consciousness the phenomena experienced by the patient. Trainees sometimes naively assume that the examiner is trying to create the actual phenomenon in his own consciousness, hallucinations for example. This is not so. What is "acutalised" are the patient's reflections upon his experience, or the experiencing of the experience, rather than the experience itself.

Difficulties in Employing the Phenomenological Method

Difficulties that arise in using the phenomenological method to identify FRS, or any other disorders of experience, can be divided into those attributable to the patient and those that are the responsibility of the examiner.

Patient Difficulties

1. Difficulty in cooperating in the general process. This may be due to (a) affective problems such as anxiety and hostility that make difficult the relationship between examiner and patient, and (b) preoccupation with explanatory delusions that prevents the patient attending to the primary phenomena.
2. Difficulty in reflecting upon the contents of consciousness. Some people are not psychologically minded and find the exercise of self-observation difficult. Such difficulties may be attributable to the premorbid personality, or their psychiatric disorder.
3. Difficulty in describing the "reflected upon" experiences to the examiner. This is most often due to cognitive problems, particularly formal thought disorder.

This is by no means an exhaustive list and sometimes a problem of symptom identification may arise because the symptomatology varies in time. When this is suspected, serial examinations are needed.

Examiner Difficulties

1. Failure to realise that the phenomenological method is used to identify FRS. This is evident when investigators indicate that they are collecting "verbal behaviours", rather than examining the contents of consciousness.
2. Inadequate training in the phenomenological method may cause difficulties in suspending preconceptions at the first stage of the examination and in the actualisation process at the later stage.
3. Reliable analysis of the actualised experiences requires well-defined criteria for the identification of FRS that are consistently applied.

Whilst patient difficulties do not have a solution, those associated with the examiner do. This solution requires a systematic and standardised approach to identifying FRS that remains true to Jasper's phenomenological method. In order to do this, a detailed analysis of what happens during the examination of a patient for FRS is required.

Identification of FRS in Clinical Practice

This explication of the process by which FRS are identified uses three concepts. These are the *typification* statement that suggests an FRS has been experienced, viewing FRS as *ideal types* and *probability* as a subjective experience. The work of Schwartz and Wiggins (1987a, b) on Weber-Jasperian methodology has helped this analysis.

Typification Statement. The patient makes a statement which indicates to the examiner that he has had an FRS-like experience. This act of typification by the examiner is similar to that described by Schutz (1962, pp. 3–47). Describing the use of typification in psychiatric diagnosis, Schwartz and Wiggins (1987a) pointed out that typification is a skill and is not governed by procedural rules. It is the immediate perception of an object as probably belonging to a particular type. Typification in itself does not involve conceptualisation, and there are no criteria that define the object as a member of a class, but it is a preliminary to the act of conceptualisation. As Gurwitsch (1974, p. 116) has stated, "... typification is certainly at the origin of conceptual consciousness, if it is not in itself conceptualisation in an incipient or at least a germinal form."

The typification statement leads the examiner to conduct a detailed phenomenological exploration of the experience. An example of such a statement might be, "I think thoughts that are not my own", which leads to the supposition that the patient has had an experience of type similar to FRS "made thoughts".

FRS As Ideal Types: Identifying the Actualised Experience. When the exploration of a patient's FRS-like experiences is completed, and these experiences are actualised in the mind of the examiner, then comes the process of identification. FRS are complex experiences in themselves, and patients' descriptions of them are intermingled with other psychopathology and are coloured by life experiences and the premorbid personality. Such complicated psychic structures are not easily reduced to the components that permit classification.

A solution to the problem of classifying highly complex human experiences was suggested by Max Weber, a founder of modern sociology, who, writing about societies in a historical context, introduced the concept of ideal types. [Examples of Weber's ideal types given by Winch (1967) are the three forms of authority – traditional, rational and charismatic.]

Weber had considerable influence upon Jaspers and Schneider, the latter employed the concept of ideal types in his study of personality disorders. It is instructive in this context to quote Jaspers (1989):

"Reality is an infinite weaving of the meaningful and the meaningless. In order to seize it, constructed concepts are necessary which developed in themselves as meaningfully consistent, serve only as standards for reality, to see how far it conforms to those concepts. Weber called these constructed concepts "ideal types". To him, they are the perceptive-technical means of approaching reality, not reality itself. They are ... meaningful concepts by which reality is measured."

Applying this concept to the identification of the FRS Made Thoughts, the ideal type would be that actualised by the perfect examiner from data gathered from the perfect patient who had experienced this particular symptom in its totality. (The perfect examiner and the perfect patient are non-human abstractions, free from the difficulties described above.) In the reality of clinical practice, the examiner decides how closely the actualised FRS measures up to the ideal one. This leads to the problem of measuring mental events which, by their nature, have no concrete reality.

Subjective Probability. Hitherto, investigators of FRS have made an arbitrary decisions that an FRS is present, or absent. It is obvious that the examiner cannot measure the actualised FRS, which is a mental event without physical existence. Subjective experiences may sometimes be quantified by asking the patient to assess their intensity, but an experience can only be measured in this way by comparing its present intensity with its intensity at some other time. Even this is denied the practitioner of the phenomenological method, who finds it difficult enough to actualise the qualitative aspects of the experience, without its quantitative attributes.

In making a clinical decision that a symptom is an FRS, I first assess may confidence that each of the attributes of the ideal symptom is present in the actualised phenomenon. Using these data, I then decide how confident I am that the total experience corresponds to the ideal FRS. In clinical practice my level of confidence is expressed as a simple yes or no, the FRS is present or absent. The level of confidence, or subjective probability, offers a method of measuring an experience which exists only in consciousness. Subjective probability is one of the three basic theories of probability discussed by Black (1967), the others being logical and frequency theories.

The logical view, which is associated with Keynes and later Carnap, is that probability represents a logical relationship between a proposition and a body of knowledge. Given a statement *S* and a body of evidence *E*, there is only one number *p*, which represents the probability of *S* relative to *E*. Frequency theories are empirical and take the position that probability statements are statements about the real world. Knowledge of the frequency of a past event allows one to predict the frequency of that event in the future.

The subjective view of probability is that the relationship between a statement and a body of evidence is a quasi-logical one, and that the number attached to it represents a degree of belief. The given statement may have any probability value between 0 and 1 assigned to it on the basis of the evidence by the person whose degree of belief is represented by that probability. Probability, in the subjectivist sense, can therefore be used to estimate how well the actualised phenomenon conforms to the examiner's concept of an FRS. Instead of the examiner's degree of belief being limited to 0, i.e. the FRS is absent, and 1, i.e. the FRS is present, it can be expressed as a number between these two values. This accords with clinical experience because, even after an exhaustive phenomenological examination of an FRS-like statement, it is often impossible to say with certainty that an FRS is present.

Construction of the FRS Rating Scale

These three concepts, the typification statement, the FRS as an ideal type and the concept of subjective probability, provide the components for constructing an FRS scale. This construction will be using the FRS Made Thoughts, the scale for which is set out in Table 1. It is assumed that anyone using such a scale would be familiar with the operational definitions of FRS, given by Mellor (1970) and Koehler (1979), and be trained in the Jasperian phenomenological method.

The six items that comprise this scale are scored 0, 1 or 2. A score of 0 means that this feature of the FRS is absent and 2 indicates that it is certainly present. A score of 1 means that it is possibly present. Item 1 is the typification statement, which, if scored as a 1 or 2, implies that an FRS-like phenomenon is present and leads the examiner to a further exploration of the phenomenon. The patient's statement should be the same as or have a similar meaning to the one in the scale. The next four items, 2 through 5, are the essential characteristics of the ideal Made Thoughts experience. They are scored only after the process of actualisation has taken place, and each score denotes the examiner's confidence that this feature of the ideal FRS is represented in the examiner's consciousness. The final item, 6, is a delusional explanation of the Made Thoughts experience. It is not a necessary attribute of the FRS, but if

Table 1. "Made thoughts" (thought insertion)

	Score (0, 1, 2)
1. I think thoughts that are not my own Patient – example:	–
2. Thoughts that I cannot even attempt to control Examiner actualised:	–
3. Thoughts in my mind that come from outside myself Examiner actualised:	–
4. Thoughts which first exist, or existed, outside myself Examiner actualised:	–
5. Thoughts passing from the outside into my mind Examiner actualised:	–
6. Delusional explanation of statement no. 1 (Substitute for any other item score that is less)	–
Total	–
Probability = Total $\times 10^{-1}$	–

such a delusion is present then it raises the examiner's level of confidence that the FRS is present.

When the individual items have been scored, then items 1 through 5 are summed. If one of the items has a lower score than item 6 (delusional explanation), then the item 6 score is substituted for it. The total score will be in the range 0–10, and the probability is obtained by dividing this score by 10 to give a value that can vary from 0 to 1 by increments of 0.1. The decision to add the individual item scores together was based upon what happens in practice. Each piece of evidence is added to the next, and, when this is complete, a judgment about the presence of the FRS is made.

Suppose a patient had a score of 0.6 on the Made Thoughts scale, what does this number represent? It is the examiner's level of confidence, or degree of belief, that the patient's Made Thoughts-like experience matches the ideal. This also means that the score 0.4 (1 minus 0.6) represents the degree to which the examiner believes the patient's symptom is unlike the ideal. A score of 0 means that the FRS is absent, any other score means that an FRS-like symptom is present. The score does not represent the examiner's degree of belief that a particular FRS is present, but its resemblance to the ideal.

Such scales can be developed for each FRS, and, once this has been achieved, then a systematic study of the diagnostic value of these symptoms can be undertaken. The probability scores will provide refined measures of the reliability of the ascertainment of the FRS. These scores can also be used to find the FRS probability levels which have the best return in diagnostic sensitivity and specificity. Such a study will be reported later, but using, for example, the FRS Made Thoughts, the product moment correlation between two independent examiner's scores was 0.95. The probability score that yielded the best return, with a specificity of 98% and a sensitivity of 52%, was 0.4. This illustrates the potential value of this approach to measuring the disorders of experience.

References

Akiskal HS, Puzantian VR (1979) Psychotic forms of depression and mania. Psychiatr Clin North Am 6:419–439
Black M (1967) Probability. In: Edwards P (ed) The encyclopaedia of philosophy, vol 6. MacMillan, London, pp 464–479
Gharagozlou H, Behin MT (1979) Diagnostic evaluation of Schneider's first rank symptoms of schizophrenia amongst three groups of Iranians. Compr Psychiatr 20:242–245
Gurwitsch A (1974) Phenomenology and the theory of science. Northwestern University Press, Evanston, IL
Hoenig J (1984) Schneider's first rank symptoms and the tabulators. Compr Psychiatr 25:77–87
Jaspers K (1968) The phenomenological approach in psychopathology. Br J Psychiatry 114:1313–1323
Jaspers K (1989) Max Weber as a scientist. In: Dreijmanis J (ed) Karl Jaspers on Max Weber. Paragon, New York
Koehler K (1979) First-rank symptoms of schizophrenia: questions concerning clinical boundaries. Br J Psychiatry 134:236–248
Marneros A (1984) The pathognomonic value of K. Schneider's first rank symptoms. Psychiatria Fennica 15:99–105
Marneros A, Tsuang MT (eds) (1986) Schizoaffective psychoses. Springer, Berlin Heidelberg New York Tokyo
Mellor CS (1970) First rank symptoms of schizophrenia. Br J Psychiatr 140:423–424
Mellor CS (1982) The present status of first-rank symptoms. Br J Psychiatr 140:423–424
Mellor CS, Sims ACP, Cope RV (1981) Change of diagnosis in schizophrenia and first-rank symptoms: an eight year follow-up. Compr Psychiatr 22:184–188
Pope HG jr, Lipinski JF (1978) Diagnosis in schizophrenia and manic-depressive illness: a reassessment of "schizophrenic" symptoms in the light of current research. Arch Gen Psychiatr 35:811–828
Ross CA, Miller SD, Reagor P, Bjornson L, Fraser GA, Anderson G (1990) Schneiderian symptoms in multiple personality disorder and schizophrenia. Compr Psychiatr 31:111–118
Schneider K (1959) Clinical psychopathology. Grune and Stratton, New York
Schwartz MA, Wiggins OP (1987a) Typifications: the first step for clinical diagnosis in psychiatry. J Nerv Ment Dis 175:65–77
Schwartz MA, Wiggins OP (1987b) Diagnosis and ideal types: a contribution to psychiatric classification. Compr Psychiatr 28:277–291
Schutz A (1962) Common-sense and scientific interpretation of human action. In: Natanson M (ed) Collected papers I: the problem of social reality. Nijhoff, The Hague
Tandon R, Greden JF (1987) Schneiderian first rank symptoms: reconfirmation of a high specificity for schizophrenia. Acta Psychiatr Scand 75:392–396
Winch P (1967) Max Weber. In: Edwards P (ed) The encyclopaedia of philosophy, vol 8. MacMillan, London, pp 282–283

Anhedonia and the Amotivational State of Schizophrenia

R. R. J. Lewine [1]

Introduction

Acedia, a condition characterized in medieval times by pathological mental or spiritual torpor, was considered one of the seven deadly sins (Gilman 1982). Some 4 centuries later, we continue to struggle with the conceptualization and operationalization of motivation and, of specific concern to psychopathologists, with its status in individuals with schizophrenia. Carpenter (1987), for example, wrote that, "It has proved humane, heuristic, and scientifically valid to view persons with the disordered functions associated with schizophrenia as having an illness. Alternative views of persons with schizophrenia as immoral, self absorbed, *unmotivated* (emphasis added), demonically possessed, criminal, socially deviant, politically dissident, representing an extreme on normal dimensions of personal functioning, or simply as the irredeemable fringe of society have led to neglect and punishment" (p. 4).

While agreeing completely with Carpenter's observation, I would like to draw attention to a conundrum, with both etiological and treatment consequences, lurking in the illness-model analysis. As emphasized by Carpenter, conceptualization of the individual with schizophrenia as unmotivated has had unfortunate consequences. Often the "unmotivated view" of schizophrenia holds that the individual does not "want" to do anything and then by a leap of logic offers that to improve (for example, get a job, clean the room, keep regular hours, exercise), the individual simply needs to "want" to get better (or get a job, clean the room, keep regular hours, exercise). The unstated implication is that such an individual stays ill because he "wants to," a view, in its moral attributions, not dissimilar to that of acedia as a deadly sin.

The conundrum inheres in the fact that it is quite correct that the individual with schizophrenia does not *want* to do many of the things that are typically expected of him. Indeed, Kraepelin (1971) went so far as to suggest that the fundamental disorder of dementia praecox was one of the "annihilation of the will." The common error, however, is in the ascription of this loss (or diminution) of the will to a process that is easily under the individual's control. What usually troubles us about the motivational damage in schizophrenia is that it often seems selective. For example, the affected person cannot remember

[1] Department of Psychiatry, Emory University School of Medicine, Atlanta, GA 30322, USA

A. Marneros / N. C. Andreasen / M. T. Tsuang (Eds.)
Negative Versus Positive Schizophrenia

to arrive on time for a family gathering but complains loudly when dinner is more than a few minutes late. While it would be naive to deny the importance of secondary gain in the maintenance of some sickness-related behaviors, it is essential, not that we deny the importance of motivation in schizophrenia, but rather that we understand that motivation is just as liable to the influence of illness as other biological mechanisms.

In instances of more conventional illness, such as that reflected in frontal lobe syndromes (Damasio 1985), loss of motivation can be more easily accepted; in fact, apathy, loss of motivation, and inability to initiate spontaneous behavior are critical clinical elements in that syndrome. Disturbance in motivation need not necessarily take the form of loss or reduction in behavior; it may also be reflected in inappropriate behavior that is a manifestation of the loss or diminution of social norms as motivating factors, a phenomenon described by Brickner (1936) as a "loss of social sentiment."

The study of motivation in schizophrenia has, of course, a long, empirical tradition (Buss and Lang 1965). Such study took many forms, including investigation of praise and punishment, arousal, and evaluation of reward schedules, the last providing the theoretical basis for most of the behavior treatment programs of the 1960s and 1970s (Paul and Lentz 1977). In what follows, I would like to examine in some detail one aspect of the many faces of motivation: anhedonia. Anhedonia has held an honored position in theoretical formulations of schizophrenia, although ironically the concept seems to have been formalized with respect to a disorder far removed from the psychiatric realm.

Anhedonia: Physical Versus Social

Ribot (1897) was the first to use the term "anhedonia" to refer to the "loss of pleasure sense": "Like pain, pleasure is separable from the complex of which it forms part, and under certain abnormal conditions may totally disappear. *Anhedonia* (if I may coin a counter-designation to analgesia) has been very little studied, but it exists" (p. 53). The case described by Ribot was that of a young girl suffering from anhedonia secondary to liver damage. Subsequently, anhedonia has been very much studied, if sporadically, with its primary importance lying in the areas of schizophrenia and depression (Peterson and Knudson 1983). As I briefly trace the contemporary history of anhedonia, I find a bifurcation in the conceptualization of the hedonic domain: physical versus social.

Myerson (1922), in his early work on anhedonia, defined "organic anaesthesia" as the "dropping out from consciousness of desire and satisfaction" (p. 87). In addition to a diminution or loss of appetite, sexual interest, and sleep, he listed the loss of feeling of energy as a core symptom of the anhedonic state that led to, among other problems, poor concentration and loss of interest. He suggested, furthermore, that organic anesthesia had multiple causes, including infections, surgery, and mental disorder, an etiological view in keeping with the original intent of Ribot. As both a concrete description and a metaphor, Myerson (1922) stated that "the hearty folk pass through life eating of the good things of life by mouthfuls while the anhedonic nibble and are constantly on the verge of disgust and dissatisfaction" (p. 99).

Myerson articulated the specific link between anhedonia and schizophrenia 2 decades later (Myerson 1944), accompanying the focus on schizophrenia with a shift from physical to social anhedonia. Myerson (1944) wrote that, "the social neurosis is a variety of the anxiety neurosis, because it is the adverse, apprehensive reaction to the most exciting objects of our environment, namely our fellows" (p. 149). Although comparable with Adler's "inferiority complex" (Adler 1926) in its phenomenological manifestation, social anxiety neurosis was, according to Myerson, primary in that the inferiority complex was an end product of the social anxiety neurosis. Continuing his emphasis on the social aspect of anhedonia, Myerson (1946) suggested that there existed a "constitutional anhedonic personality" which was determined at birth and characterized by lessened desire and an incapacity for satisfaction. "If we encompass all of desire together as the appetite for life, this man has an all embracing anorexia" (p. 777). We see here a shift in the concept of social anhedonia from the original aversive, apprehensive reaction to social intercourse to a lessened or absent desire and/or an impairment in the satisfaction derived from social relationships.

Rado (1956) was more explicit in the description of a "schizotype" that was linked etiologically to schizophrenia. He suggested that the "ensemble of psychodynamic traits... define him as a schizotype from birth to death..." (p. 275), echoing Myerson's position regarding the early determination of this type of individual. There were two primary characteristics of the schizotype proposed by Rado: an integrative pleasure deficiency and a proprioceptive diathesis. The former referred to a weakening of the motivating power of pleasure, while the latter referred to a propensity to distorted awareness of bodily self. While Myerson emphasized the social nature of the fundamental anhedonic personality, Rado tended to emphasize a primary defect in the integrative pleasure (physical) functions which cut across multiple domains of experience.

Building, in part, upon this conceptual foundation, Meehl (1962) has provided one of the most detailed accounts of the theoretical relationship between a genetic predisposition (schizotaxia), a personality type predisposed to schizophrenia (schizotype), and the clinical disorder of schizophrenia. Anhedonia was conceptualized by Meehl as a normally distributed individual differences dimension that only led to the schizophrenic syndrome under appropriate conditions. He predicted that social indices of anhedonia would have greater saliency than physical indices because social reinforcement is less consistent on average than physical reinforcement. In an impaired system (in other words, in the individual with a neurointegrative deficit), social anhedonia becomes more apparent, therefore, because the social reinforcements are that much less effective (being less consistent) than physical ones.

The 1989 revision of the schizotypy theory represents a major break from this theoretical line in that anhedonia no longer plays a key role in defining predisposing characteristics of the full clinical schizophrenia syndrome (Meehl 1989). Rather, Meehl suggests that anhedonia is a manifestation of the mixed signals to which the preschizophrenic individual is subjected because of the neurointegrative deficit. He is, therefore, far less optimistic about the social, cognitive, and personality dimensions in schizophrenia because they are far along in the causal chain; he places more emphasis now on psychophysiological measures, such as smooth pursuit eye movement abnormalities (Holzman 1987) and attentional dysfunctions (Nuechterlein and Dawson 1984; Shakow 1956) which he claims may be quasipathonomonic.

Grinker (1975), while focusing on the interpersonal nature of anhedonia, took a somewhat different position in emphasizing the incapacity to love and to relate to others. Interpersonal anhedonia was thought to have an early onset (in contrast to depression) and was "almost constant and is not related to internal or external dynamic or experiential conditions" (p. 413). Grinker was especially critical of the inappropriate use of "flat affect" in characterizing anhedonia, as he argued that anhedonia was accompanied by a very painful affect, a point made earlier by Myerson (1944).

Anhedonia, in some form, has found its way into numerous clinical conceptualizations, including "shut-in personality" (Hoch 1910), "anaesthetic schizoid" (Kretschmer 1925), "chronic state of lack of conscious pleasure" (Glauber 1949), and "aphanisis" (McGlashan 1982). Some have emphasized the saliency of social anhedonia, while others have focused on physical anhedonia by which is meant the more elementary physical needs, such as those for food, drink, and sex; this distinction is not meant to imply that the experiencing of social relationships is somehow dissociated from physical experience, but rather that the source of stimulation differs.

The Empirical Study of Anhedonia

Languishing for many years because they were thought too difficult to assess reliably, anhedonia and more generally "negative symptoms" have within the past decade and a half become a major area of empirical research in schizophrenia. The efforts to quantify anhedonia have taken two major forms: interview-based rating scales and self-report questionnaires.

Published reviews and critiques of commonly used rating scales are available (Pogue-Geile and Zublin 1988; Sommers 1985; Walker and Lewine 1988). Despite its theoretical saliency, anhedonia (not to be equated with loss of interest) is not universally assessed in these rating scales, for example, the Brief Psychiatric Rating Scale (Overall and Gorham 1962), Scale for Emotional Blunting (Abrams and Taylor 1978), and Schedule for Affective Disorders and Schizophrenia-Change Verson (Lewine et al. 1983). The Scale for the Assessment of Negative Symptoms (SANS; Andreasen 1981), probably the most commonly used instrument, does include the assessment of anhedonia which is, however, combined with asociality into a single domain and includes the specific items of recreational activities/interests, sexual activity/interest, ability for personal intimacy and peer/friend relationships. Numerous inde-

Table 1. Illustrative items from Chapman's anhedonia scales

Social:	Writing letters to friends is more trouble than it's worth (True)
	A car ride is much more enjoyable if someone is with me (False)
Physical:	Beautiful scenery has been a great delight to me (False)
	I've never cared much about the texture of food (True)
Invalidity:	I have never gone into a store (True)
	I have never combed my hair (True)

pendent studies have established unambiguously the ability to rate reliably the negative symptoms of schizophrenia, while the various aspects of the negative symptom construct's validity continue to be explored (see Pogue-Geile and Zubin 1988; Sommers 1985; Walker and Lewine 1988).

Although the self-report questionnaire format has been used to develop an extraordinarily wide range of scales, there is surprisingly very little concerning anhedonia. Watson and his colleagues (Watson et al. 1970; Watson 1972) were unsuccessful, using Veterans Administration hospital patients, in their early attempts to measure anhedonia, with a focus on apathy and social withdrawal. As pointed out by Chapman et al. (1976), two schedules for the assessment of pleasant life events (Cautela and Kastenbaum 1967; MacPhillamy and Lewinsohn 1974) approximated anhedonia scales in requiring respondents to fill out a 5-point scale reflecting the intensity of pleasure derived from the various events listed.

The most successful effort in the development of a self-report scale of anhedonia has been undertaken by Loren Chapman and colleagues following the theoretical line of Rado and Meehl. Based on a true-false format, the Chapman scales of anhedonia have been divided into separate components for physical and social anhedonia; illustrative items from each area are listed in Table 1. A set of invalid items has been incorporated into the scales, with protocols containing less than three endorsed items having been empirically determined to be acceptable.

Evidence for the validity of the physical anhedonia scales has been reported in the form of increased prevalence of psychiatric contact, history of psychiatric disorder, psychophysiological hypoactivity, and information processing deficits among normal college students having significantly elevated physical anhedonia scores (Miller 1986; Chapman et al. 1980). Discriminant validity is suggested by the finding that schizophrenic patients score higher than controls on physical anhedonia while social anhedonia, in contrast, has not proven to be as useful (Chapman et al. 1980). In conjunction with scales of perceptual aberration and magical ideation, Chapman's physical anhedonia scale has been described as identifying "hypothetical psychosis proneness."

Conceptual and Methodological Issues

As is true for the more general constructs of negative and deficit symptoms (Carpenter et al. 1985; Lewine and Sommers 1985), a distinction must be made between anhedonia as a state and as a trait condition. The brief historical review makes clear that anhedonia has been usually considered to be a life-long, constitutional trait. There is, however, little empirical evidence that supports this position. If anhedonia could be established as a constitutional trait that preceded schizophrenia onset, it then raises the possibility that it is a predisposing factor or potentiator of schizophrenia. That is, anhedonia may hold an important place in the schizophrenia spectrum. It is also logically possible that anhedonia is independent of the schizophrenic process and that its presence or absence serves primarily to modify the clinical expression of schizophrenia; it is conceivable that anhedonia and schizophrenia could combine to produce the chronic, undifferentiated, withdrawn schizophrenic, while the absence of anhedonia (or the presence of a typical hedonic capacity) in combination with schizophrenia produces the more affectively colored or schizoaffective disorders.

The issue of the relationship between physical and social anhedonia has not been adequately clarified. It has been stated that a fundamental deficit in physical anhedonia is a feature of the neurointegrative defect presumably underlying schizophrenia. This would lead us to give physical anhedonia the role of a fundamental disorder with, perhaps, social anhedonia being a secondary consequence. In contrast, other views of schizophrenia place primary emphasis on interpersonal relationships and the dysphoric state that they engender among individuals with schizophrenia (e.g., Sullivan 1962; Myerson 1944). There has been comparatively little in the way of direct comparison of the respective utility of physical and social anhedonia.

To complicate matters further, there is the practical problem in schizophrenia of untangling the effects of antipsychotic medication from that of the disorder itself. Clinical evidence suggests that these medications can produce or exacerbate negative symptoms such as apathy, poverty of speech, and loss of energy (Carpenter et al. 1985). Wise (1982) has studied systematically the effect of antipsychotic medications on hedonic capacity in mice. He found a dose-dependent relationship between antipsychotic medication (chlorpromazine) and anhedonia; that is, the higher the dose of chlorpromazine per body weight, the greater the degree of anhedonia. The generalizability of this animal model is, admittedly, limited in that anhedonia is operationalized on the basis of learning performance rather than the subjective, anhedonic states that are presumably assessed in humans. Nevertheless, there are several principles suggested by the animal model that are worth examining in the study of anhedonia in schizophrenia.

Wise has argued that the data are consistent with an impairment of the reward/reinforcement system rather than a performance impairment. This anhedonia represents what Wise calls a "rate intensity shift" (1982, p. 49), a term meant to reflect the shifting of the reward value of external stimuli such that a greater stimulus intensity is required to elicit a given behavior than had been required prior to the shift. The reduction in performance under typical circumstances that this rate intensity shift engenders is a problem of response maintenance, not one of response initiation. That is, it can be demonstrated that animals on chlorpromazine given the proper stimulating environment can initiate but not maintain responses, whereas off chlorpromazine they will both initiate and maintain performance.

To begin to address some of these issues, I undertook a short-term longitudinal study of anhedonia as part of a larger effort to examine the construct validity of negative symptoms in an inpatient sample of schizophrenic subjects. Using both self-report and interview-based rating scales, I assessed patients off medication and again after approximately 2 months on medication. Further differentiation of social and physical anhedonia is provided by contrasting their discriminative utility and temporal stability.

Methods

Patients

The subjects for this study were drawn from consecutive admissions to two 22-bed inpatient research units at Illinois State Psychiatric Institute. Written, informed consent to participate was obtained from each patient. A discharge consensus Diagnostic and Statistical Manual (DSM)-III diagnosis based on all available historical and clinical information was assigned, although none of the dependent measures analyzed in this study were included in the diagnostic process. Nineteen schizophrenic patients and 14 nonschizophrenic patients completed all of the testing both off and on medication. The nonschizophrenic group included: major depressive disorder = 4; dysthymic disorder = 1; schizoaffective, mainly depressed = 4; borderline personality disorder = 1; mania = 2; obsessive-compulsive disorder = 1; psychotic disorder not otherwise specified = 1. Of these 14 patients, 10 (71.4%) exhibited psychotic symptoms at some time during their hospitalization, and 7 (50%) were receiving antipsychotic medication.

Measures

The interview-based scale of negative symptoms was the SANS (Andreasen 1981). Intraclass correlations for the SANS component subscores as well as the global SANS total score (sum of the subcomponent global ratings; scores can range from 0 to 25) for three raters jointly rating 25 patients were excellent. They ranged from a low of 0.65 (alogia) to a high of 0.91 (global sum). The mean intraclass correlation for the five subcomponents of the SANS was 0.75. Scales for Physical and Social Anhedonia (Chapman et al. 1976) were filled out by each patient; scores are calculated as the simple sum of items ranging from 0 to 40 for physical anhedonia and 0 to 48 for social anhedonia. A validity scale allows the elimination of profiles from individuals whose responses are invalid, operationalized as the endorsement of more than two invalidity items.

Procedures

The study design called for an initial medication washout period of 2–4 weeks, at the end of which baseline measures were taken. Self-report anhedonia scales and the SANS were filled out again just prior to discharge from hospital. The data for this analysis come from all patients who completed self-report questionnaires during washout and at discharge after several weeks on medication.

Results

Validity of Self-Report Measures

Of the 19 schizophrenic patients who completed the anhedonia scales while off and on medication, 8 (42%) were invalid at either one or both times. In contrast, none of the nonschizophrenic patients produced invalid protocols at either time point. All remaining analyses of the anhedonia scales are based on those subjects who gave valid responses; the schizophrenic patients dropped because of invalid data did not differ significantly from those with valid scale responses on any of the sociodemographic variables.

Table 2 compares the basic sociodemographic and clinical features of the valid schizophrenia and nonschizophrenia groups. The schizophrenia group had a significantly lower mean SES than the nonschizophrenia group and a significantly higher proportion of black patients. Neither Socioeconomic Status (SES) nor race, however, was significantly correlated with any of the anhedonia or SANS measures.

Medication Status and Time Between Testing

Table 3 presents the means (and SD) for medication washout duration, number of days between washout and discharge assessments, and chlorpromazine equivalents for the antipsychotic medications. None of the group differences

Table 2. Characteristics of valid study samples

	Schizophrenia (n = 11)	Nonschizophrenia (n = 14)
Percentage men	81.8	78.6
Percentage black	54.5	21.4
Age, $\bar{x}$	28.9	29.7
(SD) (years)	(7.0)	(7.9)
First admission, $\bar{x}$	24.5	26.1
(SD)	(4.9)	(7.7)
SES, $\bar{x}$ [a]	111.7	79.2
(SD)	(17.6)	(34.8)

SES, socioeconomic status.

[a] Scale points for socioeconomic status range from 20 (high socioeconomic status) to 134 (low socioeconomic status).

Table 3. Duration and medication variables for patients completing valid self-report questionnaires

	Schizophrenia ($n = 11$)		Nonschizophrenia ($n = 14$)	
	$\bar{x}$	(SD)	$\bar{x}$	(SD)
Washout (days)	17.5	(6.9)	18.2	(9.5)
Time between questionnaires (days)	71.8	(28.5)	67.9	(28.9)
Chlorpromazine equivalent dose[a]	446.6	(320.2)	182.2	(256.9)[b]

[a] Honigfeld and Howard (1973).
[b] $n = 7$.

was statistically significant at conventional probability levels, although the difference in chlorpromazine mean approached significance ($P = 0.085$).

Self-Report Anhedonia

Figure 1 provides a summary of the social anhedonia scores. Among the schizophrenic patients, this increased over time (medication status), while in

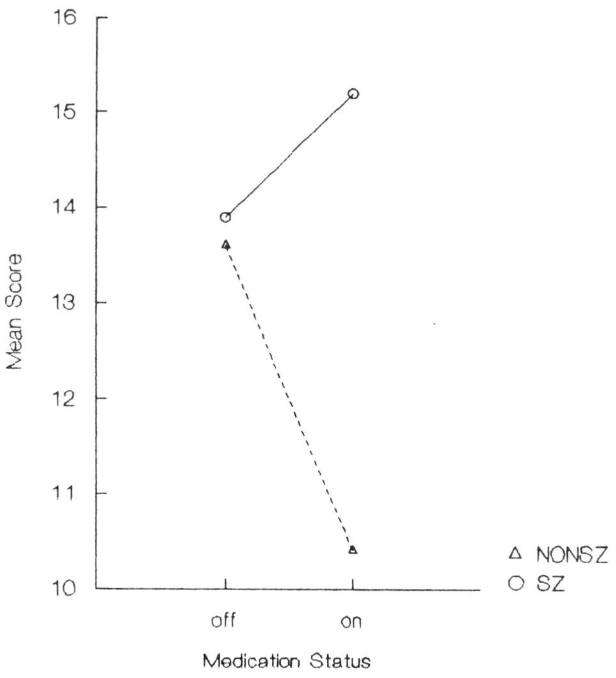

Fig. 1. Self-report social anhedonia as a function of medication status and diagnosis. *SZ*, schizophrenic patients

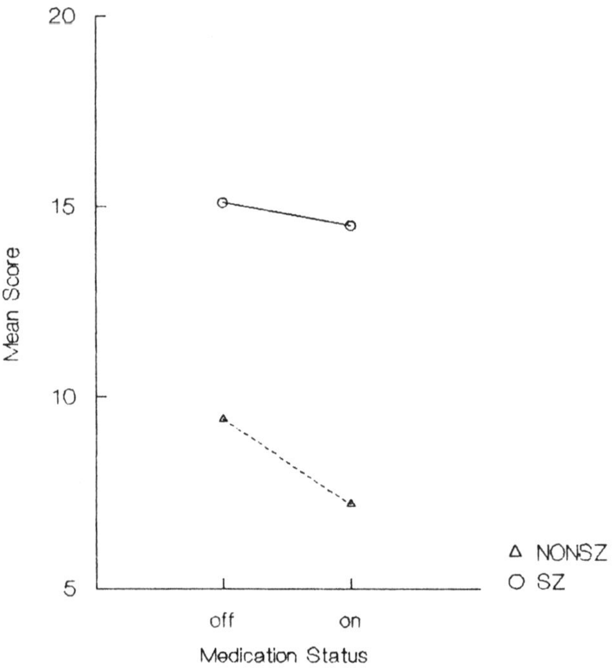

Fig. 2. Self-report physical anhedonia as a function of medication status and diagnosis. *SZ*, schizophrenic patients

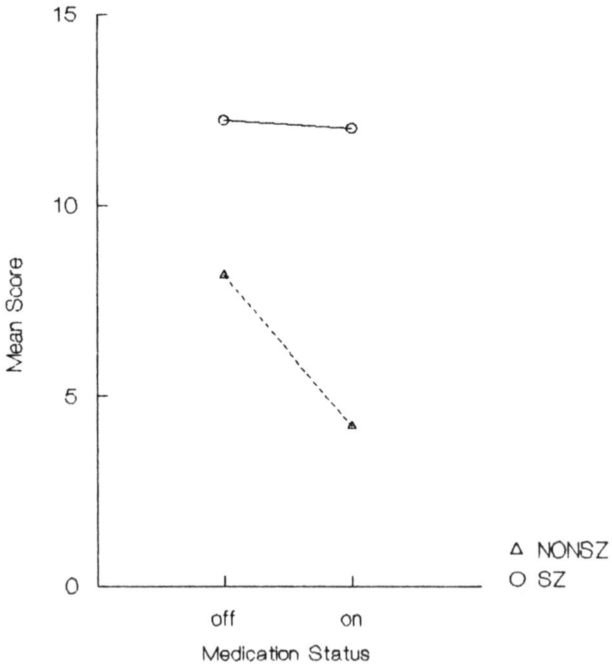

Fig. 3. Total Scale for the Assessment of Negative Symptoms global score as a function of medication status and diagnosis. *SZ*, schizophrenic patients

contrast, it decreased considerably for nonschizophrenic patients, resulting in a significant diagnosis (D) × time (T) interaction ($F_{1,23} = 4.529$, $P = 0.044$). Neither main effect of diagnosis ($F_{1,23} = 1.019$), $P = 0.323$) nor of time ($F_{1,23} = 0.812$, $P = 0.377$) was significant.

Figure 2 presents the mean physical anhedonia scores off and on medication for schizophrenic and nonschizophrenic patients. The schizophrenia group exhibited a significantly higher mean physical anhedonia score overall ($\bar{x} = 14.8$) than the nonschizophrenia group ($\bar{x} = 8.3$) as indicated by a significant main diagnosis effect ($F_{1,23} = 8.215$, $P = 0.009$); although there was a substantial decrease in physical anhedonia over time for the nonschizophrenia group and only a slight decrease among the schizophrenia patients, the main effect of time only approaches statistical significance ($F_{1,23} = 3.525$, $P = 0.073$). The $D \times T$ interaction was not significant ($F_{1,23} = 1.245$, $P = 0.276$).

Figure 3 presents total global SANS scores over time by diagnostic group. Diagnosis ($F_{1,20} = 10.283$, $P = 0.004$) was significant; time ($F_{1,20} = 4.004$, $P = 0.059$) approached significance, as did the $D \times T$ interaction ($F_{1,22} = 3.519$, $P = 0.074$). Examination of the five components of the SANS reveals considerable variability in their course over the two testing time points. (See Table 4 for means and standard deviations of component scores.)

All SANS subcomponents except attention were associated with a significant diagnosis effect: affective flattening ($F_{1,20} = 16.180$, $P = 0.001$), alogia

Table 4. Scale for the Assessment of Negative Symptoms (SANS) component scores at washout and on medication

	Schizophrenia		Nonschizophrenia	
	$\bar{x}$	(SD)	$\bar{x}$	(SD)
Affective flattening				
Washout	2.8	(1.6)	1.2	(1.4)
Medication	2.8	(1.8)	0.7	(0.9)
Alogia				
Washout	1.9	(1.2)	0.6	(1.4)
Medication	1.4	(1.7)	0.4	(0.8)
Avolition				
Washout	2.7	(1.2)	1.8	(1.5)
Medication	2.4	(1.7)	0.6	(1.0)
Anhedonia-asociality				
Washout	3.4	(1.1)	3.2	(0.9)
Medication	3.3	(1.0)	1.2	(1.5)
Attention				
Washout	1.4	(1.1)	1.4	(1.8)
Medication	2.0	(1.2)	0.7	(1.4)
SANS total				
Washout	12.2	(3.9)	8.2	(4.9)
Medication	12.0	(6.3)	4.2	(4.5)

Table 5. Test (washout)-retest (medication) correlations (Pearson) for study variables

	Schizophrenics	Nonschizophrenics
Social anhedonia	0.66	0.91
Physical anhedonia	0.81	0.75
Affective flattening	0.34	−0.02
Alogia	0.89	0.15
Anhedonia-asociality	0.85	0.33
Avolition	0.76	0.23
Attention	−0.45	0.39

($F_{1,20} = 6.263$, $P = 0.02$), avolition ($F_{1,20} = 7.036$, $P = 0.015$), and anhedonia-asociality ($F_{1,20} = 7.372$, $P = 0.013$), schizophrenic patients having the higher mean rating in all cases. The main effect of time was significant on both avolition ($F_{1,20} = 5.633$, $P = 0.028$) and anhedonia-asociality ($F_{1,20} = 14.763$, $P = 0.001$), reflecting a significant decrease in ratings (clinical improvement) in both groups. Only anhedonia-asociality revealed a significant $D \times T$ interaction ($F_{1,20} = 11.714$, $P = 0.003$), which is accounted for by the much larger decrease in ratings for the nonschizophrenia than schizophrenia group.

Table 5 summarizes the test-retest correlations for each of the measures by diagnostic group. Within schizophrenia, physical anhedonia, alogia,

Table 6. Correlations (Pearson) between anhedonia scales and SANS for schizophrenic patients

	Social		Physical	
	Washout	Medication	Washout	Medication
Affective flattening				
Washout	0.07	−0.29	0.51	0.18
Medication	−0.30	−0.47	−0.04	0.28
Alogia				
Washout	0.18	−0.19	0.48	0.27
Medication	0.49	0.03	0.68	0.51
Avolition				
Washout	0.08	−0.19	0.52	0.25
Medication	−0.16	−0.39	0.23	0.00
Anhedonia-asociality				
Washout	−0.08	0.21	0.42	0.36
Medication	−0.12	−0.03	0.35	0.12
Attention				
Washout	0.35	0.04	−0.08	−0.38
Medication	0.32	0.09	0.48	0.49
SANS total				
Washout	0.18	−0.15	0.60	0.23
Medication	0.16	−0.12	0.48	0.34

Table 7. Correlations (Pearson) between anhedonia scales and SANS for nonschizophrenic patients

	Social		Physical	
	Washout	Medication	Washout	Medication
Affective flattening				
Washout	0.32	0.25	0.02	−0.19
Medication	0.34	0.59	0.24	0.00
Alogia				
Washout	0.30	0.27	−0.03	−0.23
Medication	0.08	0.11	−0.28	−0.24
Avolition				
Washout	−0.26	−0.32	−0.42	−0.56
Medication	0.03	0.22	−0.06	−0.48
Anhedonia-asociality				
Washout	−0.29	−0.24	0.06	−0.20
Medication	−0.02	0.22	0.12	−0.36
Attention				
Washout	−0.11	−0.06	0.08	0.14
Medication	0.40	0.44	0.16	−0.14
SANS total				
Washout	0.00	0.00	−0.04	−0.23
Medication	0.19	0.38	0.00	−0.45

anhedonia-asociality and avolition emerge with the greatest stability. Only social anhedonia and physical anhedonia are substantially positively correlated over testings among the nonschizophrenic patients.

To determine further the nature of the social and physical anhedonia differences in schizophrenia, their correlational relationship to the SANS, and in particular to its subcomponents, was examined. Tables 6 and 7 summarize these correlations for schizophrenic and nonschizophrenic patients, respectively.

Among schizophrenic patients, physical anhedonia is more strongly related than social anhedonia to SANS subcomponents, with eight correlations above 0.40 (vs. only two of the social anhedonia correlations). This is revealed even more dramatically in the correlations between social/physical anhedonia and total SANS rating: The mean correlation for physical anhedonia is 0.41 vs. 0.02 for social anhedonia. Furthermore, many of the correlations between SANS variables and social anhedonia are negative, that is, opposite to expectation. In contrast, among nonschizophrenic patients, social and physical anhedonia are comparably related to the SANS and generally much more weakly than among the schizophrenic patients.

Washout duration, test-retest interval, and chlorpromazine equivalents failed to correlate significantly with social and physical anhedonia at either washout or postmedication; correlations ranged from −0.09 to 0.46 with a mean correlation of 0.16 (see Table 8). While comparable results were obtained

Table 8. Correlations (Pearson) between clinical ratings and test interval, washout duration and chlorpromazine equivalents (all patients)

	Test interval	Washout	Chlorpromazine
Social anhedonia			
Washout	−0.09	0.36	0.39
Medication	0.04	0.18	0.04
Physical anhedonia			
Washout	0.21	0.02	0.46
Medication	0.11	−0.07	0.23
Affective flattening			
Washout	0.44	0.01	0.62
Medication	0.22	−0.09	0.02
Alogia			
Washout	0.29	0.13	0.62
Medication	0.04	0.03	0.66
Avolition			
Washout	0.39	−0.23	0.10
Medication	0.17	−0.06	0.14
Anhedonia-asociality			
Washout	0.25	0.04	0.57
Medication	0.18	−0.09	0.43
Attention			
Washout	0.50	−0.19	0.26
Medication	0.33	0.10	0.44
Total			
Washout	0.55	−0.08	0.64
Medication	0.19	0.01	0.48

for the SANS scores and washout duration and test interval, chlorpromazine equivalents exhibited substantial correlations with component scores at both time points; correlations ranged from 0.02 to 0.66, with a mean of 0.42 and 5 of 12 correlations above 0.50.

Discussion

I found, not surprisingly, with the use of the Chapman self-report scales that almost one-third of the patients provided invalid profiles while off medication; this was not, however, significantly reduced with the introduction of antipsychotic agents. Another way of looking at this is that a full two-thirds of the schizophrenic patients in this sample even while off medication were able to respond in a fashion that suggests that they both understood and appropriately answered the items. This finding should both encourage us to utilize more fully self-report measures and remind us that one should not assume the response validity of all schizophrenic patients even when stabilized on medication.

With respect to both temporal stability and discriminitive validity, physical anhedonia appears in this study to be superior to social anhedonia. I think it especially noteworthy that during washout social anhedonia was equally high for both patient groups, while schizophrenic and nonschizophrenic patients were clearly distinguishable on physical anhedonia; this latter intergroup difference continued on medication. This would appear to lend weight to the greater importance of a physically based neurointegrative deficit than social anhedonia in schizophrenia; the intransiency of physical anhedonia in the face of the intensive pharmacological treatment of the schizophrenia group is consistent with a trait characteristic over the short-term.

The differential impact of medication (time) on social and physical anhedonia demands further examination in other studies. Social anhedonia actually worsened in the schizophrenia group, while nonschizophrenic patients showed significant improvement. These results are consistent with Strauss et al.'s (1974) suggestion that social withdrawal represents a process semi-independent from psychotic symptoms and premorbid competence. From a more practical point of view, one might do well not to expect that a single antipsychotic medication (with the possible exception of atypical ones) can be universally effective for the spectrum of anhedonia.

Further support for the salience of physical anhedonia is found in the generally larger magnitude of its correlations with various SANS scores than those of social anhedonia. These findings could not be attributed to the confounding effects of medication (or time), age at assessment, age at first psychiatric hospital admission, or socioeconomic status. I have reported elsewhere (Lewine 1990) that independently rated depression (Hamilton Rating Scale of Depression) did not correlate significantly with any of the negative symptom measures.

Several recent studies and reviews of drug abuse among schizophrenic patients have concluded that there is a disproportionately greater use of dopamine agonist stimulants (amphetamine and cocaine) in this group than in other psychiatric patients (Mueser et al. 1990; Lieberman et al. 1990; Schneier and Siris 1987). Siris (1990) proposes, and I would agree, that this is attributable in some patients to attempts to counteract long-standing deficits in hedonic capacity and other negative symptoms.

Taken seriously, the view that physical anhedonia is not only a long-term characteristic of schizophrenia and an integral component of prepsychotic character development but also a fundamental neurointegrative deficit leads us to explore interventions that heighten the value of physical stimuli. This is a somewhat provocative notion as it is contrary to the view of many that schizophrenia represents a state of stimulus overload and/or poor filtering (Nuechterlein and Dawson 1984). There has been, furthermore, an almost exclusive emphasis on the development of social skills training in contemporary behavioral psychiatry (Liberman 1972). The use of token economy programs fails to address adequately the problem of the "stimulus intensity shift" as the subjective (an)hedonic experience of the patient is targetted for neither assessment nor change.

This study is obviously not without fault: The medication washout period is too short, the sample size is small, there are no direct measures of hedonic capacity, the time interval (a little more than 2 months) for studying a putative trait is inadequate, and time and medication are completely confounded. Nevertheless, there appears to be some convergence on the importance of distinguishing between physical and social anhedonia in the characterization, development, and treatment of schizophrenia.

Returning to the broader concept of motivation, these preliminary data would suggest that the schizophrenic patient may quite literally and concretely not "feel" like doing many of the things expected of him or her. In addition to efforts to improve social relatedness, therefore, we need to explore innovative procedures for enhancing physical stimulus value so that the presumed stimulant "self-medication" can be replaced with less dangerous interventions.

Acknowledgements. This research was conducted at the Illinois State Psychiatric Institute (Chicago) and supported, in part, by National Institute of Mental Health grants 37898 and 42485. I would like to thank A. Sommers, B. In, and P. Walsh for data collection, J. Caudle for data management, and S. Maxwell for manuscript preparation.

References

Abrams R, Taylor MA (1978) A rating scale for emotional blunting. Am J Psychiatry 2(135):226–229
Adler A (1926) The neurotic constitution. Dodd, Mead, New York
Andreasen N (1981) Scale for the assessment of negative symptoms. Iowa City, Iowa
Brickner RM (1936) The intellectual functions of the frontal lobes. MacMillan, New York
Buss AH, Lang PJ (1965) Psychological deficit in schizophrenia. I. Affect, reinforcement and concept attainment. J Abnorm Psychol 70:2–24
Carpenter WT (1987) Approaches to knowledge and understanding of schizophrenia. Schizophr Bull 13:1–8
Carpenter WT, Heinrichs DW, Alphs LD (1985) Treatment of negative symptoms. Schizophr Bull 11:440–452
Cautela JR, Kastenbaum R (1967) A reinforcement survey schedule for use in therapy, training, and research. Psychol Rep 20:1115–1130
Chapman L, Chapman J, Raulin M (1976) Scales for physical and social anhedonia. J Abnorm Psychol 85:374–382
Chapman LJ, Edell WS, Chapman JP (1980) Physical anhedonia, perceptual aberration, and psychosis proneness. Schizophr Bull 6, 4:639–653
Damasio AR (1985) The frontal lobes. In: Heilman EM, Valenstein E (eds) Clinical neuropsychology. Oxford University Press, New York, pp 339–376
Gilman SL (1982) Seeing the insane. Wiley, New York
Glauber IP (1949) Observations on a primary form of anhedonia. Psychoanal Q 18:67–78
Grinker RR (1975) Anhedonia and depression in schizophrenia. In: Anthony EJ, Benedek (eds) Depression and human existence. Little, Brown, Boston, pp 413–424
Hoch A (1910) Constitutional factors in the dementia praecox group. Rev Neurol Psychiatry 8:463–474
Holzman PS (1987) Recent studies of psychophysiology in schizophrenia. Schizophr Bull 13:49–76
Honigfeld G, Howard A (1973) Psychiatric drugs. Academic, New York
Kraepelin E (1971) Dementia praecox and paraphrenia. Krieger, Huntington (Original 1919)
Kretschmer E (1925) Physique and character. Harcourt Brace, New York
Lewine RRJ (1990) A discriminant validity study of negative symptoms with special focus on depression and antipsychotic medication. Am J Psychiatry (in press)

Lewine RRJ, Sommers AA (1985) Clinical definitions of negative symptoms as a reflection of theory and methodology. In: Alpert M (ed) Controversies in schizophrenia: changes and constancies. Guilford, New York, pp 267–279
Lewine RRJ, Fogg L, Meltzer HY (1983) Assessment of negative and positive symptoms in schizophrenia. Schizophr Bull 9:368–376
Liberman RP (1972) Behavioral modification of schizophrenia: a review. Schizophr Bull 6:37–48
Lieberman JA, Kinon BJ, Loebel AD (1990) Dopaminergic mechanisms in idiopathic and drug-induced psychoses. Schizophr Bull 16:97–110
MacPhillamy DJ, Lewinsohn PM (1974) Depression as a function of levels of desired and obtained pleasure. J Abnorm Psychol 83:651–657
McGlashan TH (1982) Aphanisis: the syndrome of pseudo-depression in chronic schizophrenia. Schizophr Bull 8:118–134
Meehl PE (1962) Schizotaxia, schizotypy, schizophrenia. Am Psychol 17:827–838
Meehl PE (1989) Schizotaxia revisited. Arch Gen Psychiatry 46:935–944
Miller GA (1986) Information processing deficits in anhedonia and perceptual aberration: a psychophysiological analysis. Biol Psychiatry 21:100–115
Mueser KT, Yarnold PR, Levinson DF, Singh H, Bellack AS, Kee K, Morrison RL, Yadalam KG (1990) Prevalence of substance abuse in schizophrenia: demographic and clinical correlates. Schizophr Bull 16:31–56
Myerson A (1922) Anhedonia. Am J Psychiatry 2:87–111
Myerson A (1944) The social anxiety neurosis-its possible relationship to schizophrenia. Am J Psychiatry 101:149–156
Myerson A (1946) The constitutional anhedonic personality. Am J Psychiatry 102:774–779
Nuechterlein KH, Dawson ME (1984) Information processing and attentional functioning in the developmental course of schizophrenia. Schizophr Bull 10:160–203
Overall JE, Gorham DR (1962) The brief psychiatric rating scale. Psychol Rep 10:799–812
Paul GL, Lentz RJ (1977) Psychosocial treatment of chronically institutionalized mental patients. Harvard University Press, Cambridge
Peterson CA, Knudson RM (1983) Anhedonia: a construct validation approach. J Pers Assess 5:539–551
Pogue-Geile MF, Zubin J (1988) Negative symptomatology schizophrenia: a conceptual and empirical review. Int J Ment Health 16:3–45
Rado S (1956) Psychoanalysis of behavior. Grune and Stratton, New York
Ribot TH (1897) The psychology of emotions. Scott, London
Schneier FR, Siris SG (1987) A review of psychoactive substance use and abuse in schizophrenia: patterns of drug choice. J Nerv Ment Dis 175:641–650
Shakow D (1956) Adaptation in schizophrenia: the theory of segmental set. Wiley, New York
Siris SG (1990) Pharmacological treatment of substance-abusing schizophrenic patients. Schizophr Bull 16:111–122
Sommers A (1985) Negative symptoms: conceptual and methodological problems. Schizophr Bull 11:364–379
Strauss JS, Carpenter WT, Bartko JJ (1974) Speculations on the processes that underlie schizophrenic symptoms and signs. Schizophr Bull 11:61–69
Sullivan HS (1962) Schizophrenia as a human process. Norton, New York
Walker EF, Lewine RRJ (1988) The positive/negative symptom distinction in schizophrenia. Validity and etiological distinction in schizophrenia. Validity and etiological significance. Schizophr Res 1:315–328
Watson CG (1972) Relationships of anhedonia to physiological reactivity and threshold. Psychol Rep 31:43–46
Watson CG, Klett W, Lorei T (1970) Toward an operational definition of anhedonia. Psychol Rep 26:371–376
Wise RA (1982) Neuroleptics and operant behavior: the anhedonia hypothesis. Behav Brain Sci 5:39–87

Constituting Reality – Its Decline and Repair in the Long-Term Course of Schizophrenic Psychoses: The Intentionality Model

CH. MUNDT [1]

Introduction

It is often argued against the phenomenological approach that it is too vague and unreliable for empirical research, offering interpretations rather than facts. The advantage of this approach, however, can be seen in reference to the subjective world of meanings and purposes in which a human being dwells and develops moods, feelings, affects, motives and actions. This sphere is not adequately met by either biological or operational psychopathological methodology. Psychoanalysis, however, has contributed considerably to this field. Thus, non-biological therapeutic strategies may profit from this approach, and also nosological considerations.

Phenomenological psychopathology claims that the fundamental disturbance in acute schizophrenic psychosis is a loss of constituting inter-subjective reality (Blankenburg 1971). If this hypothesis is true, interpretion of the schizophrenic defect states should also be attempted from this point of view. First, a psychopathological model and term have to be found for the ability to constitute reality. Then by means of this tool the pathways must be described in which this ability is built up in pre-morbid personality, breaks down in acute psychosis and is possibly and partly restituted in the so-called defect states. Their interpretation will not be possible without a comprehensive psychopathological model which encompasses all three stages of the disease and their ontogenetic history.

In the German-speaking psychiatric world is traditional to use the term intentionality to describe the schizophrenic patient's disturbed ability to constitute reality. Beringer (1926) spoke of the reduced intentional span in order to pinpoint the underlying disturbance of some patients' vague language with an under-structured overview of a multitude of aspects. Berze and Gruhle (1929) at the same time called this a "lack of teleological discipline" in the thinking of schizophrenic subjects. The term "intentionality" was resumed then with a more specific philosophical background by Blankenburg in the 1960s (Table 1), while examining patients with simplex schizophrenia who were able to describe with fine introspection their loss of being enmeshed in all the subtle meanings and purposes of everyday life. This fundamental uncertainty

[1] Psychiatrische Universitätsklinik, Voßstraße 4, W-6900 Heidelberg, FRG

A. Marneros / N. C. Andreasen / M. T. Tsuang (Eds.)
Negative Versus Positive Schizophrenia

Table 1. Concepts of intentionality

Authors	Basic idea
Brentano (1973), Husserl (1975)	Existence of objects in the mind
Blankenburg (1971)	Constituting the world by means of transcendental organization of the Ego
Rapaport (1967)	Over-cathexis of mental representatives
Lacan (1936), Lang (1986)	Language symbols = representatives of reality
Searle (1983)	Mind as intentional state; intentionality = biological phenomenon
Dennett (1971)	Intentional systems act by referring to each other's intentionality

about anything in everyday language, acting and experiencing which seems to us perfectly natural and unquestioned can perhaps be grasped best by the English term "common sense" which was according to Blankenburg missing in his patients in a very fundamental fashion. The theoretical background to this phenomenon of a very basic uncertainty about inter-subjective reality evolved from Husserl's (1975) hypothesis of intentionality, which in turn goes back to Brentano and the philosophy of the Middle Ages. The common core idea of the term was – to put it in a very simplified way – that inter-subjective reality and even the physical reality in which we live have to be conceptualised in mind and are not simply implicated by our sensory experiences. This act of conceptionalising reality was called intentionality.

Similar constructs were used in psychoanalysis, although different terms expressed the process of constituting reality. Rapaport (1967), Lacan (1936) and, in German structuralism, Lang (1986) spoke of the mental representatives of reality. Rapaport envisaged constituting reality in a rather mechanistic way as over-cathexis of mental representatives; Lacan thought of the language structure as the basis for inter-subjectivity.

There has been a renaissance of this term in recent years in the philosophy of mind. Two directions of usage can be distinguished, one looking from inside the subject's world, one looking from outside at the objectifiable performance of intentionality. Searle (1983) concerning the former considers intentionality as an essential of mental states in the sense of the ontological dualism, a biological phenomenon of the human brain, endowing the basically meaningless puzzle of our sensory experiences with meaning. Parallels to Gestalt psychology are obvious. Dennett (1971) from the latter, objective point of view speaks of intentional systems and claims that living systems of higher complexity can be explained by the intention they ascribe to each other. He differentiated three levels of complexity according to the multitude of mutual references the systems make to each other. Thus, the term reciprocity supplements the term intentionality in Dennett's theory.

The Intentionality Model

My definition of the term intentionality reflects the interpretation of its disturbance in schizophrenics. It ought to help in developing a psychopathological disease model. Thus, we should not indulge too much in the fundamental philosophical questions which certainly will not be solved before we have to carry on dealing with schizophrenic patients. This means that the definition of intentionality on clinical grounds will necessarily be a negative one; it emphasises what disordered intentionality is whereas the undisturbed function remains in the dark. For clinical purposes I discriminate three levels of intentionality performance (Table 2).

The Sensory Level

This level concerns the processing of sensory information to a gestalt. It enables man to orientate in the physical world. Disturbances of schizophrenic patients on this level are well investigated in experimental psychopathology. To the main findings belong that the emergence of a gestalt from visual and acoustic perception is retarded, unstable and more often mistaken as compared with that of normal subjects. Building up a special perspective shows more often inconsistencies of the estimation of the magnitude and distance of objects (Meyer-Osterkamp and Cohen 1973). Also, in the artwork of schizophrenic artists disturbances of space construction can be observed (Mundt 1985), among them the vertical shift of the viewangle (Rennert 1963). Beside an attentional deficit in the continuous performance test (CPT) and similar experiments in some patients, ill-defined perceptual schemata seem to be responsible for these findings. The function of reciprocity on this level in Dennett's sense is bound to feedback mechanisms of reafferent motor-sensory circuits as described in the concepts of assimilation accommodation by Piaget (1975) or the gestalt-circle function by von Weizsäcker (1940).

Table 2. Three levels of intentionality

Level	Psychopathological examples
Sensory processing → cognitive schemata (primary cognition)	Inconsistency of perspective Basic symptoms sensu Huber (1983), disturbed Gestalt recognition (Continuous performance Test Cross-modality stimulus response)
Language, symbolization → interpersonal communication (sencondary cognition)	Loosening of associations, sign-field disturbance sensu Peters (1973), neologism
Transcendental subject	Alienation, delusional mood (Trema sensu Conrad 1958), psychotic oneiroid state

The Level of Reality Representation in the Symbols of Language and Thinking

This level of intentionality concerns the evolution of meaning in words, language and thinking structures. Evolving and maintaining meaning on this level is bound to social exchange and permanent adjustment. Any verbal exchange contains an effort at definition which operates with the halo of connotations of words or phrases. Restricting this halo by the context of a sentence can render to the communication partner suggestions of which of several possibilities is meant. In irony or humour this process becomes very complex; Gestalt psychology speaks of the altitude of a gestalt. It is known that schizophrenic patients have particular difficulties entering this process of mutual definition of the metaphoric level of a word meaning. Concretism and the opposite, an inadequate symbolism, are well-known as very specific types of schizophrenic thought disorders. The necessity of reciprocity in Dennett's sense is particularly obvious at this level. Linguistic research has developed many operationalisations which can depict a decline of reciprocity on this level, e.g. the cloze procedure (Taylor 1953), which demonstrates that texts of not-thought-disordered schizophrenic subjects are less successfully reconstructed than texts of controls if every 5th word has been skipped. The Saarbrücken group (Villenave-Cremer et al. 1989) most recently found by means of Gottschalk-Gleser language content analysis that in the dialogue between non-thought-disordered schizophrenic patients and healthy volunteers the former were regularly inclined to withdraw from attempts at definition, allocating to the other person the task to suggest a common meaning.

The Level of Complex and Comprehensive Meanings and Purposes of the Person and Existence

This level concerns the idea a person has of himself/herself in the future, relationships, place in society. Again, Gestalt psychology has coined a term which refers to the special way of well-being if the idea of the self and its societal reality coincide: the good gestalt. The typical expression for clinical disturbance of this personal existential level of intentionality is the delusional mood, "trema" (Conrad 1958) and the psychotic oneiroid state with the experience of false pretense and the recognition of disguised persons and theatre-like acting all around. Blankenburg's ontological formulation of the lack of transcendental organisation of the schizophrenic's Ego refers to this level.

This three level order is of course artificial to a certain degree. Especially between the 2nd and the 3rd level can the distinction be difficult. Moreover, there are of course manifold interactions between the disturbances of these levels. The order may imply an idea of the ontological history of schizophrenia from the more basic disturbances of frail sensory and cognitive schemata to symbolisation deficiencies and eventually existential psychopathology. Klosterkötter (1988) of Huber's group described the psychopathological transitions from basic disturbances to manifest psychosis.

The Interpretation of Clinical Phenomena

Acute Stage

Now an attempt can be made to look at the long-term course of schizophrenia by means of the psychopathological tool intentionality. Let us start with the acute stage of the illness. One should differentiate between acute loosening or dissolution of meanings on the one hand and their redefinition in an alien way for us on the other (Table 3). Examples for an acute loosening of meanings include besides hallucinations, language and thought disorders as incoherence; redefinitions are the so-called sign-field disturbances (Peters 1973) in which the common meaning of the single word or phrase has slipped and has been redefined in an autistic way very similar to neologisms. Its meaning cannot be corrected as opposite to a misunderstanding. Just arising delusional symptoms as delusional perception, delusional ideas and delusional remembrances, which may be called phenomena of nascent delusion, belong to gliding intentionality. The redefinition of meaning here concerns mainly the coherent, stable delusion. In this case meanings and purposes became stable and safe again, the subject's re-orientation is possible, the wholeness of psychic life is safeguarded but at the price of autism: reciprocity with the referential society is suspended. In this sense manifest delusion can be considered as a repair mechanism in terms of the intentionality model.

Other, less effective attempts to reorganise intentional efforts or rather to prevent their total destruction can be seen in repetitive thoughts, ruminations, obsessive-compulsive phenomena, echo phenomena and mannerisms. The obsessional looking for one's own identity in a mirror by some schizophrenic patients may be mentioned here; one of my patients kept touching objects around him, saying he needs to know whether they are real. Mannerisms and

Table 3. Types of disturbed intentionality in schizophrenia

Level	Acute	Transition acute-chronic-repair	Repair
	("Cognitive gliding")	(Habituation; disorganisation as behavioural style)	(Alleviation for intentional performance; retreat from intentional efforts)
Sensory	Acute hallucination	Chronic hallucinosis with little affective engagement	Retardation; protection from stimuli
Symbolisation	Acute thought and language disturbances	Vague speech, "woolly thinking"; schizophasia, partly controllable	Coherent delusion, neologism, poverty of speech
Transcendental	Delusional mood	Simplex schizophrenia	"Deranged structure" sensu Janzarik (1968)

the phenomena of iteration can be interpreted as clinging to remainders of formerly defined meanings, which have elapsed into an autistic world without reciprocal adjustments of definition but with either private, rigid and growingly odd definitions, or they are used as an empty cipher from a formerly lived-in world. The former content of the intended cipher may still be recognised in some mannerisms. Acute cognitive gliding and the rigid autistic re-definition of reality in delusions have in common the loss of reprocity in the sense of Dennett.

There are some transitions of phenomena between acute cognitive gliding with dissolution of meaningful contents and rigid re-definitions in an autistic fashion. As examples can be regarded chronic, in a way blunted hallucinoses without much affective impact for the patient in residual states and the schizophasia in the area of language disturbances. Especially the latter phenomenon conveys the impression that it orginally emerged from acute cognitive gliding but has been perpetuated and become a new cognitive style in which some patients feel at home in a way. Thus, schizophasic passages in the speech of schizophrenic patients often start when disputable topics are touched upon; it seems that to a certain degree for these patients the choice between desultory and understandable speech is available (see Hölderlin interpretations by Bertaux 1978 and Peters 1982). Similar processes can be observed in what Janzarik (1968) called structural distortion, which means a gradual alteration of personality. The beginning may be set off by an acute gliding of meanings and purposes, but at the end there is a new sort of security in a private world of an oddish life style with queer but firm meanings and purposes in every-day life.

These remarks on some examples of repair mechanisms for disturbed intentionality lead to the post-acute stage of the illness. For a better understanding of the patients' situation in the post-acute stage from the point of view of the intentionality model, a look should be cast back to the pre-morbid development of intentionality.

Premorbid Course

In the Weinsberg study of chronic schizophrenia (Mundt 1985) patients and their relatives were asked to depict the pre-morbid personality in terms of the affective style in contrast with siblings and friends. Patients and relatives described very heterogeneous features which, however, had something in common, what may be considered as weakened intentionality. Although these features are not specific for identifying future schizophrenic patients, they can be found in the disorder spectrum. If they are looked at retrospectively, knowing that they emerged into manifest psychosis some time later, they appear partly as a manifestation of and partly as a reaction to an instable performance of intentionality in pre-morbid life.

Asthenic features (Table 4) are those most frequently described. They go along with early social withdrawal, social fears and often symbiotic life arrangements in which the future patients are still sustained by some structured frame of meanings and purposes. The over-charge of personal intentional

Table 4. Pathways into manifest psychosis

Premorbid type	Premorbid features	Precipitating constellations	Post-acute characteristics
Asthenic	Withdrawn, sensitive, symbiotic-protected	Request of mature social role, overwhelming intentionality of others	Apathy
Tense, atactic	Well-adapted, over-structured	Predominance of a biographical main topic, clear-cut conflicts	Delusion, paraphrenia
Open	Naive, lively, popular, under-structured	Stimulation in puberty	Abandonment

efforts then happens when steps into social maturity are challenged, e.g. leaving the parents' home, taking up secondary relationships, choosing a profession and entering into working life. A special hazard seems to be the confrontation with others with strong intentionality e.g. in intimate relationships. This has been demonstrated quasi-experimentally in a study by von Held (1984) on schizophrenic first episodes triggered off in encounter groups with very intruding, revealing and aggressive interpretations of the future patients' behaviour. The intended reality of their self turned out to be the weaker one, which was overwhelmed by the stronger reality of the therapists and the other group members. Also, the expressed-emotions and life-event findings could be interpreted in this sense as well as the nature of preventative biographical factors. In my sample there were some patients with late onset who lived under such protecting life circumstances with clear but unobtrusive structures for intentions in thinking, feeling and acting, structures which did not force and overwhelm and which could be experienced as friendly and resilient.

A completely different pathway into psychosis is marked by the growth of a biographical topic which dominates the psychic life of a personality more and more until in the end this topic slips away from the reciprocity of inter-subjective intentionality in the sense of Dennett. This mechanism is bound to stronger, more clear-cut personalities, whose psychosis may be of the paranoid, late-onset type. One patient illustrates this pathway: as a student in chemistry, shortly before finishing his thesis, he developed the delusion of being a great scientist and engineer who invented new chemicals. This development had a long history of pre-occupation by the loss of his father in the last World War in the USSR. He was believed by the family to have become a great engineer in the USSR and originator of space technology there. The patient's mother contributed by her narcissistic over-involvement to the growth of the later delusional topic in the patient's life. The family and the patient remained focussed on the lost fame, wealth and grandeur attributed to the dead father.

Asthenic features were also missing in some psychopathic patients who were first hospitalised because of delinquency; they developed their psychosis only years later. They displayed a strong affective make-up of their pre-morbid personality with a sort of social ataxia, sometimes possibly parathymic, with heavy social conflicts, reduced social learning and peculiar, insensitive behaviour. Although there was a high level of activity and strong affects there was also an instable, atactic reciprocity.

Different again is the open personality's pathway into psychosis. A small group of patients was described as pre-morbidly lively, vivid but naive, too easy-going, too easily stimulated and impressed. It seemed that they did not comprehend the complexity and consequences of relationships, biographical stages, situations and decisions. The impression was that they did not develop cognitive and emotional structures on the second level, hardly any defense mechanisms, fears or social inhibitions. Obligation was lacking concerning consistency of recognition patterns and their consequences for acting, feelings and mood.

Recently Sauer et al. (1989) could find differences in personality inventories between the open personality in this sense on the one hand and the tense and atactic one on the other, which I keep together as the fragmented ones; whereas the group of asthenics seems to be more heterogeneous, mixing much more biologically based affective make-up on one side and psychological reactions and behavioural styles on the other.

These different pathways into psychosis highlight different qualities of the intentional performance which become more and more instable in the pre-morbid course of psychic development. In the delusion of fragmented personalities, intentionality shows a deflection into their private world, which is the original meaning of autism by Eugen Bleuler. Intentionality is clearly structured in these patients, but the reciprocity is given up in favour of a private framework of meanings whose changes follow different psychotic projections but not adjustments to the views of others. The characteristic of the open pre-morbid personality is vagueness, lack of structure. Intentionality remains unclear without consistency, exposed to instant influences and stimuli, only sustained by external structure. I call it "amorphous intentionality". The asthenic pre-morbid personality seems to have less vigour available in intentionality. This aspect may also be a result of reactions to the experienced risk of losing reciprocity. Marcus of the Jerusalem high-risk study group (1981) described children who displayed signs of emotional instability at early school age and developed schizoidism in mid-adolescence which was interpreted by the group as reaction.

Thus, clinical observation suggests that successful intentionality needs a minimal vigour, structure and centrifugal direction in order to enable growth of the personality structure, the possibility of emotional experience and learning from conflicts, the handling of anxiety and the exchange with the marked intentionality of others without losing one's own subjectivity. All this may fail with unstable intentionality, Pre-morbid schizoidism may ensue, autonomous over-arousal, prodromal and basic symptoms. The three qualities of intentional efforts correspond well with ego qualities as they were described by Scharfetter (1986) in the tradition of Karl Jaspers.

Post-Aaute Stage

If we look now at the apathy syndrome by means of the intentionality model, the following questions have to be discussed: What are the conditions under which the qualities of intentionality can be restituted? How can patients deal with the problem that intentional threads of pre-morbid life are cut with the acute psychosis? Can patients possibly resume these threads with insufficient intentional stability without putting themselves at risk of a relapse? This last refers to the problem of down-rehabilitation and the high suicidal risk especially in patients from ambitious, demanding families. Also, what are the conditions under which weakened intentionality can be kept stable with a minimum of reciprocity?

The reduction of the overall affectivity by neurolepsy and the clear-cut structure of the external reality in hospital are known as main factors which help the schizophrenic patient to regain wholistic experience from psychotic confusion (Table 5). High expressed emotion (EE) families produce this affective overcharge possibly combined with a strong sort of counter-intentionality which may drown the patients intentionality. Reiss (1968) could demonstrate in an experimental psychopathological study that schizophrenic patients were prone to give up correct solutions they had found in a mathematical problem solving task in order to follow wrong patterns of key relatives, which was not the case in neurotic patients and healthy controls.

Complex social fields with a high degree of freedom for definitorial acts are very difficult to master for schizophrenic patients. Such situations occur in all group situations in which hierarchy, roles, tasks and ranks are not yet distributed, be it occupational, private or therapeutic relations. Ciompi's work on the Soteria project demonstrated that clearly visible social structures correlated with the stability of the patients (Ciompi 1981). One of our

Table 5. Factors with impact on the performance of intentionality

Destabilising	Stabilising
Tension between inside and outside reality	Harmonious, "gentle", reliable outside structure
High affective charge on intentions	Reduction of affective charge
Complex intentions ("Hohe Gestalt"), humour, irony, blurred social roles	Clear-cut social roles, unambiguous communication
Overwhelming intentionality of others in intimacy, encounter groups	Flexible, tolerant, secure relationships, time enough to accommodate
Entering open social field without definition of personal goals and behavioural style	guidance by non-conflicting external structure

schizophrenic patients on a ward came into a state of excitation when he was confronted in a game with an ironic sort of aggression by another patient, who deliberately kept undetermined whether he meant what he said or whether he was joking. Game, joke, aggression, honest or pseudo-comradship were blurred to test the other patient's attitude, an unbearable situation for the schizophrenic patient who got lost inbetween these different meta-communication levels.

The special problem of how to handle the loose ends of pre-morbid intentional contents – Jung and Bleuler (cf. Jung 1973) spoke of complexes, Janzarik of "Wertgefüge" in the sense of Gestalt psychology – has produced a very rich phenomenological literature. Schindler (1960), Benedetti (1983), Minkowski (1971, 1972) and in more recent times with another language McGlashan et al. (1977) and Wing (1987) described ways which either lead astray or at least to some re-integration of pre-morbid contents. All variants can be seen, from post-psychotic maturation taking up late pre-morbid lines of development to complete standstill at the biographical situation at which the onset of the psychosis broke in. In these cases of a peculiar standstill of personality development the experience of time can be expanded afterwards. Crow and Stevens (1978) have demonstrated this in an empirical study.

Other patients live against their impaired intentionality, denying it, and thus provoking relapses. Especially in the first 2 years after the onset of illness when the suicidal risk is particularly high is this adjustment very painful for patients and their families with an ambitious, demanding attitude towards academic achievements (Schubart et al. 1986).

Therapeutic strategies should recognise and respect the reduced level of intentionality. They should support those alleviating factors which do not hamper too much social integration and facilitate an after-maturation as some patients with early onset in the Weinsberg study could achieve when they lived in a protective relationship for some years. Böker et al. (1989) collected schizophrenic patients' self-reports on auto-protective attitudes and emphasised as coping strategies shifts of acting away from stressing fields, reality testing and the development of behavioural stereotypes. Pre-requisites for the development of these coping strategies are basic symptoms and their recognition by the patients as alarm signals, which implies a certain degree of insight.

Conclusions

To sum up the main aspects of the intentionality model five hypotheses are presented (Table 6):

1. The qualitative core phenomenon of the psychopathology of schizophrenia is a disturbance of constituting reality, which can manifest on different levels of complexity, the sensory, symbolization and transcendental organisation. All three levels interact with each other.
   The three empirically found factors which organise the clinical psychopathology of schizophrenia, namely paranoid projection, disorganisation

Table 6. Hypotheses of the intentionality model of schizophrenia

- The core phenomenon of schizophrenic psychopathology is a disturbance in constituting reality
- Disturbed constitution of reality provokes psychic repair mechanisms
- Even in the pre-morbid course unstable intentionality hampers the development of a structured personality
- The pathway into psychosis is formed by expected steps into mature social roles and interactions which over-challenge unstable intentionality
- The "defect" states are an equilibrium between unstable intentionality and conditions of reduced challenge for intentional efforts

and apathy, can be interpreted as three fundamental forms of alterations of intentionality: direction, which is deflected into the autistic private world; structure; and the qualities of speed, vigor and fluidity.

2. With the disturbance of constituting reality, repair mechanisms arise instantly, among them the counter-reality of delusion and neologisms or the permanent loosening and gliding of constituting reality as a stable new behavioral style. Beside these passive, unwilling repair mechanisms on the symbolisation and person level, more active coping strategies concern the sensory level of basic symptoms with reality testing, auto-protection from too complex and too highly affect-charged stimuli.
3. Even in the pre-morbid course unstable intentionality hampers the development of a well-structured, integrated personality. Critical experiences, conflicts and life events which could facilitate ways to cope with and form strong affects cannot be lived through. Thus, the structural capacity to bind and use affects remains underdeveloped, and emotional learning remains on a low level. Schizoid personality features most often emerge. In unfavourable cases neurotic arrangements of evasion or protection from intentional efforts may weaken even further the development of the intentional organisation.
4. The pathways into manifest psychosis are marked by an over-challenge of intentional efforts, preferably due to steps of social maturation of the respective age. Typical challenges are the need for self-assertion and definition of one's own role and self in very complex situations, in very unstructured situations or in situations with very intense and adverse intentional efforts by others. Modes of the intentional break-down can be the fracture of a well-organised structure by delusion, the asthenic fading of intentional efforts or the unstructured surrender to psychotic alteration due to internal and external stimuli in the open personality.
5. The so-called defect states are the result of an enforced equilibrium between unstable intentionality and the post-acute conditions of reduced challenge for intentional efforts. The establishment of such an equilibrium is impeded by the disruption of the pre-morbid intentional lines with the onset of the psychosis. The higher the pre-morbid level of intentional organisation was, the more difficult will be the post-acute new beginning in terms of the

narcissistic balance and adaptation to a new social role. Therapeutic and rehabilitation strategies have to take into account the contributions of delusion, autism, personality alteration, symbioses to this equilibrium, the time consumption needed for the development of this equilibrium and the special hazards which put it at risk, which basically resemble the pathways into the first episode.

I would like to conclude by coming back to the introductory remarks, which should remind you of the two aims of this model: to integrate the multitude of empirical findings and to gain access to the patients' existential meanings and purposes, their destruction and loss in psychosis and the struggle for their development in pre-morbid life and their reconstruction in post-acute life. Thus, compared e. g. with the vulnerability model, the intentionality model emphasises much more the active, strategic character of constituting reality and building up inter-subjectivity.

References

Benedetti G (1983) Todeslandschaften der Seele. Vandenhøeck and Ruprecht, Göttingen
Beringer K (1926) Denkstörungen und Sprache bei Schizophrenen. Z Gesamte Neurol Psychiatr 103:185–197
Bertaux P (1978) Friedrich Hölderlin. Suhrkamp, Frankfurt
Berze J, Gruhle HW (1929) Psychologie der Schizophrenie. Springer, Berlin
Blankenburg W (1971) Der Verlust der natürlichen Selbstverständlichkeit. Ein Beitrag zur Psychopathologie symptomarmer Schizophrenien. Enke, Stuttgart
Böker W, Brenner HD, Würgler S (1989) Vulnerabilitätsverbundene Defizienzen. Psychopathologie und Bewältigungsverhalten bei Schizophrenen und deren Angehörigen. In: Böker W, Brenner HD (eds) Schizophrenie als systemische Störung. Huber, Bern, pp 283–299
Brentano F (1973) Psychologie vom empirischen Standpunkt, vol 1. Meiner, Hamburg (Original 1924)
Ciompi L (1981) Wie können wir die Schizophrenen besser behandeln? Eine Synthese neuer Krankheits- und Therapiekonzepte. Nervenarzt 52:506–515
Conrad K (1958) Die beginnende Schizophrenie. Versuch einer Gestaltanalyse des Wahns. Thieme, Stuttgart
Crow TJ, Stevens M (1978) Age disorientation in chronic schizophrenia: the nature of the cognitive defect. Br J Psychiatry 133:137–142
Dennett D (1971) Intentional systems. J Philos 68:87–106
von Held H-R (1984) Umgang mit Psychosen in Encounter- und Therapiegruppen. Gruppenpsychother Gruppendyn 19:231–242
Huber G (1983) Das Konzept substratnaher Basissymptome und seine Bedeutung für Theorie und Therapie schizophrener Erkrankungen. Nervenarzt 54:23–32
Husserl E (1975) V. Logische Untersuchung. Über intentionale Erlebnisse und ihre "Inhalte". Meiner, Hamburg (Original 1901)
Janzarik W (1968) Schizophrene Verläufe. Eine strukturdynamische Interpretation. Springer, Berlin Heidelber New York
Janzarik W (1988) Strukturdynamische Grundlagen der Psychiatrie. Enke, Stuttgart
Jung CG (1973) Zur Psychogenese der Geisteskrankheiten. Walter, Olten
Klosterkötter J (1988) Grenzen zwischen Persönlichkeitsvarianten und Schizophrenien? In: Janzarik W (ed) Persönlichkeit und Psychose. Enke, Stuttgart, pp 112–127
Lacan J (1936) Au-delà du "principe de réalité". Evol Psychiatr 3:67–86

Lang H (1986) Die Sprache und das Unbewußte. Jacques Lacans Grundlegung der Psychoanalyse. Suhrkamp, Frankfurt
Marcus J, Auerbach J, Wilkinson L, Burack C (1981) Infants at risk for schizophrenia. The Jerusalem infant developement study. Arch Gen Psychiatry 38:703–713
McGlashan TH, Wadeson HS, Carpenter WT, Levy ST (1977) Art and recovery style from psychosis. J Nerv Ment Dis 164:182–190
Meyer-Osterkamp S, Cohen R (1973) Zur Größenkonstanz bei Schizophrenen. Eine experimental-psychologische Untersuchung. Springer, Berlin Heidelberg New York
Minkowski E (1971) Die Gelebte Zeit. I. Über den zeitlichen Aspekt des Lebens. (Translation.) Müller, Salzburg
Minkowski E (1972) Die Gelebte Zeit. II. Über den zeitlichen Aspekt psychopathologischer Phänomene. (Translation.) Müller, Salzburg
Mundt Ch (1985) Das Apathiesyndrom der Schizophrenen. Eine psychopathologische und computertomographische Untersuchung. Springer, Berlin Heidelberg New York
Peters UH (1973) Wortfeldstörung und Satzfeldstörung. Arch Psychiatr Nervenkr 217:1–10
Peters UH (1982) Hölderlin. Wider die These vom edlen Simulanten. Rowohlt, Reinbek
Piaget J (1975) Der Aufbau der Wirklichkeit beim Kinde. Klett, Stuttgart
Rapaport D (1967) The theory of attention cathexis. An economic and structural attempt at the explanation of cognitive processes. The collected papers of D. Rapaport. Basic , New York
Reiss D (1968) Invidual thinking and family interaction. III. An experimental study of categorization performance in schizophrenics. J Nerv Ment Dis 146:384–403
Rennert H (1963) Eigengesetze des bildnerischen Ausdrucks bei Schizophrenie. Psychiatr Neurol Med Psychol 15:282–288
Sauer H, Richter P, Sass H (1989) Zur prämorbiden Persönlichkeit von Patienten mit schizoaffektiven Psychosen. In: Marneros A (ed) Schizoaffektive Psychosen. Springer, Berlin Heidelberg New York, pp 109–118
Scharfetter C (1986) Schizophrene Menschen. Bewußtseinsbereiche und Psychopathologie, Ich-Psychopathologie des schizophrenen Syndroms, Forschungsansätze und Deutungen, Therapiegrundsätze, 2nd edn. Urban and Schwarzenberg, Munich
Schindler R (1960) Das psychodynamische Problem beim sogenannten schizophrenen Defekt. In: Benedetti G, Müller C (eds) 2. Internationales Symposium über die Psychotherapie der Schizophrenen. Karger, Basle
Schubart C, Schwarz R, Krumm B, Biehl H (1986) Schizophrenie und soziale Anpassung. Springer, Berlin Heidelberg New York
Searle JR (1983) Intentionality. An essay in the philosophy of mind. Cambridge University Press, Cambridge
Taylor WL (1953) Cloze procedure: a new tool for measuring readability. Journalism Q 30:415–433
Villenave-Cremer S, Kettner M, Krause R (1989) Verbale Interaktion von Schizophrenen und ihren Gesprächspartnern. Z Klin Psychol Psychopathol Psychother 37:401–420
von Weizsäcker V (1940) Der Gestaltkreis. Theorie der Einheit von Wahrnehmen und Bewegen. Thieme, Leipzig
Wing JK (1987) Rehabilitation, Soziotherapie und Prävention. In: Kisker KP, Lauter H, Meyer J-E, Müller C, Strömgren E (eds) Schizophrenien. Springer, Berlin Heidelberg New York (Psychiatrie der Gegenwart, vol 4)

Negative Symptoms in Schizophrenia: Relationship to Positive Symptoms and Outcome *

J. A. LIEBERMAN [1], D. JODY [1], J. M. J. ALVIR [1], M. BORENSTEIN [1], D. I. MAYERHOFF [1], S. GEISLER [1], S. SZYMANSKI [1], A. GONZALES [1], B. BOGERTS [2], and M. ASHTARI [1]

The diagnostic criteria for schizophrenia have historically been based predominantly on the so-called positive symptoms, i.e., delusions, hallucinations, thought disorganization. This is not to say that the significance of negative symptom psychopathology, i.e., deficits of affect, drive, interest, speech, and thought, has been minimized, but rather less well characterized and understood. Reported differences between positive and negative symptoms in their pharmacologic response (Csernansky et al. 1986; Huber et al. 1980; Johnstone et al. 1983; Kay and Opler 1987) and pathobiologic correlates have been interpreted as evidence that these symptom clusters reflect different pathophysiologic processes or substrates (Andreasen 1982; Andreasen and Olsen 1982; Andreasen et al. 1982; Crow 1980a, b). In addition, follow-up studies indicating that negative symptoms are associated with a more chronic course of illness and poorer outcomes have been taken as evidence that negative symptom psychopathology may reflect a specific subtype of schizophrenia (Carpenter et al. 1988; Crow 1985; Kay et al. 1986; Pogue-Geile and Harrow 1984).

We have attempted to examine these issues utilizing the concept of primary and secondary negative symptoms as described by Carpenter (Carpenter et al. 1985) and to test certain hypotheses in a prospective longitudinal study of patients ascertained to be in their first episode of schizophrenia without prior exposure to neuroleptic medication. The methods and results of this study have previously been reported (Lieberman et al. 1989, Lieberman et al. 1991a, b). Our hypotheses were as follows:

1. Primary negative symptoms are difficult to characterize during the acute phase of the illness and in the presence of positive symptoms.
2. Primary negative symptoms are associated with a poor treatment response and outcome in patients.
3. Primary negative symptoms reflect a different pathophysiologic substrate than positive symptoms.

---

* This study was supported by NIMH grant (MH 41646) and a Research Scientist Development Award (MH 00537) to Dr. Lieberman and the Mental Health Clinical Research Center for the Study of Schizophrenia (MH 41960); MRI studies were performed in association with The Brain Morphometry and Image Analysis Center supported by a grant from the Helen and Irving Schneider Family.

[1] Hillside Hospital, Division of Long Island Jewish Medical Center, Albert Einstein College of Medicine, 75-59 263 St., Glen Oaks, NY 11004, USA

[2] Psychiatrische Klinik, Universität Düsseldorf, Bergische Landstraße 2, W-4000 Düsseldorf, FRG

A. Marneros / N. C. Andreasen / M. T. Tsuang (Eds.)
Negative Versus Positive Schizophrenia

Methods

Subject Ascertainment and Evaluation

All patients admitted to the inpatient service of Hillside Hospital were screened for the study. Eligible patients met the following criteria: no prior psychotic episodes; a diagnosis of definite or probable schizophrenia, or schizoaffective disorder, mainly schizophrenia, according to the Research Diagnostic Criteria (RDC) and based upon a structured interview (Schedule for Affective Disorders and Schizophrenia, SADS) and supplemental data from family members (Spitzer and Endicott 1977; Spitzer et al. 1978); less than 12 weeks of prior neuroleptic treatment received in their lifetimes; between the ages of 16 and 40; and no history of neuromedical illness that could influence the diagnosis or the biologic variables to be assessed in the study (e.g., endocrinopathy, hydrocephalus, seizure disorder). The purpose and procedures of the study were explained to eligible patients and their families, and informed consent was obtained.

Patients who had received neuroleptic treatment immediately prior to hospital admission were maintained drug free for at least 14 days. Prior to the initiation of neuroleptic treatment, baseline evaluations were conducted using the following assessments: the SADS Change and Psychosis and Disorganization Scale (SADS C + PD, Spitzer and Endicott 1978), the Scales for the Assessment of Negative Symptoms (SANS; Andreasen 1983), the Clinical Global Impression scale (CGI; Guy 1976), the Simpson Angus Neurologic Rating Scale (SANRS; Simpson and Angus 1970), and the Simpson Dyskinesia Scale (Simpson et al. 1979). Patients had challenge procedures with methylphenidate (METHYL) and apomorphine (APO) and underwent magnetic resonance imaging (MRI) of the brain (Lieberman et al. 1989). Patients underwent repeat METHYL and APO tests later in the study, 16 weeks after they had achieved symptom remission.

Acute Treatment

Following these baseline procedures, patients were treated openly in accordance with a standardized algorithm. They initially received 20 mg/day po fluphenazine HCl for 6 weeks. Antiparkinsonian medication was not administered prophylactically so that the incidence of acute extrapyramidal side effects (EPS) could be determined. If acute EPS developed, patients were given 2–6 mg/day benztropine. For akathisia, lorazepam was used and, if ineffective, followed by propranolol.

During the acute treatment phase, patients were evaluated for behavioral response and side effects biweekly with the SADS C + PD, SANS, CGI, and SANRS. If patients showed continuing improvement or achieved remission, they remained on the above-described regimen. Significant improvement was defined as a decrease in psychopathology to where three of the four positive psychotic symptom items (severity of delusions, severity of hallucinations, impaired understandability, bizarre behavior) were rated 3 (mild) or less, and a

CGI rating of much improved or very much improved was obtained. If unimproved after 6 weeks, the dose of fluphenazine was doubled to 40 mg/day po for an additional 4 weeks. If still unimproved, patients were switched to haloperidol 20 mg/day for 6 weeks at which point, if they still were unresponsive, the haloperidol doese was increased to 40 mg/day po for 4 weeks. If still unresponsive, a third neuroleptic from a different biochemical class, molindone at a dosage of up to 300 mg/day, was tried for 6 weeks. Treatment-esistant patients could then be considered for clozapine treatment.

Definition of Remission

Since this was a study of first-episode patients, most of whom would be expected to enjoy full recovery, we adopted a conservative definition of remission. Patients were considered to have remitted when they had no rating greater than 3 on any of the SADS C + PD positive psychotic symptom items (suspiciousness, severity of delusions, severity of hallucinations, impaired understandability, bizarre behavior), a CGI severity rating of 3 (mild) or less, and a CGI improvement item rating of 2 (much improved) or 1 (very much improved). This level of improvement was required to persist for 8 weeks (4 consecutive biweekly ratings). Barring relapse, patients then entered the stabilization and maintenance phases of this study (not described in this paper) and were followed up for up to 3 years.

Statistical Methods

Univariate comparisons were performed using χ^2 analyses with the Yates Correction. Survival analysis (Cox 1970, 1972) was used to estimate time-to-treatment outcome in the patient sample as well as to test for differential time to remission and outcome between subgroups of patients. Survival analysis is particularly useful for the treatment-outcome data because some patients still had not stabilized as of the data cut-off date, either due to their recent entry into the study or the long duration of their acute treatment.

Results

Of 268 patients screened over a 36-month period, 154 were eligible for the study. Reasons for ineligibility included inappropriate diagnosis (78%), medical contraindications (2%), and early discharges against medical advice prior to completion of study evaluation (11%). Seventy-two (47%) of the eligible patients consented to enter the study. Eighty-two eligible patients (53%) did not enter the study for the following reasons: involuntary admission status (49%)), refusal (35%), and miscellaneous clinical/administrative reasons (16%), e.g., residence outside geographic area or history of violence. These was no demographic difference between eligible patients who entered the study and those who did not.

Table 1. Baseline psychopathology ratings of first-episode schizophrenic patients, prior to treatment ($n = 56$)

	Variable mean (SD)
Psychotic symptoms at baseline[a]	
Severity of delusions	5.0 (1.0)
Severity of hallucinations	3.7 (1.9)
Impaired understandability	2.7 (1.4)
Derailment	2.7 (1.6)
Illogical thinking	2.2 (1.6)
Bizarre behavior	2.5 (1.8)
Negative symptoms at baseline[b]	
Affective flattening	2.3 (1.2)
Alogia	2.6 (1.1)
Avoliton-apathy	3.0 (1.1)
Anhedonia-asociality	3.5 (1.1)
Attention	2.3 (1.3)
CGI[c]	5.2 (1.4)
GAS rating at baseline[d]	26.2 (10.2)

[a] Positive symptom items are from the SADS C + PD which uses a 6 point severity scale (1 = none, 6 = very severe).
[b] Negative symptoms are from the SANS which uses a 5-point severity scale (0 = none, 5 = severe).
[c] The Clinical Global Impression (CGI) scale reflects overall severity of illness on a 7-point scale (1 = normal, 7 = among the most severely ill).
[d] The Global Assessment Scale (GAS) reflects overall illness and level of function on a 0–100 scale, with 90–100 being normal and 0–10 indicating extreme incapacity requiring constant supervision.

Five patients who entered the study were subsequently withdrawn for diagnostic reasons. Not included in the analyses were 11 patients since they had been in the study less than 12 weeks. Analyses were performed on data from 56 patients. The sample had a mean age of 23.9 years (SD, 5.7) and 63% were male. The sample was 50% white, 29% black, 14% Hispanic, and 7% Asian. Patients had been ill with psychotic symptoms for a mean of 53 weeks (SD, 53), and a median of 39 weeks.

Of the sample, 72% met RDC for schizophrenia (32% paranoid, 38% undifferentiated, 2% disorganized subtypes) and 28% met diagnostic criteria for mainly schizophrenic schizoaffective disorder (7% manic, 21% depressed subtypes). Psychopathology of patients at study entry is shown in Table 1. Patients were severely ill, mean CGI 5.2 (SD 1.4) with substantial positive and negative symptoms. The Global Assessment Scale Score (GAS) is a scale 0–100 in which 100 is normal and that reflects overall symptom severity and functional impairment. The group's score was 26.2 (SD 10.2).

Acute Treatment Response

Eighty-four percent (47 of 56) of the patients recovered from their first episode of schizophrenia; seven patients (13%) were considered refractory after failing

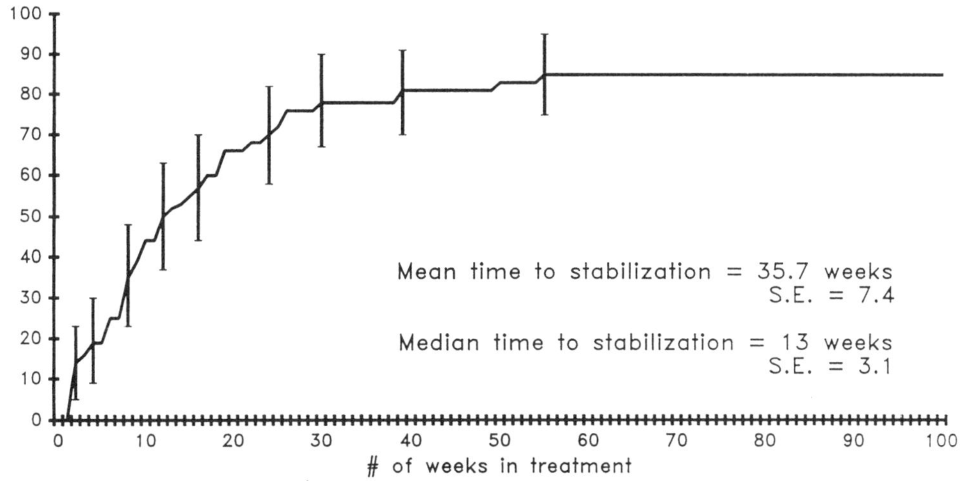

Fig. 1. Prospective study of psychobiology. Proportion (%) of patients stabilizing by week of treatment. The time course to remission for the sample is shown here. Forty-two patients (89%) responded to fluphenazine, one (2%) to haloperidol and four (9%) to molindone

to respond to the treatment protocol and ultimately were considered for clozapine; two additional patients were still undergoing acute treatment and had not yet responded. The time course to remission for the sample is shown in Fig. 1. The mean (SE) and median (SE) times to remission were 35.7 (7.4) weeks and 13 (3.1) weeks. Of the 47 patients who responded to treatment, 42 (89%) responded to fluphenazine (mean ±SD dose 20.2 ± 9.8 mg/day); 1 (2%) to haloperidol (20 mg/day); and 4 (9%) to molindone (225 ± 75 mg/day).

The effects of treatment on composite variables of positive symptom scores (delusions, hallucinations, impaired understandability, bizarre behavior) and negative ones (affective blunting, alogia, attention, anhedonia) are shown in Fig. 2. Positive symptom scores declined precipitously in the first 10 weeks of treatment, then more gradually through week 24 to a minimal severity level, while negative symptoms showed a modest gradual decline in severity levels over the first 12 weeks of treatment, and little change beyond that. To examine the relationship of positive and negative symptoms to the time course of treatment response, patients were classified into early (met remission criteria in 10 weeks or less), intermediate (remission in 11–20 weeks), and slow responders (remission after 20 weeks of treatment or failed to remit). Since remission was largely defined on the basis of positive symptoms, it is not surprising that the curves of the three groups fall in parallel, with the slope of the early responders being the steepest, and the slow and nonresponders, the most gradual (Fig. 3).

When negative symptoms were examined for the three treatment response groups, two things were apparent. First, the slow-responder group had higher negative symptom levels at baseline. And secondly, the curves for the early and intermediate groups declined in tandem to a mild level of severity over 24

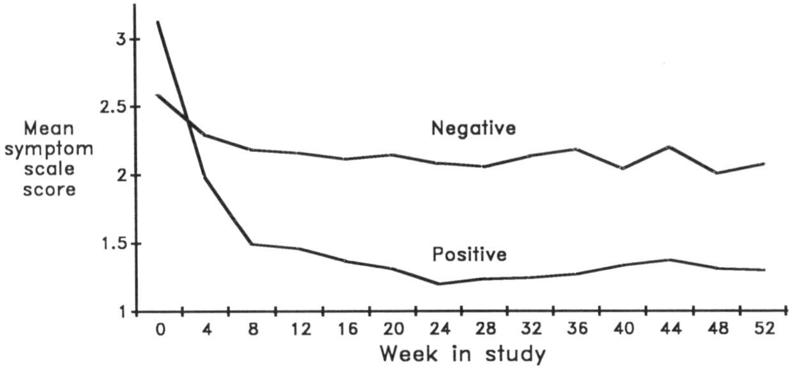

Fig. 2. Positive and negative symptom scores by week of treatment. Positive symptom scores declined precipitously in the first 10 weeks of treatment, then more gradually through week 24, while negative symptom scores showed a modest gradual decline in severity levels over the first 12 weeks of treatment and little change beyond that

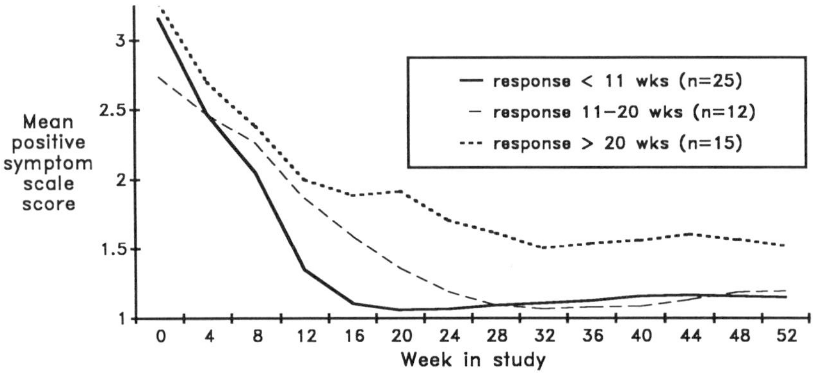

Fig. 3. Positive symptom scores by week and response to treatment. Remission is largely defined by positive symptom scores decreasing. Here the curves of the three groups are shown by week and response to treatment. The slope of the early responders is by definition the steepest, demonstrating the fastest response time

weeks, while the poor responders' negative symptoms declined minimally, remaining at a moderate level of severity over 52 weeks of treatment (Fig. 4).

Positive and negative symptoms were significantly correlated at baseline ($r = 0.58, p = 0.000$) and during acute treatment ($r = 0.55, p = 0.000$), but were not correlated following remission ($r = -0.17, p = 0.3$).

Behavioral Response to Methylphenidate

Thirty-seven patients underwent METHYL tests at baseline. METHYL produced a general worsening of psychopathology in the patients, reflected by increases in positive and negative symptoms and global severity ratings

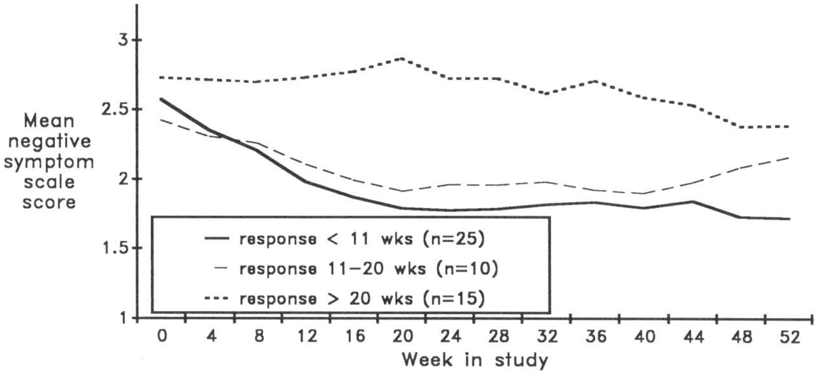

Fig. 4. Negative symptom scores by week and response to treatment. The slow-responder group had higher negative symptom levels at baseline. The curves for the early and intermediate groups declined in tandem to a mild level of severity over 24 weeks. The poor responders' negative symptoms declined minimally over 52 weeks of treatment

(Fig. 5). Of the five positive symptoms, only the increases in the delusions and hallucination items did not reach statistical significance, perhaps reflecting the fact that assessment of these symptoms depends largely on subjective report, whereas impaired understandability, bizarre behavior, and suspiciousness can be rated observationally. Acutely ill patients who became even more symptomatic after METHYL administration often could not respond to questions about their mental experiences.

Negative symptoms evaluated with the SANS global items were also significantly increased by METHYL administration; alogia and attention showed the most robust changes. Positive symptom change (severity of delusions, hallucinations, suspiciousness, bizarre behavior, impaired understandability) and negative symptom change (alogia, affective flattening, attention) were significantly correlated ($r = 0.68$, $p = 0.01$).

Patients were classified as to whether their symptoms were significantly activated by METHYL. Symptom activation was defined as an increase of four or more points over their preinfusion SADS C + PD score on the sum of the four psychotic symptom items and a CGI (global change) rating of 6 (much worse) or 7 (very much worse). Twenty-three patients (61%) were classified as demonstrating METHYL-activated symptoms. Fifteen patients (39%) showed little or no change, and no patients showed diminished psychotic symptoms.

Of the 38 patients, 13 underwent repeat METHYL tests approximately 16 weeks after their remissions, i.e., at a point when they had little or no positive symptoms. Six patients (46%) exhibited mild or moderate symptom activation with METHYL. Seven patients had no provocation of positive symptoms. As was seen in the behavioral response to METHYL at baseline, both positive and negative symptoms were increased in METHYL tests after remission albeit in lesser magnitude. For the whole group, only change in the impaired under-

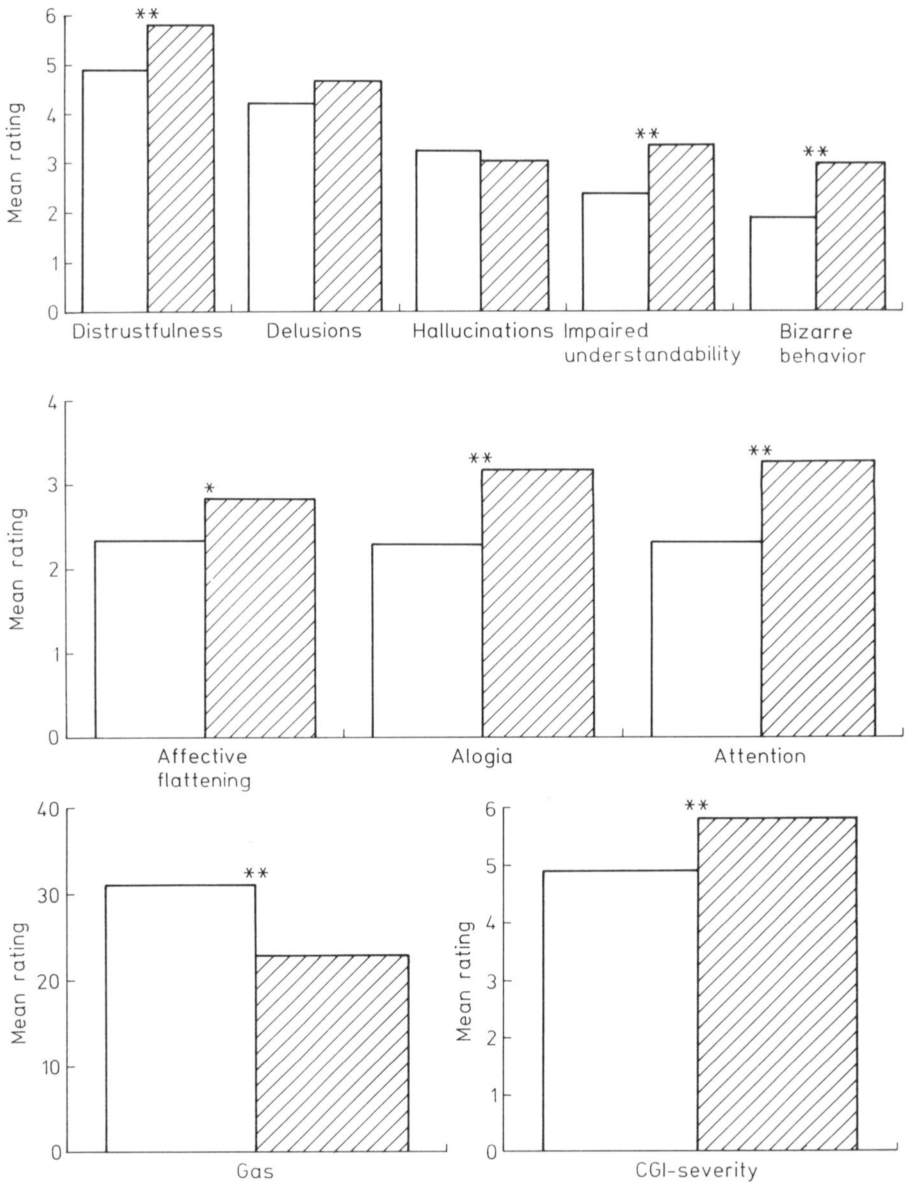

Fig. 5. Behavioral response to methylphenidate at baselin. Behavioral response to METHYL is displayed in three graphs. The *top graph* depicts positive symptom items of the SADS C + PD. Four of the five items increase in severity, three significantly. Ratings of hallucinations, which show no change, and of delusions, which increase nonsignificantly, are based on subjective reports of patients. Consequently, these items may have reduced sensitivity in acutely psychotic patients who are not fully cooperative. The *middle graph* depicts negative symptom items of the SANS. The increase in negative symptoms was significantly correlated with positive symptoms change ($r = 0.68$, $p = 0.01$) leading us to conclude that this effect consisted predominantly of secondary negative symptoms. The *bottom graph* depicts two global measures of severity (Clinical Global Impression Scale, CGI, and Global Assessment Scale, GAS) both of which showed significant worsening after METHYL. Note that for GAS, the lower the score the greater the severity, whereas for CGI, the higher score is worse (*$p = 0.05$; **$p = 0.01$)

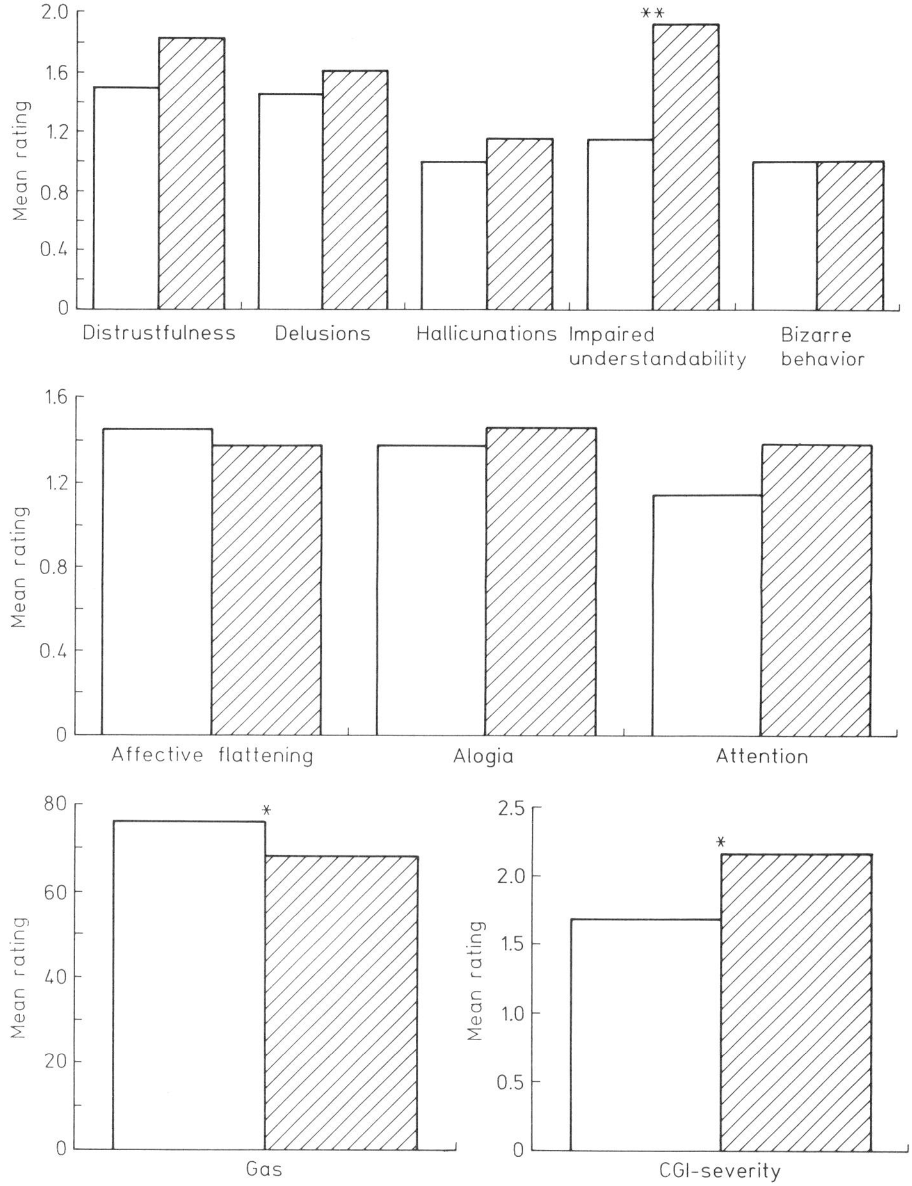

Fig. 6. Repeat METHYL tests, administered 16 weeks after remission. Behavioral response to repeat METHYL challenge is displayed in three graphs ($n = 13$). Six patients (46%) exhibited mild or moderate symptom activation with METHYL. Seven patients showed no provocation of positive symptoms. Both positive and negative symptoms were increased in METHYL tests after remission, but with less magnitude than at baseline challenge. Only change in the impaired understandability item reached statistical significance ($^{**}p < 0.05$). Positive and negative symptom change was again significantly correlated ($r = 0.62$, $p = 0.02$, $^{*}p < 0.10$)

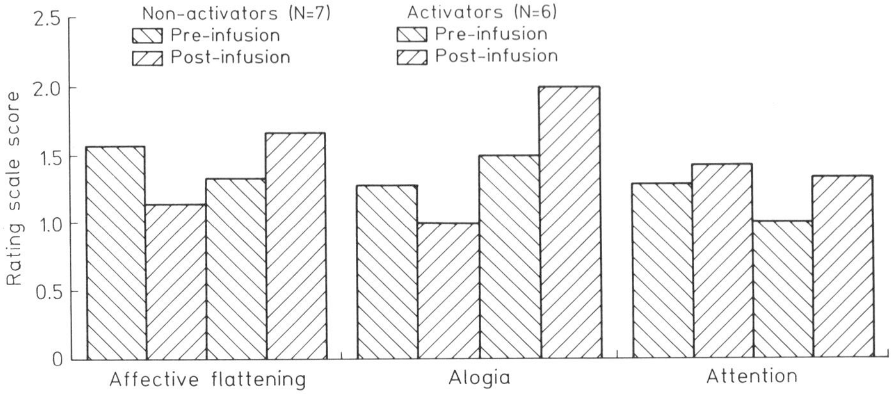

Fig. 7. Prospective study of psychobiology. Negative symptom item change in response to methylphenidate infusion during stabilization phase for patients classified as positive symptom activators and nonactivators. Activators showed corresponding increases in negative symptoms while nonactivators showed decreases or no change in negative symptoms

standability item reached statistical significance (Fig. 6). Positive and negative symptom change was again significantly correlated ($r = 0.62$, $p = 0.02$). To determine the effect of METHYL on primary negative symptoms, we separated patients into those with positive symptom activation and nonactivation and examined negative symptom response (Fig. 7). Patients with positive symptom activation had concurrent increases in negative symptoms, while patients with no positive symptom activation had a decrease in negative symptoms. This differential response in psychopathology for psychotic symptom activators and nonactivators was significant or nearly significant for an infusion by group interaction for two of the three negative symptom items assessed (Fig. 7; affective flattening, $f = 1.8$, $p = 0.19$; alogia, $f = 3.8$, $p = 0.06$; attention, $f = 4.8$, $p = 0.03$).

Negative Symptoms and Treatment Outcome

We evaluated the patient's symptom ratings at two time points, baseline pretreatment and at 20 weeks, as predictors of treatment outcome. Using the composite of positive and negative symptoms and individual symptom items of the SADS C + PD and SANS as the independent variables, the patients' time course to remission was projected using a Cox proportional hazards model. In this way, neither positive and negative symptoms nor global severity at baseline significantly predicted treatment response. Since remission was defined largely on the basis of positive symptoms, it is to be expected (and of little value) that positive symptom severity at 20 weeks would be correlated with time to remission. However, when specific negative symptoms (affective flattening, alogia) were analyzed in this way, we found that higher negative symptom levels at 20 weeks were associated with longer time to remission. Still, it could

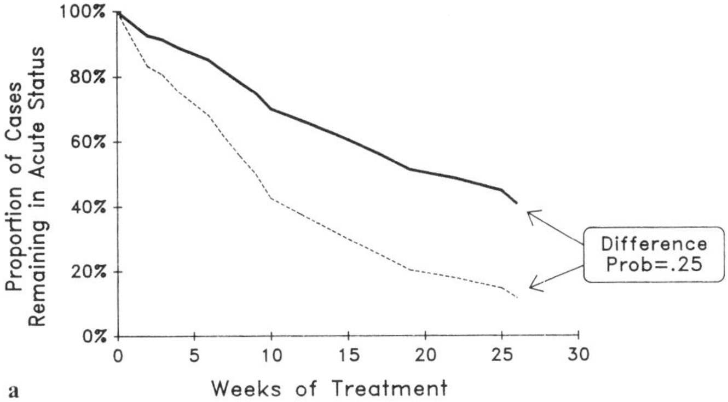

a

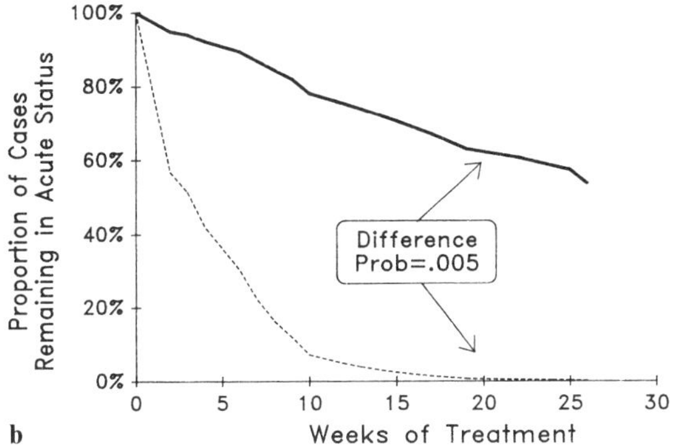

b

Fig. 8 a, b. Flat affect as a predictor of remission. **a** At baseline with positive symptoms covaried (=2). The relationship between affective flattening at baseline and the probability of remission within a given time interval when positive symptoms at baseline are covaried. *Continuous line* indicates rating 5, *dashed line* indicates rating 1. **b** After treatment with positive symptoms covaried (=1). The relationship between affective flattening at 20 weeks and the probability of remission when positive symptoms at 20 weeks are covaried (see text). *Continuous line* indicates rating 4, *dashed line* indicates rating 1

be argued that negative symptoms remained high in patients who took longer to remit due to their persisting positive symptoms. In an effort to disentangle the two symptom constellations, we repeated the analysis of time to remission by measuring negative symptom levels at 20 weeks controlling for the (change in) positive symptom severity at 20 weeks. Affective flattening and alogia remained significant predictors of time to remission ($p < 0.05$, Fig. 8, 9). Figure 8 a shows the relationship between affective flattening at baseline and the probability of remission within a given time interval. The relationship was computed by means of the Cox proportional hazards model, and positive symptoms at baseline were covaried. In this manner, a patient's level of affective flattening could be seen in the context of his positive symptoms; it is the disparity between the negative symptoms that are observed and those that

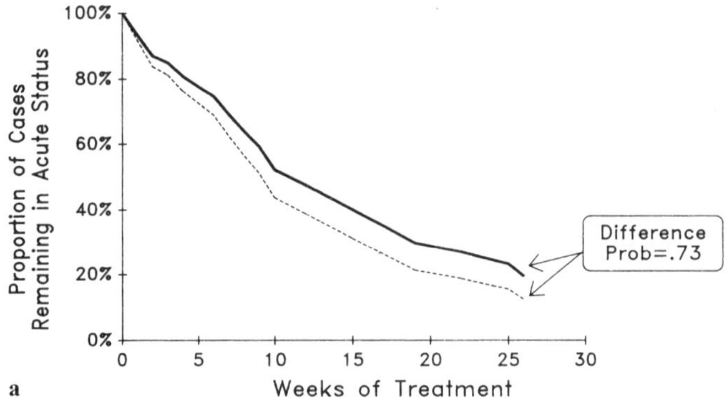

a

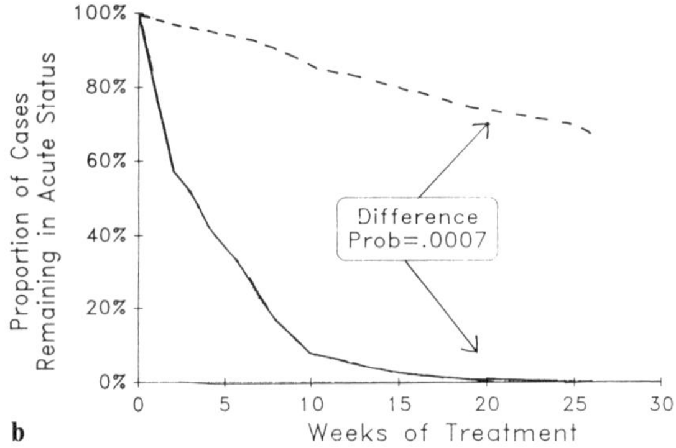

b

Fig. 9 a, b. Alogia as a predictor of remission. **a** At baseline with positive symptoms covaried (=2). The relationship between alogia at baseline and the probability of remission within a given time interval when positive symptoms at baseline are covaried. *Continuous line* indicates rating 5, *dashed line* indicates rating 1. **b** After treatment with positive symptoms covaried (=1). The relationship between alogia at 20 weeks and the probability of remission when positive symptoms at 20 weeks are covaried (see text). *Continuous line* indicates rating 5, *dashed line* indicates rating 1

would be commensurate with the positive symptoms that serves as the predictor variable. For illustrative purposes only, this graph shows the projected remission rate for patients with a positive level of two and affective flattening of one or five. The actual computations and the test of significance are, however, based on the full sample. The p value of 0.25 indicates that there is no evidence that negative symptoms at baseline, with positive symptoms covaried, may be used to predict time to remission.

Figure 8 b shows the relationship between affective flattening at 20 weeks and the probability of remission, when positive symptoms at 20 weeks are covaried. Again, by covarying the positive symptoms we are focusing on the disparity between the affective flattening that is observed and that which would have been commensurate with the positive symptoms. For example, a moderate level of affective flattening could be of little consequence in a patient

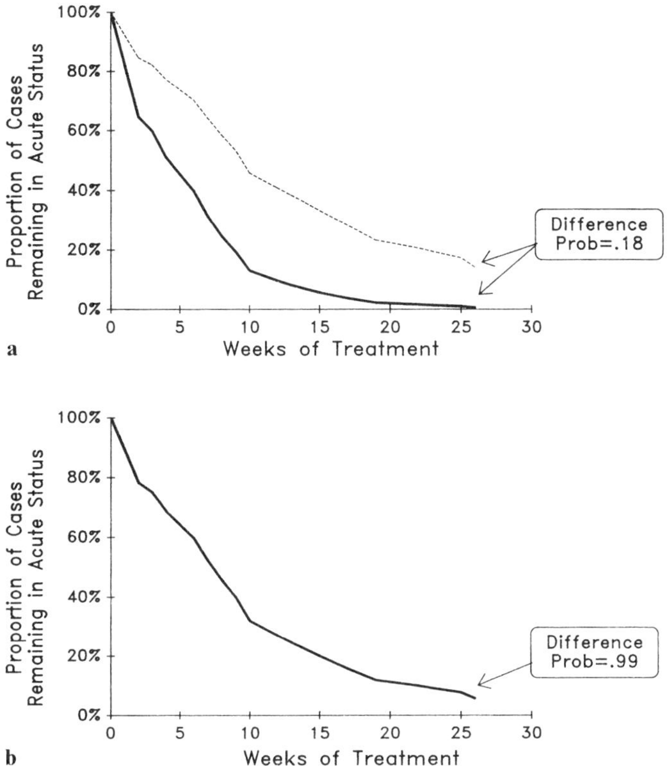

Fig. 10a, b. Attention deficit as a predictor of remission. **a** At baseline with positive symptoms covaried (= 2). The relationship between attention deficit at baseline and the probability of remission within a given time interval when positive symptoms at baseline are covaried. *Continuous line* indicates rating 5, *dashed line* indicates rating 1. **b** After treatment with positive symptoms covaried (= 1). The relationship between attention deficit at 20 weeks and the probability of remission when positive symptoms at 20 weeks are covaried (see text). *Continuous line* indicates rating 3, *dashed line* indicates rating 1

with a high level of positive symptoms, but indicative of special problems in a patient with no residual positive symptoms. The *p* value of 0.005 indicates that with positive symptoms covaried, higher levels of affective flattening are associated with a lower probability of remission within any given time interval.

The same concept can be demonstrated with the negative symptom alogia, as shown in Fig. 9a, b. Attentional impairment on the other hand (a negative symptom that is most likely to be influenced by the level of positive symptoms), was not correlated with time to remission (Figs. 10a, b).

Brain Morphology, Negative Symptoms and Treatment Outcome

In a preliminary analysis, we examined the relationship of brain morphology to negative symptoms and treatment outcome. Patients who had undergone MRI

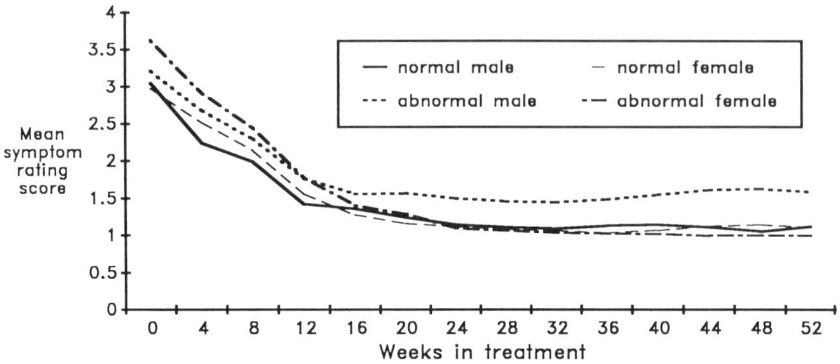

Fig. 11. Positive symptoms (SADS C + PC psychotic items) in male and female schizophrenics as a function of brain morphology and weeks in treatment. Positive symptom severity is slightly higher for abnormal male and female patients at baseline, but then declines in parallel with the positive symptom curves of the normal patient groups. The abnormal male patients exhibit slightly higher positive symptom levels throughout the follow-up period

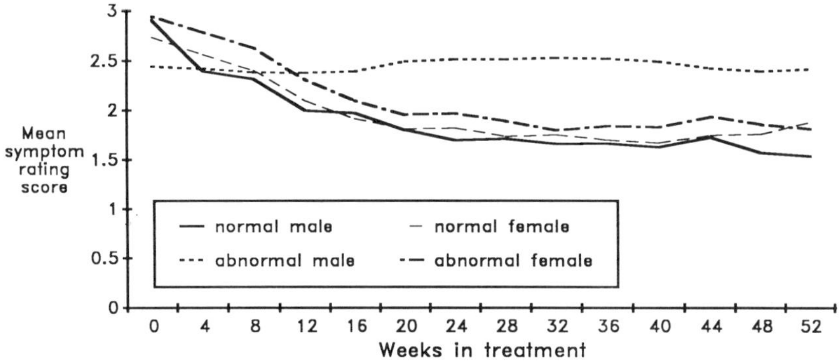

Fig. 12. Negative symptoms (mean of SANS globals) in male and female schizophrenics as a function of brain morphology and weeks in treatment. The severity levels of negative symptoms decline with treatment for the normal patients and the abnormal female patients, but remain the highest and unchanged for the abnormal male patients

of the brain were classified as having normal or abnormal brain morphology by visual qualitative inspection of MR scans under blind conditions (methods described in Lieberman et al. 1991a). Since brain pathomorphology has been found to be preferentially associated with male gender (Degreef et al. 1991; Andreasen et al. 1990; Bogerts et al. 1990), we plotted the time course of positive and negative symptom response to treatment by brain morphology status for male and female patients (Figs. 11, 12). As seen in Fig. 11, positive symptom severity is slightly higher for abnormal male and female patients at baseline, but then declines in parallel with the positive symptom curves of the normal patient groups. The abnormal male patients exhibit slightly higher positive symptom levels throughout the follow-up period. On the other hand, the severity levels of negative symptoms decline with treatment for the normal patients and the abnormal female patients, but remain the highest and unchanged for the abnormal male patients (Fig. 12). Thus, it appears that this group is accounting for most of the association between negative symptoms and slow or poor treatment response.

Discussion

It is apparent from these results that positive and negative symptoms are highly correlated during the acute phase of schizophrenia and periods of symptom exacerbation. At these times, when positive symptom levels are high, it is difficult (and may be impossible) to identify primary negative symptoms accurately, and, therefore, it may be necessary to assess negative symptoms following positive symptom remission or during the residual phase of the illness.

Primary negative symptoms appear to have prognostic importance as they are associated with a slower and possibly poorer treatment response in patients. This is not merely to say that negative symptoms are less responsive to neuroleptic treatment, but that patients in whom they occur have a poorer response in terms of their positive symptoms. The interaction between positive and negative symptoms and their different pharmacology is demonstrated by the patient responses to METHYL after remission. In the absence of positive symptom activation, negative symptoms actually declined with METHYL. This effect has been previously reported with psychostimulants (Angrist et al. 1980, 1982; Lieberman et al. 1985) and has been interpreted as negative or deficit symptomatology reflecting a condition of reduced dopaminergic activity.

The implication of these results is that primary negative symptoms are mediated through a different neurochemical process than are positive symptoms, and the process of the latter is likely located in a different anatomic region. The MRI data are interesting in this regard in that they indicate a direct relationship between enduring negative symptoms (which were also associated with poor treatment response) and abnormal brain morphology. The fact that this predominated in the male patients is consistent with prior reports and the long-observed sex differences in course of illness, treatment response, and outcome in schizophrenia (Lewine 1981; McGlashan and Bardenstein 1990; Seeman 1986).

Acknowledgements. The authors are grateful to Mrs. Sabina Meyer, Camille Valentino, Gwen Wellington and Greta Schimmel who assisted in data collection; the Lowenstein III staff who provided inpatient care to study subjects and Mrs. Maureen Ward for manuscript preparation.

References

Andreasen NC (1982) Negative symptoms in schizophrenia: definition and reliability. Arch Gen Psychiatry 39:784–788

Andreasen NC (1983) The scale for the assessment of negative symptoms (SANS). University of Iowa, Iowa City

Andreasen NC, Olsen S (1982) Negative vs positive schizophrenia: definition and validation. Arch Gen Psychiatry 39:789–794

Andreasen NC, Olsen SA, Deenert JW, Smith MR (1982) Ventricular enlargement in schizophrenia: relationship to positive and negative symptoms. Am J Psychiatry 139:297–302

Andreasen NC, Flaum M, Swayze VW II, Tyrrel G, Arndt S (1990) Positive and negative symptoms in schizophrenia. A critical reappraisal. Arch Gen Psychiatry 47:615–621

Angrist B, Rotrosen J, Gershon S (1980) Differential effects of amphetamine and neuroleptics on positive vs negative symptoms in schizophrenia. Psychopharmacology (Berlin) 72:17–19

Angrist B, Peselow E, Rubinstein M et al. (1982) Partial improvement in negative schizophrenic symptoms after amphetamine. Psychopharmacology (Berlin) 78:128–130

Bogerts B, Ashtari M, Degreef G, Alvir JM, Bilder RM, Lieberman JA (1990) Reduced temporal limbic structure volumes on magnetic resonance images in first episode schizophrenia. Psychiatry Res 35:1–13

Carpenter WT Jr, Heinrichs DW, Alphs LD (1985) Treatment of negative symptoms. Schizophr Bull 11:440–452

Carpenter WT, Heinrichs DW, Wagman AMI (1988) Deficit and nondeficit forms of schizophrenia. The concept. Am J Psychiatry 145:578–583

Cox DR (1970) The analysis of binary data. Chapman and Hall, London

Cox DR (1972) Regression model and life tables. J R Stat Soc [B] 34:187–220

Crow TJ (1980a) Molecular pathology of schizophrenia: more than one disease process? Br Med J 280:66–68

Crow TJ (1980b) Positive and negative symptoms and the role of dopamine. Br J Psychiatry 137:383–386

Crow TJ (1985) The two-syndrome concept: origins and current status. Schizophr Bull 11:471–486

Csernansky JG, Brown K, Hollister LE (1986) Is there drug treatment for negative schizophrenic symptoms? Hosp Formul 21:790–792

Degreef G, Ashtari M, Bogerts B, Bilder RM, Jody DN, Alvir JM, Lieberman JA (1991) Temporal horn volumes measured from magnetic resonance images are correlated with symptoms of schizophrenia (in press)

Guy W (1976) Clinical global impression scale. In: EDCEU Assessment Manual. US Department of Health Education and Welfare, Washington DC, pp 281–222

Huber G, Gross G, Schüttler R, Linz M (1980) Longitudinal studies of schizophrenic patients. Schizophr Bull 6:592–605

Johnstone EC, Crow TJ, Ferrier IN et al. (1983) Adverse effects of anticholinergic medication on positive schizophrenic symptoms. Psychol Med 13:513–527

Kay SR, Opler LA (1987) The positive-negative dimension in schizophrenia: its validity and significance. Psychiatr Dev 2:79–103

Kay SR, Fiszbein A, Lindenmayer JP, Opler LA (1986) Positive and negative syndromes in schizophrenia as a function of chronicity. Acta Psychiatr Scand 74:507–518

Lewine RRJ (1981) Sex differences in schizophrenia: timing or subtypes? Psychol Bull 90:432–434

Lieberman JA, Kane JM, Gadaletta D, Ramos-Lorenz J, Bergmann K, Wegner J, Novacenko H (1985) Methylphenidate challenge tests and course of schizophrenia. Psychopharmacol Bull 21(1):123–129

Lieberman J, Jody D, Geisler S, Vital-Herne J, Alvir J, Walsleben J, Woerner M (1989) Treatment outcome of first-episode schizophrenia. Psychopharmacol Bull 25:92–96

Lieberman J, Jody D, Alvir J, Ashtari M, Levy D, Bogerts B, Degreef G, Cooper T, Novacenko H (1991a) Brain morphology, dopamine and eye movement function in first episode schizophrenia (in press)

Lieberman J, Jody D, Geisler S, Szymanski S, Alvir J, Woerner M, Borenstein M (1991b) Time course and biologic correlates of treatment response in first episode schizophrenia (in press)

McGlashan TH, Bardenstein KK (1990) Gender differences in affective, schizoaffective and schizophrenic disorders. Schizophr Bull 16(2):312–329

Pogue-Geile MF, Harrow M (1984) Negative and positive symptoms in schizophrenia and depression: a follow up. Schizophr Bull 10:371–387

Seeman MV (1986) Current outcome in schizophrenia: women vs men. Acta Psychiatr Scand 73(6):609–617

Simpson GM, Angus JWS (1970) A rating scale for extrapyramidal side effects. Acta Psychiatr Scand [Suppl] 212:11–19

Simpson GM, Lee JH, Zoubek B et al. (1979) A rating scale for tardive dyskinesia. Psychopharmacology 64:171–179

Spitzer RL, Endicott J (1977) Schedule for affective disorders and schizophrenia (SADS), 3rd edn. NY State Psychiatric Institute Biometrics Division, New York

Spitzer RL, Endicott J (1978) Schedule for affective disorders and schizophrenia – change version, 3rd edn. NY State Psychiatric Institute Biometrics Division, New York

Spitzer RL, Endicott JE, Robins E (1978) Research diagnostic criteria for a selected group of functional disorders, 3rd edn. NY State Psychiatric Institute Biometrics Research, New York

Negative Symptoms: A Critique of Current Approaches

W. T. CARPENTER, R. W. BUCHANAN, B. KIRKPATRICK, G. THAKER, and C. TAMMINGA [1]

Introduction

There has been considerable interest in the negative symptoms of schizophrenia. However, the conceptual and methodologic approaches employed in most investigations have undermined the power of study designs and severely limited advances in the field.

What are the problems that have hampered progress? First, there has been an uncritical acceptance of approaches which neglect the differential diagnosis of negative symptoms. The study of schizophrenic psychopathology (whether negative symptoms or other symptom manifestations) should be concerned with that which is primary to the disease process not that which is secondary to associated conditions, e.g., neuroleptic-induced akinesia or anhedonia induced by depression. Second, reliance on proxy measures of negative symptoms, such as social withdrawal for diminished social drive, undermines the study of the latter since patients with schizophrenia may be withdrawn for many reasons (e.g., suspiciousness, autistic preoccupation, demoralization, or low drive). Third, positive vs. negative schizophrenia is a false dichotomy for the study of etiology and pathophysiology since all current approaches to diagnosis require positive symptoms for the classification of schizophrenia.

These propositions were implicit in Kraepelin's work (1971) and made explicit in 1974 (Strauss et al. 1974). However, misapplications of psychopathologic concepts and methods continue and are described below. A solution and validating data are proposed.

Background

There is heuristic value in research on schizophrenia that focuses on discrete psychopathologic processes. Such an approach serves to counter problems created by studying illness classes defined by various combinations of symptoms without evidence that these varied symptom complexes are manifestations of the same pathological process (Strauss et al. 1974; Carpenter and

[1] Maryland Psychiatric Research Center, Department of Psychiatry, University of Maryland, Baltimore, MD 21228, USA

A. Marneros/N. C. Andreasen/M. T. Tsuang (Eds.)
Negative Versus Positive Schizophrenia

Buchanan 1989). There is a long history to this approach, dating back to Kraepelin (1971), who asserted that there were two processes underlying dementia praecox: avolition and dissociative processes. Other candidate psychopathological processes have been proposed, and our suggestions are described elsewhere (Carpenter and Buchanan 1989).

Considerable attention is now given to the rubric of positive and negative symptoms. Although there is disagreement on details, a general acceptance exists of the proposition that dissociative cognition, delusions, and hallucinations define a positive symptom domain, i.e., psychosis. Avolition, restricted affect, and low social drive define a negative symptom domain. Accepting this, key questions in *each* domain are: etiology, pathophysiology, neuroanatomy, and prevention. Secondary questions are: specific treatments, associated features, and animal models of each domain. However, attempts to answer these questions have been severely limited through the application of constructs which avoid central questions of psychopathology and fail to reduce confounding.

Less confusion surrounds the positive symptom domain than the negative one since all patients meeting criteria for schizophrenia manifest positive symptoms, and researchers are familiar with other potential causes of psychosis, and these are routinely considered in differential diagnosis. Investigators studying positive symptoms in schizophrenia exclude patients in whom the psychotic symptoms are likely to be due to psychotomimetic drugs, partial complex seizures, toxic psychoses, affective disorder, etc. Differential diagnosis, *although acknowledged not to be infallible*, is recognized as necessary and sufficiently reliable. Surprisingly, such is rarely the case with negative symptoms. For example, negative symptoms in a commonly used instrument, the Schedule for Assessment of Negative Symptoms (SANS), are assessed with explicit disregard of their etiology or primacy to schizophrenia other than the fact that the patient manifesting the negative symptom has schizophrenia (Andreasen 1982)!

Briefly stated, there are three main problems in the study of negative symptoms. First is the inclusion of secondary negative symptoms when the aims of the study relate only to primary ones. Second is the definition of a negative symptom subtype by the presence or absence of criteria other than negative symptoms. In the most commonly used approaches, categorization of a patient relative to a putative negative symptom subtype is influenced by the presence or absence of positive symptoms. Third, in many studies, differences in a validating variable between the negative symptom subtype and a comparative cohort cannot be traced directly to the negative symptoms, as such comparison groups may systematically differ in age of onset, duration of illness, drug responsiveness, severity of psychosis, or other associated features. In such a situation, for example, an observation of enlarged ventricles in a putative negative symptom subtype may be attributable to any of several uncontrolled variables.

The positive vs. negative construct (Andreasen and Olsen 1982) and the associated SANS evaluation procedures illustrate the first two problems. In the

SANS procedure, the negative symptoms are not intended to represent core schizophrenic psychopathology but are rated as generic symptoms. This approach is appropriate for questions concerning the multiple causes of negative symptoms in patients with schizophrenia, but this is rarely a study aim. It is a weak approach when the questions relate to schizophrenia per se. It has long been clear that there are multiple causes of such symptoms (Carpenter et al. 1985), and Mayer et al. (1985) have recently demonstrated the same using SANS methodology. However, when determining whether or not some dependent variable is related to Kraepelin's avolitional syndrome, the investigator is not concerned with apathy and social withdrawal in response to psychosis, anhedonia secondary to depression or demoralization, or the restricted expression of affect secondary to neuroleptic drugs.

The second problem is illustrated by the positive vs. negative schizophrenia construct (Andreasen and Olsen 1982). Andreasen proposed this approach based on a single factor analysis in which positive symptoms and negative symptoms loaded on the same factor, but with opposite polarity. However, clinical observation reveals that these symptoms can concur without a tendency for one set to worsen when the other set improves. Moreover, Barnes and Liddle (1990) note that nine studies using factor analyses and correlational approaches support this independent dimension view, as does Andreasen's (this volume) second study. Second, if positive and negative symptoms are manifestations of the same pathologic process, it is difficult to imagine how a single dimension could be used as a decisive dichotomizing variable in examining dependent trait variables such as brain structure, especially considering how each patient's symptoms frequently shift depending on the exacerbation and remittance of psychosis. Third, the classification of a group of patients positive, mixed, or negative subtypes will tend to shift, over time, from more positive and mixed subtypes to more negative subtypes, with the shift in classification being based on decreasing positive symptoms rather than increasing negative symptoms. Finally, experience has shown that positive vs. negative subtyping most often results in the mixed type and is highly dependent on the severity of psychosis the patient exhibits on the day of assessment.

Even study of extreme groups (i.e., positive vs. negative, excluding mixed type) is not feasible since the proportion of patients in each is small, and patients change categories fequently. Between-group differences cannot be interpreted with precision, and between-group similarities may be misleading. For example, both groups may have impaired psychological test performance, but motivation may be the key causative factor in one group and cognitive disturbance the key factor in the other.

The third problem is illustrated by Crow's Type I/Type II construct (Crow 1985). Since multiple criteria can be used to define Type I and Type II schizophrenia, group differences cannot securely be attributed to any one defining attribute. The study hypothesis may deal with negative symptoms, but Type I and Type II differ in positive symptoms, duration of illness, neuroleptic responsiveness, brain structure, and IQ. Even though this approach uses the primary form of negative symptoms as defining criteria, Type I and Type II differences may relate to other factors. This division of the clinical syndrome into two disease entities is meritorious. The strategic question is whether the multiple defining criteria are sufficiently validated and coherent in each disease entity, or should present investigations focus on the negative symptom domain while controlling for other defining variables or treating them as dependent variables?

If the above considerations are correct, then reports testing the validity of negative symptom subtypes based on ascertainment with the Brief Psychiatric Rating Scale (BPRS) factor II, SANS, or other approaches not restricted to primary negative symptoms are problematic. Type II errors, i.e., not finding a difference between the groups when in fact a time difference exists, may be avoided as long as the negative subtype is skewed mainly toward the primary type. The nonnegative comparison group will have few false-positive cases. However, the negative symptom cohort would be expected to have many false-positives (due to secondary negative symptoms) in the first-episode cohort and fewer in chronic populations. Thus, differences between negative and nonnegative cohorts on a potential discriminating marker will vary according to sampling. This may obscure between-group differences in acute populations and weaken between-group differences in chronic populations. In any case, investigators need not leave to luck what can be resolved in design.

An Approach to Negative Symptoms

For resolution of the aforementioned problem, we recommend the following for the study of negative symptoms of schizophrenia:

1. Primary negative symptoms are likely to differ from primary positive symptoms in etiology, pathophysiology, neuroanatomy, treatment response, and course. Negative symptoms may define a different phenotype from that based on psychosis. Therefore, negative symptoms merit specific study.
2. The negative symptoms of greatest theoretical interest are the primary or core manifestations of some forms of schizophrenia. They should be distinguished from the many secondary sources of negative symptoms common in schizophrenia (Carpenter et al. 1985).
3. A differential diagnosis of cause requires a longitudinal perspective. Enduring trait forms of negative symptoms are easier to differentiate as primary than are transitory ones. Most study designs will be best served by differentiating primary, enduring negative, or deficit symptoms from secondary and/or transitory negative symptoms (Carpenter et al. 1988).
4. Until compelling evidence modifies Kraepelin's view, negative symptoms should be defined according to his description. For example, he does not place attention dysfunction and incongruity of affect in the avolitional domain. We propose the use of six negative symptoms (i.e., restricted affect, diminished emotional range, poverty of speech, curbing of interests, diminished sense of purpose, and diminished social drive) for the

purpose of defining a negative symptom subtype, the deficit syndrome of schizophrenia (Carpenter et al. 1988; Kirkpatrick et al. 1989).

5. The enduring presence of two or more of these six symptoms should be used to define the deficit symptom domain of psychopathology. This can be reliably accomplished with the Schedule for the Deficit Syndrome (Kirkpatrick et al. 1989). Researchers can no longer shy away from this crucial clinical judgment, any more than they avoid the other clinical judgments requiring primary vs. secondary distinctions that pervade contemporary diagnostic criteria, including the positive symptoms used to diagnose schizophrenia.
6. Contrast schizophrenia with the deficit syndrome to that without the deficit syndrome. Make strategic decisions based on study aim regarding the few ambiguous cases.
7. When deficit patients differ from nondeficit patients, control groups should be used to determine which group is deviant.
8. Control/match deficit and nondeficit patients on key confounding variables such as age, gender, race, duration of illness, severity of psychosis on the day of study, etc.
9. Examine the distribution of deficit symptoms in biologic relatives to test the construct as a putative phenotype. Parenthetically, the proposition that this domain does define a separate genetic entity is generally supported by data defining the schizophrenia spectrum.
10. Establish animal models specific to the deficit syndrome and distinct from models of psychosis (Kirkpatrick and Buchanan 1990b).
11. Ascertain whether neural circuits associated with deficit symptoms are different from those associated with psychotic symptoms.
12. Study the deficit syndrome in nonpsychotic, nonschizotypal populations, such as schizoid personality. Be aware that schizotypal personality has both positive and negative symptom defining criteria.

Workers at the Maryland Psychiatric Research Center have reported the following data pertaining to the reliability and validity of deficit symptoms as a method to subtype schizophrenic patients:

1. Individual deficit symptoms can be rated reliably, including differentiation from secondary negative symptoms and from an absence of negative symptoms (Kirkpatrick et al. 1989). In a group of chronic nondeficit and deficit schizophrenic patients, weighted kappas for the six negative symptoms used to define the deficit syndrome were all $\geqq 0.60$.
2. Deficit and nondeficit schizophrenic probands can be reliably classified (Kirkpatrick et al. 1989). Among a sample of chronic patients, deficit and nondeficit patients were categorized with 90% agreement (a kappa of 0.73), with all patients assigned to one of the two groups.
3. Longitudinal clinical and neuropsychological data support defining qualities of this approach (Carpenter et al. 1988; Wagman et al. 1987).
4. Social and physical anhedonia, as assessed by the Chapman Psychosis Proneness scales, distinguish deficit from nondeficit patients (Kirkpatrick

and Buchanan 1990a). The differences between the two groups were not due to depression, demographic, or medication variables. In contrast, there were no differences between the two groups on the Magical Ideation and Perceptual Aberration scales, suggesting that psychosis is orthogonally rather than inversely related to the deficit syndrome. BPRS psychosis factor scores also support this view and confirm that psychosis can be a matching variable in deficit/nondeficit comparisons (Carpenter et al. 1988; Wagman et al. 1987). In contrast, positive vs. negative (Andreasen and Olsen 1982) and Type I vs. Type II approaches (Crow 1985) predict that the negative symptom subtype has a lesser severity of positive symptoms.

5. Patients with deficit symptoms are characterized by poorer premorbid psychosocial adjustment, suggesting that asocial development is an early onset morbid feature in many deficit syndrome patients (Buchanan et al. 1990).
6. An increased impairment on neurological signs assessing sensory integration differentiates deficit from nondeficit patients. This finding is interpreted as indicating parietal lobe involvement in the deficit neural circuit (Buchanan et al. 1990). Deficit and nondeficit patients were similar for other neurologic signs which differentiate schizophrenic from control subjects. This suggests that sensory integration differences do not simply reflect severity of illness.
7. In oculomotor assessment data, an antisaccade paradigm differentiates deficit from nondeficit schizophrenic patients (Thaker et al. 1990). This paradigm requires the subjects to make a saccade in the direction opposite to the target jump. Deficit patients had more difficulties in generating such a volitional saccade away from the target, as suggested by longer latencies, compared with nondeficit patients. Other eye movement measures, including error rate on the antisaccade task, smooth pursuit eye movement score, and latencies for reflex saccades, were similar in the two groups. This study, together with the results of the study investigating neurological signs in deficit patients, suggests the involvement of the parietal and frontal cortices and their subcortical connections in the production of deficit symptoms. The frontal cortex, particularly the dorsolateral prefrontal cortex, is often hypothesized to be involved in negative symptom psychopathology (Weinberger 1987; Carpenter et al. 1985). The parietal cortex is a logical extension of this neural circuit, based on the neuroanatomy of saccadic eye movements and parietal involvement in sensory integration tasks. The plausibility of this neural circuit has been demonstrated (Alexander et al. 1986).
8. The robustness of the deficit syndrome approach is best illustrated by the results of a preliminary position emission tomography (PET) study (Buchanan et al. 1989). Patterns of glucose utilization, using PET imaging with ^{18}F-2-deoxyglucose, were examined in 11 drug-free schizophrenic patients, subtyped into deficit and nondeficit groups, and 12 normal controls. All subjects were examined at rest, with eyes covered and ears plugged. Glucose utilization was significantly lower in the thalamus and the frontal and

parietal cortices of the deficit patients compared with nondeficit patients and normal controls. There were no other differences between the two schizophrenic groups including three areas (the temporal, anterior cingulate, and hippocampal cortices) which differentiate the total schizophrenic sample from the normal controls. These preliminary findings, although based on a small sample size, are statistically significant. They illustrate the strength of a clear distinction between patients who do and those who do not have a core psychopathologic attribute. Interpretation of the data is made more straightforward since the schizophrenic groups were similar in severity of psychosis, age of onset, duration of illness, and medication status. A psychosis circuit including the aforementioned limbic cortical areas is postulated for psychosis in all forms of schizophrenia, while a sensory motor circuit involving the thalamus, parietal cortex, and frontal cortex is proposed for the deficit psychopathology found in some patients with schizophrenia.

Conclusions

It is heuristic to define specific psychopathological attributes as targets for the study of the etiology and pathophysiology of schizophrenia. Assessment approaches which undermine the assumptions of discrete psychopathology, cohort definition which systematically skew confounding variables, and topologies based on ephemeral states measured cross-sectionally are to be avoided. A reliable, valid, and practical approach has been developed. It is critical to note that the psychopathological process can be contrasted between groups while holding other major sources of variance constant between study cohorts. This approach is inspired by Kraepelin's distinction of two psychopathological processes of dementia praecox. We anticipate further modifications in our approach as data collect and welcome alternative approaches. However, the principles for psychopathological inquire articulated above are essential if the field is to move from weak hypotheses to the process of strong inference falsification (Platt 1964).

References

Alexander GE, DeLong MR, Strick PL (1986) Parallel organization of functionally segregated circuits linking basal ganglia and cortex. Annu Rev Neurosci 9:357–381

American Psychiatric Association (1987) Diagnostic and statistical manual of mental disorders, 3rd edn. APA, Washington

Andreasen NC (1982) Negative symptoms in schizophrenia. Arch Gen Psychiatry 39:784–788

Andreasen NC, Olsen S (1982) Negative versus positive schizophrenia: definition and validation. Arch Gen Psychiatry 39:789–794

Barnes TRE, Liddle PF (1990) Evidence for the validity of negative symptoms. In: Andreasen NC (ed) Schizophrenia: positive and negative snydromes. Karger, Basle, pp 43–72 (Modern problems of pharmacopsychiatry, vol 24)

Buchanan RW, Kirkpatrick B, Tamminga CA (1989) Differential patterns of glucose metabolism in deficit and non-deficit schizophrenia. Biol Psychiatry 27(A):99 A–100 A
Buchanan RW, Kirkpatrick B, Heinrichs DW, Carpenter WT (1990) Clinical correlates of the deficit syndrome of schizophrenia. Am J Psychiatry 147:290–294
Carpenter WT, Buchanan RW (1989) Domains of psychopathology relevant to the study of etiology and treatment in schizophrenia. In: Schulz SC, Tamminga CA (eds) Schizophrenia: scientific progress. Oxford University Press, New York, pp 13–23
Carpenter WT, Heinrichs DW, Wagman AMI (1985) Deficit and non-deficit forms of schizophrenia: the concept. Am J Psychiatry 145:578–583
Crow TJ (1985) The two-syndrome concept: origins and current status. Schizophr Bull 11:471–486
Kirkpatrick B, Buchanan RW (1990 a) Anhedonia and the deficit syndrome of schizophrenia. Psychiatry Res 31:25–30
Kirkpatrick B, Buchanan RW (1990 b) The neural basis of the deficit syndrome. J Nerv Ment Dis (in press)
Kirkpatrick B, Buchanan RW, McKenney PD, Alphs LD, Carpenter WT (1989) The schedule for the deficit syndrome: an instrument for research in schizophrenia. Psychiatry Res 30:119–124
Kraepelin E (1971) Dementia praecox and paraphrenia. Krieger, New York (Original 1919)
Mayer M, Alpert M, Stastny P, Perlick D, Empfield M (1985) Multiple contributions to clinical presentation of flat affect in schizophrenia. Schizophr Bull 11:420–426
Platt JR (1964) Strong inference. Science 146(3642):347–353
Strauss JS, Carpenter W, Bartko J (1974) The diagnosis and understanding of schizophrenia. III. Speculations on the processes that underlie schizophrenic symptoms and signs. Schizophr Bull 11:61–69
Thaker GK, Buchanan RW, Kirkpatrick B, et al. (1988) Eye movements in schizophrenia: clinical and neurobiological correlates. Abstr Soc Neurosci 14:339
Thaker CK, Kirkpatrick B, Buchanan RW, Ellsberry R, Lahti A, Tamminga CA (1990) Oculomotor abnormalities and their clinical correlates in schizophrenia. Psychopharmacol Bull 25:491–497
Wagman AMI, Heinrichs DW, Carpenter WT (1987) The deficit and non-deficit forms of schizophrenia: neuropsychological evaluation. Psychiatry Res 22:319–330
Weinberger DR (1987) Implications of normal brain development for the pathogenesis of schizophrenia. Arch Gen Psychiatry 44:660–669

Are There Two Types of Schizophrenia? True Onset and Sequence of Positive and Negative Syndromes Prior to First Admission

H. Häfner and K. Maurer [1]

Historical Development of the Concept of Positive and Negative Schizophrenia

The distinction between positive and negative symptoms, which has been postulated in different contexts by Fish (1962), Wing and Brown (1970), Andreasen and Olsen (1982), Crow (1980a, b, 1985) and others, dates back to Reynolds (1858). Jackson (1889) applied it to his speculative system of a hierarchical structure of brain functions. He assumed that negative symptoms were due to functional losses of the brain caused by the illness, whereas positive symptoms were the expression of still healthy brain tissues activated by functional deficits of the higher levels. Kraepelin's (1909–1915) assumption that there are four sub-types of schizophrenia, from dementia simplex with purely negative symptomatology and proceeding continuously towards the defect, to paranoid-hallucinatory schizophrenia with mainly positive symptomatology, paved the way for various dichotomous concepts of schizophrenia.

The Norwegian psychiatrist Langfeldt (1937, 1939), for example, only classified as schizophrenia the core state of the process psychoses with mainly negative symptoms, whereas episodes triggered by exogenous factors with mainly positive symptomatology and a good prognosis he called "schizophreniform". Færgeman (1945) called the group of acute psychotic episodes precipitated by stressful life events the "psychogenic psychoses". Subsequently, several longitudinal studies revealed that the majority of psychogenic psychoses also display negative symptoms and show the typical course of schizophrenia (Achté 1967; Astrup and Noreik 1966; Noreik and Ödegaard 1967; Noreik et al. 1967).

Meanwhile, the observations of the old clinicians have been improved upon by new methodologies. Based on standardised symptom assessment, i.e. of the positive syndrome by means of the Schedule for Affective Disorders and Schizophrenia (SADS, Bilder et al. 1985; Endicott and Spitzer 1978) or the Present State Examination (PSE, Wing et al. 1974) and of the negative Syndrome by means of the Scale for the Assessment of Negative Symptoms (SANS, Andreasen 1981; Andreasen and Olsen 1982; Lewine et al. 1983; Lenzenweger et al. 1989) or the Psychological Impairments Rating Schedule

[1] Zentralinstitut für Seelische Gesundheit, Postfach 122120, J 5, W-6800 Mannheim, FRG

A. Marneros / N. C. Andreasen / M. T. Tsuang (Eds.)
Negative Versus Positive Schizophrenia

(PIRS, Biehl et al. 1989), various statistical analyses of correlations seem to provide some evidence for the independence of the two syndromes (Strauss et al. 1974; Crow 1980a, b; Liddle 1987; Biehl et al. 1988). Most of these results are problematic for methodological reasons (Kay et al. 1986); in particular, cross-sectional findings do not allow one to define truly independent syndromes if no attention is paid to the fact that the samples are composed of individuals in different phases of the illness.

Contemporary "Dichotomy" Models

Kraepelin (1909–1915) in his early publications advocated a phenotypically dichotomous but aetiologically unitarian point of view: the florid or positive syndrome determining the symptomatology of the acute psychosis is an expression of the same illness as the negative syndrome, also called "schizophrenic defect". The differences between the acute psychosis and the residual state become obvious during the course of the disorder. To quote Andreasen (1985), "Delusions, hallucinations, and disorganised speech tend to occur early in the illness. As it progresses, these symptoms sometimes burn out. The patient is then left only with prominent negative or defect symptoms."

When attempting to set up two types of schizophrenia on the basis of symptom clusters or dimensions, there remains a category of mixed types presenting symptoms from both, the size of which depends on the inclusion criteria for the "pure" types. It amounts to approximately 30% in the study of Andreasen and Olsen (1982). Their bipolar model of schizophrenia assumes that the maxima of negative and positive symptoms occupy opposite poles of a common symptom scale, whereas the mixed type occupies the area inbetween. For an epidemiological validation on a pure symptom level, the distinction of Strauss et al. (1974; Carpenter, this volume) between deficit and non-deficit symptoms and the definition of sub-groups of schizophrenia based on this distinction can be put alongside Andreasen's model. Over the course of the illness it comes near to the Kraepelinian model of a temporal sequence of positive and negative symptomatology.

The genetically based severity-liability model of Farmer et al. (1984) and McGuffin (1990) is also very similar to the bipolar model of Andreasen from a phenomenological point of view. At the genotypic level it assumes a multifactorial continuum of liability, and at the phenotypic level it defines certain sub-types at certain positions on this dimension. The negative syndrome in this context is associated with maximum genetic load and severity of the illness. Farmer et al. (1984) developed their sub-types on the basis of multi-variate statistical analyses of symptomatic and anamnestic data. By means of a cluster analysis they found two groups of schizophrenic patients who were not significantly intercorrelated and could thus be easily discriminated (Farmer et al. 1983, 1984). The "H-type" is similar to the Kraepelinian hebephrenia or negative syndrome. It is characterised by poor pre-morbid work adjustment, blunting of affect and other negative symptoms as well as onset before 25 years of age. Farmer's paranoid-like syndrome "P-type", characterised by later onset, poor pre-morbid social adjustment and well-organised delusions, is described as showing less severity (Farmer et al. 1984). Based on a re-analysis of the Maudsley twin series (1948–1964), McGuffin et al. (1987) demonstrated that three different systems giving dichotomous definitions of schizophrenia (Tsuang and Winokur 1974; Crow 1980a, b; Farmer et al. 1984) lead to higher concordance rates in monozygotic twin pairs of the "negative" versus "positive" sub-type for all forms of schizophrenia but not for the same sub-type, thus signalling a slightly higher genetic liability of the "negative" sub-type within the group of schizophrenic syndromes.

Crow's (1980a, b) type I–type II model occupies a special position. The considerations are based on a dichotomous aetiology and thus virtually on two illnesses. Type I schizophrenia is characterised by the prominence of positive symptoms; negative symptoms and cognitive impairments are practically non-existent, and there is a good response to neuroleptic agents. Type II schizophrenia is characterised mainly by negative symptoms, cognitive impairments, poor pre-morbid functioning and neuroleptic agent non-responsiveness. Whereas type I only rarely shows cranial computed tomography (CCT) and magnetic resonance imaging (MRI) findings, type II is assumed to be associated with enlarged lateral cerebral ventricles, above all of the rear part of the temporal horn in the brain scan (Crow 1985; Andreasen et al. 1982; van Kammen et al. 1988). A neuro-anatomical cause of negative symptoms and functional impairments is assumed also by other authors, e.g. on the basis of neurophysiological findings. Lewine (1984) and Weinberger (1987, 1990) suggest a frontal lobe dysfunction. Other possibilities in the aetiology of the negative syndrome are greater frequency of obstetric complications and neurodevelopmental deviance (Lewis and Murray 1987; Lewis et al. 1988; McNeil 1988; Nimgaonkar et al. 1988; O'Callaghan et al. 1988; Owen et al. 1988, 1989). Contrary to the mainly exogenous aetiology of type II, type I is regarded to be based on a genetically transmitted dysfunction of the brain dopaminergic system and thus to be associated more often with a family history of schizophrenia.

Crow's aetiological dichotomy assumes not only – some overlapping conceded – that there is a comparative independence of the positive and negative syndromes in cross-section but also that there are two largely independent processes in the course: the negative symptomatology of type II, which is due to neuro-anatomic changes, is not supposed to disappear but rather to persist or increase over longer periods, whereas the positive syndrome is thought to exhibit an irregular, episodic course.

Possibilities of Testing the Validity of Dichotomy Models

As we do not know any external markers, the first steps towards validating the dichotomy models must be made on the basis of observable phenomena in the field of epidemiology. The following three elements forming the basis of the different dichotomy models of schizophrenia are also the three levels at which an attempt at empirical validation of the assumptions is possible:

1. The analysis of unbiased cross-sectional data to identify fairly separate symptom clusters or factors that are widely independent and can therefore be used to discriminate the two schizophrenia syndromes precisely enough.
2. The study of correlations between the assumed syndromes on the one hand and further factors of e.g. a genetic or environmental nature on the other hand. This approach is not the object of the study presented here.
3. The test for stability, trends and longitudinal correlations of the two syndromes, which are formulated either implicitly or explicitly as in Crow's two-process hypothesis or in Kraepelin's progressive-defect hypothesis. Marneros and Deister (this volume) have tested the stability of Andreasen's positive, negative and mixed types of schizophrenia in a retrospective study of 148 schizophrenic patients covering an average of 23 years. They found high probabilities of change between the three types.

Methodological Requirements

Kay et al. (1986) have already criticised that most studies on the validation of positive vs. negative syndromes of schizophrenia "have generally been limited by small samples and unstandardised rating methods, lack of long range follow-up and no control for extrapyramidal side effects". Both ways of validating (cross-sectional and longitudinal) require a standardised and comprehensive assessment of all the relevant symptoms in a sufficiently large and representative sample. The supposed longitudinal independence of symptom measures (dimensional) or types (categorial) can be studied over short periods, provided a sufficiently large number of cross-sections at short intervals allows the detailed modelling of the course. The study of long-term trends and the correlations of time-dependent measures also have greater validity if not only two but several cross-sections are considered.

The first cross-sectional assessment should be carried out at approximately the same stage of the illness, favourably during the acute episode, a rule which is neglected in many studies. However, a significant correlation between positive and negative syndromes, provided it exists, can only be proven if the study sample comprises a sufficiently large number of patients exhibiting symptoms of both dimensions. A high proportion of chronic cases in the sample displaying only negative symptoms increases the probability of finding a non-correlation between the two syndromes (van Kammen et al. 1990). This condition is usually more or less true for follow-up measures in studies with first admission samples. Nonetheless, many studies of the course of schizophrenia either do not mention the time of first admission (e.g. Huber et al. 1979; Ciompi 1980) or are based on samples comprising both acute and chronic cases.

Models and Hypotheses

For empirical validation we will translate the various dichotomy models into extremely simplified hypotheses. These hypotheses will be demonstrated graphically as course models.

Model 1 (Crow 1980a, b)

The positive syndrome (type I schizophrenia) and the negative syndrome (type II schizophrenia) are separate illness processes with discernible symptomatology and different courses. Concerning cross-sectional combinations of the syndromes, most obviously one can assume a zero correlation. Over the course, however, the positive syndrome is allowed to be unstable, whereas the negative syndrome must be persistent once it has occurred (Fig. 1).

Testing Hypotheses. For cross-sectional measurements positive and negative symptoms are not correlated. During the course, only consistent patterns of persistent negative symptoms are allowed after first onset of this syndrome. This means that the conditional probability of minus symptomatology has to be extremely high over time.

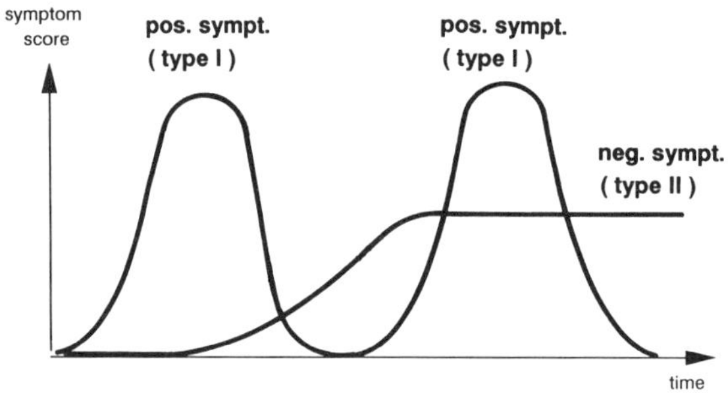

Fig. 1. Hypothesis 1 (Crow 1980a, b): the positive and negative syndromes are pathogenetically independent subtypes with different symptomatology and course

Model 2 (Andreasen and Olsen)

On the basis of a bipolar syndrome dimension of schizophrenia negative correlations of the two syndromes are expected. As individuals are classified in accordance with this typology as positive, negative or mixed, sub-types must prove as stable over the course; "pure" types as well as the mixed type have to exhibit sufficient stability (Fig. 2).

Testing Hypotheses. Schizophrenics at the same stage of illness, e.g. a population of first-onset patients, can be quite precisely classified into the two categories according to the score of negative or positive symptomatology. Between the two syndrome scores, negative correlations are expected. If a patient who developed symptoms of schizophrenia is classified as belonging to one of the sub-types, this categorisation must be stable over time.

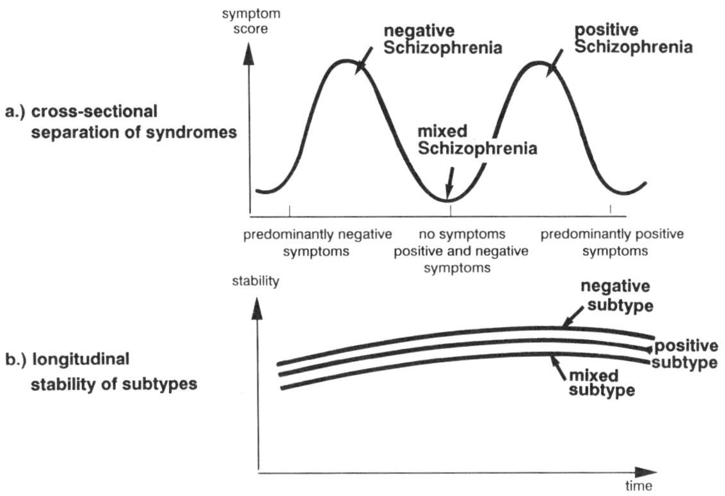

Fig. 2. Hypothesis 2 (Andreasen and Olsen 1982): negative and positive symptoms are ordered on a bipolar dimension, and the three subtypes, "negative", "positive" and "mixed", are stable over time

Model 3 (Kraepelin)

The positive syndrome expresses the acute state of the illness; the negative syndrome is the residual or defect syndrome, which emerges increasingly from the episodes with positive symptomatology (Fig. 3).

Testing Hypotheses. Positive symptoms usually precede the negative symptoms. Over the long-term course the score of positive symptoms decreases and that of negative symptoms increases.

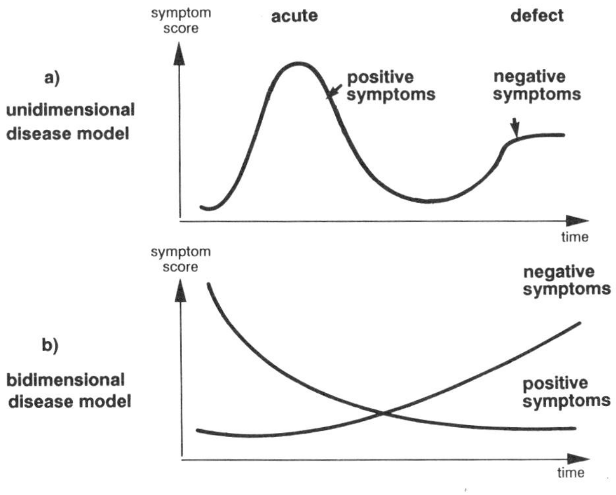

Fig. 3. Hypothesis 3 (Kraepelin 1909–1915): the positive syndrome is prevalent in acute episodes and the negative syndrome in the schizophrenic defect state or residual schizophrenia

Model 4 (Huber 1983)

The negative syndrome is an expression of the schizophrenic basic disorder from which the positive syndrome emerges at a later date (Fig. 4).

Testing Hypothesis. The negative syndrome precedes the positive syndrome which does not arise until the negative symptoms have been present for some time and reach a certain threshold level.

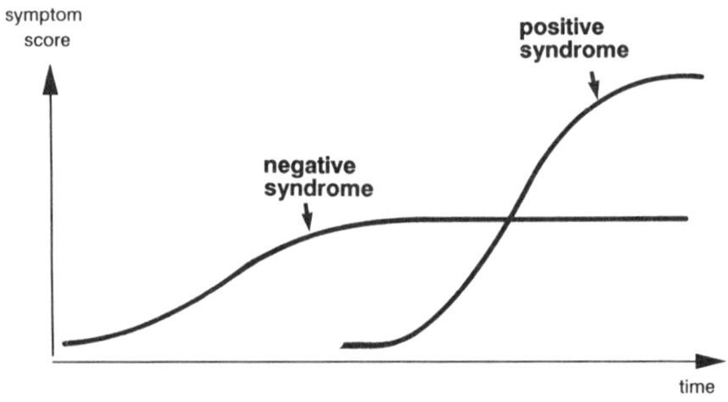

Fig. 4. Hypothesis 4 (Huber 1983): the negative syndrome is a manifestation of the schizophrenic basic disorder, which precedes the positive syndrome

Model 5 (own assumption and van Kammen et al. 1990)

Both positive and negative symptoms are simultaneously an expression of the same disease process and possibly of the same basic aetiology (Fig. 5).

Testing Hypothesis. Increase and decrease of positive and negative symptomatology are almost parallel.

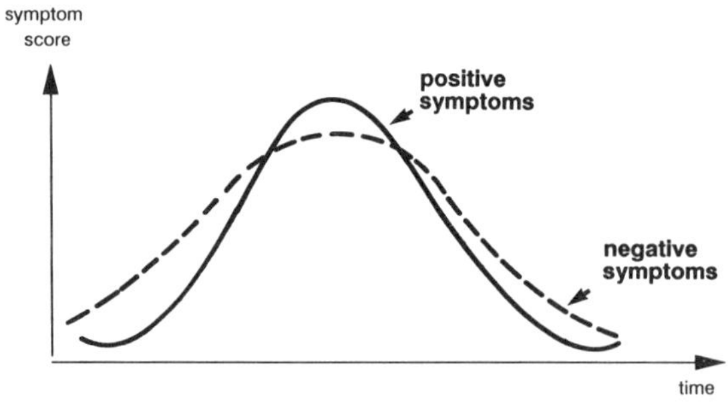

Fig. 5. Hypothesis 5 (van Kammen et al. 1990): positive and negative symptoms are part of the same disease process

Model 6 (additional assumption to model 5)

The construct "negative" syndrome consists of three components. Two of them are directly illness-related, the first component occurring in the early and acute stages of the illness process, visible for example in a purely negative prodromal stadium of a positive or mixed type of schizophrenia, and the second one is the residual or scar component due to direct biopsychological consequences of episodes of the disease. The third component is caused by coping with the illness itself and its consequences for the patient's life and environment, including long-term institutionalisation (Fig. 6).

Testing Hypothesis. There are significant time differences in the maxima and minima of positive symptomatology and at least two distinguishable items of the negative symptomatology, the directly illness-related and the illness-behaviour-related components, in the course of schizophrenia.

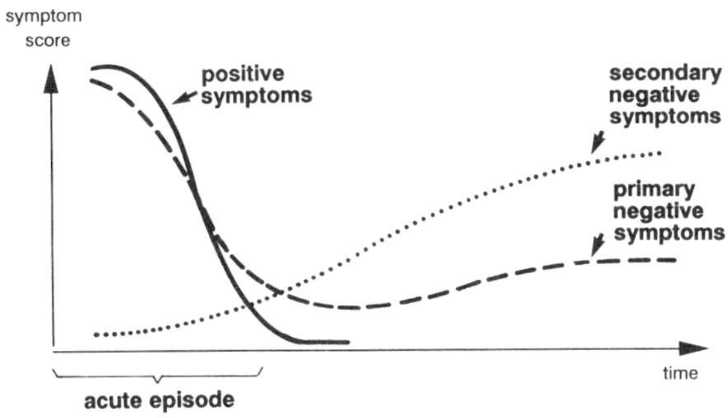

Fig. 6. Hypothesis 6: part of the negative symptoms is a direct consequence of the disease process ("primary negative symptoms"), another part is the consequence of other factors like coping behaviour ("secondary negative symptoms")

The reasons for constructing model 6 include the lack of specificity of essential parts of the negative syndrome (e.g. social withdrawal and avolition are also present in chronic depression), the frequency of depressive episodes in the course of schizophrenia (Hirsch 1982; Hirsch and Jolley 1989), the high frequency of depressive symptoms in the negative syndrome (Biehl et al. 1988) and the overlapping of the negative syndrome with secondary impairments due to social under-stimulation (Wing and Brown 1970). In addition, the coping efforts of schizophrenic patients must be considered, such as attempts to prevent relapse by avoiding social contact (Thurm and Häfner 1987; Straube 1980; Strauss 1987; Wing 1975; Carpenter et al. 1988; Nuechterlein 1990).

The degree or severity of the directly illness-related component, the "primary negative symptoms", varies largely in parallel with the positive symptomatology. The illness-behaviour-related component, the "secondary negative symptoms", will increasingly develop due to its scar element, depending on the number and severity of episodes. In subsequent relapses they could precede the increase in productive symptomatology as an indicator of intensified coping efforts. A syndrome associated with illness behaviour should also exhibit higher variability between the sexes and between individuals than the symptom components directly connected with the disease. The validation of model 6, which is one of the most interesting models, is not the topic of this paper.

Data and Operationalisation of Positive and Negative Syndromes

The validation of the models 1–5 is performed with different methodology in three individual studies:

1. Part of the models and hypotheses can be tested in the early course of positive and negative symptomatology. Hypotheses that assume a certain succession of positive and negative symptoms must be tested from the time point of first onset of symptoms, for example by data collected from a representative first-admission sample of 236 schizophrenic patients, 12–59 years of age, 112 males and 124 females from a population of 1.5 millions (Rhine-Neckar District and Palatinate), who reported to have had continuously persisting positive or negative symptoms before their first hospitalisation with a diagnosis of schizophrenia.
2. In order to demonstrate the changes during individual episodes, Maurer et al. (1989) and Krumm et al. (1990) of our group studied and modelled the course of PIRS and PSE measures in 15 first-onset and 15 chronic schizophrenic patients by means of 7 cross-sections at 2-week intervals (PIRS) and of 4 cross-sections at 4-week intervals (PSE).
3. The third study is based on data of the Mannheim cohort of the WHO Disability Study (Biehl et al. 1986; Maurer and Biehl 1990), which was carried out in 7 cross-sections over 5 years of observation of patients after first hospitalisation for schizophrenia.

The results of the first two data sets will be given in this chapter; the results of the Disability Study are presented in Maurer and Häfner (this volume). The validation of the models will be based mainly on retrospective data of the first study. On the basis of approved instruments (see Table 1) we developed a semi-structured Instrument for the Retrospective Assessment of the Onset of Schizophrenia (IRAOS; Table 1) (Häfner et al. 1990).

To operationalise positive and negative syndromes, in the first study we identified in accordance with accepted psychopathology scales the corresponding items in our research instrument IRAOS, in order to define positive and negative symptom scores. By interviewing each patient and one key person, usually a relative, the first onset and the continuity of the course of positive and negative symptoms could be registered to derive a course pattern from earliest occurrence until the time point of first hospitalisation.

For the second and the third studies we used two operationalised constructs of the negative and the positive symptomatology based on the PSE (Wing et al. 1974) and the PIRS (Biehl et al. 1989). The PSE registered mainly symptoms experienced by the patient himself, while the PIRS measured psychological functional impairments rated by experienced interviewers through direct observation.

A factor analysis of 32 predominant PSE symptoms in two independent samples and in 7 cross-sections of the Mannheim cohort of the WHO Disability Study revealed three largely stable psychopathology factors: a positive, a

Table 1. Relevant aids for the development of the Instrument for the Retrospective Assessment of the Onset of Schizophrenia

Acute Schizophrenia Diagnostic Checklist (ASDC)	Fish (1969)
AMDP system, manual	Arbeitsgemeinschaft für Methodik und Dokumentation in der Psychiatrie (1983)
Bonner Scale for the Assessment of Basic Symptoms (BSABS)	Gross (1985)
Brief Psychiatric Rating Scale (BPRS)	Overall and Gorham (1962)
Disability Assessment Schedule (DAS)	WHO (1988), Jung et al. (1989)
Frankfurter Beschwerde-Fragebogen (FBF)	Süllwold (1977, 1981)
Fragebogen zur Erfassung subjektiv erlebter Störungen der Schizophrenie (FEB)	Langer et al. (1985)
Goldstein Premorbid Attainment Scale	Rodnick and Goldstein (1974)
Paranoid-Depressivitäts-Skala (PD-S)	von Zerssen and Koeller (1976)
Past History and Sociodemographic Description Schedule (PHSD)	WHO (1973), Jablensky et al. (1980)
Perceptual Aberration Scale	Chapman et al. (1978)
Physical Anhedonia Scale	Chapman et al. (1978)
Premorbid Adjustment Scale (PAS)	Cannon-Spoor et al. (1982)
Premorbid Asocial Adjustment Scale (PAAS)	Gittelman-Klein and Klein (1969)
Present State Examination (PSE)	Wing et al. (1973)
Prognostic Scale (PS)	Strauss and Carpenter (1974)
Psychiatric and Personal History Schedule (PPHS)	WHO (1978)
Scale for the Assessment of Negative Symptoms (SANS)	Andreasen (1982)
Scales for Assessing Social Adjustment (SSA)	Isele et al. (1985)
Schizophrenia Assessment	Salokangas (1978)
Social Behaviour Assessment Schedule (SBAS)	Platt et al. (1980)

negative and an anxiety-dysphoria factor (Table 2) (Biehl et al. 1988). In this three-factor solution it is remarkable that the negative one includes not only the typical symptoms of the negative syndrome but also depressive symptoms, e.g. depressed mood, hopelessness and morning depression. This result indicates that the depressive syndrome in schizophrenia must be considered as a partial aspect of the whole complex of negative symptomatology. In order to operationalise plus and minus symptomatology, those items which showed high factor loadings were in either case added together.

For the definition of a positive and a negative "functional impairment" measure, the relevant characteristic PIRS items were summed without applying a statistical procedure by the members of our research group (Biehl et al. 1989) and listed in two sub-scores, "POSY" and "NESY" (Table 3).

The object of the analysis is, according to a categorial-typological model, the alternative classification of individuals by positive, negative or mixed type

Table 2. Factor loadings of 32 PSE symptoms used to operationalise additive positive and negative symptom scores (PSE data of 62 schizophrenics 3 years after onset) (from Biehl et al. 1988)

	Symptom	Factor I delusional	Factor II residual	Factor III anxiety
6	Tiredness or exhaustion	0.01	0.57[a]	0.11
11	Free-floating autonomic anxiety	−0.02	0.10	0.49[a]
12	Anxious foreboding	−0.06	0.21	0.33[a]
13	Autonomic anxiety due to delusions	0.77[a]	0.08	−0.07
15	Situational autonomic anxiety	0.23	0.08	0.65[a]
16	Autonomic anxiety on meeting people	−0.07	0.02	0.70[a]
18	Avoidance of anxiety-provoking situations	0.09	−0.02	0.42[a]
19	Subjectively inefficient thinking	0.15	0.58	0.07
20	Poor concentration	0.50[a]	0.28	−0.06
21	Neglect due to brooding	0.39	0.48[a]	0.07
22	Loss of interest	0.37	0.51[a]	0.24
23	Depressed mood	0.02	0.53[a]	−0.08
24	Hopelessness	0.00	0.69[a]	−0.16
25	Suicidal plans or acts	−0.11	0.35[a]	0.18
27	Morning depression	−0.01	0.62[a]	−0.16
28	Social withdrawal	0.27	0.23[a]	0.18
29	Self-depreciation	−0.04	0.60[a]	0.08
30	Lack of self-confidence in social relations	−0.04	0.53[a]	0.14
31	Simple ideas of reference	0.02	0.03	0.35[a]
36	Subjective anergia and retardation	0.31	0.64[a]	0.01
38	Loss of libido	0.16	0.65[a]	0.31
49	Delusional mood	0.71[a]	0.17	0.16
54	Lost emotions	0.40	0.52[a]	0.18
59	Delusions of thought being real	0.51[a]	−0.06	−0.26
72	Delusions of reference	0.65[a]	0.14	0.09
73	Delusional misinterpretations	0.78[a]	−0.06	0.19
74	Delusions of persecution	0.47[a]	0.01	−0.26
80	Delusions explicable in terms of physical forces	0.44[a]	0.10	−0.01
93	Systematization of delusions	0.91[a]	−0.06	0.15
94	Evasiveness	0.43[a]	−0.06	0.35
95	Preoccupation with delusions and hallucinations	0.92[a]	0.02	0.19
96	Acting out delusions	0.99[a]	0.03	−0.01

[a] PSE symptom used for factor scoring.

PSE, Present State Examination.

as well as, according to the dimensional model, the respective score of negative or positive symptomatology. The dimensionally quantifying procedure is necessary to study possible correlations between the two syndromes cross-sectionally and longitudinally and the categorial procedure, in order to make statements about those patients with changing categories over time.

Table 3. PIRS items which constitute the positive (POSY) and negative (NESY) impairment score (from Biehl et al. 1989, p. 76)

POSY		NESY	
Item no.	Item label	Item no.	Item label
004	Stupor	001	Slowness and underactivity
006	Distractability	002	Reduction of facial movements
007	Hallucinatory behaviour	003	Slow speech
008	Blank spells	019	Loss of initiative
018	Over-initiative	020	Reduced quantity of facial expression
021	Increased facial expression	022	Reduced range of facial expression
023	Inappropriate facial expression	025	Gaze avoidance
036	Agitation	029	Facial mannerisms or stereotypies
038	Catatonic movements	035	Limited use of gesture
042	Observed anxiety	037	Mannerisms and posturing
043	Observed depression	039	Stereotypies
044	Hypomanic affect	047	Blunted affect
045	Hostile irritability	055	Unmodulated and flat tone of voice
048	Incongruity of affect		
049	Gross excitement and violence	061	Lack of "non-verbal grammar"
050	Lability of mood	062	Restricted quantity of speech
053	Abnormally loud voice	067	Poverty of content of speech
057	Incoherence	069	Lack of humour
058	Neologisms, idiosyncrasies	070	Lack of listener feedback
060	Talking out of turn	080	Lack of "presence"
063	Pressure of speech	085	Over-compliance
066	Flight of ideas		
068	Perseveration		
074	Embarrassing behaviour		
076	Disturbed reasoning		
077	Bizarre appearance		
078	Irreverent behaviour		
079	Histrionic behaviour		
082	Suspiciousness		
083	Hostility to interviewer		

PIRS, Psychological Impairments Rating Schedule.

Results

Models 1 and 2: Independence of Dependence of Early Positive and Negative Symptoms (Crow vs. Andreasen and Olsen)

At the time point of first hospitalisation, the patients had a mean number of 4.2 for negative and of 3.6 for positive symptoms. On average, negative symptoms date back 6.5 years before first admission (with a maximum of 38

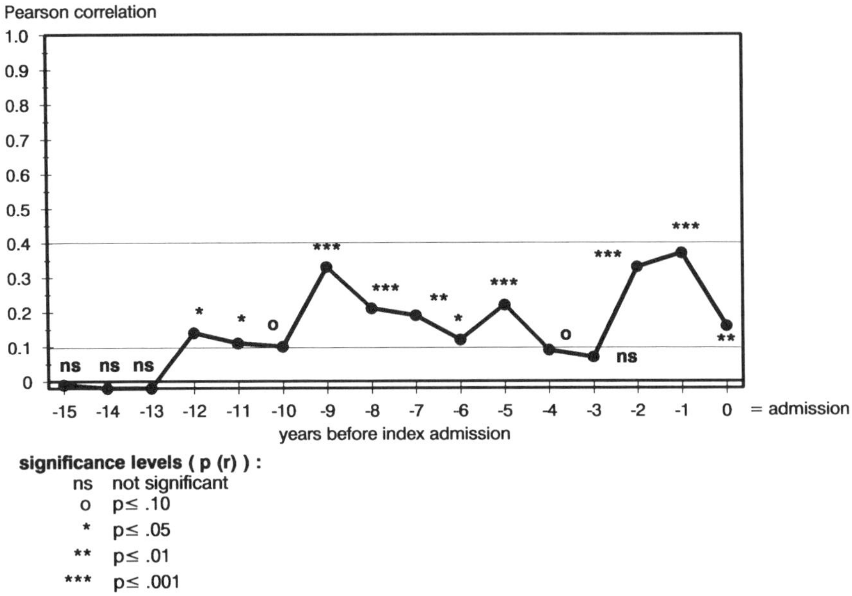

Fig. 7. Correlations of positive and negative symptoms during the development of schizophrenia over 15 years until first hospital admission

years), and the earliest positive symptom reported dates back about 2 years on average (maximum 24 years). To decide between model 1 and model 2 concerning the question of dependence or independence of the two syndromes, the total number of positive and negative symptoms was correlated: for the time point of first admission the two syndromes have a low but significant correlation ($r = 0.16$, $P \leqq 0.01$), a result that contradicts the hypotheses of both Crow and Andreasen and Olsen.

Looking at the years before first admission, it seems to be reasonable to test the dependence of the two syndromes at different time points during the early development of the disease. For each monthly cross-section dating back up to 15 years from the time point of the interview, the number of positive and negative symptoms were correlated. For each year the correlation coefficients are presented graphically in Fig. 7. At 13 years before first admission the correlations between the two syndrome scores are zero, because the variance of acute symptomatology is extremely reduced. After that, we normally find low positive correlations between 0.10 and 0.40. This analysis clearly demonstrates the interdependence of developing positive and negative symptoms. Even if the biological processes producing positive and negative syndromes are independent, this does not exclude interactive development of these syndromes, as indicated by positive correlations.

To test the Andreasen and Olsen (1982) typology of positive, negative and mixed sub-types, we decided to which sub-type the individuals belong at 7 time points and whether or not these sub-types prove to be stable over at least 2-year

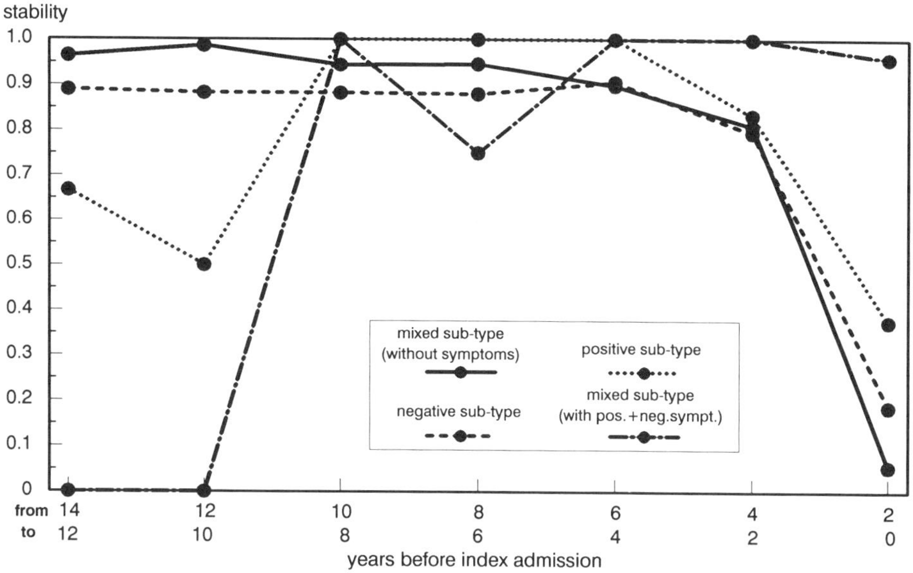

Fig. 8. Stability (conditional probabilities) of sub-types (positive, negative and mixed) within 2-year intervals over 14 years before first hospital admission ($n = 236$)

intervals (Fig. 8). We distinguished two "pure" sub-types – those patients who developed early positive symptoms without negative symptoms and patients with a beginning schizophrenia manifested only by negative symptoms – and a mixed one with simultaneous onset of both syndromes. Before symptom onset, all patients belonged to the favourable mixed form.

The conditional probability functions of the sub-types are quite stable. Patients with a beginning schizophrenia of the pure form will have a high probability of belonging to this sub-type between two subsequent measures with the exception of the time interval before the admission episode. Then, of course, the pure negative type develops positive symptoms, while the pure positive type develops negative symptoms as well. The vanishing favourable "mixed type" at index admission is a consequence of developing psychotic symptoms beforehand. On the other hand, the remaining stability of the unfavourable mixed type until the index episode is also trivial: probably a higher intensity of already existing acute symptoms leads to the admission, accompanied by negative symptoms so that no categorial change will be observed.

On the whole, the stability of the Andreasen sub-types during the phase of the early development of schizophrenia is quite good, at least if we limit our stability analysis to the intermediate time range of 2 years. A prolongation of time intervals or looking at the time period from symptom onset until first admission in total would result in a much higher proportion of categorial changes. For the last 2-year segment, characterised by the intensification of symptoms before admission, the stability of the pure sub-types becomes rather low. Therefore, to validate these sub-types, it is debatable whether the transmission into or out of a psychotic episode should be excluded. It should be tested if the patients after discharge return back to their earlier sub-type class, to which they belonged before the first hospitalisation. Only if we can identify the patients as belonging to the same sub-type from early onset over a long time period, with just short category changes during acute episodes, can this typology be accepted as valid.

Models 3 and 4: Negative Symptomatology as "Preceding Defect" (Huber) or as "Residual State" (Kraepelin)

The validation of the hypothesis that the negative symptomatology precedes the positive requires not only the (retrospective) assessment of behavioural changes prior to first admission but also of positive and negative symptoms from their first occurrence. The validation of Huber's model (no. 4) indirectly invalidates that of Kraepelin (no. 3), because they are incompatible.

For 17 positive and 13 negative items contained in the IRAOS (see Fig. 9), the mean time values between first occurrence and the interview are computed. To this list of symptoms one depression item was added, because the first occurrence of depressive symptoms could give a hint as to whether or not depressive symptoms belong to the negative syndrome or if they have to be seen as a separate syndrome.

Figure 9 shows a surprising result: the first occurrence of the whole range of positive symptoms but only one partly negative symptom – disturbed speech – can be dated back to a period of 2 years before index admission. Since the item "disturbed speech" also includes incoherent speech, neologisms etc., it cannot be fully attributed to the positive or the negative syndrome.

The mean values of the first occurrence of the purely negative symptoms are between 2 and approximately 4 years prior to index admission. Only the depressive syndrome is exceptional with a mean value of first manifestation of more than 5 years prior to first admission.

The mean time values of the first occurrence of positive symptoms extend from approximately 2 years (thought block, delusions of influence) to 6 months (verbal and other hallucinations, delusions not specified further) prior to first admission. The earliest negative symptoms, presumably the first indicators of the psychosis (incongruity of affect, disturbed communication and loss of energy – all of them typical disturbances as listed in the approved scales of negative symptomatology), date back 3.5 years on average. They are followed soon afterwards by social withdrawal and loss of interest in leisure activities as first disabilities in social roles.

This result clearly supports the hypothesis of the preceding negative symptoms (model 4, Huber). The assumption, however, that negative symptoms occur only as a consequence of positive symptoms (model 3, Kraepelin) cannot be maintained.

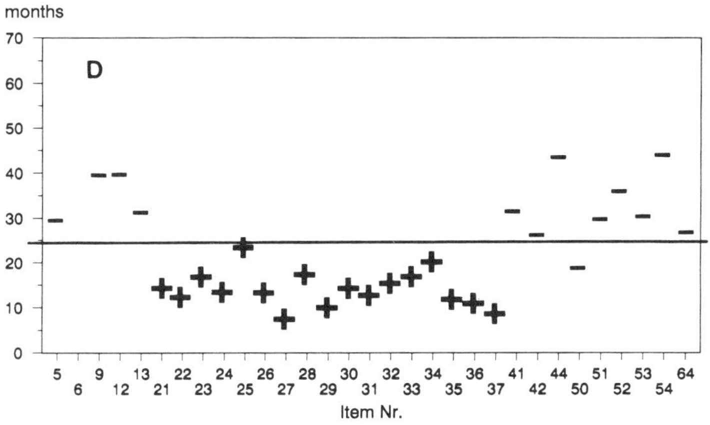

Negative symptoms (-)

5 = poor concentration
9 = social withdrawal
12 = anergia and retardation
13 = loss of libido
41 = increased distractability
42 = weakness of intentional thinking
44 = disturbance of affect
50 = disturbance of speech
51 = self-care
52 = underactivity
53 = slowness
54 = social withdrawal
64 = loss of interest

Depression

6 = depressed mood

Positive symptoms(+)

21 = thought disorders
22 = thought insertion
23 = thought broadcast
24 = thought echo
25 = thought block or withdrawal
26 = auditory hallucinations
27 = verbal hallucinations
28 = visual hallucinations
29 = other hallucinations
30 = delusions of control
31 = delusions of reference
32 = delusions of persecution
33 = expansive delusions
34 = delusions of influence
35 = primary delusions
36 = delusions concerning appearance
37 = other delusions

Fig. 9. Positive and negative symptoms: time differences from first onset of symptoms until first hospitalisation with schizophrenia diagnosis

No statements can be made about the developmental pattern of the psychosis based merely on the sequence of the first occurrence of symptoms, neither concerning whether positive symptoms occur after the "purely" negative symptoms have reached a threshold value, nor concerning whether both trends take a parallel course with a time lag for the positive symptoms. On the basis of IRAOS data, however, the course can be revealed in the form of the cumulation of persisting symptoms from their first onset until first hospitalisation.

Figure 10 shows the almost parallel, continuous rise in symptoms over 15 years. In order to demonstrate clearly the rapid increase of both negative as well as positive symptoms immediately before index admission, we listed the year preceding first hospitalisation at the bottom of Fig. 10 in monthly intervals. At the time of index admission we find an average of 3.7 negative and 2.5 positive continuous symptoms.

a.) within 15 years (per year)

b.) within 12 months during the year before index admission

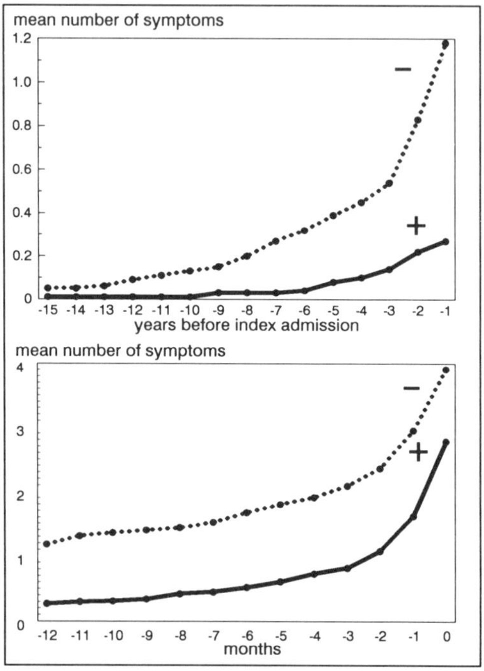

Fig. 10. Cumulative values of persistent positive and negative symptoms until first hospital admission for schizophrenia ($n = 236$)

Both syndromes display an exponential increase with a 5-year time lag of the positive and a somewhat higher growth rate of the negative symptoms. The beginning of the schizophrenic psychosis, with the sequence of negative symptoms and social disability on the one hand and positive symptoms on the other, therefore takes place according to a defineable course pattern: from the first onset the negative and the positive syndromes both proceed in a linear progressive way, the positive syndrome with a time lag and both with a clearly accelerating increase about 1 year prior to first admission. This result again confirms model 4 (Huber). There is currently no evidence for a temporal precedence of the positive syndrome (model 3, Kraepelin) or for the independence of either syndrome.

The demonstration of the developmental sequence of negative symptoms followed by positive ones leaves open the question whether or not all patients develop negative symptoms in a first step, followed by positive symptoms with a temporal delay. For example, the mean time difference of the cumulative functions could also result if a chronic sub-group with negative symptoms and acute onset and a second sub-group developing acute symptoms over a longer time period without negative symptoms existed. Therefore, the total sample was split up by possible developmental schemes of the negative and the positive syndrome, differentiating each dimension into an acute (symptoms within

Table 4. Developmental types of schizophrenia syndromes – acute, subacute or chronic development of positive and negative symptomatology

Development of the earliest positive symptom	Development of the earliest negative symptom			Total
	Acute (within 1 month)	Subacute (within 1 year)	Chronic (over several years)	
Acute (within 1 month)	21 (8.9)	14 (5.9)	56 (23.7)	91 (38.5)
Subacute (within 1 year)	4 (1.7)	20 (8.5)	37 (15.7)	61 (25.9)
Chronic (over several years)	3 (1.3)	2 (0.8)	79 (33.5)	84 (35.7)
n (Percentage)	28 (11.9)	36 (15.2)	172 (72.9)	236

1 month before hospital admission), subacute (within 1 year) and chronic development (more than 1 year), and combining these 3 types of onset into 9 sub-types, as shown in Table 4.

Concerning the negative syndrome, 73% of the patients have a chronic development and 15% subacute, and only 12% show negative symptoms primarily in the month before hospitalisation. On the other hand, the most frequent developmental type of positive symptoms is acute in 39% of the cohort. Some 26% of patients have the first persistent positive symptom within 1 year before hospitalisation and 36%, even longer.

Looking at the combinations of the syndromes, the development of positive symptoms before negative ones can be widely excluded. Also the pure positive subtype postulated by Andreasen and Olsen (1982) is quite rare, whereas a chronic subtype without acute symptoms before the inclusion episode (about 30%) cannot be denied. The most frequent combination leads to the mixed type: about 59% of the patients belong to this category.

Table 4 was constructed by the identification of the earliest positive and negative symptom per patient. This procedure is influenced by extreme values. To compensate for this, the data were re-analysed for mean time differences of all positive and negative symptoms exhibited by each patient until the time of first hospital admission: the result of this alternative tabulation is not as pronounced compared with Table 4 but leaves our conclusions unchanged.

Finally, for each patient the time difference between the earliest negative symptom and the earliest positive symptom was determined (Fig. 11). In general, earlier positive symptoms occur in about 10% of patients. In another 20% both syndromes emerge at exactly the same time point, but in most cases (70%) negative symptoms develop before the positive ones. For 50% of the patients with earlier negative symptoms the time difference until the first positive symptom is 2 years or more.

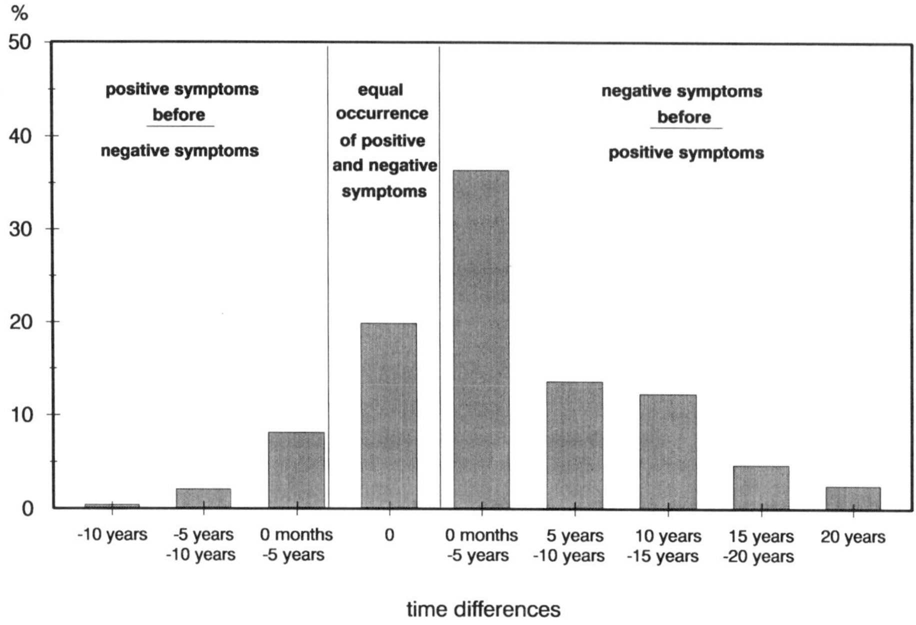

Fig. 11. Distribution of time differences between the first negative and the first positive symptom in 236 schizophrenic patients at first admission

Models 5 and 6: Negative Symptoms as Concomitant or Consequent to Positive Symptoms

The results presented so far relate to the development of the positive and negative syndromes from first onset until first hospitalisation. What can be said about the course of an episode from the time point of admission until the remission of acute symptoms? According to model 5, a parallel decline of positive and negative symptoms is expected. The phenomenon can be demonstrated only by means of data from rapidly changing states in acute episodes assessed at very short intervals. Then it is possible to test the alternative assumptions of whether the decrease of negative symptoms is linked to the remission of acute symptoms or whether it is an independent process. Ratings of a single episode from hospital admission until 6 weeks after discharge were conducted by Maurer et al. (1989) with 30 schizophrenic in-patients, 15 first-onset patients and 15 patients with the onset of the disease dating at least 10 years back. Figure 12 shows in the upper part the average PSE scores for positive and negative symptoms of the 30 patients and in the lower part, the course of positive and negative impairments, as rated by the interviewer. The short-term courses exhibit a largely parallel decrease of positive and negative symptoms. The increase of symptoms dates back before admission, which could not be assessed here. The IRAOS data given above showed – like a reflected image – a parallel increase of both syndromes before

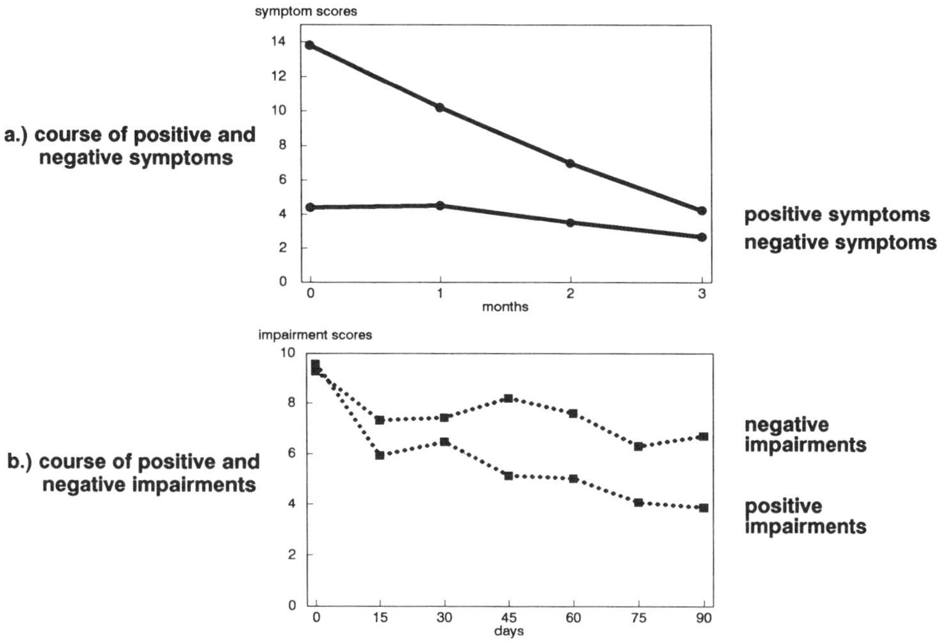

Fig. 12. Short-term course of a psychotic episode (15 first-onset patients; 15 chronic patients)

first admission. The interviewer-rated impairments (PIRS) also display a rather parallel and continuous decrease of the positive and negative impairments from the beginning of in-patient treatment until 6 weeks after discharge.

These results further contribute to the rebuttal of the hypothesis of a growing defect and support model 5, suggesting a parallel development (increasing and decreasing) of positive and negative symptoms.

The alternative models 1, 2, 3 and 5 must be further tested on their course following first hospitalisation. To this end, the data can be used of the representative cohort of 70 first-hospitalised schizophrenic patients who were examined regularly in 7 cross-sections over 5 years by Biehl et al. (1986) and by Maurer and Biehl (1990) from our research unit. In previous publications these authors have already determined that the mean values of negative symptoms exhibit a course virtually parallel to that of the positive symptoms. Both values culminate during the index episode. The decrease of the positive symptoms over the course can be explained easily: at the beginning, practically all patients were in an acute state, and afterwards the proportion of acutely ill naturally decreased. The parallel decrease of negative symptoms or the absence of comparatively high values of negative symptoms developing after the reduction of positive symptoms contradicts the Kraepelinian hypothesis of negative symptoms being only a consequence of positive symptoms in the sense of the defect syndrome. What determined the beginning – the parallel growing of both syndromes with a "preceding defect" (Janzarik 1968) – therefore also characterises the further course of the psychosis: negative and positive symptoms are obviously not independent phenomena. Negative symptoms as the direct expression of the disease process seem to announce the occurrence of positive symptoms. Furthermore, they rise steeply and concomitantly with them and recede again clearly after the acute state, although not always to the initial level before the "true" onset of the disease.

This may be an indicator for model 6: negative symptoms will develop before an acute episode and will also be reduced after it, but this is only one of their aspects. After one or more episodes there may be a growing risk of chronicity of negative symptoms as described by Kraepelin, which can only be demonstrated over the long-term course. Therefore, a more complex model of the course of schizophrenia is needed, which allows us to separate different sources of negative symptoms, e.g. those indicating beginning or remitting episodes, those determining long-term processes leading to scars and chronicity and lastly the "secondary" or illness-behaviour-related components.

Discussion and Conclusions

Several contemporary dichotomy models of schizophrenia are available, but there is a lack of empirical effort to decide between competing or contradictory aspects and to explain the interplay of positive and negative schizophrenia. It is amazing that in the large amount of literature on positive-negative schizophrenia there is an extreme shortcoming of longitudinal research. Most work is done with cross-sectional data of hospitalised patients, although many longitudinal studies on schizophrenia were performed in the past decades (see Olbrich and Strauss 1988). Our opinion is that the dichotomy models of schizophrenia have to take the developmental aspect explicitly into consideration. For example, the dependence or independence of the syndromes not only relates to the simultaneous occurrence of positive and negative symptoms but also to the interaction of the syndromes over time. Also, the postulation of sub-types (like the positive, negative or mixed ones suggested by Andreasen and Olsen 1982) only makes sense if it leads to stable sub-types and not to often changing categorisations over time.

To analyse dichotomy models of schizophrenia under the developmental or longitudinal view, 6 different models and possible testing hypotheses were formulated and related to the early development of schizophrenia from first onset of symptoms until first hospitalisation. Some of these models have to be tested for the long-term course as well (see Maurer and Häfner, this volume); others can only be tested by data concerning the beginning psychosis before first admission or by the course of a single episode.

The mean values presented to describe the first occurrence of all positive and negative symptoms of schizophrenia and the cumulative pattern of illness development from the first indicator of the beginning psychosis until the first hospitalisation theoretically could also be influenced by a broad individual fluctuation of symptoms and the dependence of the time point of hospital admission on the amount of symptoms in both dimensions. In fact, only 10% of the patients developed positive symptoms before negative symptoms. The mean number of symptoms at the time point of hospitalisation is comparable for the different sub-types, defined by type of symptom onset.

The nearly parallel course of both syndromes with a delay in the development of positive symptoms is not compatible with the assumption of independent syndromes as proposed by model 1: if the negative syndrome precedes the positive one, then there is clearly a temporal relation between them. The interpretation of this finding speaks rather for a common aetiological basis for at least part of the syndromes. Not only the correlations between the amount of positive and negative symptoms at the same time point demonstrate an association between them but also the mostly positive correlations between earlier and later negative and positive symptoms.

The parallel development of the syndromes supports the assumption of Huber (1983) and Janzarik (1968) of "schizophrenic basic symptoms" or the "preceding defect". On the other hand, surprisingly, it does not confirm one of the central statements of classic psychiatry made by Kraepelin that negative features do not develop over the long-term course to the maximum value but rather during the acute episode. After a very long course – which needs to be replicated in a prospective longitudinal study – negative symptomatology seems to decline while positive one increases or at least persists. It is only for an intermediate course over 5 years that Maurer and Häfner (this volume) found some evidence for the schizophrenic defect.

Whether depressive symptoms – regarded as the earliest signs, on average more than 5 years prior to first admission – are a predictor of the psychosis or only an unspecific consequence of frequent pre-morbid abnormalities cannot be answered here. But the early occurrence of negative symptoms and impairments casts a light on studies of the predictive value of pre-morbid social adjustment and other behavioural, emotional and cognitive parameters, when assessed retrospectively at the time point of first hospitalisation. These studies take a risk in validating the late course by data from the early course. Presumably, the essential source of the predictive power of pre-morbid measures as reported in many studies must be attributed to the negative syndrome or be very close to it, because this syndrome influences later-occurring negative symptoms, social outcome and partially positive symptomatology as well. The much lower predictive power of positive symptoms (see Schubart et al. 1987) for later core symptoms of schizophrenia and above all for negative symptoms and social outcome leads to the assumption that the core symptomatology is the – unfortunately mostly unspecific – negative syndrome. This is apparently supported by the fact that the negative symptomatology on average precedes the positive symptomatology by several years and will together with the acute syndrome increase exponentially before the first hospital admission. This interpretation is by no means imperative, however, as the further course does not support the classic hypothesis of Kraepelin's progressive defect. As for many diseases, it could be that schizophrenia begins with a mainly lengthy, unspecific, prodromal phase. The later-occurring positive symptoms seem to be characteristic but have no clear relation to the severity of the disease. Therefore, they have predictive power for the persistence or reappearence of this illness but not for measures of course and outcome that correlate with the severity of the disease. These latter obviously will be better predicted – similar to some physical diseases – by the unspecific negative syndrome, provided the illness is identified by characteristic, positive symptoms.

Acknowledgements. The part of the study concerning the early development of schizophrenia was conducted in the Sonderforschungsbereich 258 (SFB 258) "Indikatoren und Risikomodelle für Entstehung und Verlauf psychischer Störungen" (University of Heidelberg) with financial support from the Deutsche Forschungsgemeinschaft (DFG). We thank B. Fätkenheuer and W. Löffler for preparing the IRAOS-data and conducting the statistical analysis of this instrument.

References

Achté K (1967) On prognosis and rehabilitation in schizophrenia and paranoid psychosis. A comparative follow-up study of two series of patients first admitted to hospital in 1950 and 1960 respectively. Acta Psychiatr Scand [Suppl] 196

Andreasen NC (1981) Scale for the assessment of negative symptoms (SANS). University of Iowa, Iowa City

Andreasen NC (1982) Negative symptoms in schizophrenia. Arch Gen Psychiatry 39:784–788

Andreasen NC (1985) The broken brain. Harper and Row, New York

Andreasen NC, Olsen S (1982) Negative vs. positive schizophrenia. Arch Gen Psychiatry 39:789–794

Andreasen NC, Smith NR, Jacoby CG, Dennert JW, Olsen SA (1982) Ventricular enlargement in schizophrenia: definition and prevalence. Am J Psychiatry 139:292–296

Arbeitsgemeinschaft für Methodik und Dokumentation in der Psychiatrie (1983) Das AMDP-System. Manual zur Dokumentation psychischer Befunde, 4th edn. Springer, Berlin Heidelberg New York

Astrup C, Noreik K (1966) Functional psychoses: diagnostic and prognostic models. Thomas, Springfield

Biehl H, Maurer K, Schubart C, Krumm B, Jung E (1986) Prediction of outcome and utilization of medical services in a prospective study of first onset schizophrenics. Eur Arch Psychiatry Neurol Sci 236:139–147

Biehl H, Maurer K, Jung E, Krüger G, Bauer-Schubart C (1988) Reported symptoms in schizophrenic patients within five years of the onset of illness. In: Dencker SJ, Kulhanek F (eds) (1988) Treatment resistance in schizophrenia: an approach for research and clinical routine together with a reconnaissance paper. Vieweg, Braunschweig

Biehl H, Maurer K, Jung E, Krumm B (1989) The WHO psychological impairments rating schedule (WHO/PIRS). II. Impairments in schizophrenics in cross-sectional and longitudinal perspective – the Mannheim experience in two independent samples. Br J Psychiatry [Suppl 7] 155:71–77

Bilder RM, Mukherjee S, Rieder RO, Pandurangi AK (1985) Symptomatic and neuropsychological components of defect states. Schizophr Bull 11:409–419

Cannon-Spoor HE, Potkin SG, Wyatt RJ (1982) Measurement of premorbid adjustment in chronic schizophrenia. Schizophr Bull 8:470–484

Carpenter WT, Heinrich DW, Wageman AMI (1988) Deficit and nondeficit forms of schizophrenia: the concept. Am J Psychiatry 195:578–583

Chapman LJ, Chapman JP, Raulin ML, Edell WS (1978) Schizotypy and thought disorder as a high risk approach to schizophrenia. In: Serban G (ed) Cognitive defects in the development of mental illness. Bruner/Mazel, New York
Ciompi L (1980) The natural history of schizophrenia in the long term. Br J Psychiatry 136:413–420
Crow TJ (1980a) Molecular pathology of schizophrenia: more than one disease process. Br Med J 260:66–68
Crow TJ (1980b) Positive and negative schizophrenic symptoms and the role of dopamine. Br J Psychiatry 137:383–386
Crow TJ (1985) The two syndrome concept: origins and current status. Schizophr Bull 11:471–486
Endicott J, Spitzer RLA (1978) A diagnostic interview. The schedule for affective disorders and schizophrenia. Arch Gen Psychiatry 35:837–844
Færgeman PM (1945) Psychogenic psychoses (in Danish). Munksgaard, Copenhagen
Farmer AE, McGuffin P, Spitznagel E (1983) Heterogeneity in schizophrenia. A cluster analytic approach. Psychiatry Res 8:1–12
Farmer AE, McGuffin P, Gottesman II (1984) Searching for the split in schizophrenia: a twin study perspective. Psychiatry Res 13:109–118
Fish F (1969) The diagnosis of acute schizophrenia. Instructions on the use of acute schizophrenia diagnostic checklist (ASDC). Psychiatr Q 43:35–45
Fish TJ (1962) Schizophrenia. Williams and Wilkins, Baltimore
Gittelman-Klein R, Klein DF (1969) Premorbid asocial adjustment and prognosis in schizophrenia. J Psychiatr Res 7:35–53
Gross G (1985) Bonner Untersuchungsinstrument zur standardisierten Erhebung und Dokumentation von Basissymptomen (BSABS). In: Huber G (ed) Basisstadien endogener Psychosen und das Borderline-Problem. Schattauer, Stuttgart
Häfner H, Riecher A, Maurer K, Meissner S, Schmidtke A, Fätkenheuer B, Löffler W, an der Heiden W (1990) Ein Instrument zur retrospektiven Einschätzung des Erkrankungsbeginns bei Schizophrenie (Instrument for the retrospective assessment of the onset of schizophrenia – "IRAOS") – Entwicklung und erste Ergebnisse. Z Klin Psychol 19: 230–255
Hirsch SR (1982) Depression "revealed" in schizophrenia. Br J Psychiatry 140:421–423
Hirsch SR, Jolley AG (1989) The dysphoric syndrome in schizophrenia and its implications for relapse. Br J Psychiatry 155:46–50
Huber G (1983) Das Konzept substratnaher Baisissymptome und seine Bedeutung für Theorie und Therapie schizophrener Erkrankungen. Nervenarzt 54:23–32
Huber G, Gross R, Schüttler R (1979) Schizophrenie. Eine verlaufs- und sozialpsychiatrische Langzeitstudie, Springer, Berlin Heidelberg New York
Isele R, Merz J, Malzacher M, Angst J (1985) Social disability in schizophrenia: the controlled prospective Burghölzli study. II. Premorbid living situation and social adjustment - comparison with a normal control sample. Eur Arch Psychiatry Neurol Sci 234:348–356
Jablensky A, Schwarz R, Tomov T (1980) WHO collaborative study on impairments and disabilities associated with schizophrenic disorders. Acta Psychiatr Scand [Suppl 285] 62:152–163
Jackson JH (1889) On postepileptic states: a contribution to the comparative study of insanities. J Ment Sci 34:490–500
Janzarik W (1968) Schizophrene Verläufe. Springer, Berlin Heidelberg New York
Jung E, Krumm B, Biehl H, Maurer K, Bauer-Schubart C (1989) DAS-M: Mannheimer Skala zur Einschätzung sozialer Behinderung. Beltz, Weinheim
Kay SR, Opler LA, Fiszbein A (1986) Significance of positive and negative syndromes in chronic schizophrenia. Br J Psychiatry 149:439–448
Kraepelin E (1909–1915) Psychiatrie, vols 1–4, 8th edn. Barth, Leipzig
Krumm B, an der Heiden W, Biehl H, Ditton U (1990) Die schizophrene Episode. Ein einfaches mathematisches Modell. Z Klin Psychol (submitted)
Langer H, Oldigs J, Rey ER (1985) Vorstellung und Analyse einer empirisch begründeten Itemselektion von Fragebögen zur Erfassung subjektiv erlebter Störungen der Schizo-

phrenie. In: Hehl FJ, Ebel VP, Ruck VP (eds) Diagnostik psychischer und psychophysiologischer Störungen, Deutscher Psychologen-Verlag, Bonn, pp 112–153
Langfeldt G (1937) The prognosis in schizophrenia and the factors influencing the course of the disease. Melford, London
Langfeldt G (1939) The schizophreniform states. Munksgaard, Copenhagen
Lenzenweger MF, Dworkin RH, Wethington E (1989) Models of positive and negative symptoms in schizophrenia: an empirical evaluation of latent structures. J Abnorm Psychol 98:62–70
Lewine RRJ, Fogg L, Meltzer HY (1983) Assessment of negative and positive symptoms in schizophrenia. Schizophr Bull 9:368–376
Lewine S (1984) Frontal lobe dysfunction in schizophrenia. II. Impairments of psychological and brain functions. J Psychiatr Res 14:241–253
Lewis SW, Murray RM (1987) Obstetric complications, neurodevelopmental deviance and risk of schizophrenia. J Psychiatr Res 21:413–421
Lewis SW, Murray RM, Owen M (1988) Obstetric complications in schizophrenia, methodology and mechanisms. In: Tamminga CA, Schulz SC (eds) Schizophrenia, a scientific focus. Oxford University Press, Oxford
Liddle PF (1987) The symptoms of chronic schizophrenia: a reexamination of the positive-negative dichotomy. Br J Psychiatry 151:145–151
Maurer K, Biehl H (1991) Models for the development of symptomatology and course of schizophrenia. In: Häfner H, Gattaz WF (eds) Search for the causes of schizophrenia II. Springer, Berlin Heidelberg New York, pp 77–93
Maurer K, Biehl H, Kühner C, Löffler W (1989) On the way to expert systems. Comparing DSM-III computer diagnoses with CATEGO (ICD) diagnoses in depressive and schizophrenic patients. Eur Arch Psychiatry Neurol Sci 239:127–132
McGuffin P (1991) Models of heritability and genetic transmission. In: Häfner H, Gattaz WF (eds) Search for the causes of schizophrenia II. Springer, Berlin Heidelberg New York, pp 109–125
McGuffin P, Farmer AE, Gottesman II (1987) Modern diagnostic criteria and genetic studies of schizophrenia. In: Häfner H, Gattaz WF, Janzarik W (eds) Search for the causes of schizophrenia I. Springer, Berlin Heidelberg New York, pp 143–156
McNeil TF (1988) Obstetric factors and perinatal injuries. In: Nasrallah HA (ed) Handbook of schizophrenia, vol 3. Elsevier, Amsterdam, pp 319–344
Nimgaonkar VL, Wessely S, Murray RM (1988) Prevalence of familiality, obstetric complications and structural brain damage in schizophrenic patients. Br J Psychiatry 153: 191–197
Noreik K, Ödegaard Ö (1967) Age at onset of schizophrenia in relation to socio-economic factors. Br J Soc Psychiatry 1:243–249
Noreik K, Astrup C, Dalgaard OS, Holmboe R (1967) A prolonged follow-up of acute schizophrenic and schizophreniform psychoses. Acta Psychiatr Scand 43:432–443
Nuechterlein KH, Dawson ME, Ventura J, Fogelson D, Gitlin M, Mintz J (1991) Testing vulnerability models: Stability of Potential Vulnerability Indicators Across Clinical State. In: Häfner H, Gattaz WF (eds) Search for the causes of schizophrenia II. Springer, Berlin Heidelberg New York, pp 177–191
O'Callaghan E, Larkin C, Waddington IC (1988) Clinical correlates of obstetric complications in schizophrenia. Schizophr Res 1:125
Olbrich RK, Strauss E (1988) Prospektive Verlaufsuntersuchungen zur Schizophrenie seit dem 2. Weltkrieg: Eine Literaturrecherche. In: Olbrich RK (ed) Prospektive Verlaufsforschung in der Psychiatrie. Springer, Berlin Heidelberg New York, pp 11–19
Overall JE, Gorham DR (1962) The brief psychiatric rating scale. Psychol Rep 10:799–812
Owen MJ, Lewis SW, Murray RM (1988) Obstetric complications and schizophrenia: a computo-tomographic study. Psychol Med 18:331–339
Owen MJ, Lewis SW, Murray RM (1989) Family history and cerebral ventricular enlargement in schizophrenia. A case control study. Br J Psychiatry 154:629–634
Platt S, Weyman A, Hirsch S, Hewett S (1980) The social behaviour assessment schedule (SBAS): rationale, contents, scoring and reliability of a new interview schedule. Soc Psychiatry 15:43–55

Reynolds JR (1858) On the pathology of convulsions, with special reference to those of children. Liverpool Med Chir J 2:1–14
Rodnick EH, Goldstein MJ (1974) Premorbid adjustment and the recovery of mothering function in acute schizophrenic women. J Abnorm Psychol 83:623–628
Salokangas RK (1978) Psychosocial prognosis in schizophrenia. Turun Yliopisto, Turku
Schubart C, Krumm B, Biehl H, Maurer K, Jung E (1987) Factors influencing the course and outcome of symptomatology and social adjustment in first-onset schizophrenics. In: Häfner H, Gattaz WF, Janzarik W (eds) Search for the causes of schizophrenia I. Springer, Berlin Heidelberg New York, pp 98–106
Straube ER (1980) Reduced reactivity in psychopathology – examples from research in schizophrenia. In: Koukkou M, Lehmann D, Angst J (eds) Functional states of the brain: their determinants. Elsevier, Amsterdam
Strauss JS (1987) Processes of healing and chronicity in schizophrenia. In: Häfner H, Gattaz WF, Janzarik W (eds) Search for the causes in schizophrenia I. Springer, Berlin Heidelberg New York, pp 75–87
Strauss JS, Carpenter WT (1974) The prediction of outcome in schizophrenia. Arch Gen Psychiatry 31:37–42
Strauss JS, Carpenter WT, Bartko JJ (1974) The diagnosis and understanding of schizophrenia. III. Speculations on the processes that underlie schizophrenic symptoms and signs. Schizophr Bull 11:61–69
Süllwold L (1977) Symptome schizophrener Erkrankungen. Springer, Berlin Heidelberg New York
Süllwold L (1981) Basisstörungen: Ergebnisse und offene Fragen. In: Huber G (ed) Schizophrenie: Stand und Entwicklungstendenzen der Forschung. Schattauer, Stuttgart
Thurm I, Häfner H (1987) Perceived vulnerability, relapse risk and coping in schizophrenia. An explorative study. Eur Arch Psychiatry Neurol Sci 237:46–53
Tsuang MT, Winokur G (1974) Criteria for sub-typing schizophrenia. Arch Gen Psychiatry 31:43–47
van Kammen DP, Peters J, Yao J, van Kammen WB, Neylan T, Shaw D, Linnoila M (1990) Norepinephrene in acute exacerbations of chronic schizophrenia. Arch Gen Psychiatry 47:161–168
van Kammen DP, van Kammen WB, Peters J, Goetz K, Neylan T (1988) Decreased slow wave sleep and enlarged lateral ventricles in schizophrenia. Neuropsychopharmacology 1:265–271
von Zerssen D, Koeller DM (1976) Klinische Selbstbeurteilungs-Skalen (KSb-S) aus dem Münchener Psychiatrischen Informations-System (PSY-CHIS München). Manuale. Beltz, Weinheim
Weinberger DR (1987) Implications of normal brain development for the pathogenesis of schizophrenia. Arch Gen Psychiatry 44:660–669
Weinberger DR (1991) Brain anatomy in schizophrenia: discussion. In: Häfner H, Gattaz WF (eds) Search for the causes of schizophrenia II. Springer, Berlin Heidelberg New York, pp 275–281
Wing JK (1975) Impairments in schizophrenia. In: Wist R, Winokur G, Roff M (eds) Life history research in psychopathology, vol 4. University of Minnesota Press, Minneapolis
Wing JK, Brown GW (1970) Institutionalism in schizophrenia. Cambridge University Press, London
Wing JK, Cooper JE, Sartorius N (1973) Present state examination (PSE). Medical Research Council, Cambridge University Press, London
Wing JK, Cooper JE, Sartorius N (1974) The measurement and classification of psychiatric symptoms. Cambridge University Press, Cambridge
World Health Organization (ed) (1973) The international pilot study of schizophrenia, vol 1. WHO, Geneva
World Health Organization (ed) (1978) Psychiatric and personal history schedule. WHO, Geneva (5365 MNH)
World Health Organization (ed) (1988) Psychiatric disability assessment schedule (WHO/DAS). WHO, Geneva

Dependence, Independence or Interdependence of Positive and Negative Symptoms

K. MAURER and H. HÄFNER [1]

Present Studies Concerning the Correlations of Positive and Negative Symptoms

Concerning the correlations of positive and negative symptoms of schizophrenia, three competing hypotheses exist, i.e. the severity-liability model of Gottesman et al. (1987) assuming positive associations between the two syndromes, Andreasen's one-dimensional, bipolar model (Andreasen and Olsen 1982) with negatively correlated dimensions and Crow's (1980, 1985) independency or dual-process model. Lenzenweger's confirmatory factor analysis (Lenzenweger et al. 1989) about the goodness-of-fit of empirical data of 220 patients corresponds best with Crow's dual-process model. Andreasen's model of a bipolar dimension with factor loadings of opposite signs of positive and negative symptoms could not be confirmed.

Kay et al. (1986a) are right in saying that most studies about the positive-negative dichotomy of schizophrenia "have generally been limited by small samples, unstandardised rating methods, lack of long range follow-up, and no control for extrapyramidal drug side-effect" (p. 439). According to the correlation of positive and negative scores Kay et al. (1986a) found that "the positive and negative scales have a modest but significant inter-relationship (Pearson's $r = +0.27$, $p < 0.01$)" (p. 442).

Lindenmayer et al. (1986) carried out a follow-up with 19 of 37 schizophrenic patients 2 years after the index study. The Pearson's correlation coefficients between positive and negative symptoms were not significant either at index measurement ($r = -0.04$ for the whole group and $r = 0.11$ for the follow-up sample) or at second follow-up ($r = 0.29$). According to the opinion of Lindenmayer et al. (1986), these results support the position that both syndromes have no direct association. Nevertheless, the relationship at the second follow-up can also be understood as a low positive correlation, as found by others (e.g. Kay et al. 1986a), which could not reach statistical significance due to the small sample size. Lewine et al. (1983), selecting their items by the Rasch scaling technique with existing instruments in order to determine positive and negative symptoms, could not prove a correlation between the scores. This might also be due to the method used for scaling which leads to

[1] Zentralinstitut für Seelische Gesundheit, Postfach 122120, J 5, W-6800 Mannheim, FRG

A. Marneros / N. C. Andreasen / M. T. Tsuang (Eds.)
Negative Versus Positive Schizophrenia

homogeneity: symptoms which could correspond with both syndromes have a reduced chance of being considered by this technique of scale construction. Lewine et al. (1983) also interpret the result of uncorrelated symptom dimensions in correspondence with the hypothesis that positive and negative schizophrenia are two independent processes (Strauss and Carpenter 1974; Crow 1980).

Some factor analytic studies also support the hypothesis of independence: if a principal component analysis is done with a pool of positive and negative items of schizophrenia, several independent factors are found in most cases, one of which shows a high number of acute-psychotic (positive) symptom loadings, another a correspondingly high number of negative symptoms. Bilder et al. (1985), Liddle (1987) and Biehl et al. (1988) give examples for this procedure.

Bilder et al. (1985) operationalised positive symptomatology by the Schedule for Affective Disorders and Schizophrenia (SADS; Endicott and Spitzer 1978) and negative symptomatology by the Scale for the Assessment of Negative Symptoms (SANS; Andreasen 1981). The sample consisted of 32 consecutively hospitalised schizophrenic patients. Most of the positive symptoms were correlated as well as the negative ones. With the exception of the positive correlations between alogia and attentional impairment with bizarre behaviour and positive formal thought disorders, the symptoms of both syndromes were not correlated. The authors stated explicitly that "There were no significant ($p < 0.05$) negative correlations between positive and negative symptoms" (p. 413), which is in contrast to the bipolarity model of Andreasen and Olsen (1982). The factor analysis leads to three factors: the first has high loadings of items of both syndromes, the second has loadings of negative symptoms and the third, of positive symptoms. Liddle (1987) carried out a study with 40 schizophrenic patients and made independent factor analyses with the data received from the Present State Examination (PSE; Wing et al. 1974), Comprehensive Assessment of Symptoms and History (CASH; Andreasen 1983) and SANS (Andreasen 1981). In each factors arose which could be interpreted as "psychomotoric poverty syndrome", "disorganisation syndrome" and "reality distortion syndrome".

In an extensive review of the literature concerning negative symptoms in schizophrenia, Pogue-Geile and Zubin (1988) came to the conclusion that in most studies dealing with the question of dependence or independence of positive and negative symptoms, independence of both dimensions was found at least for cross-sectional measurements, because no significant correlations between the scales could be demonstrated.

Operationalisation of Positive and Negative Symptoms by Research Instruments Applied in the WHO Schizophrenia Studies

The following results on the course of positive and negative symptoms and the dependence vs. independence of these syndromes are based on data of the

World Health Organization (WHO) Disability Study. Seven WHO collaborative centres participated in this study. One of them was Mannheim, assessing 7 cross-sectional measurements over 5 years with complete data of 62 schizophrenic patients from the 70 patients initially included. It is not necessary to go into more detail here, because the study is described in a series of publications by Schubart et al. (1986 a, b) and Biehl et al. (1986, 1988). It was fundamental to the design of the Disability Study to distinguish symptoms as reported by the patient, observable impairments (or "signs") and disabilities in social performance.

For these three levels of assessment:

- the PSE (Wing et al. 1974) was used to measure symptomatology.
- the Psychological Impairments Rating Schedule (PIRS); Biehl et al. 1989 a, b) was rated by the interviewer after the semistructured clinical PSE interview.
- the Disability Assessment Schedule (DAS; WHO 1988; Jung et al. 1989) was assessed after an interview with a key informant.

Concerning the question of measuring positive and negative symptoms as two well-defined syndromes of schizophrenia, it should be brought mind that the Disability Study "was initiated in 1977/78, before this duality had again become a main focus of attention in research" (Biehl et al. 1989 b, p. 71) by the attempts of Andreasen (1982), Andreasen and Olsen (1982) and Crow (1980, 1985).

For the data analysis, one important question was how to compress the available information to positive or negative syndromes and to what degree the main constructs of the study, symptomatology, impairment and disability, represent these syndromes.

How to Measure Negative Symptoms with the PSE?

Maurer (1990) suggested several possibilities to define negative schizophrenia based on PSE data. As the CATEGO programmme does not consider a special sub-score of negative symptoms and the "CATEGO residual syndrome" is too narrowly defined, the following attempts were tested (Table 1):

- To model several well-known scales of negative symptoms using PSE items.
- Factor analytical studies on PSE data identified a 3-factor solution. One factor was interpreted as a residual syndrome or negative-symptom factor (s. Häfner and Maurer, this volume, Table 1; Biehl et al. 1988).
- A DSM-III computer programmme was developed based on PSE data, supplemented by 22 additional DSM-III-specific items. Among other diagnoses, the algorithm evaluates sub-types of schizophrenia, including the "residual type" (Maurer et al. 1989), primarily marked by negative symptoms.

Table 1. Important instruments for the measurement of negative symptoms (according to Pogue-Geile and Zubin 1988) and the number of corresponding items in the Present State Examination, PSE (Wing et al. 1974)

Reference/scale	Number of items	Number contained in the PSE with comparable meaning
Venables (1957) Activity Withdrawal Scale	10	8
Wing (1961) Rating Scale for Chronic Schizophrenia	8	7
Overall and Gorham (1962) Brief Psychiatric Rating Scale	3	3
Krawiecka et al. (1977) Manchester Rating Scale	4	4
Abrams and Taylor (1978) Rating Scale for Emotional Blunting	3	3
Andreasen (1982) Scale for the Assessment of Negative Symptoms	21	9
Lewine et al. (1983) Schedule for Affective Disorders and Schizophrenia C	11	10
Pogue-Geile and Harrow (1984) Negative Symptom Behaviour Rating Scales	3	3
Iager et al. (1985) Negative Symptom Behaviour Rating Scale	10	4
Kay et al. (1987) Positive and Negative Syndrome Scale	7	4

How to Measure Negative Symptoms with the PIRS?

Biehl et al. (1989b) suggested an additive aggregation of 20 PIRS items to evaluate negative impairments in a score called "NESY". A corresponding score "POSY" for the positive syndrome was also defined (s. Häfner and Maurer, this volume, Table 2). More sophisticated statistical analyses on PIRS data were done by the WHO: a principal component analysis on the PIRS items of all cases ($n = 513$) of the first cross-section of the Disability Study with more than 10% of positive resulted in a first factor with 13 high item loadings, defined as "psychomotor inhibition factor". A 2-item factor was called "non-assertiveness". All items defining these factors are also included in the PIRS score (Biehl et al. 1989b).

How to Measure Negative Symptoms by the DAS?

With the exception of the DAS item "friction in inter-personal relationships", the items of the disability scale (section 1 which assesses general social behaviour and section 2 concerning specific social role performance) define a one-dimensional, homogenous scale of social deficiencies, according to aspects of the negative syndrome of schizophrenia, like deficits in self-care, underactivity, slowness, social withdrawal, loss of interest or poor work performance (WHO 1988; Jung et al. 1989).

An Attempt to Validate WHO Instruments to Assess Negative Symptoms

In a recent research project on gender differences in schizophrenic patients (Häfner et al. 1989, 1990; Riecher et al. 1989), besides the PSE, PIRS and DAS, the SANS was also assessed for quantifying negative symptoms by using a well-accepted scale. It is possible to validate the procedures and instruments described so far to measure negative symptoms and also to define a negative symptom score based on WHO instruments analogous to the SANS.

In a first step for each SANS item, corresponding PSE, PIRS or DAS items were selected. It was possible to find at least one corresponding item for 20 of the 21 SANS items. In a second step, by cross-tabulating SANS and PSE, PIRS and DAS items, the most corresponding one was selected (see Table 2).

Some 13 (65%) times an impairment (PIRS) had the closest relation to the SANS item, 4 times (20%) a reported symptom (PSE) and 3 times (15%) a social disability item (DAS). The agreement of the SANS item and the corresponding item was between 45% and 88%, and not acceptable discrepancies achieved a maximum of only 12%. The correlation coefficient of the additive overall value of negative symptoms derived from WHO research instruments with the SANS sum score was 0.60. For the section sum scores these correlations reached values of 0.82 for section 1 (affective flattening or blunting), and with the exception of section 5, which could not be adequately represented by WHO instruments, all correlations were larger than 0.55.

Therefore, it seems to be adequate to select items from different WHO instruments to build scores for positive and negative symptoms in a way comparable to those instruments specifically constructed for this purpose. For the following analysis, the additive PSE and PIRS scores introduced by Häfner and Maurer (this volume) are used to operationalise positive and negative symptoms.

Results of the Mannheim Disability Study

The following presentation of results of the Mannheim disability cohort firstly concentrates on the question of the dependence or independence of positive and negative symptoms measured cross-sectionally. After the determination of positive, negative and zero correlation coefficients for positive and negative symptoms and symptom scores, the frequency distribution of an overall symptom score is discussed as an indicator of two distinguishable schizophrenia sub-types.

For the sub-types positive, negative and mixed as suggested by Andreasen and Olsen (1982), the relative frequencies per cross-section and their stability

Table 2. Correspondence of items of WHO research instruments and SANS items

SANS items	Best correspondence		$P(\chi^2)$	Contingency coefficient	Agreement (%)	Disagreement (%)
	Instrument and item number	Item label				
Affective flattening or blunting						
Unchanging facial expression	PIRS 2.1.1	Reduced quantity of facial expression	***	0.63	70.7	0.8
Decreased spontaneous movements	PIRS 1.1.1[a]	Slowness and under-activity	***	0.57	63.0	1.5
Paucity of expressive gestures	PIRS 2.2.5	Abnormally limited use of gesture	***	0.40	67.4	5.4
Poor eye contact	PIRS 2.1.6[a]	Gaze avoidance	***	0.58	88.3	1.2
Affective non-responsivity	PIRS 2.3.6[a]	Blunted affect	***	0.57	74.0	2.2
Inappropriate affect	PIRS 2.3.7[a]	Incongruity of affect	***	0.50	88.3	1.2
Lack of vocal inflections	PIRS 2.4.3	Abnormally unmodulated expressionless and flat tone of voice	***	0.49	78.9	1.5
Alogia						
Poverty of speech	PIRS 2.4.10[a]	Restricted quantity of speech	***	0.59	88.0	0.4
Poverty of content of speech	PIRS 2.4.15[a]	Poverty of content of speech	***	0.41	85.0	1.5
Blocking	PIRS 1.2.3[a]	Blank spells	***	0.59	82.5	0.0
Increased latency of response	PIRS 1.1.3[a]	Slow speech	***	0.46	73.9	3.1

Table 2 (Continued)

SANS items	Best correspondence		$P(\chi^2)$	Contingency coefficient	Agreement (%)	Disagreement (%)
	Instrument and item number	Item label				
Avolition-apathy						
Grooming and hygiene	PIRS 2.5.1[a]	Self-neglect	***	0.62	80.2	0.8
Impersistence at work or school	DAS 2.7/2.8	Occupational role	***	0.45	55.6	11.1
Physical anergia	PSE 36	Subjective anergia and retardation	***	0.35	45.0	11.6
Anhedonia-asociality						
Recreational interests and activities	DAS 1.2	Under-activity	***	0.54	58.5	4.1
Sexual interest and activity	PSE 38	Loss of libido	***	0.45	58.0	9.4
Ability to feel intimacy and closeness	PSE 54	Lost emotions	**	0.26	52.0	11.1
Relationships with friends and peers	DAS 1.4	Social withdrawal	***	0.53	54.8	4.2
Attentional impairment						
Work and social inattentiveness	PSE 28	Social withdrawal	*	0.20	44.5	11.8
Inattentiveness during mental status testing	PIRS 1.2.1[a]	Distractability	***	0.28	60.2	6.8
Subjective complaints of inattentiveness	–	–	–	–	–	–

Significance level: * $P \leqq 0.05$; ** $P \leqq 0.01$; *** $P \leqq 0.001$.

[a] This item is also contained in the Present State Examination (PSE); SANS, Scale for the Assessment of Negative Symptoms.

over the course are determined. Additionally, a typical course pattern of negative symptoms derived from Crow's (1980, 1985) type I/type II distinction is tested.

As the stability of schizophrenia sub-types could not be proved, the positive and negative syndrome scores were analysed as two separate dimensions. Using this, a further correlational analysis demonstrated the dependencies of positive and negative symptoms over time. The course of a negative and positive symptom score over 5 years is interpreted in the view of Kraepelin's notion of a residual syndrome. Overall, it will be shown that the definition of sub-types is insufficient, whereas the use of two independently defined dimensions of the course leads to fewer difficulties of interpretation.

Relationship Between Positive and Negative Symptoms in Cross-Sectional Measurements

For the Mannheim data of the Disability Study, it can be stated that most positive and negative symptoms (see Biehl et al. 1988) are not correlated (Table 3). However, approximately one-third of the correlation coefficients deviates significantly from zero, 30% in the positive and only 3% in the negative direction. This result based on item level is also supported on the level of symptom scores (Table 4).

With the exception of the time point of inclusion, at which the syndromes are not correlated, for all the cross-sections low positive correlations between 0.22 and 0.41 resulted, which are statistically significant at least at the 5% level. A general trend of growing or step-wise reduction of the correlation coefficients over time could not be proved.

The operationalisation of syndromes at the level of impairments (see Biehl et al. 1989a, b) leads to a (not yet significant) reduction of the relationships.

Another indication for a relationship between positive and negative symptomatology is (as shown in Fig. 1) the fact that in cross-section all patients with acute symptomatology have a partially significantly higher occurrence of minus symptomatology than the non-acute probands.

Table 3. Number of significant positive, significant negative and non-significant correlations between 12 positive and 9 negative symptoms in 7 cross-sectional measurements

	Cross-section							Over all cross-sections
	1	2	3	4	5	6	7	
Positive correlations	31	45	34	41	32	34	12	229 (30.3%)
Zero correlations	73	63	71	65	73	73	87	505 (66.8%)
Negative correlations	4	0	3	2	3	1	9	22 (2.9%)

Table 4. Correlations of positive and negative schizophrenia scores in 7 cross-sectional measurements (WHO Disability Study, Mannheim centre, $n = 62$)

	Cross-sections						
	1	2	3	4	5	6	7
positive × negative symptoms	0.14	0.33**	0.25*	0.35**	0.22*	0.23*	0.41**
positive × negative impairments	−0.14	0.15	0.12	0.20•	0.10	0.20•	0.20•

Significance values for Pearson's correlation coefficients: • $P \leqq 0.10$; * $P \leqq 0.05$; ** $P \leqq 0.01$; *** $P \leqq 0.001$.

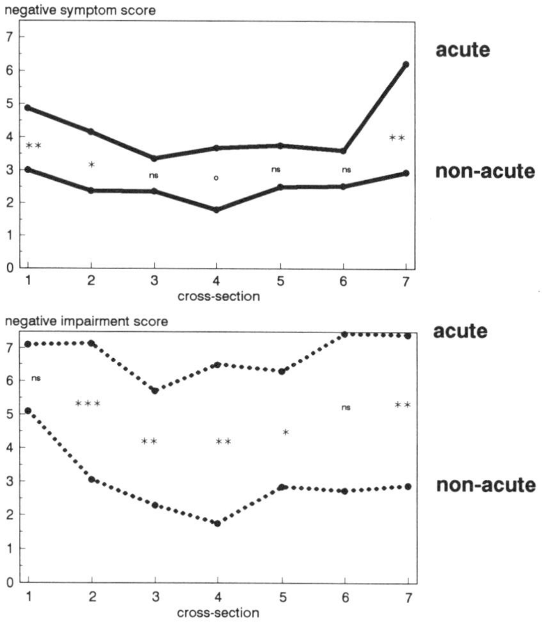

Fig. 1. Negative symptoms in acute and non-acute probands in seven cross-sectional measurements. Significance of t-values: *ns*, non-significant; *o*, $p < 0.10$; *, $p < 0.05$; **, $p < 0.01$; ***, $p < 0.001$

Due to the information missing between the cross-sections, it is impossible to decide by means of the cohort study whether the patients suffer only a temporary increase of their negative symptoms as a side-effect of the acute phase or whether constantly higher negative symptoms raise the risk for acute episodes in general.

Frequency Distributions of the Symptomatology Scores

If all negative symptoms were weighted negatively (weight = − 1), according to the model of negative correlated syndromes, the total sum of positive and negative symptom ratings should lead to a bimodal distribution. The purely positive sub-type would be characterised by high positive values, the purely negative one by high negative values, and in between we would expect the mixed types (see also Kay et al. 1986b), because negative and positive partial sums cancel each other.

From our data the bimodality of the distribution of symptom scores can only be insinuated (Fig. 2). As during the course a great part of the patients who belong to the mixed type had no symptoms, the calculations were made without them, which makes falsification of the model more difficult. Under this condition no bimodal distributions result. In fact, none was expected, because this model is based on negative correlations of the cross-sectional scores, which, as already shown, is not true for any of the 7 cross-sections.

Frequency and Stability of the Positive, Negative and Mixed Type over the Course

The differentiation of positive and negative schizophrenia is based on the idea that a schizophrenic patient belongs clearly to one of both types, perhaps with a more or less rough change during the course. After an acute episode, in which the patient suffers from the type I syndrome, the type II syndrome develops after remission. Andreasen and Olsen (1982) additionally introduce a mixed type to abolish the rigid dichotomy of this model. This category comprises those cases with both syndromes or when no symptoms appear at all. In their study 18 (35%) of the patients belong to the mixed, 16 (30%) to the negative and 18 (35%) to the positive type. If we take into consideration that the negative cases are not completely free of positive symptoms as well as that the positive ones can also have some negative symptoms, the classification into types seems to be somewhat arbitrary. Andreasen (1985) herself considers the mixed type as one of the unsolved problems, as is the stability of the types over the course. If types should vary considerably over time, this would bring into doubt the validity of the cross-sectionally derived classification.

Sub-dividing the sample into three groups may be correct for the clinical utilisation sample examined by Andreasen and Olsen (1982), in which each patient has probably been hospitalised because he or she suffered from a certain degree of symptoms. This classification was developed on the basis of cross-sectional measurements and needs validation in a longitudinal study. Using the Mannheim data of the WHO Disability Study we examined how the three subtypes are distributed over the 7 cross-sections. Furthermore, it must be evaluated whether a considerable proportion of the patients belongs to the "pure" types. Then the stability of the types during the course can be tested.

According to Andreasen and Olsen (1982) the patients are divided into negative, positive and mixed sub-types. In the following, the mixed type is distinguished into cases without any symptoms and those with remarkable symptoms in both dimensions. This seems to be adequate because it contributes to the separation of a favourable and an unfavourable sub-group.

Figure 3 shows that the "rest category" of the mixed type consists of more than 50% of the cases in each cross-section and that the purely positive type

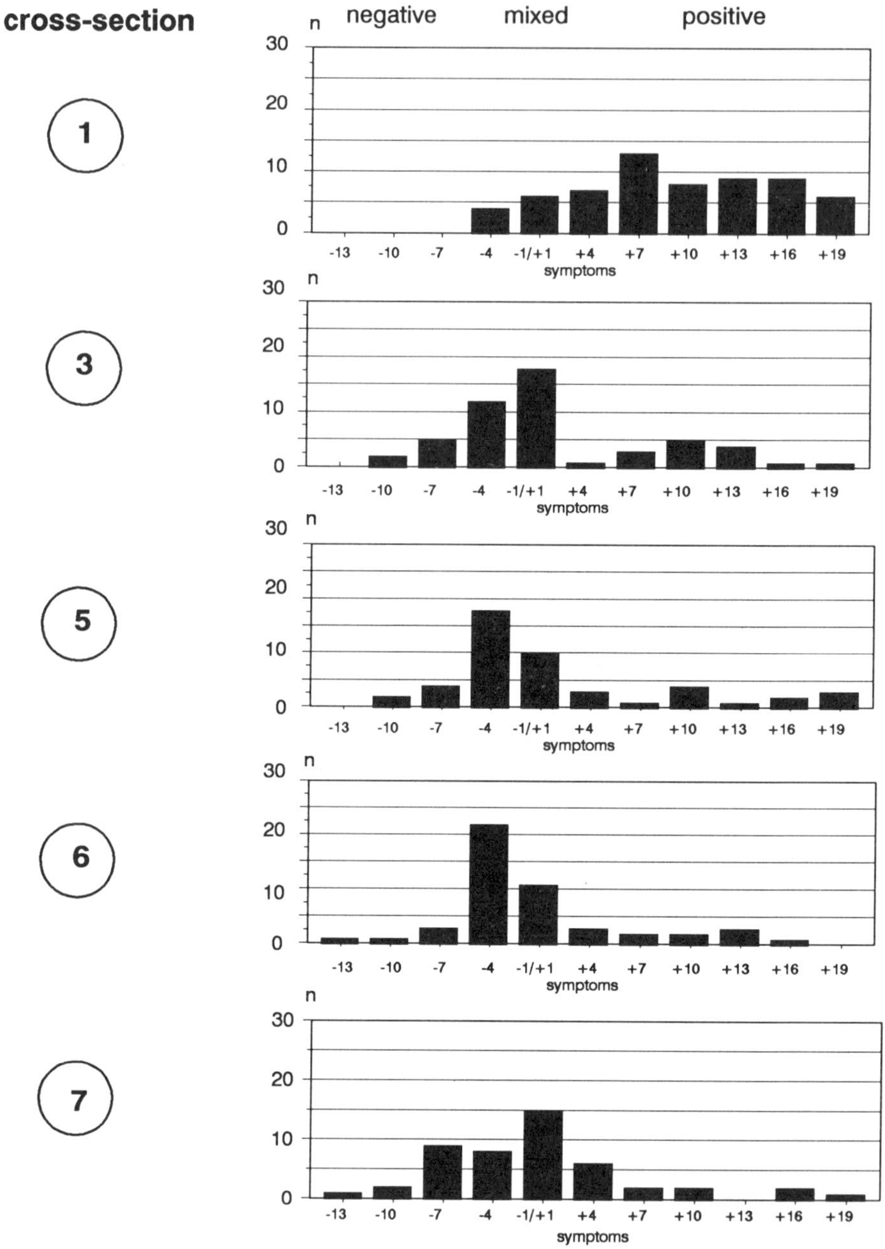

Fig. 2. Distribution of positive, negative and mixed schizophrenia over 5 years (test for "bimodality")

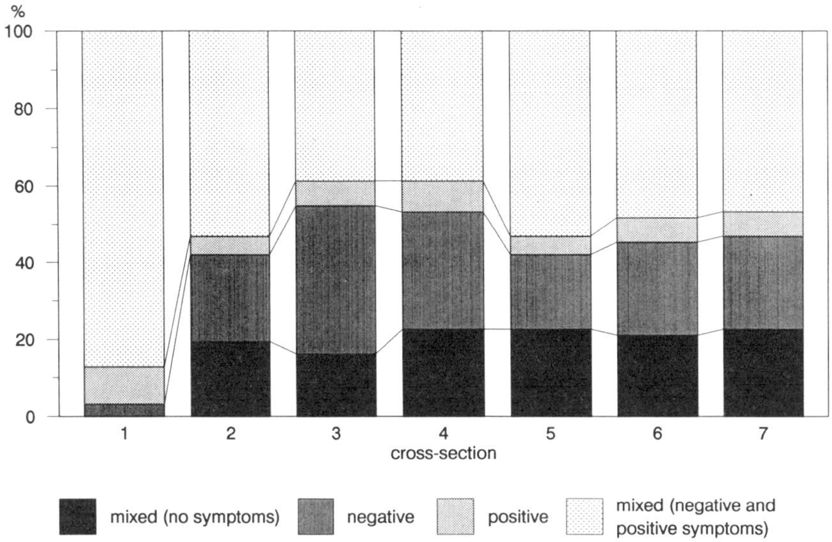

Fig. 3. Distribution of negative, positive and mixed types of schizophrenia in 7 cross-sectional measurements

appears extremely seldom, i.e. between 3 (4.8%) and 6 (9.7%) times per cross-section. The unfavourable mixed type with symptoms of both syndromes defines the modal class in all cross-sections. If the justification of a syndrome needs more than only one typical symptom, it is useful to presume a certain number of positive or negative symptoms before the application of a classification rule. The introduction of such threshold values leads to a significant increase of the positive type at the beginning but overall to no clear change of the percentage of pure types. Only the proportion of mixed types without considerable symptomatology increases, at the cost of a corresponding reduction of the unfavourable mixed type.

Also, the stability of the types from one point of measurement to the next is not sufficiently high (Fig. 4): the highest conditional probability, always over 50%, is found for the unfavourable mixed type. After the 4 cross-section the stability for the favourable mixed type also reaches at least 50%. The instability of the purely positive type is compatible with short episodes, but it contradicts the idea of stable types during the course. However, due to the small sample size of the positive sub-type no further conclusions should be drawn. If a threshold is introduced, allowing patients with a small number of symptoms not to be categorized into the pure or unfavourable sub-types, an improvement of stability values is seen, but it is insufficient.

As the stability of the sub-types was weak from one cross-section to the next, an attempt was made to classify the patients on the basis of an interval of 1 year in the early phase and to see whether this classification remained stable for the later phase of the course, from the 2- to the 5-year follow-up. This typology was based on the following classification rules. Patients who at 1 of the 3 time

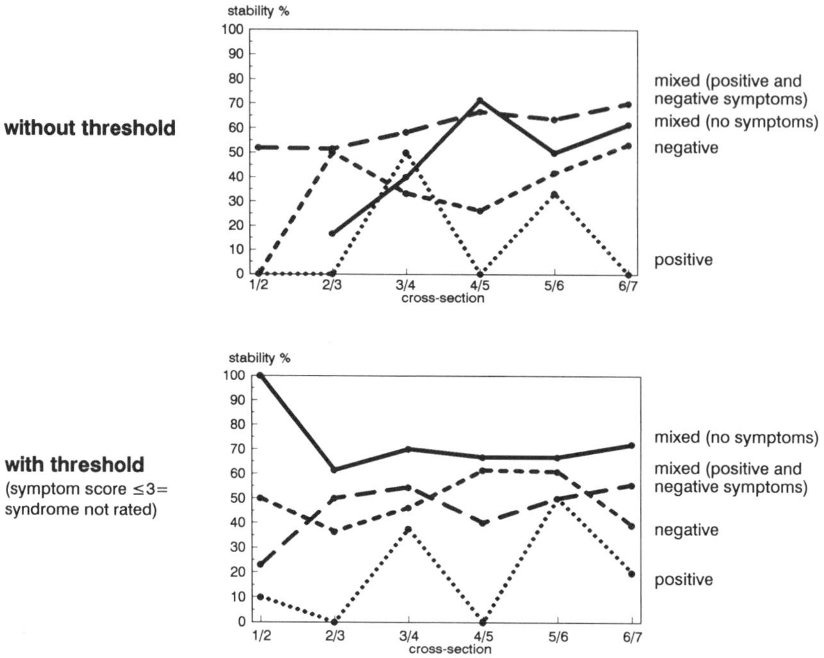

Fig. 4. Stability of positive, negative and mixed types over 5 years

Table 5. Stability of positive, negative and mixed schizophrenia from an early to a late phase of the course

Type	Early phase (6–18 months)		Stability		Late phase (24–60 months)	
	n	(%)	*n*	(%)	*n*	(%)
Without threshold						
Mixed (no symptoms)	9	14.5	5	55.6	13	21.0
Negative	23	37.1	7	30.4	15	24.2
Positive	4	6.5	1	25.0	4	6.5
Mixed (positive and negative)	26	41.9	20	76.9	30	48.4
With threshold						
Mixed (no symptoms)	36	58.1	22	61.1	28	45.2
Negative	11	17.7	7	63.6	23	37.1
Positive	4	6.5	1	25.0	3	4.8
Mixed (positive and negative)	11	17.7	4	36.4	8	12.9

points have mostly positive or negative symptoms belong to the favourable mixed type, while patients who are disturbed in both dimensions in 2 or 3 of the cross-sections belong to the unfavourable mixed type. Patients with disturbances in only one dimension at 2 or 3 time points form the group of the purely "positive" or "negative" types.

Table 5 shows the distribution of the types in an early and a late phase of the study. This distribution could be influenced by the construct (symptomatology or impairment) used and by possible threshold values for the definition of positive and negative syndromes in the cross-section. One important result not affected by these factors is the rare occurrence of the positive sub-type. The pure types, essential for the bipolar model, consist of less than 50% of patients. They are less stable than the mixed types. Only 30% of the negative sub-type in the early phase still belongs to this type in the second part of the study. For the positive sub-type this proportion is even smaller. Only for the unfavourable mixed type is the stability over 75%. Taking into consideration a threshold value for the classification of types, the stability of negative schizophrenia is improved but at the expense of a reduced stability of the unfavourable mixed type.

To sum up, the stability test questions the validity of sub-types derived in cross-sectional measurement because they are not sufficiently stable, and the proportion of cases belonging to the "purely" positive and negative categories were much too low.

Are Negative Symptoms Stable over the Course?

One essential aspect of Crow's model of type I/type II schizophrenia is the irreversibility of negative symptoms, because they are understood to be a behavioural correlate of degenerative processes in the brain (Crow 1980, 1985). On this basis, a specific pattern of negative symptoms in successive measurements should be identifiable (Table 6).

Once negative symptoms have occurred, they should be demonstrable at all the following time points. A patient with negative symptoms beginning in the 3rd cross-section and lasting until the end of the study is considered a consistent case. If the disturbance is present only from the 3rd to the 5th cross-section and not in the 6th one, this would be an inconsistent pattern.

Table 6. Examples of consistent and inconsistent course patterns of negative symptoms concerning Crow's (1980, 1985) type I/type II model

	Cross-sections						
	1	2	3	4	5	6	7
Consistent pattern	0	0	1	1	1	1	1
Inconsistent pattern	0	0	1	1	0	0	1

0, no negative symptoms; 1, negative symptoms.

Table 7. Percentage of patients with consistent (type II) course patterns of negative symptoms

	Without threshold	Negative symptom score ≧ 3	Negative symptom score ≧ 5
All cross-sections			
Consistent patterns	35.5	4.8	9.7
Inconsistent patterns	65.5	92.0	64.5
No negative symptoms/ below threshold	0.0	3.2	25.5
Without first cross-section			
Consistent patterns	48.4	21.0	16.1
Inconsistent patterns	51.6	70.9	40.4
No negative symptoms/ below threshold	0.0	8.1	43.5

For patients of the Disability Study it was tested whether or not the course pattern conformed to this model (Table 7). The result of calculating the proportion of conformity is disappointing. Inconsistent course patterns are clearly more frequent than consistent ones. This result is not influenced by defining negative schizophrenia by reported symptoms or observed impairments. If Crow's model is tested independently from the amount of the negative symptoms, we find two-thirds of courses are inconsistent. Among the consistent patterns, nearly 80% belong to the sub-group with negative symptoms in all 7 cross-sections.

This procedure can be criticised because a negative syndrome should include more than just one symptom. Therefore, the analysis was repeated for different threshold values, but the result was not improved: in more than 90% with the low threshold inconsistent patterns resulted, and using the higher threshold value did not change the proportion of inconsistent patterns at all, while the proportion of consistent patterns decreased to less than 10%. If the 1st cross-section, in which nearly all patients have both positive and negative symptoms, is not taken into consideration, then the proportion of consistent patterns increases, but it is still lower than the proportion of inconsistent ones.

Does this analysis disprove Crow's model? Crow (1985) attributes a higher value to primary negative symptoms, which occur as a consequence of structural changes in the brain, than to secondary ones, which are due to other conditions and may be remittent. Unfortunately, we do not find any difference between primary and secondary negative symptoms on the basis of psychopathology in the article of Carpenter et al. (1985), except when considering causal conditions. Therefore, should a secondary form of negative symptoms always be presumed when inconsistencies of Crow's model are observed, when there are no computed tomography data? Furthermore, a 5-year follow-up may be too short to lead to a schizophrenic defect, which can also be concluded by Crow's (1985) hint to Huber's longitudinal study of the course (Huber et al. 1979).

Table 8. Correlations within negative and positive symptom scores over 7 time points

	Negative Cross-section						
Negative	1	2	3	4	5	6	7
Cross-section 1		–	–	–	–	–	–
2			0.40***	0.49***	0.30**	0.21•	0.31**
3				0.61***	0.56***	–	0.35*
4					0.58***	–	0.22*
5						0.32**	0.31**
6							0.39**
7							
	Positive Cross-section						
Positive	1	2	3	4	5	6	7
Cross-section 1		–	–	–	–	0.25*	–
2			0.46***	0.27*	0.25*	–	–
3				0.37***	0.41***	0.18•	–
4					0.38***	–	0.24*
5						0.34**	–
6							0.21•
7							

Significance levels of Pearson's correlation coefficients: •, $P \leqq 0.10$; *, $P \leqq 0.05$; **, $P \leqq 0.01$; ***, $P \leqq 0.001$.

Relationship of Positive and Negative Symptoms over the Course

The results concerning the question of dependence or independence of positive and negative symptoms suggest – as already shown – low but significant correlations. This is based on cross-sectional measurements. If we have to distinguish sub-types of positive and negative schizophrenia, earlier negative symptoms should correlate with later ones, and the same relation must be true for positive symptoms. If the two forms of schizophrenia influence each other, early negative symptoms must predict late positive symptoms and vice versa (Table 8).

Negative symptoms at the beginning do not show any significant correlation with later negative symptomatology, but the time point half a year after

Table 9. Correlations between negative and positive symptoms over 7 time points

	Positive Cross-section						
Negative	1	2	3	4	5	6	7
Cross-section 1		—	0.31**	—	0.36**	—	—
2			$0.20^{\bullet}$	0.34**	0.24*	0.21*	0.22**
3				—	0.18*	—	—
4					0.25*	0.24*	—
5						—	—
6							$0.18^{\bullet}$
7							

	Negative Cross-section						
Positive	1	2	3	4	5	6	7
Cross-section 1		—	—	—	$-0.17^{\bullet}$		$-0.20^{\bullet}$
2			—	0.23	—	—	—
3				0.27*	0.17*	—	0.25*
4					0.29**	—	—
5						$0.20^{\bullet}$	—
6							—
7							

Significance levels of Pearson's correlation coefficients: $^{\bullet}$, $P \leqq 0.10$; *, $P \leqq 0.05$; **, $P \leqq 0.01$; ***, $P \leqq 0.001$.

inclusion is most important: the negative symptoms measured here show significant correlations with later negative symptoms and positive symptoms as well. Negative symptoms 5 years after onset are positively related to all earlier measurements of negative symptoms beginning with the half-year follow-up. With increasing intervals between measurements the significance level decreases. Significant correlations also can be demonstrated between positive symptoms; in most cases, however, they are lower and less significant than for negative symptoms.

Table 9 demonstrates that negative symptoms at the beginning correlate with positive symptoms 1 and 2 years later. Negative symptoms at the half-year follow-up correlate with positive symptoms at each following time point. The relationship of an earlier positive syndrome with later negative symptoma-

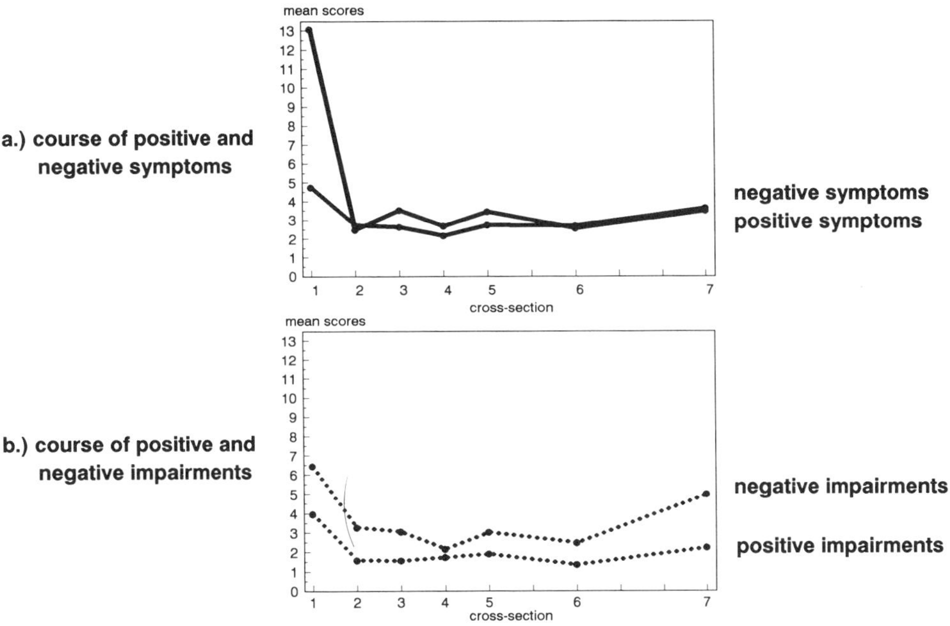

Fig. 5. Means of positive and negative symptoms and impairments over 5 years

tology is not as significant as that between acute episodes and the preceding negative syndrome. For the determination of positive symptoms by negative symptoms, significant product-moment correlations are found for 9 of the 21 possible combinations, but for the determination of negative symptoms following acute phases, only 4 of the correlations are significant. The negative (tendential) correlations of earlier acute symptomatology and later negative symptomatology should be mentioned, which coincides with the experience of an acute beginning and no chronic course.

Kraepelin's Hypothesis of a Schizophrenic Residual Syndrome

From Kraepelin's assumption that during the course of schizophrenia negative symptoms manifest as a residual syndrome or a schizophrenic defect state, an increase of negative symptoms should follow after one or more episodes. Figure 5 shows more a corresponding course of both syndromes, with a decrease at the beginning and a similar increase at the end.

However, two other results emphasise Kraepelin's hypothesis: first, the growing stability of the negative syndrome over time (Fig. 6) and second, the shift of the mean value of the total symptom score from the positive to the negative direction (Fig. 7).

If positive symptoms are considered as a temporary syndrome which leads at least to a transitory remission while negative symptoms are a more persistent disturbance, the coefficient of stability determined from one point of measure-

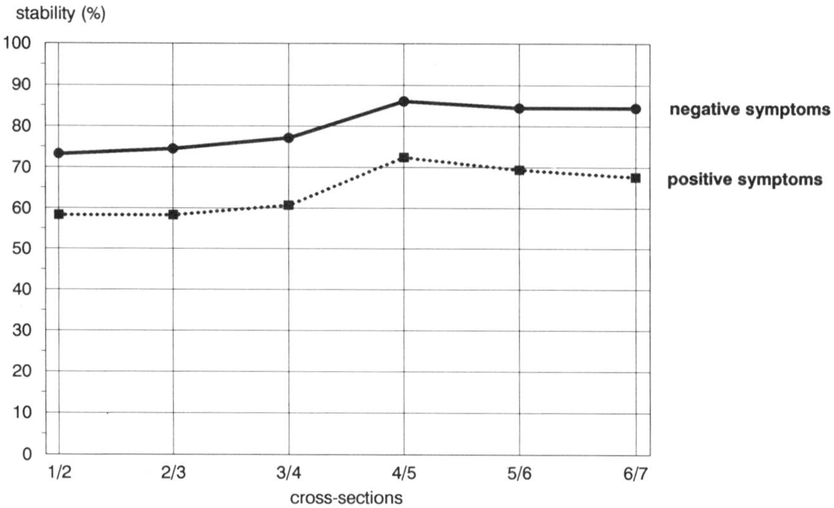

Fig. 6. Stability of positive and negative symptoms over 5 years

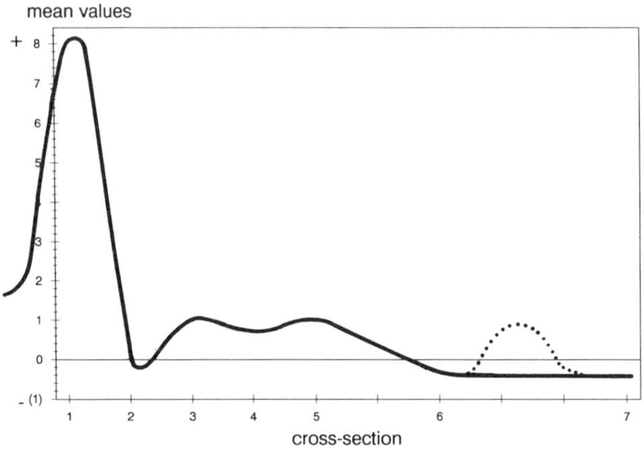

Fig. 7. Mean values of weighted sum scores of positive (weight = + 1) and negative (weight = − 1) symptoms over 5 years

ment to the next should be higher for the negative syndrome than for the positive one. This is found to be true: if we consider the stability of negative symptoms independently of the number of symptoms, for all changes between the time points of measurement the minus symptomatology occurs again (or remains) more probably in comparison with the positive symptomatology. The stability of negative symptomatology amounts to 73% from the initial measurement to the half-year follow-up and increases to 86% at the 2-year follow-up. Afterwards, the transition probability reaches 84%, a quite convincing result because the time span between the last two measurements is doubled from the initial half-year intervals to 1 or 2 years. The stability for negative symptoms is acceptable, but also for the acute symptomatology surprisingly high coefficients appear, which increase from 58% at the beginning to 72% at the 2-year follow-up and amount to 68% from the 3- to the 5-year follow-up. Not only the stability of the negative symptoms is higher than that of the positive symptoms, the proportion of the patients involved per cross-section is also greater for the minus symptomatology.

The distribution of total symptoms are characterized by a shift of the mean values from the positive to the negative pole of the scale (Fig. 7). The connection of the means remains a weak oscillation with a decreasing axis of oscillation. This shift of the mean also validates the Kraepelinian model of a relative increase of negative symptoms over the course.

Conclusions and Discussion

Using the data of a 5-year follow-up study, the relation of positive and negative symptoms was analysed for 7 cross-sectional measurements and for the entire course. In a first step, the cross-sectional correlations of the syndromes were computed. This part of the analysis suggested low but significant correlations between positive and negative symptoms, a result not compatible with the bipolar model of Andreasen and Olsen (1982). It was also impossible to identify convincing proportions of pure positive and negative sub-types. Moreover, these sub-types did not prove stable over the course. An attempt to identify consistent, unremitting course patterns of negative symptoms analogous to Crow's model of type I/type II schizophrenia was also not satisfying.

The discrepancy between the negative correlations of the syndromes reported by Andreasen and Olsen (1982) and our data could be due to the selection of cases. In the Mannheim study an epidemiologically defined and complete cohort was used, while Andreasen and Olsen (1982) worked with a sample of patients being treated in a hospital. In the former study most of the patients had no or only a small number of symptoms at follow-up compared with in-patients, who seek treatment because they suffer from positive or negative symptoms or both. The selection of in-patients as shown in Fig. 8 could explain the negative correlation between the syndromes in an utilization sample.

The Mannheim study data support a dimensional concept of schizophrenia syndromes rather than a typological one. The stability of the dimensions is higher than that of the sub-types. The results are in good agreement with Kraepelin's notion of a schizophrenic defect, which is concluded from the shift of a total symptom score from the positive to the negative axis of the symptom scale.

To sum up, it is strongly recommended to replicate our analysis with the data of other studies on the course of schizophrenia. It seems to be necessary to

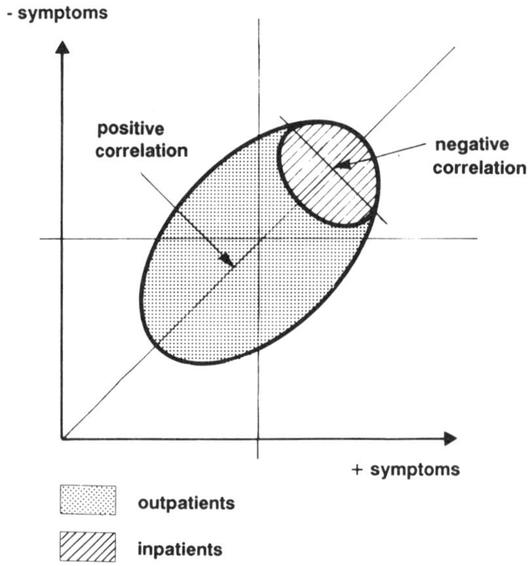

Fig. 8. Selection hypothesis to explain positive and negative correlations between positive and negative schizophrenia

develop models of positive and negative schizophrenia which take the longitudinal aspect of the disease into consideration. Most of the studies on negative symptoms are characterised by non-representative samples, by too-small sample sizes, by patients in different developmental states of the disease and by a lack of follow-up data. All these factors and limitations can lead to inadequate conclusions, which means that existing relations between positive and negative symptoms will not be recognised or artificial relations taken as true.

References

Abrams R, Taylor MA (1978) A rating scale for emotional blunting. Am J Psychiatry 135:226–229

Andreasen NC (1981) Scale for the assessment of negative symptoms (SANS). University of Iowa, Iowa City

Andreasen NC (1982) Negative symptoms in schizophrenia. Definition and reliability. Arch Gen Psychiatry 39:784–788

Andreasen NC (1983) Comprehensive assessment of symptoms and history (CASH). University of Iowa, Iowa City

Andreasen NC (1985) Positive vs. negative schizophrenia: a critical evaluation. Schizophr Bull 11:380–389

Andreasen NC, Olsen S (1982) Negative vs. positive schizophrenia. Arch Gen Psychiatry 39:789–794

Biehl H, Maurer K, Schubart C, Krumm B, Jung E (1986) Prediction of outcome and utilization of medical services in a prospective study of first onset schizophrenics. Eur Arch Psychiatry Neurol Sci 236:139–147

Biehl H, Maurer K, Jung E, Krüger G, Bauer-Schubart C (1988) Reported symptoms in schizophrenic patients within five years of the onset of illness. In: Dencker SJ, Kulhanek F (eds) (1988) Treatment resistance in schizophrenia: an approach for research and clinical routine together with a reconnaissance paper. Vieweg, Braunschweig

Biehl H, Maurer K, Jablensky A, Cooper JE, Tomov T (1989a) The WHO psychological impairments rating schedule (WHO/PIRS). I. Introducing a new instrument for rating observed behaviour and the rationale of the psychological impairment concept. Br J Psychiatry 155:68–70

Biehl H, Maurer K, Jung E, Krumm B (1989b) The WHO psychological impairments rating schedule (WHO/PIRS). II. Impairments in schizophrenics in cross-sectional and longitudinal perspective – the Mannheim experience in two independent samples. Br J Psychiatry 155:71–77

Bilder RM, Mukherjee S, Rieder RO, Pandurangi AK (1985) Symptomatic and neuropsychological components of defect states. Schizophr Bull 11:409–419

Carpenter WT, Heinrichs DW, Alphs LD (1985) Treatment of negative symptoms. Schizophr Bull 11:440–452

Crow TJ (1980) Positive and negative schizophrenic symptoms and the role of dopamine. Br J Psychiatry 137:383–386

Crow TJ (1985) The two-syndrome concept: origins and current status. Schizophr Bull 11:471–486

Endicott J, Spitzer RL (1978) A diagnostic interview: the schedule for affective disorders and schizophrenia. Arch Gen Psychiatry 35:837–844

Gottesman II, McGuffin P, Farmer A (1987) Clinical genetics as clues to the "real" genetics of schizophrenia (a decade of modest gains while playing for time). Schizophr Bull 13:23–47

Häfner H, Riecher A, Maurer K, Löffler W, Munk-Jørgensen P, Strömgren E (1989) How does gender influence age at first hospitalisation for schizophrenia? A transnational case register study. Psychol Med 19:903–918

Häfner H, Riecher A, Maurer K, Meissner S, Schmidtke A, Fätkenheuer B, Löffler W, an der Heiden W (1990) Ein Instrument zur retrospektiven Einschätzung des Erkrankungsbeginns bei Schizophrenie (Instrument for the retrospective assessment of the onset of schizophrenia – "IRAOS") – Entwicklung und erste Ergebnisse. Z Klin Psychol 19:230–255

Huber G, Gross R, Schüttler R (1979) Schizophrenie. Eine verlaufs- und sozial-psychiatrische Langzeitstudie. Springer, Berlin Heidelberg New York

Iager AC, Kirch DG, Wyatt RJ (1985) A negative symptom rating scale. Psychiatr Res 16:27–36

Jung E, Biehl H, Krumm B, Maurer K, Bauer-Schubart C (1989) DAS-M. Mannheimer Skala zur Einschätzung sozialer Behinderung. Beltz, Weinheim

Kay SR, Opler LA, Fiszbein A (1986a) Significance of positive and negative syndromes in chronic schizophrenia. Br J Psychiatry 149:439–448

Kay SR, Fiszbein A, Lindenmayer J-P, Opler LA (1986b) Positive and negative syndromes in schizophrenia as a function of chronicity. Acta Psychiatr Scand 74:507–518

Kay SR, Fiszbein A, Opler LA (1987) The positive and negative syndrome scale (PANSS) for schizophrenia. Schizophr Bull 13:261–273

Krawiecka M, Goldberg D, Vaughan M (1977) A standardized psychiatric assessment scale for rating chronic psychotic patients. Acta Psychiatr Scand 55:299–308

Lenzenweger MF, Dworkin RH, Wethington E (1989) Models of positive and negative symptoms in schizophrenia: an empirical evaluation of latent structures. J Abnorm Psychol 98:62–70

Lewine RRJ, Fogg L, Meltzer HY (1983) Assessment of negative and positive symptoms in schizophrenia. Schizophr Bull 9:368–376

Liddle PF (1987) The symptoms of chronic schizophrenia: a reexamination of the positive-negative dichotomy. Br J Psychiatry 151:145–151

Lindenmayer J-P, Kay SR, Friedman C (1986) Negative and positive schizophrenic syndromes after the acute phase: a prospective follow-up. Compr Psychiatry 27:276–286

Maurer K (1990) PSE-standardisierte Verlaufsdaten zur Minussymptomatik. In: Möller H-J, Pelzer E (Hrsg.) Neuere Ansätze zur Diagnostik und Therapie schizophrener Minussymptomatik. Springer, Berlin Heidelberg New York London Paris Tokyo Hong Kong Barcelona

Maurer K, Biehl H, Kühner C, Löffler W (1989) On the way to expert systems. Comparing DSM-III computer diagnoses with CATEGO (ICD) diagnoses in depressive and schizophrenic patients. Eur Arch Psychiatry Neurol Sci 239:127–132

Overall JE, Gorham DR (1962) The brief psychiatric rating scale. Psychol Rep 10:799–812

Pogue-Geile MF, Harrow M (1984) Negative and positive symptoms in schizophrenia and depression: a follow-up. Schizophr Bull 10:371–385

Pogue-Geile MF, Zubin J (1988) Negative symptomatology and schizophrenia: a conceptual and empirical review. Int J Ment Health 16:3–45

Schubart C, Krumm B, Biehl H, Schwarz R (1986a) Measurement of social disability in a schizophrenic patient group. Definition, assessment and outcome over 2 years in a cohort of schizophrenic patients of recent onset. Soc Psychiatry 21:1–9

Schubart C, Schwarz R, Krumm B, Biehl H (1986b) Schizophrenie und soziale Anpassung – Eine prospektive Längsschnittuntersuchung. Springer, Heidelberg Berlin New York

Strauss JS, Carpenter WT (1974) Characteristic symptoms and outcome in schizophrenia. Arch Gen Psychiatry 30:429–434

Riecher A, Maurer K, Löffler W, Fätkenheuer B, an der Heiden W, Häfner H (1989) Schizophrenia – a disease of young single males? Eur Arch Psychiatry Neurol Sci 239:210–212

Venables PH (1957) A short scale for rating "activity-withdrawal" in schizophrenics. J Ment Sci 103:197–199

Wing JK (1961) A simple and reliable subclassification of chronic schizophrenia. J Ment Sci 107:862–875

Wing JK, Cooper JE, Sartorius N (1974) The measurement and classification of psychiatric symptoms. Cambridge University Press, Cambridge

World Health Organization (1988) WHO psychiatric disability assessment schedule (WHO/DAS). WHO, Geneva

Long-Term Monomorphism of Negative and Positive Schizophrenic Episodes

A. MARNEROS, A. DEISTER, and A. ROHDE [1]

Introduction

As Berrios (1985, 1991) pointed out, "positive" and "negative" symptoms of mental disorders were already described in the 19th century, especially by Reynolds (1858) and Jackson (1889). Their relevance in schizophrenia research increased, however, after the descriptions of Bleuler's "Grundsymptome" ("fundamental Symptoms") and Kurt Schneider's "first rank symptoms". In the 1960s and 1970s, however, the interest of clinicians and researchers focused on positive symptoms, especially on schizophrenic first rank symptoms (Koehler 1979, Marneros 1984a, b, Mellor 1970, 1991, Taylor 1972). As Andreasen (1990a) pointed out, the emphasis on positive symptoms, and especially Schneiderian symptoms, derived from several concerns: The first was that Bleulerian symptoms were difficult to define and to rate reliably. They are often continuous with normality, while positive symptoms are clearly abnormal. In addition, stressing florid psychotic symptoms, particularly Schneiderian symptoms, was a useful way to achieve a narrow concept of schizophrenia, since it appeared that schizophrenia was often diagnosed on the basis of mild Bleulerian negative symptoms (Andreasen 1990). The Schneiderian first rank symptoms, the core of positive symptoms, proved to be reliable, easy to be detected and independent of cultural and social factors (Marneros 1984a, b, Mellor 1970, Taylor 1972). That was one of the most important factors leading to the incorporation of first rank symptoms in many diagnostic instruments like Research Diagnostic Criteria (RDC, Spitzer et al. 1978), DSM-III and DSM-III-R (APA 1980, 1987), Present State Examination (PSE, Wing et al. 1974, 1982) etc.

Paradoxically enough, the focus of interest on positive symptoms caused an increasing interest in negative symptoms: The opinion of Kraepelin that negative symptoms could be the central symptoms of the disease, as well as Bleuler's view of them as fundamental symptoms, experienced a renaissance. Huber completed his life-time investigation in schizophrenia by identifying and describing the so-called basic symptoms (Huber 1983, Süllwold and Huber 1987, Gross 1989, Gross et al. 1987), assumed to be the basis of the so-called productive schizophrenic symptoms, which are almost identical with relevant positve symptoms. In the USA, Andreasen demonstrated that – using an

[1] Psychiatrische Universitätsklinik, Sigmund-Freud-Straße 25, W-5300 Bonn 1, FRG

A. Marneros / N. C. Andreasen / M. T. Tsuang (Eds.)
Negative Versus Positive Schizophrenia

empirical approach that emphasized objective phenomena – reliable definitions could be achieved (Andreasen 1979a–c, 1990b). Her investigation led to the meanwhile internationally broadly used Scale for the Assessment of Negative Symptoms (SANS, Andreasen 1982). Since the operational assessment of positive and negative symptoms much work has been done to relate the two groups of symptoms to different etiopathogenesis (Crow 1980, 1985, 1991), therapeutic response (Angrist et al. 1980, Meltzer 1991) and prognosis (Carpenter et al. 1978, Johnstone et al. 1979, Pogue-Geile and Harrow 1984, 1985, Strauss et al. 1974).

Expanding the relevance of positive and negative symptoms, some authors described "types" or "subtypes" of schizophrenia (Andreasen 1990a, Andreasen and Olsen 1982) or "syndromes" (Crow 1985). Andreasen distinguished between positive, negative and mixed subtypes of schizophrenia (Andreasen 1982, 1985a, b, 1987, 1990a, b, Andreasen and Olsen 1982, Andreasen et al. 1991). She described first of all phenomenological-psychopathological subtypes. Crow (1980) went over the borderlines of phenomenology and linked the clinical phenomenology with external factors, such as premorbid functioning underlying etiopathological mechanisms and treatment (Crow 1980, 1985a, b, 1989). In spite of some essential differences from Andreasen's dichotomy into negative and positive schizophrenia, Carpenter's dichotomy into "deficit" vs "non-deficit" schizophrenia also has many basic similarities (Carpenter and Stephens 1979, Carpenter et al. 1985, 1988, 1991). In some way similar to the positive and negative distinction is the dichotomic model of Farmer and McGuffin (Farmer et al. 1983, 1984, McGuffin et al. 1991) of a "H-type", similar to negative syndromes, and a "P-type", similar to positive type or type II.

Since the distinction of a negative, a positive and a mixed form of schizophrenia much work has been done to identify external validators for the subtyping (Andreasen 1990a, 1991, Barnes and Liddle 1990, Marks and Luchins 1990). However, the distinction made between negative, positive and mixed schizophrenia is based mainly on cross-sectional, not on longitudinal criteria (Andreasen and Olsen 1982, Andreasen 1990a, Crow 1985). One of the external validators of the above-mentioned distinction could be the longitudinal course of positive, negative and mixed schizophrenic episodes regarding their stability or monomorphism (Andreasen 1990, Barnes and Luchins 1990). Investigating the longitudinal stability of negative and positive symptomatology, we have to distinguish between stability of symptoms and stability of syndromes (or episodes). Investigations by Andreasen (1990a) make it quite clear that none of the symptoms used to describe and define patients suffering from schizophrenia are specific in these disorders when patients are evaluated cross-sectionally. It seems that negative symptoms are more resistant against neuroleptic treatment, so their stability during one and the same episode can be higher than that of positive symptoms. But the stability of symptoms regarding a relatively short course, despite the euphemistic term "longitudinal", does not say anything about the stability of type of episode or syndromes. As we have already shown (Deister et al. 1990, Marneros et al.

1991), the distinction of subtypes of schizophrenia, like positive, negative or mixed, is only possible with high stability of positive, negative and mixed episodes during a long period, i.e. if the course is monomorphous.

This basic condition for the acceptance of positive/negative subtypes is quite important, considering that syndrome shift in mental diseases is a relatively common affair (Angst 1986, Marneros et al. 1988, 1991). The given frequencies of the so-called "diagnostic change" or "syndrome shift" vary from more than 50% (Cutting et al. 1978, Horgan 1981, Lewis and Piotrowski 1954) to less than 10% (Angst et al. 1978, Clark and Mallett 1963, Coryell and Winokur 1980, Lee and Murray 1988, Winokur 1974). The frequency of such changes is a function partly of the length of the observation time and partly of the diagnostic criteria (Angst 1986, Marneros et al. 1988). The stability of diagnosis over many years and even decades is an important factor for defining homogeneous diagnostic groups. Homogeneity and reliable definition of a group is a conditio sine qua non for subtyping mental disorders. In former work we showed that for patients diagnosed as having schizophrenia based on the first episode of illness, the probability of unchanging initial diagnosis during the long-term course is high: 90% of the patients remained schizophrenic during a very long course (more than 25 years), so the long-term diagnosis remained unchanged, namely "schizophrenic disorders" (Marneros et al. 1991a). But even in the cases of schizophrenia with stable course over decades, i.e. cases without syndrome shift into schizoaffective or affective or other psychotic disorders, the richness and changeableness of schizophrenic phenomenology is impressive, as long-term investigations of the phenomenological aspects of schizophrenic course show (M. Bleuer 1972, Ciompi and Müller 1976, Huber et al. 1979, Janzarik 1968, Marneros et al. 1991). Clinical experience and long-term studies demonstrate a frequent change of positive to negative schizophrenic symptomatology and vice versa.

Test Hypotheses

If positive and negative cross-sectional phenotypes of schizophrenia were distinct subtypes they would have to be monomorphous during long-term course, i.e. even also after many years or even decades and after many remanifestations of illness. "Ideal" monomorphism means that all patients in a study either have only positive or only negative episodes of schizophrenia throughout the observation time.

The aim of the present study was to investigate:

a) The stability/instability of positive and negative schizophrenic episodes of illness – not of single symptoms – during the long-term course of schizophrenia
b) Whether there are relevant correlations between the type of initial episode and several aspects of long-term outcome
c) Whether there are relevant correlations between the type of initial episode and premorbid adaption and other sociodemographic data

In this paper the results on the stability of types of episodes during course will be presented. In a second paper (Rohde et al. 1991) the correlation of positive, negative or mixed beginning of illness to sociodemographic and premorbid data will be described, and in a third paper (Deister et al. 1991) the correlation to the long-term outcome.

Material and Methods

The present study is part of the Cologne study on the long-term course and outcome of functional psychotic disorders, based on the investigation of 402 patients after a mean duration of illness of more than 25 years (Marneros et al. 1986a, 1988a, b, 1991). Considering the longitudinal aspect and using narrow definitions, 148 of these patients were diagnosed as having schizophrenia, 106 as having affective disorders, and 101 as having schizoaffective disorders at the end of the observation time. Forty-seven cases did not fulfill the criteria of any of these diagnoses, but were instead classified as "personality disorder", "exogeneous psychosis" etc.

The diagnosis of schizophrenia was made if during the whole observation time only episodes fulfilling the criteria of a schizophrenic episode were present, i.e. no affective or schizoaffective episodes. The diagnostic criteria for an episode were based on slightly modified DSM-III criteria (Marneros et al. 1988a; for more details and diagnostic criteria of episodes and disorders see Marneros et al. 1986, 1988, 1991), i.e. all 148 investigated patients fulfilled the psychopathological DSM-III criteria of schizophrenia. In order to make the statistical investigations more reliable, an *episode of illness* was defined as the manifestation or remanifestation of psychopathological symptoms needing either inpatient or inpatient-like treatment. Inpatient-like treatment was defined as the treatment of manifest symptoms when (a) intensive medical care was needed and (b) the symptoms necessitated the interruption of usual work or duties.

At the end of the observation time all patients were interviewed personally. The exploratory framework used was the German translation of the PSE (Wing et al. 1974, 1982) and a pool of questions based on some instruments of the WHO (FU-HSD, PHSD etc.). Additionally the status at the end of the observation time was evaluated using some standardized instruments assessing positive and negative symptomatology (SANS, SAPS, NSRS), global functioning (GAS), psychological deficits (WHO/PIRS), social impairments and social disability (WHO/DAS) and social consequences of the illness (for details see Deister et al. 1991). Additionally the case records of all episodes of illness during the whole course were evaluated and cross-sectionally diagnosed. Psychopathological parameters were evaluated as well as all relevant extra-symptomatological features like sociodemographic variables, life events, treatment, prophylaxis etc.

Table 1 shows some *features of the schizophrenic study population*. The female to male ratio was 0.7:1, the mean follow-up period 23.0 years.

Table 1. Features of study population (n = 148)

Sex distribution	Male	86 (58.1%)
	Female	62 (41.9%)
Age at first manifestation		
Arithmetic mean		27.7 years
Median		24.0 years
Standard deviation		10.6 years
Minimum		14 years
Maximum		64 years
Duration of follow-up period		
Arithmetic mean		23.0 years
Median		25.0 years
Standard deviation		9.9 years
Minimum		10 years
Maximum		50 years
Age at the end of observation time		
Arithmetic mean		50.7 years
Median		51.0 years
Standard deviation		13.2 years
Minimum		27 years
Maximum		84 years

Thirty-five of the patients had been permanently hospitalized during the course of the illness (> 3 years) and were therefore excluded from all calculations regarding syndrome shift during course. Another 13 patients with only one manifestation of illness (monoepisodic cases) were also excluded from these statistical procedures.

Each single episode during the course of illness was classified according to the criteria of Andreasen and Olsen (1982) as positive, negative or mixed (Table 2), that means all investigated episodes are DSM-III schizophrenic episodes fulfilling also Andreasen's criteria of positive, negative or mixed episodes.

In this context, it has to be pointed out that the classification of the schizophrenic episodes into positive, negative and mixed was made according to the *most prominent symptomatology* rather than the absolute existence or otherwise of symptomatology. That means that a positive episode could include some negative symptoms which were not prominent, intensive or severe, and a negative episode could include some positive symptoms. Episodes in which both kinds of symptoms were prominent were classified as mixed.

"*Preepisodic alterations*" (i.e. states usually called "prodromal state") were excluded from the evaluation, as were as "*persisting alterations*" (usually called "residual state"); theoretical considerations on both these terms can be found in Marneros et al. 1991. The aim of these exclusions was the achievement of states fulfilling all criteria of an episode. Preepisodic alterations having a prodromal character – although showing some symptoms which can be identified as schizophrenic ones – (Häfner and Maurer 1991, Huber et al. 1979,

Table 2. Criteria of positive, negative and mixed schizophrenia according to Andreasen and Olsen (1982)

Negative symptoms Alogia Affective flattening Anhedonia-asociality Avolition-apathy Attentional impairment	Negative schizophrenic episode 1. At least two of the negative symptoms are present to a marked degree 2. None of the positive symptoms dominate the clinical picture
	Mixed schizophrenic episode Criteria neither for positive nor for negative episode are fulfilled, or criteria for both types of episodes are fulfilled
Positive symptoms Hallucinations Delusions Positive formal thought disorders Bizarre or disorganized behavior	Positive schizophrenic episode 1. At least one of the positive symptoms is a prominent part of the episode 2. None of the negative symptoms is present to a marked degree

Marneros et al. 1991) do not yet fullfill the criteria of an episode mentioned above. Persisting alterations in the sense of residual states can consist of positive and negative symptoms, without fulfilling the criteria of an episode in the sense of manifestation, remanifestation or exacerbation of illness and discontinuity of life style or interruption of existing social interactions.

That means that the present work differs from that of Häfner and Maurer (1991) and Maurer and Häfner (1991) in the sense that our investigations concerned the criteriologically defined episodes of the illness, but not the preepisodic symptoms or the residual states.

The question treated in the presented paper is whether the illness schizophrenia is *monomorphous* during a long-term course (i.e. with only one kind of episode of illness) or *bimorphous* (i.e. with both types of schizophrenic symptomatology, positive and negative). The Mannheim group of Häfner and co-workers investigated the models of development of positive and negative symptomatology, their interactions and the parallel stability of *symptoms*, while the present work deals with the stability of *episodes*, i.e. with the monomorphism of the longitudinal course of schizophrenic disorders.

Results

Type of Initial Episode

The application of the criteria of positive, negative and mixed schizophrenic symptomatology to the initial episodes of illness showed that 44% of the 148 schizophrenic patients had positive, 32% negative and 24% mixed schizophren-

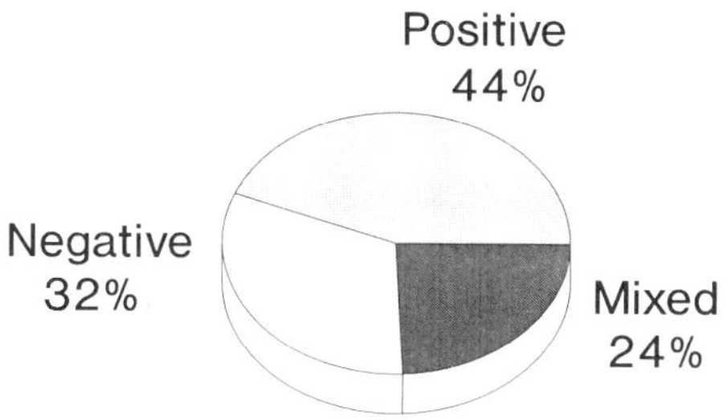

Fig. 1. Type of initial episode ($n = 148$)

ic symptomatology (Fig. 1). Eight (23%) of the 35 patients who had been living continuously in mental hospitals for at least 3 years at the end of the observation time (median 20 years, maximum 36 years) and who were therefore excluded from the statistical evaluations had had a positive initial episode, 16 (46%) a negative first episode and 11 (31%) a mixed schizophrenic syndrome at onset.

Initial Episode and Type of Subsequent Episodes During Course

For the 100 schizophrenic patients (permanently hospitalized and monoepisodic patients excluded) a total number of 458 episodes was evaluated; 100 initial episodes and 358 subsequent episodes. Table 3 shows the frequency of the various types of episodes during course in relation to the type of initial episode. In cases with a *positive initial episode* 53% of the subsequent episodes were also positive, while 23% were categorized as negative and 23% as mixed schizophrenic episodes. Patients with *initial negative schizophrenic syndrome* had predominantly negative symptoms in 46% of the episodes during the course; the remaining episodes of illness were positive and mixed in 27% of cases each. In patients with *mixed schizophrenic onset* only 29% of all following episodes were also mixed; the most frequent type of episodes in these cases was the negative schizophrenic episode (55%).

Monomorphous and Bimorphous Course of Schizophrenic Disorders

After an observation time of 23 years on average, most patients were found to have an "unstable" course (74%), i.e. more than one type of schizophrenic

Table 3. Type of episodes during course by type of initial episode (permanently hospitalized and monoepisodic patients excluded; $n = 100$)

Type of initial episode	Type of episodes during course			Total
	Positive	Mixed	Negative	
Positive ($n = 50$)	87 (53.4%)	38 (23.3%)	38 (23.3%)	163
Mixed ($n = 20$)	15 (16,5%)	26 (28.6%)	50 (54.9%)	91
Negative ($n = 30$)	28 (26.9%)	28 (26.9%)	48 (46.2%)	104

episode had occurred. Only 18 of the 100 schizophrenic disorders had remained "purely" positive, only 6 "purely" negative and in 2 cases the course was a stable mixed schizophrenic one (Fig. 2).

Figure 3 shows the frequency of homogeneous courses always having the same type of schizophrenic episode (monomorphous type of course) in relation to the duration of the illness. It is evident that the frequency of cases with monomorphous type of course ("stable" course) is a function of the duration of the illness: the number of patients with a pure positive, a pure negative or a pure mixed course becomes lower continuously in proportion to the length of course.

The first syndrome shift occurred very early after the onset of illness, i.e. in the majority of cases in the first 5 years (on average 6.1 years) after onset.

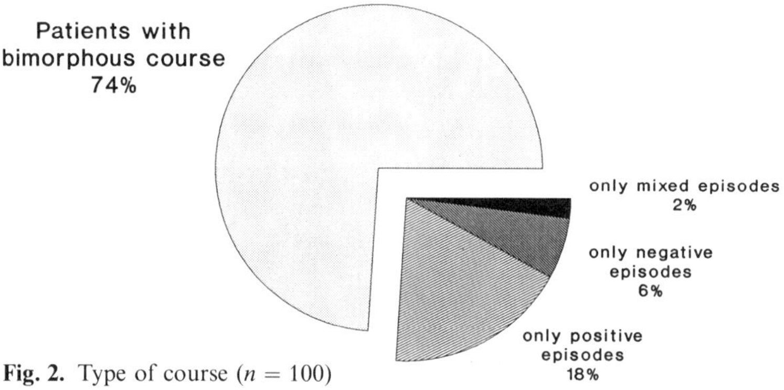

Fig. 2. Type of course ($n = 100$)

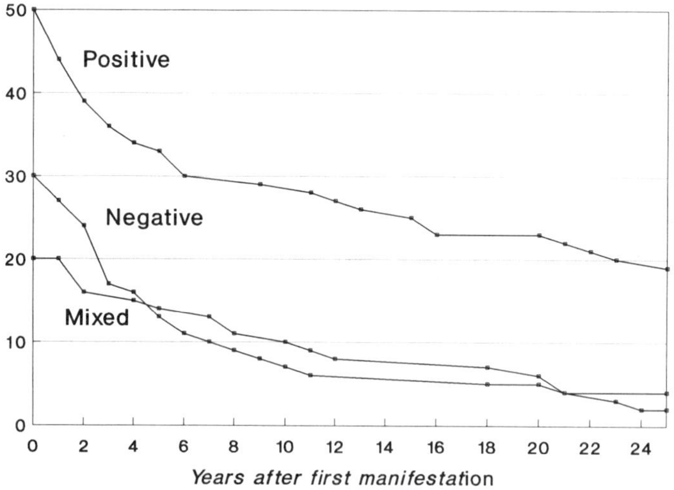

Fig. 3. Patients with only one type of episode during course in relation to years after first manifestation

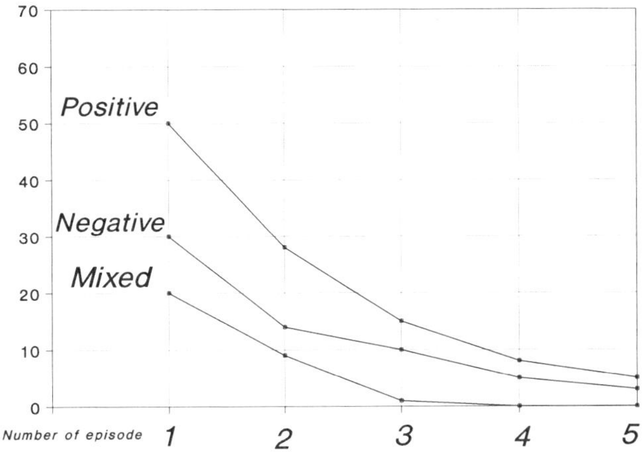

Fig. 4. Number of patients with only one type of episode during the first five episodes

In more than 50% of the schizophrenic disorders the shift from one type of schizophrenic episode to another took place already with the second episode of illness (mean 2.8 episodes, median 2 episodes; Fig. 4).

Direction of First Syndrome Shift Within the Course of Schizophrenic Disorders

As shown in Fig. 5, the first change from one type of schizophrenic episode to another occurred in any direction, without a clear pattern. In the majority of cases with positive schizophrenic onset the first change was to a negative schizophrenic episode; the same was true in an even higher percentage of cases with mixed schizophrenic onset (56% and 67%). From a negative initial episode the first change took place in 58% in cases to a positive and in 42% to a mixed schizophrenic episode.

Conclusions and Discussion

Dividing schizophrenia into a positive and a negative type could be meritorious: the creation of homogeneous subtypes increases the possibility to find correlations between narrowly defined subtypes and premorbid and sociodemographic data, course and outcome parameters, and biological and genetic findings. Some investigations seem to provide evidence of some correlations (Andreasen 1990a, Barnes and Liddle 1990, Crow 1985, Markes and Luchins 1990, Pickar 1990), but most of these results are problematic because of some shortcomings (Carpenter et al. 1991, Häfner and Maurer 1991, Kay et al. 1986): (a) there is insufficient differentiation between negative symptoms which are core symptoms of the disease (i.e. primary negative symptoms) and those negative symptoms which are secondary to illness-associated conditions

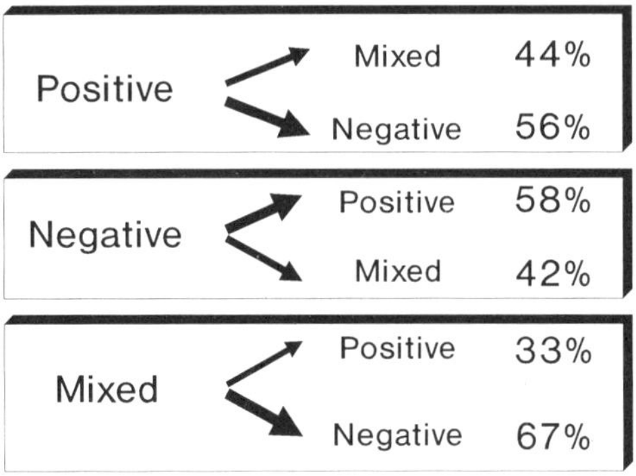

Fig. 5. Direction of first syndrome shift

(Carpenter and Buchanan 1988, Carpenter et al. 1988, Strauss et al. 1974) or psychologically understandable reactions of the patients (Brenner 1987, Brenner et al. 1991, Mundt 1985, 1991); (b) small samples do not allow consideration of many possible combinations of psychopathological phenomena (Huber et al. 1979, Janzarik 1968, Marneros et al. 1991); (c) cross-sectionally diagnosed samples have the shortcoming that they do not take into consideration the syndrome shift, the interaction between positive and negative symptomatology or the proportion of changes between negative and positive symptomatology during long-term course (Carpenter et al. 1991, Deister and Marneros 1990, Eggers 1991, Häfner and Maurer 1991, Huber et al. 1979, Marneros et al. 1988, 1991, Remschmidt 1991).

In conclusion, it can be stated that *the results of the present study do not support the assumption of "pure" positive or "pure" negative schizophrenic disorders, longitudinally defined.* Positive schizophrenic episodes were followed by negative ones and vice versa; negative symptoms were found to be in longitudinal interaction with positive ones. In this respect, the findings of the present study are compatible with the findings of Häfner and Maurer (1991) and Maurer and Häfner (1991): these authors found, in 5 years' follow-up investigation, significant correlations between positive and negative symptoms, a result not compatible with the bipolar model of Andreasen and Olsen (1982). In the Mannheim study it was also impossible to identify convincing proportions of pure positive and negative subtypes (Maurer and Häfner 1991). The authors could not identify consistent, unremitting course patterns of negative symptoms analogous to Crow's model of type I versus type II schizophrenia; moreover, they found – similar to the present study – that the positive and negative subtypes of schizophrenia did not prove stable during course, thus supporting the observations of earlier European long-term studies of schizophrenia using different definitions, terms and designs (M. Bleuler 1972, Ciompi und Müller 1976, Huber et al. 1979, Janzarik 1968).

Positive and negative subtypes of schizophrenia remaining stable over several years are the exception. It can be concluded that the course of schizophrenic disorders is *bimorphous*, i.e. involves both groups of schizophrenic symptoms, negative and positive. A monomorphous schizophrenic course, with only positive or only negative schizophrenic episodes of illness, is the very rare exception.

But, nevertheless, the question remains: What are positive and negative schizophrenia? Are they forms of schizophrenic disease beginning with a positive or negative episode respectively, independently of the fact that other types of schizophrenic episodes occur more or less frequently during the course? The results of the present study show a high frequency of syndrome shift in the course of schizophrenia without any special pattern. This investigation on the long-term course of schizophrenic disorders does not support the assumption of distinct subtypes of schizophrenia.

The results regarding premorbid and sociodemographic features and long-term outcome are presented elsewhere in this volume (see Rohde et al. 1991 and Deister et al. 1991).

References

American Psychiatric Association (APA) (1980) Diagnostic and Statistical Manual of Mental Disorders (3rd edition). American Psychiatric Press, Washington D.C.

American Psychiatric Association (APA) (1987) Diagnostic and Statistical Manual of Mental Disorders (3rd edition – revised). American Psychiatric press, Washington D.C.

Andreasen NC (1979a) Thought, Language, and Communication Disorders. I. Clinical Assessment, Definition of Terms, and Evaluation of Their Reliability. Arch Gen Psychiatry 36, 1315–1321

Andreasen NC (1979b) Thought, Language, and Communication Disorders. II. Diagnostic Significance. Arch Gen Psychiatry 36, 1325–1330

Andreasen NC (1979 c) Affective flattening and the criteria for schizophrenia. Am J Psychiatry 136, 944–947

Andreasen NC (1982) Negative Syndromes in Schizophrenia: Definition and Reliability. Arch Gen Psychiatry 39, 784–788

Andreasen NC (1985a) Positive vs. Negative Schizophrenia. A Critical Evaluation. Schizophrenia Bull 11, 380–389

Andreasen NC (1987) The diagnosis of schizophrenia. Schizophr Bull 13, 9–22

Andreasen NC (1990b) Positive and Negative Symptoms: Historical and Conceptual Aspects. In: Andreasen NC (ed.). Schizophrenia: Positive and Negative Symptoms and Syndromes (Mod Probl Pharmacopsychiatry, Vol. 24). Basel, Karger

Andreasen NC (1990c) Methods for Assessing Positive and Negative Symptoms. In: Andreasen NC (ed.). Schizophrenia: Positive and Negative Symptoms and Syndromes (Mod Probl Pharmacopsychiatry, Vol. 24). Basel, Karger

Andreasen NC, Olsen S (1982) Negative vs. Positive Schizophrenia. Arch Gen Psychiatry 39, 789–794

Andreasen NC, Flaum M, Arndt S, Alliger R, Swayze VW (1991) Positive and Negative Symptoms: Assessment and Validity. In: Marneros A, Andreasen NC, Tsuang MT (eds.). Negative vs. Positive Schizophrenia. Springer, Berlin Heidelberg New York

Angrist B, Rotrosen J, Gershorn S (1980) Differential Effects of Amphetamine and neuroleptics on Negative vs. Positive Symptoms in Schizophrenia. Psychopharmacology 72, 17–19

Angst J (1986) The course of affective disorders. Psychopathology 119, Suppl 2, 47–52

Angst J, Felder W, Frey R, Stassen HH (1978) The Course of Affective Disorders. I. Change of Diagnosis of Monopolar, Unipolar, and Bipolar Illness. Arch Psychiatr Nervenkr 226, 57–64

Barnes TRE, Liddle PF (1990) Evidence for the Validity of Negative Symptoms. In: Andreasen NC (ed.). Schizophrenia: Positive and Negative Symptoms and Syndromes (Mod Probl Pharmacopsychiatry, Vol. 24). Basel, Karger

Berrios GE (1985) Positive and Negative Symptoms and Jackson. Arch Gen Psychiatry 42, 95–97

Berrios GE (1991) Positive and Negative Signals: A Conceptual History. In: Marneros A, Andreasen NC, Tsuang MT (eds.). Negative vs. Positive Schizophrenia. Springer: Berlin Heidelberg New York

Bleuler M (1972) Die schizophrenen Geistesstörungen im Lichte langjähriger Kranken- und Familiengeschichten. Springer, Berlin Heidelberg New York

Brenner HD, Hodel B, Merlo MCG (1991) Nonpharmacological Treatment Concepts of Negative Symptomatology. In: Marneros A, Andreasen NC, Tsuang MT (eds.). Negative vs. Positive Schizophrenia. Springer, Berlin Heidelberg New York

Carpenter WT, Buchanan RW (1988) Domains of psyhopathology relevant to the study of etiology and treatment in schizophrenia. Schizophrenia: Scientific Progress. Oxford University Press, New York

Carpenter WT, Stephens JH (1979) An attempted integration of formation relevant to schizophrenic subtypes. Schizophr Bull 490–506

Carpenter WT, Bartko JJ, Strauss JS, Hawk AB (1978) Signs and symptoms as predictors of outcome: A report from the International Pilot Study of Schizophrenia. Am J Psychiatry 135, 940–945

Carpenter WT Jr., Heinrichs DW, Wagman AMI (1985) On the Heterogeneity of Schizophrenia. In: Alpert M (ed.). Controversies in Schizophrenia. Guilford Press, New York London

Carpenter WT, Heinrichs DW, Wagman AMI (1988) Deficit and Nondeficit Forms of Schizophrenia: The Concept. Am J Psychiatry 145, 578–583

Carpenter WT, Buchanan RW, Kirkpatrick B, Thaker G, Tamminga C (1991) Negative Symptoms: A Critique of Current Approaches. In: Marneros A, Andreasen NC, Tsuang MT (eds.). Negative vs. Positive Schizophrenia. Springer, Berlin Heidelberg New York

Ciompi L, Müller C (1976) Lebensweg und Alter der Schizophrenen. Eine katamnestische Langzeitstudie bis ins Senium. Springer, Berlin Heidelberg New York

Clark JA, Mallett BL (1963) A follow-up study of schizophrenia and depression in young adults. Br J Psychiatry 109, 491–499

Coryell W, Winokur G (1980) Diagnosis, Family, and Follow-up Studies. In: Belmaker RH, van Praag HM (eds.). Mania. An Evolving Concept. Spectrum Publ. Inc., Jamaica N. Y.

Crow TJ (1980) Molecular pathology of schizophrenia: More than one disease process? Br Med J Clin Res 280, 66–68

Crow TJ (1985) The two syndrome concept: origins and current status. Schizophr Bull 11, 471–486

Crow TJ (1991) The Demise of the Kraepelinian Binary Concept and the Etiological Unity of the Psychoses. In: Marneros A, Andreasen NC, Tsuang MT (eds.). Negative vs. Positive Schizophrenia. Springer, Berlin Heidelberg New York

Cutting J, Clare A, Mann A (1978) Cycloid psychosis: an investigation of the diagnostic concepts. Psychol Med 8, 637–648

Deister A, Marneros A, Rohde A (1990) Zur Stabilität negativer und positiver Syndromatik. In: Möller HJ, Pelzer E (eds.). Neuere Ansätze zur Diagnostik und Therapie schizophrener Minussymptomatik. Springer, Berlin Heidelberg New York

Deister A, Marneros A, Rohde A (1991) Long-term outcome of patients with a positive initial episode versus patients with a negative initial episode. In: Marneros A, Andreasen NC, Tsuang MT (eds.). Negative Versus Positive Schizophrenia. Springer, Berlin Heidelberg New York

Farmer AE, McGuffin P, Spitznagel E (1983) Heterogeneity in Schizophrenia. A cluster analytic approach. Psychiatry Res 8, 1–12

Farmer AE, McGuffin P, Gottesman II (1984) Searching for the Split in Schizophrenia. A Twin Study Perspective. Psychiatry Res 13, 109–118

Gross G (1989) The "Basic" Symptoms of Schizophrenia. Br J Psychiatry 155 (Suppl. 7), 21–25

Gross G, Huber G, Klosterkötter J, Linz M (1987) BSABS. Bonner Skala für die Beurteilung von Basissymptomen. Springer, Berlin Heidelberg New York

Häfner H, Maurer K (1991) Are there two types of schizophrenia? – True onset and sequence of positive and negative syndromes prior to first admission. In: Marneros A, Andreasen NC, Tsuang MT (eds.). Negative vs. Positive Schizophrenia. Springer, Berlin Heidelberg New York
Horgan D (1981) Change of diagnosis to manic-depressive illness. Psychol Med 11, 517–523
Huber G (1983) Das Konzept substratnaher Basissymptome und seine Bedeutung für Theorie und Therapie schizophrener Erkrankungen. Nervenarzt 54, 23–32
Huber G, Gross G, Schüttler R (1979) Schizophrenie. Eine verlaufs- und sozialpsychiatrische Langzeitstudie. Springer, Berlin Heidelberg New York
Jackson JH (1889) On postepilepsie states: A contribution to the comparative study of insanities. J Ment Sci 34, 490–500
Janzarik W (1968) Schizophrene Verläufe. Eine strukturdynamische Interpretation. Springer, Berlin Heidelberg New York
Johnstone EC, Frith CD, Gold A, Stevens M (1979) The outcome of severe acute schizophrenic illness after one year. Br J Psychiatry 134, 28–33
Kay SR, Opler L, Fiszbein A (1986) The Positive and Negative Syndrome Scale (PANSS) for Schizophrenia. Schizophr Bull 13, 261–276
Koehler K (1979) First-rank symptoms of schizophrenia: questions concerning clinical boundaries. Br J Psychiatry 134, 236–248
Lee AS, Murray RM (1988) The long-term outcome of Maudsley depressives. Br J Psychiatry 153, 741–751
Lewis NDC, Pietrowski ZA (1954) Clinical diagnosis of manic-depressive psychosis. Am Psychopathol Ass 25–38
Marks RC, Luchins DJ (1990) Relationship between Brain Imaging Findings in Schizophrenia and Psychopathology. In: Andreasen NC (ed.). Schizophrenia: Positive and Negative Symptoms and Syndromes (Mod Probl Pharmacopsychiatry, Vol. 24). Basel, Karger
Marneros A (1984) The Pathognomonic Value of K. Schneider's First Rank Symptoms in Schizophrenia. Psychiatria Fennica 15, 99–105
Marneros A (1984) Frequency of occurrence of Schneider's first rank symptoms in schizophrenia. Eur Arch Psychiatr Neurol Sci 234, 78–82
Marneros A, Deister A, Rohde A (1986) The Cologne Study on schizoaffective disorders and schizophrenia suspecta. In: Marneros A, Tsuang MT (eds.). Schizoaffective Psychoses. Springer, Berlin Heidelberg New York
Marneros A, Deister A, Rohde A (1988) Syndrome in the long-term course of schiozoaffective disorders. Eur Arch Psychiatr Neurol Sci 238. 97–104
Marneros A, Deister A, Rohde A (1991) Affektive, schizoaffektive und schizophrene Psychosen. Eine vergleichende Langzeitstudie. Springer, Berlin Heidelberg New York
Maurer K, Häfner H (1991) Dependence, Independence or Interdependence of Positive and Negative Symptoms. In: Marneros A, Andreasen NC, Tsuang MT (eds.). Negative vs. Positive Schizophrenia. Springer, Berlin Heidelberg New York
Mellor CS (1970) First rank symptoms of schizophrenia. Br J Psychiatry 140, 423–424
Mellor CS (1991) Methodological Problems in Identifying and Measuring First-Rank Symptoms of Schizophrenia. In: Marneros A, Andreasen NC, Tsuang NC (eds.). Negative vs. Positive Schizophrenia. Springer, Berlin Heidelberg New York
Meltzer HY (1991) Pharmacologic Treatment of Negative Symptoms. In: Greden JF, Tandon R (eds.). Negative schizophrenic symptoms: pathophysiology and clinical implications. American Psychiatric Press, Washington DC
Mundt C (1985) Das Apathiesyndrom der Schizophrenen. Eine psychopathologische und computertomographische Untersuchung. Springer, Berlin Heidelberg New York
Mundt C (1991) Constituting Reality – Its Decline and Repair in the Long-Term Course of Schizophrenic Psychoses. In: Marneros A, Andreasen NC, Tsuang MT (eds.). Negative vs. Positive Schizophrenia. Springer, Berlin Heidelberg New York
Pickar D, Litman RE, Konicki PE, Wolkowitz OM, Breier A (1990) Neurochemical and Neural Mechanisms of Positive and Negative Symptoms in Schizophrenia. In: Andreasen NC (ed.). Schizophrenia: Positive and Negative Symptoms and Syndromes (Mod Probl Pharmacopsychiatry, Vol. 24). Basel, Karger

Pogue-Geile MF, Harrow M (1984) Negative and positive symptoms in schizophrenia and depression. Schizophr Bull 10, 371–387
Pogue-Geile M, Harrow M (1985) Negative symptoms in schizophrenia: their longitudinal course and prognostic importance. Schizophr Bull 11, 427–439
Reynolds JR (1858) On the pathology of convulsions, with special reference to those of children. Liverpool Med Chir J, 1–14
Rohde A, Marneros A, Deister A (1991) Premorbid and Sociodemographic Features of Initially Positive and Initially Negative Schizophrenia. In: Marneros A, Andreasen NC, Tsuang NC (eds.). Negative vs. Positive Schizophrenia. Springer, Berlin Heidelberg New York
Spitzer RL, Endicott J, Robins E (1978) Research Diagnostic Criteria: Rationale and reliability. Arch Gen Psychiatry 35, 773–782
Strauss JS, Carpenter WT jr, Bartko JJ (1974) The diagnosis and understanding of schizophrenia: Part III. Speculations on the processes that underlie schizophrenic symptoms and signs. Schizophr Bull, 61–69
Süllwold L, Huber G (1987) Schizophrene Basisstörungen. Springer, Berlin Heidelberg New York
Taylor MA (1972) Schneiderian first-rank symptoms and clinical prognostic features in schizophrenia. Arch Gen Psychiatry 26, 64–67
Wing JK, Cooper JE, Sartorius N (1974) Measurement and classification of psychiatric symptoms. Cambridge University Press, Cambridge
Wing JK, Cooper JE, Sartorius N (1982) Die Erfassung und Klassifikation psychiatrischer Symptome: Beschreibung und Glossar des PSE (Present State Examination). Beltz, Weinheim
Winokur G (1974) Genetic and clinical factors associated with course in depression. Contributions to genetic aspects. Pharmakopsychiatr 7, 122–126

Premorbid and Sociodemographic Features of Schizophrenia with Positive and Negative Initial Episodes

A. ROHDE, A. MARNEROS, and A. DEISTER [1]

Introduction

Psychiatric diagnoses remain "psychopathological compromises" (Janzarik 1976) if no external validators can be found. Having no concrete agents, morphological alterations, biochemical findings, or similar "hard" validators of schizophrenia, we are compelled to determine some other external "soft" validators such as age at onset, sex distribution, social factors, premorbid personality, etc. This way proved to be correct. Several and relevant differences were found between the various kinds of mental disorders, for example, among the so-called functional disorders like schizophrenia, schizoaffective and affective disorders (Marneros and Tsuang 1986, 1990; Marneros et al. 1991a). External, nonsymptomatological variables, which differed among the various types of functional disorders, were found to be: sex distribution, age at onset, premorbid personality and premorbid social interactions, marital status and stable heterosexual partnership before onset, education, occupation at onset, social class, and social mobility (Marneros et al. 1991a).

The comparative research found that *female patients* are more frequently represented than male patients in groups of affective and schizoaffective disorders, but that is not the case in narrowly defined schizophrenic groups (Angst 1980, 1986, 1987; Berner and Lenz 1986; Dohrenwend and Dohrenwend 1976; Goodwin and Jamison 1990; Häfner 1987; Marneros et al. 1991; McGlashan and Bardenstein 1990; Lewine 1988). The investigations which found that female patients are overrepresented in the group of schizophrenics are those which apply broad criteria in defining schizophrenia, and those which also include schizoaffective and other disorders. Such investigations are, for instance, the studies of Bleuler (1972), Ciompi and Müller (1976), and Huber et al. (1979).

Differences among the various types of psychoses were also found regarding *age at onset*. Schizophrenic patients usually become ill for the first time in their life earlier than patients with affective disorders, while patients with schizoaffective disorders occupy a position in between (Angst 1986, 1988a, b; Goodwin and Jamison 1990; Häfner 1987, 1990; Lewine 1988; Loranger 1984; McGlashan and Bardenstein 1990; Marneros et al. 1991; Möller and von Zerssen 1986).

[1] Psychiatrische Universitätsklinik, Sigmund-Freud-Straße 25, W-5300 Bonn 1, FRG

A. Marneros / N. C. Andreasen / M. T. Tsuang (Eds.)
Negative Versus Positive Schizophrenia

Another possible external validator of functional psychoses could be the *premorbid personality* and *premorbid social interactions* of the patients. Relevant differences were found among the various groups of functional disorders (Angst and Clayton 1986; Goodwin and Jamison 1990; Hirschfeld and Gross 1982; Marneros et al. 1991; Möller and von Zerssen 1986; von Zerssen and Pössl 1990).

Differences in *educational level* between the various types of endogenous psychoses (Achté and Tuulio-Henriksson 1983; Dohrenwend et al. 1987; Marneros et al. 1991) seem to be caused not only by the different age at onset (i.e., early manifestation of schizophrenic disorders), but also by other parameters such as premorbid personality and original social class.

Schizophrenic patients also differ from affective and schizoaffective patients with regard to *stable heterosexual relationships* and *marital status* before onset of the illness (Angst 1966; Bland and Orn 1978; Dohrenwend et al. 1987; Eaton et al. 1988; Marneros et al. 1991; Munk-Jorgenssen 1985).

Differences between schizophrenic, schizoaffective, and affective patients are also found with regard to some aspects of *social mobility*, i.e., negative social mobility (Angermeyer and Klusmann 1987; Dilling and Weyerer 1987; Dohrenwend and Dohrenwend 1964; 1969; Eaton et al. 1988; Marneros et al. 1991a).

Interesting for the present investigation is the finding that functional disorders other than schizophrenia, i.e., affective and schizoaffective disorders, are inhomogeneous with regard to the above-mentioned premorbid and sociodemographic parameters. This means that there are differences among different subgroups of these disorders: unipolar and bipolar affective disorders, and unipolar and bipolar schizoaffective disorders differ significantly regarding most of the above-mentioned parameters (Angst 1987; Goodwin and Jamison 1990; Marneros et al. 1990a, b, c, 1991a).

The question that arises for schizophrenic disorders is whether there are also differences regarding some relevant social and premorbid features between distinct subtypes of schizophrenia, i.e., between a "positive schizophrenic subtype" versus a "negative schizophrenic subtype." In order to answer this question, a definition of the negative and positive subtypes of schizophrenia is required. As the results in our previous paper showed (Marneros et al. 1991b), the long-term course of schizophrenia is usually bimorphous regarding positive and negative symptomatology, and definitively polymorphous regarding psychopathological and psychological symptomatology. This means that a longitudinal distinction between positive and negative schizophrenia is only possible in exceptional cases.

But how can findings in the literature which differences between positive and negative subtypes be explained? According to the positive/negative dichotomy, the negative subtype of Andreasen (1990), the type II of Crow (1980), or the H-type of Farmer and co-workers (1983, 1984) represents a syndrome in young people with poor premorbid adjustment and other deficits. The question is how these reported correlations can be prooven if the long-term distinction between positive and negative subtypes is only possible in exceptional cases? For the present investigation we decided to categorize subtypes following the initial episode into *initially positive*, *initially negative*, and *initially mixed schizophrenia*. These categories are considered independently of the types of schizophrenic episodes occurring later during the course of the illness. The assumption behind this distinction is the following: negative symptomatology achieving the criteriological status of an episode – as defined in our earlier paper (Marneros et al., 1991 b) – may be more severe symptomatology corresponding with preepisodic psychosocial dysfunctions.

Material and Methods

Material, methods, and definitions have already been described in our earlier paper (Marneros et al., 1991b). There, initial symptomatology fulfilling the criteria of an episode is categorized according to the criteria of Andreasen and Olsen; that is, as "positive," "negative", or "mixed" initial episodes.

Of the patients referred to in Table 1, 65 (44%) had a positive initial episode, 47 patients (32%) a negative initial episode, and 36 patients (24%) a mixed initial episode. The three groups of patients were compared with regard to the following variables:

- Sex distribution
- Age at onset
- Premorbid personality
- Premorbid social interactions
- Stable heterosexual partnership
- Marital status at onset
- Educational level
- Occupation at onset
- Social class

Results

Sex distribution

There was no statistically significant difference in the female-to-male ratio in the three groups investigated (Table 1). Male patients were found in 56%–60% of the total in all three groups.

Age at Onset

The patients with a negative initial episode had the lowest age at onset, on average 22.4 years (minimum 14 years, maximum 37 years; Table 1). There was significant difference in comparison to both other groups: the mean age at onset of the patients with a mixed schizophrenic initial episode was 28.2 years (minimum 15 years, maximum 48 years); and 31.3 years (minim 14 years,

Table 1. Sex, age at onset, and premorbid personality

		Positive initial episode ($n = 65$)	*p*1	Mixed initial episode ($n = 36$)	*p*2	Negative initial episode ($n = 47$)	*p*3
Sex			–		–		–[a]
Male	(*n*)	38		20		28	
	(%)	58.5		55.6		59.6	
Female	(*n*)	27		16		19	
	(%)	41.5		44.4		40.4	
Sex distribution (f:m)		1:1.41		1:1.25		1:1.47	
Age at onset (years)							
Arithmetical mean		31.3	–	28.2	**	22.4	**[b]
Median		26.0	–	24.0	**	21.0	**[c]
Standard deviation		12.1		10.0		5.9	
Minimal value		14		15		14	
Maximal value		64		48		37	
Premorbid personality (global categories)							
Not classifiable	(*n*)	35		11		10	
	(%)	53.8		44.0		27.0	
Classifiable	(*n*)	30		25		37	
Obsessoid	(*n*)	0		0		1	
	(%					2.7	
Sthenic/	(*n*)	5		4		7	
high self-confidence	(%)	16.7		16.0		18.9	
Asthenic/	(*n*)	25		21		29	
low self-confidence	(%)	83.3		84.0		78.4	
Premorbid social interactions							
Not classifiable	(*n*)	7		3		0	
	(%)	10.8		8.3			
Classifiable	(*n*)	58	–	33	–	47	*[a]
Tendency to isolation	(*n*)	30		23		35	
	(%)	51.7		69.7		74.5	
No tendency to isolation	(*n*)	28		10		12	
	(%)	48.3		30.3		25.5	

[a] χ^2 test.
[b] *t*-test.
[c] Mann-Whitney U test.
*p*1, significance of positive initial episode versus mixed initial episode; *p*2, significance of mixed initial episode versus negative initial episode; *p*3, significance of positive versus negative initial episode; * = $p < 0.05$; ** = $p < 0.01$; – = not significant.

maximum 64 years) in the group of patients with a positive schizophrenic onset of illness. While the minimal values are nearly identical in all three groups, there is a wide spread of maximal values over the three groups: from 37 years in the group of patients with a negative onset to 64 years in the group of patients with a positive initial episode.

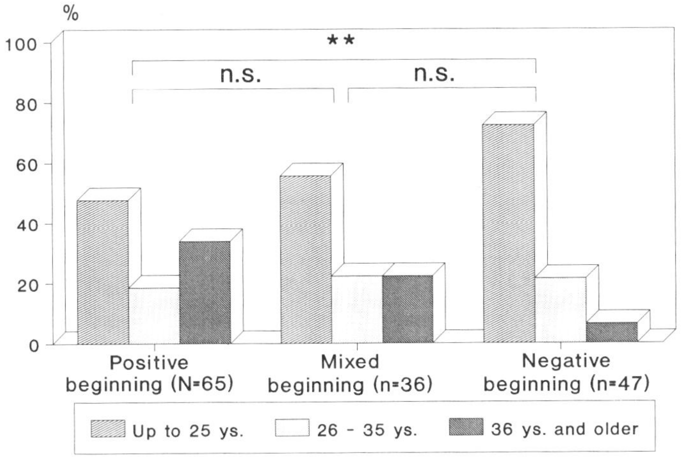

Fig. 1. Age at onset (3 categories)

The classification of age at onset into three categories (25 years or younger, 26–35 years, 36 years and older; Fig. 1) demonstrates that especially the frequency of young patients (up to 25 years of age) and of patients with a higher age at onset (36 years and older) differs between the group with a positive schizophrenic onset and the group with a negative initial episode (Fig. 1).

Premorbid Personality and Social Interactions

Methodological shortcomings regarding the evaluation of the premorbid personality structure in functional psychoses have been pointed out repeatedly (Marneros et al. 1989a, b, 1990a, 1991a). Particularly in schizophrenic disorders there is a risk of confusing "premorbid" and "postmorbid" features (Marneros et al. 1990). Because of these limitations, no standardized instruments were used for the present investigations. In order to estimate the premorbid personality the interviewer instead relied on information provided by patients and their families case records, etc. Three global categories of premorbid personality were used (Marneros et al. 1989a):

- *Obsessoid personality*, showing similarities to the "obsessive-compulsive personality" of DSM-III.
- *Asthenic/low-self-confident personality* (oriented on the "dependent personality" of DSM-III).
- *Sthenic/high-self-confident personality* (which is the opposite of the former type).

Because of the above-mentioned methodological problems, in 56 cases (37.8% of all the schizophrenic patients investigated) the premorbid personality was not classifiable (Table 1). The majority of patients in all three groups (78%–84%) had an asthenic/low-self-confident personality. Only one patient was categorized as having an obsessoid personality. Comparing the cases with a classifiable "premorbid" personality, there was no statistically significant difference among the three groups with positive, negative, and mixed schizophrenic onset.

The same methodological problems as for the premorbid personality arise in the retrospective evaluation of premorbid social interactions of schizophrenic patients. The patients were therefore classified into two global categories, again considering all the information available:

- Patients with a premorbid tendency to social isolation.
- Patients with no premorbid tendencies to social isolation and good premorbid contacts.

Patients with a negative initial episode were found to have a higher premorbid tendency to social isolation (74.5%) than patients with positive initial symptomatology (52%). Patients with a mixed schizophrenic episode at onset showed a tendency to social isolation in 70% of cases (Table 1).

Marital Status and Stable Heterosexual Partnership Before Onset

Closely connected with premorbid personality and premorbid social interactions is the ability to have "stable heterosexual relationships" (married, engaged, or with a steady girlfriend/boyfriend for at least 6 months). Significantly more patients with a positive initial episode were married or had a stable heterosexual partnership at onset (Table 2). This finding remains stable even if all patients younger than 25 years at onset are excluded. Further statistical analysis demonstrates that these significant differences were caused by the female patients with either a positive or a negative initial episode, while for male patients no differences were found among the three groups.

Educational Level

The educational level was evaluated using four global categories (Marneros et al. 1989a):

- *Very low educational level* (uncompleted elementary school, or special education for children with learning difficulties).
- *Low educational level* (completed elementary school, or uncompleted intermediate school).
- *Middle educational level* (completed intermediate/vocational school, or high school, not completed).
- *High educational level* (completed high school or university study).

There was no significant difference regarding the educational level (in some cases completed after the first manifestation of illness) among the three groups, although the group with a positive schizophrenic episode at onset had the highest percentage of patients with a very low educational level (Table 2).

Table 3. Marital status, stable sexual partnership, educational and occupational levels

		Positive initial episode ($n = 65$)	$p1$	Mixed initial episode ($n = 36$)	$p2$	Negative initial episode ($n = 47$)	$p3$
Married at onset							
All patients	(n)	22/65	–	10/36	–	8/47	*
	(%)	33.8		27.8		17.0	
Patients older than 25 years at onset	(n)	20/34	–	8/16	–	5/13	*
	(%)	58.8		50.0		38.5	
Stable heterosexual partnership before onset (> 6 months)							
All patients	(n)	29/65	–	13/36	–	9/47	**
	(%)	44.6		36.1		19.1	
Patients older than 25 years at onset	(n)	25/34	–	10/16	–	5/13	*
	(%)	73.5		62.5		38.5	
Educational level			–		–		–
Very low level	(n)	15		5		6	
	(%)	23.1		13.9		12.8	
Low level	(n)	33		16		23	
	(%)	50.8		44.4		48.9	
Intermediate level	(n)	8		8		7	
	(%)	12.3		22.2		14.9	
High level	(n)	9		7		11	
	(%)	13.8		19.4		23.4	
Occupation at onset (excluding housewives)		($n = 50$)	–	($n = 32$)	–	($n = 44$)	–
Without paid occupation	(n)	15		12		16	
	(%)	30.0		37.5		36.4	
No vocational training	(n)	17		12		15	
	(%)	34.0		37.5		34.1	
Skilled laborer	(n)	9		4		5	
	(%)	18.0		12.5		11.4	
White collar worker	(n)	8		1		8	
	(%)	16.0		3.1		18.2	
Top white collar worker	(n)	0		2		0	
	(%)			6.3			
Self-employed	(n)	1		1		0	
	(%)	2.0		3.1		0	

Significance (χ^2 test): $p1$, significance of positive initial episode versus mixed initial episode; $p2$, significance of mixed initial episode versus negative initial episode; $p3$, significance of positive versus negative initial episode; – = not significant; * = $p < 0.05$; ** = $p < 0.01$.

About one-quarter of the group of patients with a positive onset and more than one-third of the patients with a negative or a mixed onset had a middle or high educational level.

Occupation at Onset

There were no significant differences among the three groups regarding occupation at onset (Table 2). Most of the patients in all three groups had rather a low-level occupation (unskilled or skilled labourer), while fewer than 20% of the patients were white-collar workers or top white collar workers.

Social Class

The social class was estimated according to the criteria of Kleining and Moore (1968) and transferred to the classification of Hollingshead and Redlich (1958).

Table 3. Social class

		Positive initial episode ($n = 65$)	*p*1	Mixed initial episode ($n = 36$)	*p*2	Negative initial episode ($n = 47$)	*p*3
Parents' social class			–		–		–
Upper classes	(*n*)	1		4		4	
	(%)	1.6		11.4		8.7	
Middle middle class	(*n*)	8		7		5	
	(%)	12.7		20.0		10.9	
Lower middle class	(*n*)	11		3		15	
	(%)	17.5		8.6		32.6	
Higher low class	(*n*)	24		10		11	
	(%)	38.1		28.6		23.9	
Lower low class	(*n*)	19		11		11	
	(%)	30.2		31.4		23.9	
Patientś social class at onset			–		–		–
Upper classes	(*n*)	1		2		1	
	(%)	1.5		5.6		2.1	
Middle middle class	(*n*)	9		6		6	
	(%)	13.8		16.7		12.8	
Lower middle class	(*n*)	10		2		10	
	(%)	15.4		5.6		21.3	
Higher low class	(*n*)	15		10		10	
	(%)	23.1		27.8		21.3	
Lower low class	(*n*)	30		16		20	
	(%)	46.2		44.4		42.6	

Significance (χ^2 test): *p*1, significance of positive initial episode versus mixed initial episode; *p*2, significance of mixed initial episode versus negative initial episode; *p*3, significance of positive versus negative initial episode; – = not significant.

There were no differences among the three groups investigated regarding the social class of the parents (original social class; Table 3). Similarlys no differences were found in the social class of the patient at the onset of the illness. Nevertheless, the comparison of the original social class and the patient's social class at onset shows an interesting result. There is already a shift to the lowest social classes before the onset of illness. This finding is not only caused by the young age of the patients who are at the beginning of their occupational career. Individual case analysis showed that there were several patients who had suffered an occupational downward drift (negative occupational mobility) leading to negative social mobility some time before the first manifestation of the illness when no obvious signs of prodromal symptoms were present.

Discussion and Conclusions

The present study shows that no differences were found in relevant premorbid and sociodemographic features (i.e., for parameters like sex distribution, premorbid personality, educational level, occupational level at onset, parents' social class, and social class at onset of the illness) among the three groups investigated (positive, negative, or mixed schizophrenic episode at onset of the illness).

On the other hand, some parameters were found to show significant differences between the groups of patients with a positive and a negative initial episode. The most impressive difference seems to be the difference in age at onset: patients with a negative initial episode were significantly younger at onset than patients with a positive or mixed initial episode.

It could be argued that the age at onset is more a variable of the course than a direct sociodemographic variable. For the present study this variable was included because of a possible interference between age at onset and other parameters.

Patients with a negative initial episode showed a premorbid tendency to social isolation more frequently than patients with a positive initial episode, and they were married at onset at a significantly lower frequency. Further analysis showed that the lower age at onset in the group of patients with a negative schizophrenic onset does not seem to be the most relevant reason for these differences in premorbid adjustment as they were also found between patients with a negative and a positive schizophrenic onset who were older than 25 years at onset of the illness.

It can therefore be concluded that the type of onset of schizophrenic disorders (positive, negative, or mixed schizophrenic episodes) is correlated to some, but not all, relevant sociodemographic parameters. The correlations in the age at onset seem to be easily explained following the thesis of Huber (1982) and Häfner and Maurer (1991), i.e., that positive and negative symptoms are not independent but interdependent with an earlier beginning of symptomatology and later development of positive symptoms. However, that means that in narrowly defined schizophrenic disorders all the groups of symptoms – positive and negative – are an expression of one and the same disease.

References

Achté K, Tuulio-Henriksson A (1983) Schizophrenia and schizoaffective psychosiss. Psychiatr Clin 16:126–140

Andreasen NC (1990) Positive and negative Symptoms: historical and conceptual aspects. In: Andreasen NC (eds) Schizophrenia: Positive and negative symptoms and syndromes. Basel, Karger

Angermeyer MC, Klusmann D (1987) From social class to social stress: new developments in psychiatric epidemiology. In: Angermeyer MS (eds) From social class to social stress. Springer, Berlin Heidelberg New York

Angst J (1966) Zur Ätiologie und Nosologie endogener depressiver Psychosen. Eine genetische, souiologische und klinische Studie. Springer, Berlin Heidelberg New York

Angst J (1980) Verlauf unipolarer depressiver, bipolar manisch-depressiver und schizoaffektiver Erkrankungen und Psychosen. Fortschr Neurol Psychiatr 48:3–30

Angst J (1986) The course of schizoaffective disorders. In: Marneros A, Tsuang MT (eds) Schizoaffective psychoses. Springer, Berlin Heidelberg New York

Angst J (1987) Epidemiologie der affektiven Psychosen. In: Kisker KP, Lauter H, Meyer JE, Müller C, Strömgren E (eds) Psychiatrie der Gegenwart, Vol. 5. Springer, Berlin Heidelberg New York

Angst J (1988a) Clinical course of affective disorders. In: Helgason T, Daly RJ (eds) Depressive illness: prediction of course and outcome. Springer, Berlin Heidelberg New York

Angst J (1988b) European long-term follow-up studies of schizophrenia. Schizophr Bull 14:501–513

Angst J, Clayton PJ (1986) Premorbid personality of depressive, bipolar and schizophrenic patients with special reference to suicidal issues. Compr Psychiatry 27:511–532

Berner P, Lenz G (1986) Definitions of schizoaffective psychosis: mutual concordance and relationship to schizophrenia and affective disorder. In: Marneros A, Tsuang MT (eds) Schizoaffective psychoses. Springer, Berlin Heidelberg New York

Bland RC, Orn H (1978) 14-year outcome in early schizophrenia. Acta Psychiatr Scand 58:327–338

Bleuler M (1972) Die schizophrenen Geistesstörungen im Lichte langjähriger Kranken- und Familiengeschichten. Springer, Berlin Heidelberg New York

Ciompi L, Müller C (1976) Lebensweg und Alter der Schizophrenen. Eine katamnestische Langzeitstudie bis ins Senium. Springer, Berlin Heidelberg New York

Crow TJ (1980) Molecular pathology of schizophrenia: more than one disease process? Br Med J (Clin Res) 280:66–68

Dilling H, Weyrerer S (1987) Social class and mental disorders: results from upper bavarian studies. In:Angermeyer MS (eds) From social class to social stress. Springer, Berlin Heidelberg New York

Dohrenwend BP, Dohrenwend BS (1969) Social status and psychological disorder: a causal inquiry. Wiley, New York

Dohrenwend BP, Dohrenwend BS (1974) Social and cultural influences on psychopathology. Annu Rev Psychol 25:417–452

Dohrenwend BP, Dohrenwend BS (1976) Sex differences and psychiatric disorders. Am J Soc 81:1447–145

Dohrenwend BP, Shrout PE, Link BG, Martin JL, Skodol AE (1987) Overview and initial results of a risk factor study of depression and schizophrenia. In: Angermeyer MS (eds) From social class to social stress. Springer, Berlin Heidelberg New York

Eaton WW, Day R, Kramer M (1988) The use of epidemiology for risk factor research in schizophrenia: an overview and methodologic critique. In: Nasrallah HA (eds) Handbook of Schizophrenia, vol. 3. Elsevier, Amsterdam

Farmer AE, McGuffin P, Spitznagel E (1983) Heterogeneity in schizophrenia. A cluster analytic approach. Psychiatry Res 8:1–12

Farmer AE, McGuffin P, Gottesman II (1984) Searching for the split in schizophrenia: a twin study perspective. Psychiatry Res 13:109–118

Goodwin FK, Jamison KR (1990) Manic-depressive illness. Oxford University Press, New York
Häfner H (1987) Epidemiology of schizophrenia. In: Häfner H, Gattaz WF, Janzarik W (eds) Search for the causes of schizophrenia. Springer, Berlin Heidelberg New York
Häfner H (1990) New perspectives in the epidemiology of schizophrenia. In: Häfner H, Gattaz WF (eds) Search for the causes of schizophrenia II. Springer, Berlin Heidelberg New York
Häfner H, Maurer K (1991) Are there two types of schizophrenia? True onset and sequence of positive and negative syndromes prior to first admission. In: Marneros A, Andreasen NC, Tsuang MT (eds) Negative vs. positive schizophrenia. Springer, Berlin Heidelberg New York
Hirschfeld RMA, Cross CK (1982) Epidemiology of affective disorders. Psychosocial risk factors. Arch Gen Psychiatry 39:35–46
Hollingshead AB, Redlich FC (1958) Social class and mental illness. Wiley, New York
Huber G, Gross G, Schüttler R (1979) Schizophrenie. Eine verlaufs- und sozialpsychiatrische Langzeitstudie. Springer, Berlin Heidelberg New York
Janzarik W (1976) Die Krise der Psychopathologie. Nervenarzt 47:73–80
Kleining G, Moore H (1968) Soziale Selbsteinstufung (SSE) – Ein Instrument zur Messung sozialer Schichten. Köln Z Sozialpsychol 20:502–552
Lewin RRJ (1988) Gender and schizophrenia. In: Nasrallah HA (ed) Handbook of Schizophrenia, vol. 3: Nosology, epidemiology and genetics of schizophrenia. Elsevier, Amsterdam
Loranger AW (1984) Sex difference in age at onset of schizophrenia. Arch Gen Psychiatry 41:157–161
Marneros A, Tsuang MT (eds) (1986) Schizoaffective psychoses. Springer, Berlin Heidelberg New York
Marneros A, Tsuang MT (eds) (1990) Affective and schizoaffective disorders. Similarities and differences. Springer, Berlin Heidelberg New York
Marneros A, Deister A, Rohde A, Steinmeyer EM, Jünemann H (1989a) Long-term outcome of schizoaffective and schizophrenic disorders: a comparative study. Part I: Definitions, methods, psychopathological and social outcome. Eur Arch Psychiatry Neurol Sci 238:118–125
Marneros A, Deister A, Rohde A (1989b) Prämorbide and soziale Merkmale von Patienten mit schizoaffectiven Psychosen. Fortschr Neurol Psychiatr 57:205–212
Marneros A, Deister A, Rohde A (1990a) The concept of distinct but voluminous bipolar and unipolar diseases. I: the bipolar diseases. Eur Arch Psychiatry Clin Neurosci 240:77–84
Marneros A, Rohde A, Deister A (1990b) The concept of distinct but voluminous bipolar and unipolar diseases. II: the unipolar diseases. Eur Arch Psychiatry Clin Neurosci 240:85–89
Marneros A, Deister A, Rohde A (1990c) The concept of distinct but voluminous bipolar and unipolar diseases. III: unipolar and bipolar comparison. Eur Arch Psychiatry Clin Neurosci 240:90–95
Marneros A, Deister A, Rohde A (1991a) Affektive, schizoaffektive und schizophrene Psychosen. Eine vergleichende Langzeitstudie. Springer, Berlin Heidelberg New York
Marneros A, Deister A, Rohde A (1991b) Long-term investigations in stability of negative/positive distinction. In: Marneros A, Andreasen NC, Tsuang NC (eds) Negative versus positive schizophrenia. Springer, Berlin Heidelberg New York
McGlashan TH, Bardenstein KK (1990) Gender differences in affective, schizoaffective, and schizophrenic Disorders. Schizophr Bull 16:319–330
Möller HJ, von Zerssen D (1986) Der Verlauf schizophrener Psychosen unter den gegenwärtigen Behandlungsbedingungen. Springer, Berlin Heidelberg New York
Munk-Jorgensen P (1985) The schizophrenia diagnosis in Denmark. A register-based investigation. Acta Psychiatr Scand 72:266–273
von Zerssen D, Pössl M (1990) Structures of premorbid personality in endogenous psychotic disorders. In: Sarteschi P, Maggini C (eds) Personalitá e psicoatologia. Personality and psychopathology. Edizioni Tecnico Scientifiche, Pisa

Long-Term Outcome of Patients with a Positive Initial Episode Versus Patients with a Negative Initial Episode

A. DEISTER, A. MARNEROS, and A. ROHDE [1]

Introduction

The dichotomy of schizophrenic disorders into positive and negative subtypes (Andreasen and Olsen 1982; Andreasen 1990; Andreasen et al., 1991) and other dichotomies close to this distinction – such as Crow's (1980) dichotomy into type I and type II schizophrenia or Farmer's dichotomy (Farmer et al. 1983, 1984) into H-type and P-type of schizophrenia – goals to identify (additional to other correlations) also different degrees of severity of the illness. The negative subtype is said to be more severe than the positive (Andreasen et al., 1991); but the discussion reagarding the prognostic value of negative and positive symptoms is much older than the modern concept of negative and positive symptomatology in schizophrenia. More than 50 years ago Langfeldt (1937) found that blunted affect during an acute episode was prognostically unfavorable (see also Berrios 1991; Häfner and Maurer 1991; Lieberman et al. 1991; Meltzer 1991).

However, up to now, the results regarding the relationship between the type of symptomatology and the long-term outcome are contradictory. Some studies have found correlations between negative symptomatology and an unfavorable outcome (Astrup et al. 1962; Carpenter et al. 1978; Pogue-Geile and Harrow 1985), other studies have not (Bland et al. 1978; Gift et al. 1980; Knight and Roff 1985; Lindenmayer and Kay 1989).

It has been repeatedly pointed out that most studies on the prognostic value of positive or negative symptomatology are plagued by severe methodological shortcomings, such as the use of different criteria of negative and positive symptomatology, short observation time, no distinction between acute and chronic symptomatology, insufficient distinction of primary and secondary negative symptoms, etc. (Deister et al. 1990a; Häfner and Maurer 1991; Pogue-Geile 1989). As we have already shown (Marneros et al. 1991), the long-term course of schizophrenic psychoses is usually *bimorphous* regarding positive/negative symptomatology, i.e., with changes between positive and negative symptomatology during the long-term course, and the majority of schizophrenic disorders are even *polymorphous* regarding symptomatology in general. Therefore, considering longitudinal aspects of the course, it is not possible to compare the outcome of "positive" or "negative" subtypes of schizophrenic disorders.

[1] Psychiatrische Universitätsklinik, Sigmund-Freud-Straße 25, W-5300 Bonn, FRG

A. Marneros / N. C. Andreasen / M. T. Tsuang (Eds.)
Negative Versus Positive Schizophrenia

Under the same conditions as regards material and methods as in our previous papers (Marneros et al. 1991; Rohde et al. 1991), we tried to prove the hypothesis whether a negative initial episode could be an indicator of a greater severity of the illness. For these purposes, various aspects of long-term outcome (global functioning, psychological deficits, disability, and social consequences of the illness) were compared among three groups of schizophrenic patients categorized according to their initial episode (i.e., negative, positive, or mixed schizophrenic episode). Only the symptomatology of the first "episode of illness" (for the criteria of an episode, see next section) was considered, while the symptomatology of "pre-episodic alterations" (prodromal states) or "persisting alterations" (residual states) does not fulfill the criteria of an "episode" and therefore did not influence the categorization into positive, negative, or mixed onset.

Subjects, Methods, and Instruments

Subjects and Methods

The present investigation is part of the Cologne Study of Marneros and co-workers (Marneros et al. 1986a, b, c, 1989a, b, 1990a, b, 1991a, b; Rohde et al. 1991). The study population and follow-up methods have already been described (Marneros et al. 1991). The 148 patients longitudinally diagnosed as having a schizophrenic disorder had a mean follow-up period of 23 years and a mean age at the end of the observation time of 50.7 years. As already shown (Marneros et al. 1991), 65 patients (44%) had a positive schizophrenic episode at the onset of illness, 36 patients (24%) a mixed one, and 47 patients (32%) a negative one. An "episode of illness" was defined as the time between the beginning and end of inpatient or inpatient-like treatment. Inpatient-like treatment had to fulfill the following criteria: (a) intensive medical care (treatment with pyschotropic drugs and frequent consultation with a psychiatrist); and (b) interruption of usual work or duties.

Instruments of Evaluation

The evaluation of the long-term outcome is based on personal follow-up investigations. The various aspects of outcome were evaluated using the following instruments.

Global Assessment Scale. The Global Assessment Scale (GAS) (Spitzer et al. 1976; Endicott et al. 1976) is a rating scale for the evaluation of the overall functioning of a subject during a specified period on a continuum from psychological or psychiatric illness to health.

Disability Assessment Schedule. The Disability Assessment Schedule (WHO/DAS) was developed by the World Health Organization (WHO 1979, 1988) for the assessment of social behavior and disability during or after mental illness. In this study we used the German version of the WHO/DAS, developed by the Central Institute of Mental Health in Mannheim (Jung et al. 1989). Because of sample-dependent specificities, only the items of the section "Overall Behavior" were used for statistical purposes. The items of the section "Social Role Performance" were not compared because of the high frequency of permanently hospitalized patients or the absence of the necessary conditions for the performance of the social roles rated by these items, especially parental or occupational roles (Marneros et al. 1989a). For each item the interviewer had to rate both intensity and duration. The scores finally assigned were the sum totals of the scores for intensity and duration.

Psychological Impairments Rating Schedule. The Psychological Impairments Rating Schedule (WHO/PIRS) was developed by the WHO (1979) for the assessment of psychological impairment after mental illness. It reflects the opinion of the observing expert. The WHO/PIRS is strongly related to the Present State Examination (PSE) (Biehl et al. 1986, 1989; Schubart et al. 1986b). Seventy-five single items – representing observed behavior – were rated for each patient, and these items were grouped into ten sections. Additionally, an overall impression was evaluated for every section.

Instruments for the Evaluation of Social Consequences of the Illness. The following variables were selected from the group of evaluated factors reflecting social consequences of the illness (Marneros et al. 1989b) as being the most representative and at the same time reliable: (a) negative occupational mobility; (b) negative social mobility; (c) premature retirement; (d) non-achievement of the expected social development; and (e) impairment of autarky.

Results

Level of Global Functioning

The level of global functioning was estimated using GAS (Table 1). Regarding the arithmetic mean and the median of GAS scores, there were no significant differences among the three groups investigated. Patients with a positive initial episode had a mean score of 44.8 at the time of follow-up, patients with a mixed onset 39.8, and patients with a negative schizophrenic onset 40.0 (Table 1).

A significant difference was found between patients with a positive schizophrenic onset and patients with a negative onset when the scores were grouped into the following categories: (a) no difficulties (score 91–100); (b) slight difficulties (score 71–90); (c) moderate difficulties (score 51–70); (d) severe difficulties (score 31–50); and (e) very severe difficulties (score 1–30) (Table 1).

In all three groups more than two-thirds of the patients had severe or very severe difficulties. Patients without any impairment of global functioning (score 91–100) were very rare (ten patients, 6%). However, a striking

Table 1. Global functioning and social adjustment at the end of the observation time

	Positive initial episode ($n = 65$)	$p1$	Mixed initial episode ($n = 36$)	$p2$	Negative initial episode ($n = 47$)	$p3$
Global Assessment Scale	(GAS)	–		–		* [a]
No difficulties						
(score 91–100) (n)	8		1		1	
(%)	12.3		2.8		2.1	
Slight difficulties						
(score 71–90) (n)	7		5		6	
(%)	10.8		13.9		12.8	
Moderate difficulties						
(score 51–70) (n)	4		4		9	
(%)	6.2		11.1		19.1	
Severe difficulties						
(score 31–50) (n)	16		7		5	
(%)	24.6		19.4		10.6	
Very severe difficulties						
(score 1–30) (n)	30		19		26	
(%)	46.2		52.8		55.3	
Arithmetical mean	44.8	–	39.8	–	40.0	– [b]
Median	40	–	30	–	30	– [c]
Standard deviation	28.5		24.8		23.7	
Minimum	10		5		10	
Maximum	100		95		100	
Disability Assessment Schedule (WHO/DAS)		–		–		– [a]
Excellent social adjustment						
(score 0) (n)	9		1		1	
(%)	13.8		2.8		2.1	
Good social adjustment						
(score 1) (n)	6		4		3	
(%)	9.2		11.1		6.4	
Fair social adjustment						
(score 2) (n)	16		6		7	
(%)	24.6		16.7		14.9	
Poor social adjustment						
(score 3) (n)	11		8		11	
(%)	16.9		22.2		23.4	
Very poor social adjustment						
(score 4) (n)	15		9		16	
(%)	23.1		25.0		34.0	
Severe social maladjustment						
(score 5) (n)	8		8		9	
(%)	12.3		22.2		19.2	

[a] χ^2 test. [b] t test. [c] Mann-Whitney U test.

$p1$, significance of positive versus mixed initial episode; $p2$, significance of mixed versus negative initial episode; $p3$, significance of negative versus positive initial episode. Asterisk, $p < 0.05$.

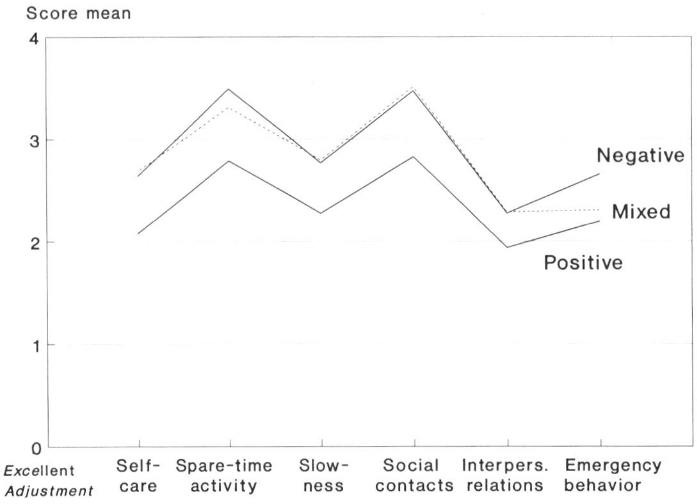

Fig. 1. Disability Assessment Schedule (WHO/DAS): profiles of disability

relationship was found between the category score 91–100 and a positive schizophrenic onset of illness: eight of the patients without any difficulties had a positive initial episode, only in one patient had the illness started with a negative and in another patient with a mixed schizophrenic episode (Table 1).

Level and kind of Disability

The level and kind of disability were assessed using the WHO/DAS. In this instrument "disability" is defined as "a disturbance or loss of the ability to perform specific social functions and roles in the family, at work, and/or in social groups, according to the normal expectations of the community" (Schubart et al. 1986a). Table 1 shows the global evaluation of WHO/DAS, considering all information recorded and rated in the schedule. No significant differences were found among the three groups, but as in GAS the majority of patients with excellent social adjustment were found to have a positive schizophrenic episode at the onset of illness.

Using section 1 of the WHO/DAS, overall behavior was rated by evaluating six items. The arithmetic mean of the scores of all patients in a group was calculated for each of these items. Figure 1 shows the profile of these items for the three groups. In all the items, patients with a negative initial episode had a worse social adjustment than patients with a positive onset, but only in the categories spare-time activity and social withdrawal were the differences statistically significant. Patients with a mixed initial episode had nearly identical scores to patients with a negative onset. Despite the numerical differences, there seem to be impressive parallels in all three profiles.

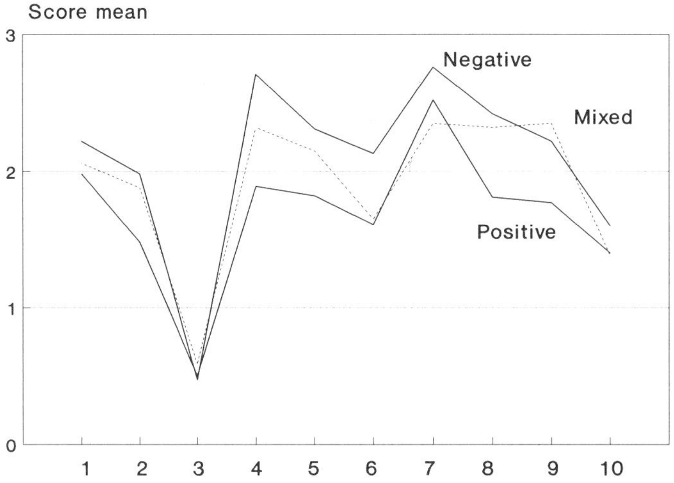

Fig. 2. Psychological Impairments Rating Schedule (WHO/PIRS): profiles of psychological deficits (global assessment). *1*, slowness; *2*, attention withdrawal; *3*, fatiguability; *4*, initiative; *5*, facial expression; *6*, body language; *7*, affect display; *8*, conversational skills; *9*, self-presentation; *10*, cooperation

Psychological Deficits

The psychological deficits were assessed using WHO/PIRS. For each section of the WHO/PIRS an "overall impression" was rated. The profiles of these ten sections are shown in Fig. 2. The three profiles – representing the different types of onset – were very similar. Only the item "initiative" showed a significant difference between negative and positive onsets: patients with a negative onset had less initiative at the end of the observation time than patients with a positive onset.

Social Consequences of the Illness

Negative Occupational Mobility

Occupational mobility is defined in this paper as the difference in occupational status between the beginning of occupational life and the time of the follow-up investigation or, for retired patients, the time of retirement. Only those patients were considered for statistical purposes for whom a negative occupational drift was possible, the other patients – mainly housewives as a result of marriage or childbirth – were excluded. In all three groups about 70% of the patients had suffered a downward occupational drift, without any significant difference among the groups (Table 2).

Negative Social Mobility

The social drift was evaluated by comparing the patient's original class (parents' social class) with the patient's social class at the end of the observation

Table 2. Social consequences

	Positive initial episode ($n = 65$)	$p1$	Mixed initial episode ($n = 36$)	$p2$	Negative initial episode ($n = 47$)	$p3$
Negative occupational mobility (n)	36/50	–	22/32	–	32/44	–
(%)	72.0		68.8		72.7	
Negative social mobility (n)	27/38	–	13/20	–	23/32	–
(%)	71.1		65.0		71.9	
Premature retirement (because of mental illness) (n)	21/49	–	17/32	–	25/44	–
(%)	42.9		53.1		56.8	
Non-achievement of the expected social development (n)	37/65	–	26/36	*	40/47	**
(%)	56.9		72.2		85.1	
Autarky		–		–		*
Autark (n)	32/62		12/36		15/46	
(%)	51.6		33.3		32.6	
Not autark (because of mental illness) (n)	22/62		13/36		15/46	
(%)	35.5		36.1		32.6	
Permanently hospitalized (n)	8/62		11/36		16/46	
(%)	12.9		30.6		34.8	

χ^2 test. $p1$, significance of positive versus mixed initial episode; $p2$, significance of mixed versus negative initial episode; $p3$, significance of negative versus positive initial episode. One asterisk, $p < 0.05$; two asterisks, $p < 0.01$.

time. The social class was estimated according to the criteria of Kleining and Moore (1968), transferred to the classification of Hollingshead and Redlich (1958). All patients for whom a negative social drift was impossible, i.e., because their original social class was already the lowest one, were excluded for statistical purposes. In all three groups more than two-thirds of the remaining patients had experienced a negative social mobility, but there were no significant differences among the three groups (Table 2).

Premature Retirement

With regard to premature retirement, no significant differences were found among patients with a positive, a mixed, and a negative schizophrenic episode at onset (Table 2).

Achievement of the Expected Social Development

In addition a parameter called the "achievement of the expected social development" was evaluated. This parameter reflects the opinion of the expert as to whether the patient is fulfilling his or her expected social role and whether he or she has achieved the social status which would be expected on the basis of the status of the family, education, possibilities of positive social mobility, and so on (Marneros et al. 1989b). This parameter can be evaluated for all patients independently of occupational status or social class and it seems to be very sensitive.

In the group of patients with a positive schizophrenic episode at onset, 57% had not achieved the expected social development; in the group of patients with a mixed onset the frequency of non-achievement was 72%; and in the group of patients with a negative initial episode the frequency was 85%. Statistically significant differences were found between patients with a positive and patients with a negative onset, and also between patients with a mixed and patients with a negative initial episode of illness (Table 2).

Impairment of Autarky

Autarky has been defined as the ability of the patient to take care of him- or herself and meet the needs of dependent family members. In practice autarky means the ability of a person to provide for him- or herself and other persons living in the same family, for instance, by working and earning money or by keeping house, without any outside support (Marneros et al. 1990b). The patients were categorized into three groups regarding their autarky status:

- Patients with no autarky limitations, i.e., patients were able to take care of the needs of their family or of their own needs.
- Patients who continuously needed help for their daily life, but were nevertheless able to live outside a psychiatric clinic.
- Patients who were permanently hospitalized in a psychiatric clinic because of their mental illness (> 3 years).

Significant differences were found between patients with a positive and patients with a negative schizophrenic episode at onset. In the group of patients with a negative onset, more than one-third of the patients had to be permanently hospitalized because of their mental illness, but in the group of patients with a positive initial episode only 13% had to be permanently hospitalized. About one-half of the patients with a positive initial episode had no limitations of the autarky at the end of the observation time (Table 2).

Discussion and Conclusions

Investigations regarding the impact of the positive/negative distinction in schizophrenic disorders on the long-term outcome – "long-term" in the real meaning of the word and not only in an euphemistic sense – have so far been very rare. Most of the studies are plagued by some relevant methodological shortcomings (Pogue-Geile 1989) and are therefore not comparable. In some studies, a positive correlation between negative symptomatology and some aspects of an unfavorable outcome were found (Astrup et al. 1962; Carpenter et al. 1978; Pogue-Geile and Harrow 1985), while in other studies there was no correlation or a correlation between negative symptomatology and a more favorable outcome (Lindenmayer and Kay 1989; Singh and Kay 1988).

The present study investigated the long-term course and outcome of schizophrenic patients with a positive, a negative, and a mixed schizophrenic episode at onset according to the criteria of Andreasen and Olsen (1982). Only symptomatology of the initial episode was considered; pre-episodic alterations (prodromal symptomatology) or persisting alterations (residual states) were not included. The majority of patients in all three subgroups showed an unfavorable outcome after a duration of illness of about 23 years on average.

In evaluating the long-term outcome, it has to be considered that "outcome" is not a monolithic term. The "outcome" of an illness is only a compromise, characterizing the present psychopathological, psychological, and social state of the patient, usually some months or years after onset of the illness (Angst 1980; Marneros et al. 1989a; Deister et al. 1990b). In investigating these various aspects of outcome, some differences were found between patients with a positive and patients with a negative schizophrenic onset: 80% of the patients who had no persistent alterations at the end of the observation time had had a positive schizophrenic episode at the onset of illness; on the other hand, about one-third of the patients with a negative initial episode had to be permanently hospitalized.

The type of initial symptomatology may have a predictive value with regard to long-term outcome – probably not as an isolated factor but in combination and interaction with premorbid and sociodemographic features such as age at first manifestation, premorbid social interactions, and so on (Pogue-Geile and Harrow 1985; Rohde et al. 1991).

References

Andreasen NC (1990) Positive and negative symptoms: historical and conceptual aspects. In: Andreasen NC (ed) Schizophrenia: positive and negative symptomes and syndromes. Karger, Basel

Andreasen NC, Olsen S (1982) Negative vs. positive schizophrenia. Arch Gen Psychiatry 39:789–894

Andreasen NC, Flaum M, Arndt S, Alliger R, Swayze VW (1991) Positive and negative symptoms: assessment and validity. In: Marneros A, Andreasen NC, Tsuang MT (eds) Negative vs. positive schizophrenia. Springer, Berlin Heidelberg New York

Angst J (1980) Verlauf unipolar depressiver, bipolar manisch-depressiver und schizoaffektiver Erkrankungen und Psychosen. Fortschr Neurol Psychiatr 48:3–30

Astrup C, Fossum A, Holmboe R (1962) Prognosis in functional psychoses. Thomas, Springfield

Berrios GE (1991) Positive and negative signals: a conceptual history. In: Marneros A, Andreasen NC, Tsuang MT (eds) Negative vs. positive schizophrenia. Springer, Berlin Heidelberg New York

Biehl H, Maurer K, Schubart C, Krumm B, Jung E (1986) Prediction of outcome and utilization of medical services in a prospective study of first onset schizophrenics – results of a prospective 5-year follow-up study. Eur Arch Psychiatry Neurol Sci 236:139–147

Biehl H, Maurer K, Jablensky A, Cooper JE, Tomov T (1989) The PIRS/WHO. I: introducing a new instrument for rating observed behaviour and the rationals of the psychological impairment concept. Br J Psychiatry 155 (Suppl 7): 68–70

Bland RC, Parker JH, Orn H (1978) Prognosis in schizophrenia. Arch Gen Psychiatry 35:72–77

Carpenter WT, Bartko JJ, Strauss JS, Hawk AB (1978) Signs and symptoms as predictors of outcome: a report from the International Pilot Study of Schizophrenia. Am J Psychiatry 135:940–944

Crow TJ (1980) Molecular pathology of schizophrenia: more than one disease process? Br Med J (Clin Res) 280:66–68

Deister A, Marneros A, Rohde A (1990a) Zur Stabilität negativer und positiver Syndromatik. In: Möller HJ (ed) Neuere Ansätze zur Diagnostik und Therapie schizophrener Minussymptomatik. Springer, Berlin Heidelberg New York

Deister A, Marneros A, Rohde A, Staab B, Jünemann H (1990b) Long-term outcome of affective, schizoaffective, and schizophrenic disorders: a comparison. In: Marneros A, Tsuang MT (eds) Affective and schizoaffective disorders: similarities and differences. Springer, Berlin Heidelberg New York

Endicott J, Spitzer RL, Fleiss JL, Cohen J (1976) The Global Assessment Scale. A Procedure for Measuring Overall Severity of Psychiatric Disturbance. Arch Gen Psychiatry 33:766–771

Farmer AE, McGuffin P, Spitznagel E (1983) Heterogeneity in schizophrenia. A cluster analytic approach. Psychiatry Res 8:1–12

Farmer AE, McGuffin P, Gottesmann II (1984) Searching for the split in schizophrenia: a twin study perspective. Psychiatry Res 13:109–118

Gift TE, Strauss JS, Kokes RF et al. (1980) Schizophrenia: affect and outcome. Am J Psychiatry 137:580–585

Häfner H, Maurer K (1991) Are there two types of schizophrenia? True onset and sequence of positive and negative syndromes prior to first admission. In: Marneros A, Andreasen NC, Tsuang MT (eds) Negative vs. positive schizophrenia. Springer, Berlin Heidelberg New York

Hollingshead AB, Redlich FC (1958) Social class and mental illness. Wiley, New York

Jung E, Krumm B, Biehl H, Maurer K, Bauer-Schubart C (1989) Disability Assessment Schedule. DAS-M Mannheimer Skala zur Einschätzung sozialer Behinderung. Beltz, Weinheim

Kleining G, Moore H (1968) Soziale Selbsteinstufung (SSE) – Ein Instrument zur Messung sozialer Schichten. Köln Z Soziol Sozialpsychol 20:502–552

Knight RA, Roff JD (1985) Affectivity in schizophrenia. In: Alpert M (ed) Controversies in schizophrenia. Guilford, New York

Langfeldt G (1937) The prognosis in schizophrenia and the factors influencing the course of the disease. Acta Psychiatr Scand (Suppl) 13

Lieberman JA, Jody D, Alvir JM, Borenstein M, Mayerhoff DI (1991) Negative symptoms in schizophrenia. Relationship to positive symptoms and outcome. In: Marneros A, Andreasen NC, Tsuang MT (eds) Negative vs. positive schizophrenia. Springer, Berlin Heidelberg New York

Lindenmayer JP, Kay SR (1989) Depression, affect and negative symptoms in schizophrenia. Br J Psychiatry 155 (Suppl 7):108–114

Marneros A, Deister A, Rohde A (1986a) The Cologne Study on schizoaffective disorders and schizophrenia suspecta. In: Marneros A, Tsuang MT (eds) Schizoaffective psychoses. Springer, Berlin Heidelberg New York

Marneros A, Rohde A, Deister A (1986b) Features of schizoaffective disorders: the "cases-in-between". In: Marneros A, Tsuang MT (eds) Schizoaffective psychoses. Springer, Berlin Heidelberg New York

Marneros A, Rohde A, Deister A, Risse A (1986c) Schizoaffective disorders: the prognostic value of the affective component. In: Marneros A, Tsuang MT (eds) Schizoaffective psychoses. Springer, Berlin Heidelberg New York

Marneros A, Deister A, Rohde A, Steinmeyer EM, Jünemann H (1989a) Long-term outcome of schizoaffective and schizophrenic disorders: a comparative study. Part I. Definitions, methods, psychopathological and social outcome. Eur Arch Psychiatry Neurol Sci 238:118–125

Marneros A, Steinmeyer EM, Deister A, Rohde A, Jünemann H (1989b) Long-term outcome of schizoaffective and schizophrenic disorders: a comparative study. Part III. The social consequences. Eur Arch Psychiatry Neurol Sci 238:135–139

Marneros A, Deister A, Rohde A (1990a) Sociodemographic and premorbid features of schizophrenic, schizoaffective and affective disorders. In: Marneros A, Tsuang MT (eds.) Schizoaffective and affective disorders: similarities and differences. Springer, Berlin Heidelberg New York

Marneros A, Deister A, Rohde A (1990b) Autarkie und Autarkiebeeinträchtigung bei schizophrenen Patienten. Nervenarzt 61:503–508

Marneros A, Deister A, Rohde A (1991a) Affektive, schizoaffektive und schizophrene Psychosen. Eine vergleichende Langzeitstudie. Springer, Berlin Heidelberg New York

Marneros, Deister A, Rohde A (1991b) Long-term investigations in stability of negative/positive distinction. In: Marneros A, Andreasen NC, Tsuang MT (eds) Negative vs. positive schizophrenia. Springer, Berlin Heidelberg New York

Meltzer HY (1991) The effect of clozapine and other atypical antipsychotic drugs on negative symptoms. In: Marneros A, Andreasen NC, Tsuang MT (eds) Negative vs. positive schizophrenia. Springer, Berlin Heidelberg New York

Pogue-Geile MF (1989) The prognostic significance of negative symptoms in schizophrenia. Br J Psychiatry 155 (Suppl 7):123–127

Pogue-Geile MF, Harrow M (1985) Negative symptoms in schizophrenia: their longitudinal course and prognostic importance. Schizophr Bull 11:427–439

Rohde A, Marneros A, Deister A (1991) Premorbid and sociodemographic features of initially positive and initially negative schizophrenia. In: Marneros A, Andreasen NC, Tsuang MT (eds) Negative vs. positive schizophrenia. Springer, Berlin Heidelberg New York

Schubart C, Schwarz R, Krumm B, Biehl H (1986a) Schizophrenie und soziale Anpassung. Springer, Berlin Heidelberg New York

Schubart C, Krumm B, Biehl H, Schwarz R (1986b) Measurement of social disability in a schizophrenic patient group. Soc Psychiatry 21:1–9

Singh MM, Kay SR (1988) Is the positive-negative distinction in schizophrenia valid? Br J Psychiatry 150:879–880

Spitzer RL, Gibbon M, Endicott J (1976) The global assessment scale. Arch Gen Psychiatry 33:768

World Health Organization (WHO) (1979) Schizophrenia. An international follow-up study. Wiley, New York

World Health Organization (WHO) (1988) WHO Psychiatric Disability Assessment Schedule (WHO/DAS). WHO, Geneva

The Concept of Positive and Negative Schizophrenia in Child and Adolescent Psychiatry

H. REMSCHMIDT, M. MARTIN, E. SCHULZ, C. GUTENBRUNNER, and C. FLEISCHHAKER [1]

Introduction

Psychoses in Childhood and Adolescence

Schizophrenic psychoses in childhood are important but rare disorders within the spectrum of psychoses. They had been delineated as specific psychotic disorders only at the end of the 1930s (Lutz 1937/1938). At the end of the 1950s and 1960s, it became evident that age and developmental stage may be looked upon as important criteria for the classification of childhood psychoses (GAP 1966; Stutte 1969), which was demonstrated by several empirical studies (Rutter et al. 1967; Kolvin et al. 1971 a–d). Finally, these studies confirmed the notion of Kanner (1943, 1957) who subdivided psychoses in childhood into three groups: early infantile autism, childhood schizophrenia, and disintegrative psychoses of childhood, the last comprising disorders such as dementia infantilis (Heller 1908) and psychoses related to different kinds of brain damage. These aspects have also influenced the multiaxial classification system on the basis of the International Classification of Diseases (ICD-9) (Rutter et al. 1976) and the Diagnostic and Statistical Manual (DSM-III and DSM-III-R) of the American Psychiatric Association (APA 1980, 1987). Both classification systems differentiate between early infantile autism, childhood schizophrenia, and early childhood dementia.

Several studies have shown that age and developmental stage are those factors that influence most the clinical picture of childhood psychoses (Anthony 1958, 1962; Bettes and Walker 1987, Stutte 1960, 1969; Kolvin et al. 1971 a–d; Werry 1979). Most researchers agree that with respect to them at least four groups of psychoses in childhood and adolescence can be differentiated. This subdivision was first proposed by Anthony (1958, 1962) and is demonstrated in Table 1.

The first group of psychoses (Group I) comprises different psychotic syndromes with slow beginning, chronic course, and manifestation before the 3rd year of life. All except early infantile catatonia have no connection to schizophrenia.

The second group includes different psychotic states, most of them with acute beginning and different regressive behaviors that manifest themselves

[1] Abteilung für Kinder- und Jugendpsychiatrie, Philipps-Universität, Hans-Sachs-Straße 6, W-3550 Marburg, FRG

A. Marneros / N. C. Andreasen / M. T. Tsuang (Eds.)
Negative Versus Positive Schizophrenia

Table 1. Different psychotic syndromes in childhood and adolescence and their relation to schizophrenia

Clinical syndrome	Age of manifestation and course	Relation to schizophrenia
Group I (Anthony 1958, 1962)	Early manifestation until 3rd year of life and chronic course	No relation to schizophrenia
– Autism Kanner (Kanner 1943)		
– Pseudodefective psychosis (Bender 1947, 1959)		
– "No-onset-type" (Despert 1938)		
– Early infantile catatonia (Leonhard 1986)	Manifestation before 3rd year of life possible	Relation to schizophrenia likely
Group II (Anthony 1958, 1962)	Manifestation between 3rd and 5th year of life with acute course and regressive behavior	Relation to schizophrenia questionable
– Dementia infantilis (Heller 1908)		
– Dementia praecocissima (de Sanctis 1908)		
– Pseudoneurotic schizophrenia (Bender 1947, 1959)		
– "Acute-onset-type" (Despert 1938)		
– Symbiotic psychosis (Mahler et al. 1949; Mahler 1952)		
– Asperger syndrome (1944, 1968)		
– Early infantile catatonia (Leonhard 1986)	Most frequent manifestation within the first 6 years of life	Relation to schizophrenia likely
Group III (Anthony 1958, 1962)	Late-onset psychoses (late childhood and prepuberty) with fluctuating, subacute course	With a relation to schizophrenia of adolescence and also adulthood (Anthony 1958, 1962; Eisenberg 1957; Rimland 1964; Rutter 1967)
Psychoses (late-onset psychoses) (Kolvin et al. 1971 a–d)		
– Pseudopsychopathic schizophrenia (Bender 1959)		
– Prepuberal schizophenia (Stutte 1969; Eggers 1973)	Manifestation in prepuberty	Clear relation to schizophrenia
Group IV		
Adolescent schizophrenia	Manifestation during puberty and adolescent age	Clear relation to schizophrenia

from Remschmidt (1988).

between the 3rd and 5th year of life. The connection with schizophrenia is questionable, again with the exception of early infantile catatonia described by Leonhard (1986). According to him, the connection to schizophrenia is likely.

The third group of psychoses is characterized as late-onset psychoses with a manifestation in late childhood until prepuberty, fluctuating or subacute course, and a clear relationship to schizophrenia of adolescence and adulthood. This applies especially for prepubertal schizophrenia as described by Stutte (1969) and Eggers (1973).

The fourth group finally is adolescent schizophrenia with manifestation at puberty and adolescence and a very clear relationship to schizophrenia. Psychoses in adolescence belong to the type of newly manifested disorders (Rutter et al. 1976; Remschmidt 1975a, b). Some of them do and some do not have precursor symptoms in childhood. This subdivision according to premorbid personality and adaptation seems to be important also with respect to the concept of positive and negative schizophrenia in adolescence, because there is a relationship between poor premorbid adjustment and negative schizophrenia in adulthood (Andreasen and Olsen 1982).

The Concept of Positive and Negative Schizophrenia

As Angst et al. (1989) have pointed out, the terms "negative" and "positive" symptoms go back to a description of the British neurologist Jackson (1884) who used them in connection with a hierarchical model of cerebral functions. The concept was then applied by Strauss et al. (1974) using positive and negative symptoms as predictors. Before this time, the main elements of the deficit syndrome had already been described by Bleuler (1911) as "core symptoms schizophrenia" and by Huber (1957) as "basic syndrome of schizophrenia." These clinical descriptions have been elaborated since by many authors who developed special methods for their evaluation in schizophrenic patients (Andreasen 1982; Andreasen and Olsen 1982; Koehler and Sauer 1984; Ban et al. 1982; Carpenter et al. 1985; Johnstone et al. 1986; Walker and Lewine 1988). However, two important aspects have to be stated:

1. Positive and negative symptoms are not specific for schizophrenia. Negative symptoms, for instance, can occur also in other psychiatric syndromes outside of the schizophrenic spectrum, for instance in drug-induced depression, neurotic and personality disorders, organic brain syndromes (Angst et al. 1989).
2. Within the schizophrenic spectrum, negative symptoms can occur in different stages of the schizophrenic disorder (Angst et al. 1989), for example, in the prepsychotic period (Conrad 1958), during the productive psychotic period, and during the post-psychotic period, e.g., as "post-psychotic depression" (Mayer-Gross 1920) or as post-remissive exhaustion (Heinrich 1967).

These observations show very clearly that positive and negative symptoms are not stable conditions but fluctuate in relation to the course of schizophrenia and also in relation to neuroleptic treatment (Angst et al. 1989). Negative symptoms may be concealed by positive symptoms and may reappear, if the positive symptoms are influenced by therapy. Also, the correlation between premorbid difficulties in adaptation and negative symptoms has to be mentioned here.

While there is a rich literature on positive and negative schizophrenia in adults, we found only one study that applied this concept to childhood schizophrenia. Bettes and Walker (1987) analyzed a sample of 1084 children diagnosed as psychotic selected from a total sample of 11 478 children and adolescent aged 5–18 years from all state-supported inpatient and outpatient facilities in the Erie county and New York City area. For all these patients, the presence or absence of 31 symptoms including psychotic ones was recorded at intake by a psychiatrist, a psychologist, and a social worker. The authors found a strong effect of age on the manifestation of positive and negative symptoms. Positive symptoms increased linearly with age, while negative symptoms were most common in early childhood and late adolescence. This result applied for the total sample of children and also for the subsample of children diagnosed as psychotic. There were only a few sex differences concerning the rate of symptoms. A further result was a correlation between symptomatology and IQ in the sense that children with a high IQ showed more positive and fewer negative symptoms than children with a low IQ. Bettes and Walker (1987) offer three interpretations of their results:

1. The two types of symptoms could represent different psychiatric conditions related to *different underlying causes*. This association has been proposed by Crow (1980) for adult schizophrenia.
2. The two symptom types are associated with *different stages of the course* of schizophrenia. For instance, negative symptoms could be associated with advanced stages. As the authors state, however, this interpretation could not explain the simultaneous increase of both positive and negative symptoms during adolescence.
3. "The clinical manifestation of psychosis in the vulnerable child varies as a function of environmental demands as well as characteristics of the individual. Positive symptoms, particularly those that are based on ideational access (e.g. paranoia, delusion, grandiosity), may increase in likelihood as cognitive capacity increases. This would explain the linear increase in positive symptoms with age, as well as the lower rate of positive symptomatology in low-IQ children. Alternatively, positive symptoms may be subserved by certain biochemical processes that are triggered during puberty" (p. 565).

This investigation underlines the notion of earlier studies that age and developmental stage are decisive variables for the symptomatology of psychotic states in childhood (see Table 1).

With regard to the concept of positive and negative schizophrenia in child and adolescent psychiatry, we carried out two studies during the past years that will be described in the following section of this paper.

Positive and Negative Symptoms in Adolescent Schizophrenia

Aims of the Study

The main aim of the study was to evaluate the concept of positive and negative schizophrenia in a sample of schizophrenic adolescents who had been treated as inpatients in our clinical department between 1983 and 1988. For this study, we could rely on our basic documentation including a standardized list of symptoms that are recorded as a matter of routine for each patient at intake. As also a change of symptomatology during inpatient treatment was recorded, we were able to compare the psychopathological state of each patient at the beginning of the inpatient treatment episode and also at the end. With regard to this possibility, our aim was to objectify the shift of symptoms during inpatient treatment.

Sample

A data set of clinical documentation from the Department of Child and Adolescent Psychiatry, Philipps-University, Marburg, FRG, was used including the data of all patients who had been referred for inpatient treatment between 1 January 1983 and 31 December 1988. From a total of 1351 patients, 154 were referred with the diagnosis "schizophrenia." A careful examination at intake and during the first weeks of treatment revealed that 41 patients did not suffer from schizophrenia but from endogenous depression ($n = 14$), neurotic disorders ($n = 12$), adjustment reactions ($n = 3$), personality disorders ($n = 3$), brain damage ($n = 4$), autism ($n = 3$), and drug-induced psychosis ($n = 2$). These patients were excluded from the analysis.

The remaining 113 patients (58 male, 55 female; mean age 18.3 ± 2 years) were diagnosed as schizophrenic according to the multiaxial classification scheme (ICD-9) (Rutter et al. 1976). Table 2 gives an overview of the different

Table 2. Different subtypes and sex distribution of schizophrenic psychoses in the total sample ($n = 113$) according to ICD-9

	Total		Male		Female	
	(*n*)	(%)	(*n*)	(%)	(*n*)	(%)
Simple type (295.0)	1	0.9			1	1
Hebephenic type	35	31	19	32	16	29
Catatonic type (295.2)	2	1.8	1	1	1	1
Paranoid type (295.3)	52	46	26	44	26	47
Acute schizophrenic episode (295.4)	3	2.7	1	1	2	3
Residual schizophrenia (295.6)	3	2.7	2	3	1	1
Schizoaffective type (295.7)	17	15	9	15	8	14
	113		58		55	

Table 3. Different subtypes and sex distribution of the schizophrenic psychoses in the total sample (n = 113) according to DSM-III-R at intake

	Sex				Total	
	Male		Female			
	(n)	(%)	(n)	(%)	(n)	(%)
295.1 Disorganized type	18	31	16	29	34	30
295.2 Catatonic type	1	1	1	1	2	1
295.3 Paranoid type	27	46	26	47	53	46
295.4 Schizophreniform disorder	1	1	2	3	3	2
295.6 Residual type	2	3	2	3	4	3
295.7 Schizoaffective disorder	9	15	8	14	17	15
Total	58		55		113	

subtypes of schizophrenia in the total sample. As the table demonstrates, the most frequent types of schizophrenia are the paranoid type, the hebephrenic type, and the schizoaffective psychoses. There are no remarkable sex differences. With regard to the sample, it has to be mentioned that it is rather mixed, including patients with first manifestation of schizophrenia and others who had already been hospitalized several times. We always examined the last episode of each patient within the 6 years from 1983 to 1988.

Table 3 shows the different subtypes and sex distribution of the schizophrenic psychoses in the total sample according to DSM-III-R. As the table demonstrates, there are not many differences between this classification and the ICD-9 classification.

The symptomatology was also classified according to the ICD-10 criteria, but this classification will not be discussed here.

Methodology

The following instruments were used for the analysis:

1. The standardized basic documentation including a symptom list which is as a matter of routine administered in our department for each patient at intake.
2. A special rating of positive and negative symptoms and of inconsistently classified symptoms according to positive and negative symptom scales. This rating was done by an experienced child psychiatrist in that way that typical positive symptoms (e.g., hallucinations, delusions) received the value + 1 and clearly negative symptoms (e.g., affective flattening, anergia, anhedonia, and withdrawal) received the value − 1. These ratings are demonstrated in Tables 4 and 5. The symptoms of each patient were rated according to this scale at the beginning and at the end of the treatment episode. This score will be referred to as type according to score. With

Table 4. Rating of positive vs. negative symptoms

Symptom	Severity criteria
Hallucinations	+1
Delusion	+1
Positive formal thought disorder	+1
Excitement	+1
Pressure of speech	+1
Aggressiveness	+0.75
Bizarre behavior	+0.5
Affective flattening	−1
Anergia	−1
Anhedonia/social withdrawal	−1
Thought blocking	−0.5
Poverty of speech or speech content	−0.5
Attentional impairment	0

Table 5. Inconsistently classified symptoms according to positive and negative symptom scales

Symptom	Severity criteria
Loose associations (derailment)	+1
Delusional idea	+1
Idea of reference or idea of being influenced	+0.75
Neologisms	+0.75
Euphoria	+0.5
Autistic	−1
Foolish	−0.75
Depression	−0.5
Compulsion	−0.5
Obsessive/compulsive	−0.5
Inappropriate affect	0
Dysphoria	0
Suicidal or attempted suicide or suicidal thought	0
Anxiety	0

respect to it, a positive type of schizophrenia was defined from + 0.33 to + 1, a negative type from − 0.33 to − 1, and a mixed type from − 0.33 to + 0.33.

3. Finally, a clinical rating of each case according to the criteria of Andreasen (1982) was carried out by the same child psychiatrist who had also rated the symptom loadings (see Tables 4 and 5). We refer to the results of this rating as type I (positive schizophrenia), type II (negative schizophrenia), and type III (mixed type).

In terms of these symptom ratings, the symptomatology of each patient at the beginning and at the end of the inpatient episode was classified into three types: I (positive schizophrenia), II (negative schizophrenia), or III (mixed).

With respect to positive and negative symptomatology, an index was calculated for each patient, so that all patients could be placed with respect to their psychopathology on a continuous scale with the extremes $+1$ and -1 representing the positive and the negative end of the schizophrenic symptomatology spectrum, respectively.

For data analysis, several group comparisons were administered, including χ^2 and Fisher's exact test, and several explorative cluster analyses were carried out.

Results

Symptomatology at the Beginning of the Episode

Table 6 demonstrates the distribution of positive and negative symptoms at the beginning of the inpatient treatment episode with respect to the three types of schizophrenia. As it shows, some symptoms differentiate very clearly between type I and type II schizophrenia (e.g., hallucinations, delusions, excitement, pressure of speech), but the mixed type cannot be clearly delineated from the others.

Table 7 shows the distribution of inconsistently classified symptoms according to positive and negative schizophrenia at the beginning of the episode.

Symptomatology at the End of the Episode

As far as symptomatology at the end of the episode is concerned, highly significant differences can be observed with respect to several symptoms. This is demonstrated in Table 8, which shows the distribution of positive and negative symptoms at the end of the last inpatient treatment episode. From 113 patients, only 14 achieved complete remission, only 8 remained type I, as many as 38 were classified as type II and only 8 as mixed.

All in all, there is a clear shift in the direction of type II schizophrenia.

Symptom Shift During Inpatient Treatment

Figure 1 demonstrates the positivity/negativity score in relation to the number of symptoms at the beginning of the episode. The figure shows very clearly that the patients were classified into two clusters with respect to positivity/negativity. Only a few patients represent the "pure type" of positive and negative schizophrenia. Most of them are more or less positive or negative.

Figure 2 demonstrates the same score at the end of the episode. It includes two different points of information: first, a reduction of the number of symptoms can be observed, and second, there is a clear shift of symptomatology in the direction of negativity. There are only a few patients who show a symptom shift in the other direction (from negativity to positivity).

Table 6. Distribution of positive and negative symptoms at the beginning of the inpatient treatment episode in relation to the three types of schizophrenia

	Type at the beginning						Total	
	Type I		Type II		Mixed			
	(*n*)	(%)	(*n*)	(%)	(*n*)	(%)	(*n*)	(%)
Hallucinations	13	43	1	2	13	27	27	23
Delusion	29	96	0	0	34	70	63	55
Positive formal thought disorder	16	53	7	20	21	43	44	38
Bizarre behavior	1	3	2	5	2	4	5	4
Aggressiveness	3	10	5	14	6	12	14	12
Excitement	24	80	15	42	28	58	67	59
Pressure of speech	5	16	0	0	5	10	10	8
Affective flattening	5	16	14	40	23	47	42	37
Poverty of speech or speech content	7	23	12	34	15	31	34	30
Anergia	25	83	30	85	39	81	94	83
Anhedonia/social withdrawal	11	36	18	51	24	50	53	46
Thought blocking	6	20	11	31	17	35	34	30
Attentional impairment	30	100	29	82	47	97	106	93
Total	30		35		48		113	

Table 7. Distribution of inconsistently classified symptoms in relation to the three types of schizophrenia at the beginning of the episode

	Type at the beginning						Total	
	Type I		Type II		Mixed			
	(*n*)	(%)	(*n*)	(%)	(*n*)	(%)	(*n*)	(%)
Loose associations (derailment)	14	46	2	5	6	12	22	19
Inappropriate affect	6	20	5	14	5	10	16	14
Neologisms	1	3	2	5	3	6	6	5
Delusional idea	29	96	0	0	34	70	63	55
Idea of reference/being influenced	12	40	0	0	12	25	24	21
Depression	5	16	5	14	3	6	13	11
Euphoria	3	10	3	8	6	12	12	10
Dysphoria	6	20	3	8	4	8	13	11
Anxiety	3	10	0	0	3	6	6	5
Autistic	0	0	5	14	1	2	6	5
Suicidal	6	20	6	17	13	27	25	22
Suicidal thought	3	10	5	14	10	20	18	15
Attempted suicide	2	6	2	5	8	16	12	10
Obsessive/compulsive	3	10	3	8	4	8	10	8
Compulsion	1	3	2	5	2	4	5	4
Foolish	5	16	7	20	8	16	20	17
Total	30		35		48		113	

Table 8. Distribution of positive and negative symptoms at the end of the treatment episode in relation to the three types of schizophrenia

	Type at the end								Total	
	Remission		Type I		Type II		Mixed			
	(*n*)	(%)	(*n*)	(%)	(*n*)	(%)	(*n*)	(%)	(*n*)	(%)
Hallucinations	0	0	2	25	0	0	1	12	3	2
Delusion	0	0	7	87	1	1	4	50	12	10
Positive formal thought disorder	0	0	7	87	2	2	4	50	13	11
Bizarre behavior	0	0	0	0	7	8	0	0	7	6
Aggressiveness	0	0	2	25	7	8	2	25	11	9
Excitement	0	0	7	87	2	2	5	62	14	12
Pressure of speech	0	0	0	0	0	0	0	0	0	0
Affective flattening	0	0	1	12	70	84	5	62	76	67
Poverty of speech or speech content	0	0	0	0	9	10	1	12	10	8
Anergia	0	0	0	0	80	96	8	100	88	77
Anhedonia/social withdrawal	0	0	0	0	67	80	3	37	70	61
Thought blocking	0	0	1	12	44	53	4	50	49	43
Attentional impairment	0	0	8	100	56	67	6	75	70	61
Total	14		8		83		8		113	

Finally, Fig. 3 demonstrates the positivity/negativity scores at the beginning in comparison with the end of the episode. It shows 4 quadrants in which the different patients are located with regard to the change of their symptomatology, the diagonal representing patients whose symptomatology did not change. The upper right quadrant describes patients who remained positive to a different extent during the episode. The lower left quadrant represents patients who remained with a more or less negative symptomatology. The upper left quadrant includes the few patients who emerged from a more or less negative symptomatology into a positive one, and the lower right quadrant includes a relatively high number of patients who revealed a somewhat positive symptomatology at the beginning of the episode but shifted into negativity by the end.

Success of Therapy and Type of Schizophrenia

Table 9 shows a comparison of the three types of schizophrenia at the beginning of the episode as compared with the end. It becomes evident that from 30 patients belonging to type I at the beginning, 12 (40%) go into remission, 8 (26%) remain type I, 9 (30%) shift over to type II, and 1 (3%) shifts over to the mixed type. As far as type II is concerned, only 1 patient was remitted at the end of the episode, none shifted over to type I, and the remaining 34 patients (97%) stayed as type II. Finally, of the 48 patients whose symptomatology had been classified at the beginning as mixed type, only 1 went into remission, and 7

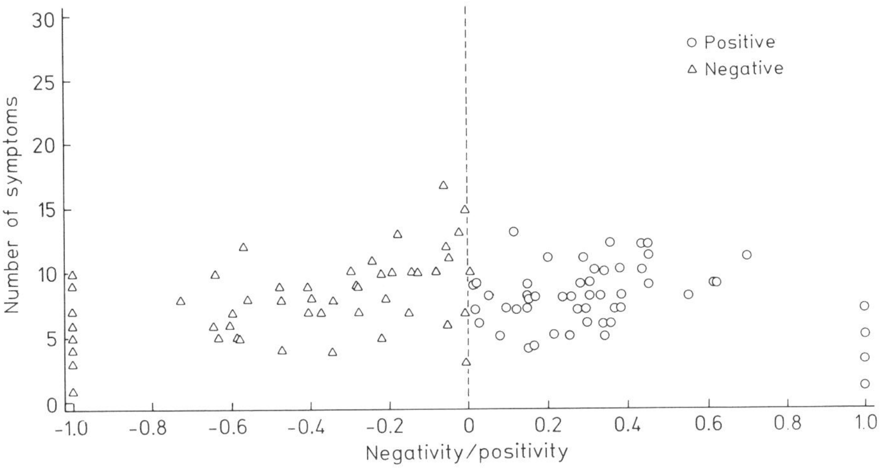

Fig. 1. Positivity/negativity score versus number of symptoms at the beginning of the episode

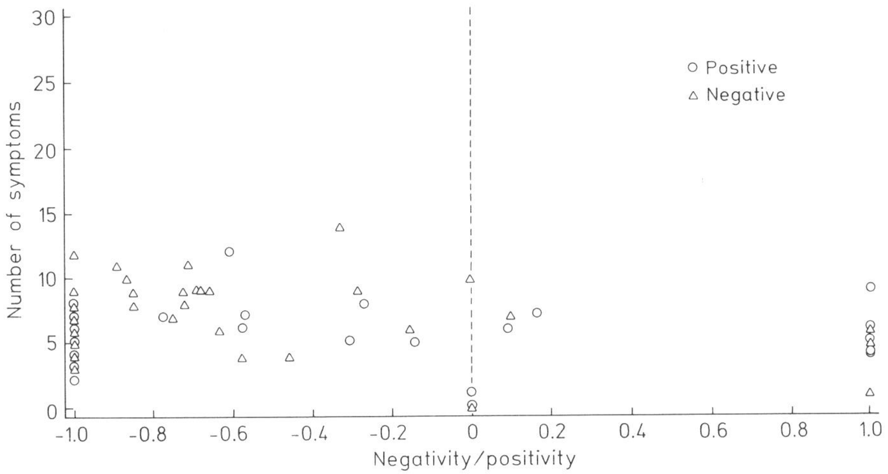

Fig. 2. Positivity/negativity score versus number of symptoms at the end of the episode

(14%) remained in the class of mixed type while the rest (40 patients; 83%) shifted over into type II schizophrenia. This is not an optimistic result, but one has to consider that many patients had already been hospitalized several times; in other words, they had become chronic.

Conclusions

The study was carried out with 113 adolescent schizophrenic patients whose last clinical episode could be analyzed in terms of symptomatology and

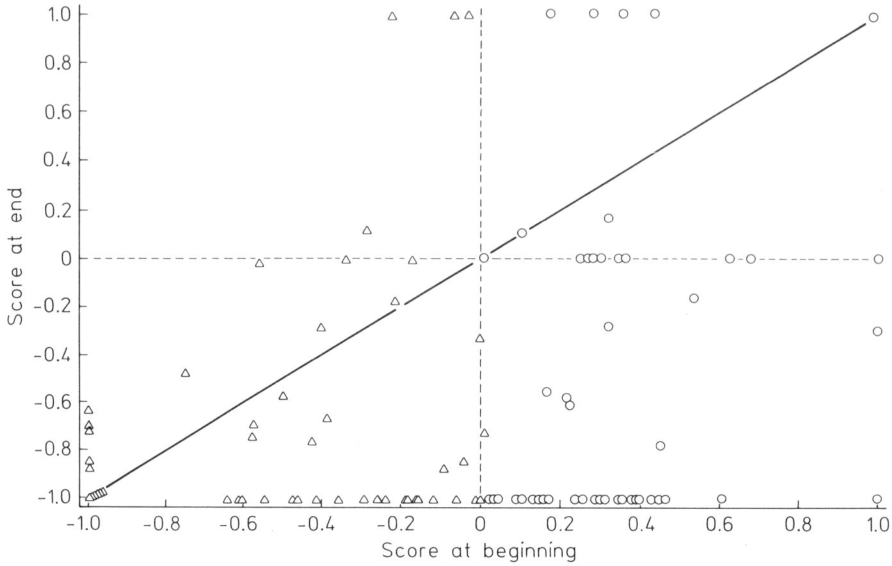

Fig. 3. Positivity/negativity scores at beginning versus end of episode

Table 9. Comparison of the frequency of the three types of schizophrenia at the beginning and at the end of the treatment episode

	Type at the beginning						Total	
	Type I		Type II		Mixed			
Type at the end	(*n*)	(%)	(*n*)	(%)	(*n*)	(%)	(*n*)	(%)
Remission	12	40	1	2	1	2	14	12
Type I	8	26	0	0	0	0	8	7
Type II	9	30	34	97	40	83	83	73
Mixed	1	3	0	0	7	14	8	7
Total	30		35		48		113	

symptom shift from the beginning of inpatient treatment to the end. A differentiation into three types of schizophrenia (I, II, and mixed) according to positive and negative symptomatology (Andreasen 1982) was possible. According to a weighted symptom score, the symptomatology of each patient could be positioned on a continuous scale reaching from the extreme pole of negativity (− 1) to the extreme pole of positivity (+ 1). The patients were classified at the beginning and at the end with respect to the severity of their symptoms. A comparison of positive and negative symptomatology revealed a reduction of the number of symptoms with time but also a clear symptom shift in the direction of negativity. This may due to the fact that negative symptoms at the beginning of the episode could be hidden by positive symptoms and probably become evident after the disappearance of the positive symptoms due to neuroleptic therapy. This notion was put forward by Angst et al. (1989). Another interpretation is, however, that a high proportion of our patients became chronic. An argument for the latter interpretation is the fact that only among type I schizophrenic patients did a higher proportion (40%) reach the state of remission.

Further, our study could demonstrate a symptom shift during inpatient treatment from type I to II and III, but not in the opposite direction. Both observations are in line with the relevant literature.

The 1-Year Course of Adolescent Schizophrenia Under Conditions of a Rehabilitation Program

Introduction and Aims of the Study

In contrast to schizophrenia in adulthood, there are not many studies concerning schizophrenic adolescents, taking into account the course of their disease. According to Weiner (1982), the prognosis of schizophrenia starting at prepuberty and adolescence is unfavorable as compared with schizophrenic disorders with a first manifestation in adulthood. About the same rate of schizophrenic adolescents and adults reach full remission (23% vs. 25%), but only 25% of adolescent schizophrenic subjects achieve a partial remission that takes place in about 50% of adult schizophrenic patients. Finally, in 52% of adolescent schizophrenic subjects, a chronic course of the disorder can be observed in contrast to only 25% in adult schizophrenic individuals.

Weiner (1982) has also pointed out some variables that are associated with a chronic long-term course of adolescent schizophrenia. The most important are:

- Slow manifestation of the disorder with continuous impairment of cognitive functions.
- Deficient adaptation before manifestation of the disorder.
- Development of symptom tolerance.
- Premorbid behavior disorders and personality characteristics.

Several investigators (most of them in adult psychiatry) have tried to predict the long-term course of schizophrenia from premorbid variables and from variables during inpatient treatment. A review of these studies shows that three factors seem to be of importance (Martin 1989):

1. Premorbid personality, including social adaptation and individual personality characteristics.
2. Characteristics of the schizophrenic disorder, including symptomatology, type of first manifestation, reaction to initial treatment, subtype of schizophrenia. There is a general rule saying that the prognosis is better in the case of acute positive symptomatology in a premorbidly inconspicuous patient.

3. Age at onset of the disorder in the sense that the later the manifestation, the better the prognosis (Retterstøl 1987).

The aim of this study was to answer two general hypotheses:

1. Schizophrenic adolescents reveal at the beginning of their disorder cognitive and emotional disturbances. It was expected that these would diminish during the rehabilitation program in the sense that adolescents with a favorable course of rehabilitation would show better cognitive achievements, lower self-ratings concerning their mental health status and less psychopathology after 1 year of rehabilitation. This hypothesis focusses on the cognitive and emotional disturbances.
2. The second hypothesis is related to prediction. It was expected that patients with premorbid disturbances of adaptation would show a less favorable prognosis after 1 year of the rehabilitation program and that patients showing a higher score of depression at the beginning of the rehabilitation program would have a less favorable prognosis than those patients who were not depressed at the same time. This expectation was derived from an earlier study (Remschmidt et al. 1988) with the first 32 patients of this study's sample in which a higher score of depression at the beginning of the rehabilitation program was associated with a poor prognosis after 1 year according to the scores of the Global Assessment Scale.

Sample

The sample comprised 88 adolescents (50 male and 38 female, aged 12–22 years) suffering from schizophrenic psychoses. Some 64 of them could be included in a 1-year longitudinal study during which each patient was examined at 3-month intervals by means of a standardized test battery, an individual psychopathological investigation, and several rating scales.

All patients were participants of a special rehabilitation program followed outside the clinic in a remedial home for schizophrenic adolescents. Of course, this group of patients is a selection including all schizophrenic adolescents who could not be discharged after inpatient clinical treatment to their families, because their condition had become more or less chronic.

Concerning the subtypes of schizophrenia according to the multiaxial classification scheme (ICD-9), 1 patient had the diagnosis "schizophrenia simplex" (295.0), 23 suffered from the hebephrenic type (295.1), 47 from the paranoid type (295.3), and 17 from the schizoaffective type (295.7).

As far as social class is concerned, a majority of the patients belonged to the lower social classes (56.4%), 42.3% to the middle classes, and only 1 patient (1.3%) to the higher social classes.

The distribution of intelligence is shown in Fig. 4. As the figure demonstrates, there is a trend in the direction of lower IQs which is in line with results in the literature. In 3 patients, intelligence testing was not carried out.

As far as family history is concerned, 12 patients (15.6% out of 77 from whom reliable data were available) had a schizophrenic mother and 8 patients

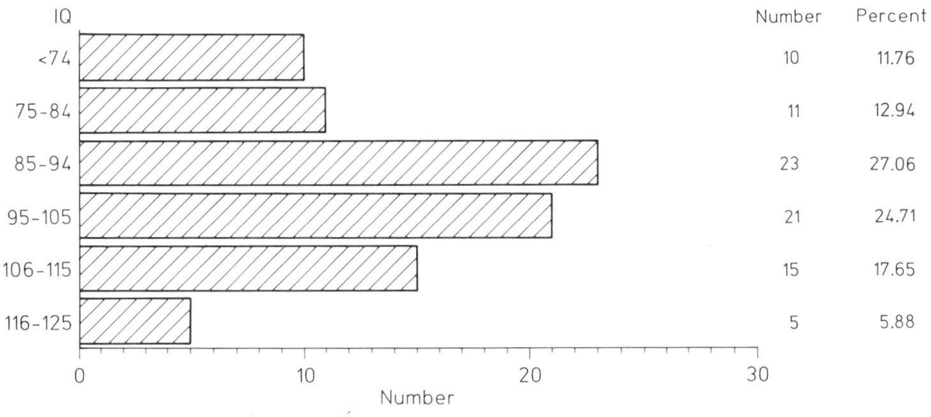

Fig. 4. Distribution of IQ in the sample of schizophrenic patients

out of 70 (11.4%), a schizophrenic father. A total of 14 patients out of 45 (31%) had other schizophrenic relatives. For the rest of the patients, reliable data on family history were not available.

Methodology

All patients ($n = 88$) were investigated by a test battery and several other methods, including self-rating scales and psychopathological examination, and underwent special ratings with respect to the rehabilitation process. Table 10 gives an overview over the areas of investigation and the instruments that were employed. As it demonstrates, four areas of investigation were used during the study:

1. Investigation of cognitive functions by objective testing
2. Subjective measures of the state of mental health by means of self-rating scales
3. An independent psychopathological investigation by a psychiatrist who was not informed about the results of the other measures
4. Measures concerning the course of rehabilitation, including the level of psychosocial functioning and a special behavior rating scale with subscales on practical abilities, social abilities, emotional behavior, and remarkable psychopathological disturbances.

All of the measures listed in Table 10 were administered at the beginning of the study to all 88 patients. In a subsample of 64 patients, all of the measures except the Global Assessment Scale were administered at intervals of 3 months (i.e., four times) until the end of the 1st year of the rehabilitation program. At that time for each patient the Global Assessment Scale (Shaffer et al. 1983; Steinhausen 1985) was administered independently.

Table 10. Areas of investigation and instruments used

Areas of investigation	Tests and scales
Cognitive functions (objective testing)	
Attention/concentration	Attention test d2 (Brickenkamp 1975)
Memory	Memory subtest Wechsler test (Wechsler 1964)
Intelligence (language-independent)	Achievement test (LPS), subtest 3 (Horn 1983)
Intelligence (language-dependent)	Achievement test, subtest 6 (Horn 1983)
Subjective state of mental health	
Paranoia self-rating scale	Paranoia depression scale, Paranoia scale (PDS-P) (von Zerssen 1976b)
Depression self-rating scale	Paranoia depression scale, Depression scale (PDS-D) (von Zerssen 1976b)
Somatic complaints self-rating scale	List of complaints (von Zerssen 1976a)
Uncharacteristic deficits (schizophrenic basic disturbance)	Frankfurt complaints questionnaire (Süllwold 1977)
Psychopathology (independent rating)	
Thinking disorders	Independent psychopathological investigation thinking disorders scale
Affective disorders	Independent psychopathological investigation affective disorders scale
Course of rehabilitation (independent rating)	
Level of psychosocial functioning	Global assessment scale for children and adolescents (Shaffer et al. 1983; Steinhausen 1985)
Behavior rating scale	Behavior rating scale of educators (EFB-P) (Rühl 1988)

Results

Cross-Sectional Analysis

The cross-sectional analysis including all 88 patients showed the following results: As a group, schizophrenic patients revealed remarkable deficiencies concerning attention and language-independent intelligence as compared with normal controls ($P < 0.0001$). This did not apply to language-dependent intelligence and to memory. There were also remarkable differences concerning all self-rating scales (as described in Table 10). All differences in comparison with normal controls were highly significant ($P < 0.0001$).

However, there were only two parameters that differentiated between the three subgroups of schizophrenic patients: paranoid ($n = 47$), hebephrenic ($n = 23$), and schizoaffective ($n = 17$) types. These were activation (motivation;

independent psychopathological investigation) and practical abilities (Behavior Rating Scale for Educators). The subgroup of hebephrenic patients revealed the most pronounced deficiencies in both variables.

We also carried out factorial analyses according to the maximum-likelihood method, involving five scales (attention test, language-independent intelligence, Paranoia Scale, Depression Scale, and Frankfurt Complaints Questionnaire). The result was a two-factor solution explaining 65.4% of the total variance. Factor 1 showed high positive loadings concerning the variables paranoid tendencies, depression, and uncharacteristic deficits in the Frankfurt Complaints Questionnaire. This factor could be interpreted as "subjective psychopathological symptoms and complaints."

Factor 2 was characterized by high loadings concerning the variables attention and language-independent intelligence. It can be interpreted as impairment of cognitive abilities.

Longitudinal Analyses

The longitudinal analyses could be carried out for 64 patients who had been followed up for 1 year, the investigation taking place four times after intervals of 3 months. The following results were obtained:

- There was a significant improvement concerning attention, language-independent intelligence, and memory with time.
- An improvement concerning the subjective psychopathological symptoms could be observed.
- The same improvement applied to psychopathological symptoms and to practical abilities rated by the educators during the course of the rehabilitation program.
- However, there was again *no difference* concerning all the measures with respect to the three subgroups of schizophrenia (paranoid, hebephrenic, and schizoaffective).

Results Concerning Subgroups

In order to derive subgroups as a special method, the latent-class analysis (LCA; Lazarsfeld and Henry 1968) was administered that allows us to derive independent groups. For this analysis, four variables were chosen that had already been relevant during the analyses described so far. The four variables were: attention score, language-independent intelligence, depression score, and paranoia score.

As Fig. 5 shows, the LCA delivers a remarkable hierarchy of the four variables. The depression score is decisive for the two classes arising as a result of this analysis. Class 1 can be described by the following items: low depression score, low paranoid tendencies, good achievement in the attention test, and high scores concerning language-independent intelligence. Beyond these differences, the first group is also different from the second one with respect to

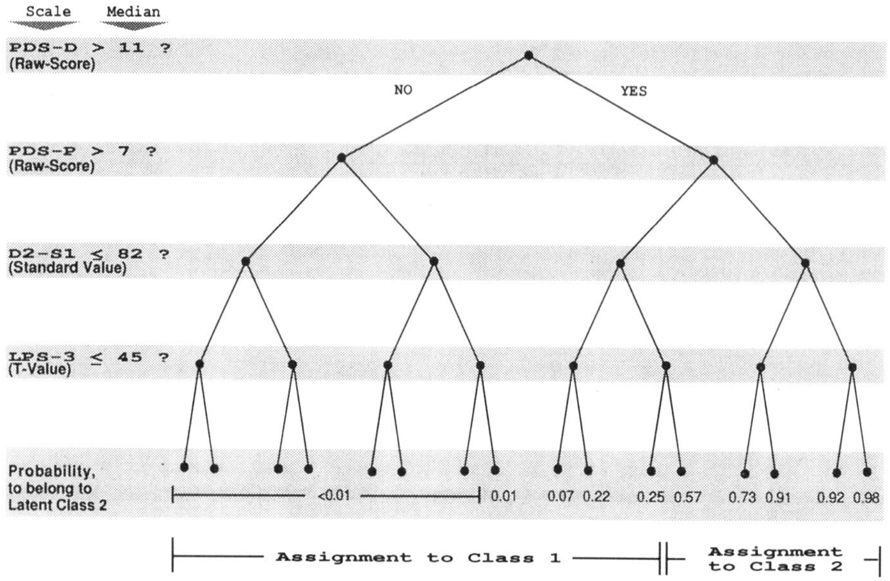

Fig. 5. Latent class analysis: hierarchy of the scales PDS-D, PDS-P, D2-S1, and LPS-3. Probability to belong to latent classes 1 or 2. The figure illustrates the importance of the different scales for the assignment to the LCA-classes

many other variables such as: older age at start of the rehabilitation program, higher education level, greater language-dependent intelligence, lower scores of subjective complaints, and higher scores in the behavior rating scale with respect to practical abilities and social abilities.

Class 2 can be characterized by the complementary features: high depression score, greater paranoid tendencies, disturbances of attention, and impairment of language-independent intelligence. Beyond these differences, there are also other characteristics such as: more subjective complaints, higher scores concerning psychopathological symptoms, etc.

Results on Prediction

Finally, we tried to predict the success after 1 year by investigating several variables at the beginning of the rehabilitation program. For that purpose, we administered a special type of discriminant analysis called Classification and Regression Trees (CART) described by Breiman et al. (1984). As criterion variable, the Global Assessment Score (German abbreviation: SGKJ) was used, subdivided dichotomously into two categories: 70–100 points as good prognosis, and 0–69 points as poor and intermediate prognosis. All the other variables (cognitive variables, self-rating scales, psychopathological variables, and variables of the behavior rating scale) were used to predict the course of rehabilitation after 1 year as measured by the Global Assessment Scale.

Figure 6 shows the decision tree according to the CART analysis including 16 variables. The depression score (PDS-D) is again of decisive importance for

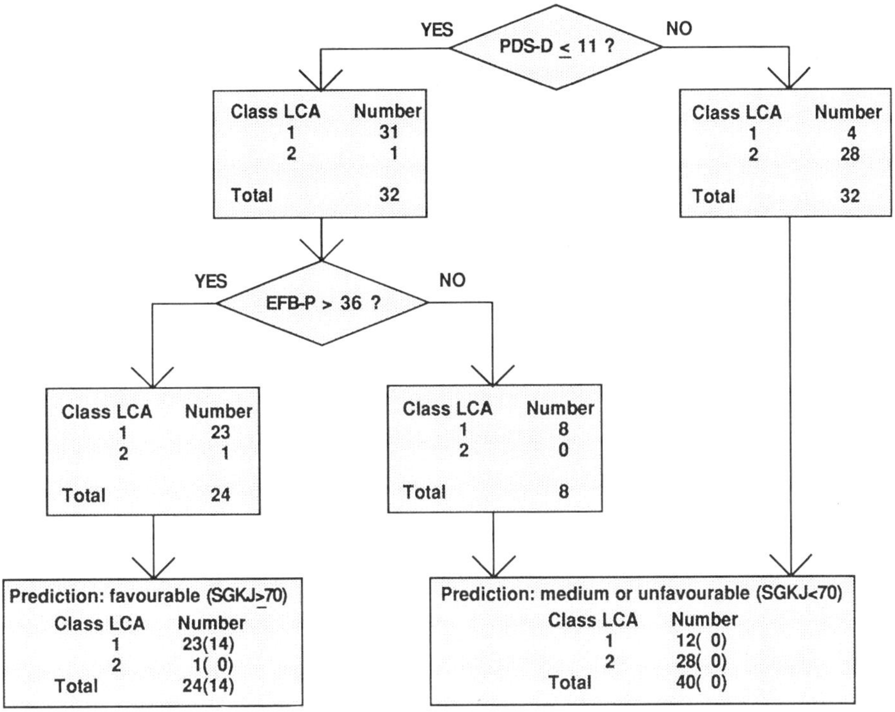

Fig. 6. Decision-tree of the CART analysis. Misclassifications of the learning sample in brackets

the subclassification of the two groups. According to this method, all patients with a good prognosis (scores over 70) could be predicted in all cases ($n = 10$, 100%), whereas an intermediate or poor prognosis could be predicted only in 74% ($n = 40$). As the CART program has an inbuilt cross-validation, it was possible to check the probability of the classification by this procedure. Under the conditions of the cross-validation, 80% of those with good prognosis could be predicted correctly and 72% with intermediate or poor prognosis.

Conclusions

1. It could be demonstrated that schizophrenic adolescents who attend a rehabilitation program are characterized by several deficits concerning cognitive functions, subjective complaints, and psychopathological symptoms.
2. During a 1-year rehabilitation program, most of these deficiencies improved remarkably.
3. This improvement does not apply to all patients, however. It is possible to subdivide the patients into two groups: Schizophrenic adolescents with higher cognitive abilities and fewer somatic and psychiatric complaints and

those with lower cognitive abilities and a higher rate of somatic and psychiatric complaints.

4. This subdifferentiation is independent of the classic subdivision of schizophrenia into hebephrenic, paranoid, and schizoaffective types.
5. The status at the end of the 1-year rehabilitation program could best be predicted by the depression score at the beginning of the rehabilitation program, which is in line with our results in an earlier study (Remschmidt et al. 1988). Further studies should therefore examine very carefully the emotional parameters and not only the cognitive ones.

Discussion

The concept of positive and negative schizophrenia can also be applied in childhood and adolescent schizophrenia. However, the data basis in support of this conception is very small. Bettes and Walker (1987) have shown that positive and negative symptoms can be observed in psychotic children and adolescents, aged 5–18 years, but can also be detected in other psychiatric conditions. In this respect, positive and negative symptoms are not characteristic of schizophrenic disorders in childhood and adolescence. This notion is in line with the observations of Angst et al. (1989) in adult psychiatry.

A further and very decisive aspect can be seen in the fact that psychotic disorders in childhood and adolescence show a clear dependence on age and developmental stage as far as symptomatology is concerned. For example, systematized delusions are not observed before the 12th year of life, but there are delusions also at an earlier age (Stutte and Dauner 1971). Further, several follow-up studies of early manifested psychotic states in childhood did not show any relationship to schizophrenia. There are, however, exceptions: Early infantile catatonia as described by Leonhard (1986) has a relation to schizophrenia, while other types of early manifested psychotic states do not (see Table 1). In general, we can say that the later the manifestation of the psychotic state, the closer the relationship to schizophrenic psychoses if one leaves out psychoses due to organic conditions. In this sense, prepuberal schizophrenic psychoses show already a clear relationship to schizophrenia in adolescents and adults. The same applies to adolescent schizophrenia.

Studies have shown that the concept of positive and negative schizophrenia is also useful in differentiating schizophrenic psychoses in late childhood and adolescence. One cannot look upon positive and negative symptomatology as stable traits of schizophrenic psychoses. They are rather dynamic symptoms that change remarkably during treatment and during the course of the schizophrenic disorder. However, the change of symptomatology seems to occur more or less in one direction only: the negative one. This was shown very clearly in our *first study*. If one compares the symptomatology at the beginning and at the end of the inpatient treatment episodes, a shift into negative symptomatology occurs significantly. At least in our sample of inpatient schizophrenics, there is more or less a one-way street from type I schizophrenia to type II and also from mixed schizophrenia to type II schizophrenia. We have to remember, however, that our sample is not representative of schizophrenic adolescents with the first manifestation of their disorders. It includes a remarkable group of patients who had already been hospitalized several times. So the result of our first study has to be controlled by a group of schizophrenic adolescents who come into treatment after the first manifestation of their disorder.

Within our *second study*, we tried to predict the success of a 1-year rehabilitation program by several conditions at the entrance. As this group of patients was investigated at regular intervals of 3 months and as we have made many observations on these patients during their stay in the rehabilitation program, we could clearly delineate two types of schizophrenic disorders. Type I could be characterized by the absence of premorbid adjustment disorders, a stable premorbid personality, a low depression score, low paranoid tendencies, and good achievements in several measures that were administered. The patients could also be characterized by higher education level, higher language-dependent intelligence, lower scores of subjective complaints, and higher scores in several behavior ratings.

Type II, however, could be described by higher depression score, greater paranoid tendencies, remarkable disturbances of attention, and impairment of language-dependent intelligence. Beyond these differences, we also found more subjective complaints and higher scores concerning psychopathological symptoms, most in the direction of negative schizophrenia. It was also remarkable that these patients had premorbid deficiencies in adaptation.

These two types could be delineated by several methods and were also found in an earlier study comprising the first 32 consecutively investigated patients (Remschmidt et al. 1988). This result was confirmed in the total sample of longitudinally investigated patients ($n = 64$). We feel therefore that this subdivision has empirical support. As the better prognosis in the rehabilitation program belonged to the patients of the first group and the decisive variable for the prediction was the depression score, we therefore conclude that we should pay more attention in the treatment of schizophrenia to the emotional conditions and not only to the cognitive ones.

References

American Psychiatric Association (1980) Diagnostic and statistical manual of mental disorders (DSM-III). APA, Washington

American Psychiatric Association (1987) Diagnostic and Statistical manual of mental disorders, 3rd edn, revised (DSM-III-R). APA, Washington

Andreasen NC (1982) Negative symptoms in schizophrenia. Definition and rehabilitation. Arch Gen Psychiatry 39:784–788

Andreasen NC, Olsen S (1982) Negative vs. positive schizophrenia. Definition and validation. Arch Gen Psychiatry 39:789–794

Angst J, Stassen HH, Woggon B (1989) Effects of neuroleptics on positive and negative symptoms and deficit state. Psychopharmacology (Berlin) 99:41–46

Anthony EJ (1958) An experimental approach to the psychopathology of childhood autism. Br J Med Psychol 31:211–225
Anthony EJ (1962) Low-grade psychosis in childhood. In: Richards BW (ed) Proceedings of London conference on scientific study of mental deficiency, vol 2. May and Baker, Dagenham
Asperger M (1944) Die "autistischen Psychopathen" im Kindesalter. Arch Psychiatr Nervenkr 117:76–136
Asperger M (1968) Zur Differentialdiagnose des kindlichen Autismus. Acta Paedopsychiatrica 35:136–146
Ban TA, Guy W, Wilson WH, Kelwala S (1982) Psychopharmacology and Leonhard's classification of chronic schizophrenias. Int Pharmacopsychiatry 17:153–162
Bender L (1947) Childhood schizophrenia: clinical study of one hundred schizophrenic children. Am J Orthopsychiatry 17:40–56
Bender L (1959) The concept of pseudopsychopathic schizophrenia in adolescence. Am J Orthopsychiatry 29:491–509
Bettes BA, Walker E (1987) Positive and negative symptoms in psychotic and other psychiatrically disturbed children. J Child Psychol Child Psychiatry 28:555–568
Bleuler E (1911) Dementia praecox oder Gruppe der Schizophrenien. In: Aschaffenburg G (ed) Handbuch der Psychiatrie, special part, fasc 4. Deuticke, Vienna
Breiman L, Friedman J, Olshen A, Stone GJ (1984) CART: classification and regression trees. Wadsworth, Belmont
Brickenkamp R (1975) Test d2. Aufmerksamkeits-Belastungs-Test. Hogrefe, Göttingen
Carpenter WT Jr, Heinrichs DW, Alphs LD (1985) Treatment of negative symptoms. Schizophr Bull 11:440–452
Conrad K (1958) Die beginnende Schizophrenie. Versuch einer Gestaltanalyse des Wahns. Thieme, Stuttgart
Crow TJ (1980) Molecular pathology of schizophrenia: more than one disease process? Br Med J 280:66–68
De Sanctis S (1908) Dementia praecocissima catatonica. Folia Neurobiol 2:9
Despert JL (1938) Schizophrenia in children. Psychiatr Q 12:366–371
Eggers C (1973) Verlaufsweisen kindlicher und präpuberaler Schizophrenien. Springer, Berlin Heidelberg New York
Eisenberg L (1957) The course of childhood schizophrenia. Arch Neurol Psychiatry 78:69–83
Group for the Advancement of Psychiatry (1966) Psychopathological disorders in childhood: theoretical considerations and a proposed classification. GAP, New York
Heinrich K (1967) Zur Bedeutung des postremissiven Erschöpfungs-Syndroms für die Rehabilitation Schizophrener. Nervenarzt 38:487–491
Heller T (1908) Über Dementia infantilis. Z Erforsch Beh Jugendl Schwachsinns 2:17
Horn W (1983) Leistungsprüfsystem LPS, 2nd edn. Hogrefe, Göttingen
Huber G (1957) Pneumencephalographische und psychopathologische Bilder bei endogenen Psychosen. Springer, Berlin Göttingen Heidelberg
Jackson JH (1958) Evolution and dissolution of the nervous system. In: Taylor J (ed) Various papers, addresses and lectures. Basic, New York (Selected writings of John Hughlings Jackson, vol 2) (original 1884)
Johnstone EC, Owens DGC, Frith CD, Crow TJ (1986) The relative stability of positive and negative features in chronic schizophrenia. Br J Psychiatry 150:60–64
Kanner L (1943) Autistic disturbances of affective contact. Nerv Child 2:217–250
Kanner L (1957) Child psychiatry, 3rd edn. Blackwell, Oxford
Koehler K, Sauer H (1984) Huber's basic symptoms: another approach to negative psychopathology in schizophrenia. Compr Psychiatry 25:174–182
Kolvin E, Ounsted C, Humphrey M, McNay A (1971a) Six studies in the childhood psychoses. II. The phenomenology of childhood psychoses. Br J Psychiatry 118:385–395
Kolvin E, Ounsted C, Richardson LM, Garside RF (1971b) Six studies in the childhood psychoses. III. The family and social background in childhood psychoses. Br J Psychiatry 118:396–402

Kolvin E, Garside RF, Kydd JSH (1971 c) Six studies in the childhood psychoses. IV. Parental personality and attitude and childhood psychoses. Br J Psychiatry 118:403–406
Kolvin E, Ounsted C, Roth M (1971 d) Six studies in the childhood psychoses. V. Cerebral dysfunction and childhood psychoses. Br J Psychiatry 118:407–417
Lazarsfeld PF., Henry NW (1968) Latent structure analysis. Houghton Mifflin, Boston
Leonhard K (1986) Aufteilung der endogenen Psychosen und ihre differenzierte Ätiologie, 2nd edn. Akademie, Berlin
Lutz J (1937/1938) Über Schizophrenie im Kindesalter. Schweiz Arch Neurol Neurochir Psychiatr 39:335–372; 40:141–163
Mahler MS (1952) On child psychosis and schizophrenia: autistic and symbiotic infantile psychosis. Psychoanal Study Child 7:286–305
Mahler MS, Ross JR, de Fried Z (1949) Clinical studies in benignant and malignant cases of childhood psychosis (schizophrenic-like). Am J Orthopsychiatry 19:295–304
Martin M (1989) Der Verlauf der Schizophrenie im Jugendalter unter Rehabilitationsbedingungen. Habilitationsschrift, University of Marburg
Mayer-Gross W (1920) Ueber die Stellungnahme zur abgelaufenen akuten Psychose. Eine Studie über verständliche Zusammenhänge in der Schizophrenie. Z Gesamte Neurol Psychiatr 60:160–212
Remschmidt H (1975 a) Neuere Ergebnisse zur Psychologie und Psychiatrie der Adoleszenz. Z Kinder Jugendpsychiatr 3:67–101
Remschmidt H (1975 b) Psychologie und Psychopathologie der Adoleszenz. Monatsschr Kinderheilkd 123:316–323
Remschmidt H (1988) Schizophrene Psychosen im Kindesalter. In: Kisker KP, Lauter H, Meyer J-E, Müller C, Strömgren E (eds) Kinder- und Jugendpsychiatrie, Springer, Berlin Heidelberg New York (Psychiatrie der Gegenwart, vol 7)
Remschmidt H, Martin M, Albrecht G, Gerlach G, Rühl D (1988) Der Voraussagewert des Initialbefundes für den mittelfristigen Rehabilitationsverlauf bei jugendlichen Schizophrenen. Nervenarzt 59:471–476
Retterstøl N (1987) Schizophrenie – Verlauf und Prognose. In: Kisker KP, Lauter M, Meyer JE, Strömgren E (eds) Schizophrenien. Springer, Berlin Heidelberg New York (Psychiatrie der Gegenwart, vol 4)
Rimland B (1964) Infantile autism. Appleton-Century-Crofts, New York
Rühl D (1988) Untersuchungen zur Basisstörung schizophrener Jugendlicher. Dissertation, University of Marburg
Rutter M (1967) Psychotic disorders in early childhood. In: Coppen AJ, Walk A (eds) Recent developments in schizophrenia. Royal Medico-Psychological Association, Headley, Ashford
Rutter M, Lockyer L (1967) A five to fifteen-year follow-up study of infantile psychosis. I. Description of sample. Br J Psychiatry 113:1169–1182
Rutter M, Lockyer L, Greenfield D (1967) A five to fifteen-year follow-up study of infantile psychosis. II. Social and behavioral outcome. Br J Psychiatry 113:1183–1199
Rutter ML, Shaffer D, Sturge C (1976) A guide to a multi-axial classification scheme for psychiatric disorders in childhood and adolescence. Frowde, London
Shaffer D, Gould MS, Brasic J, Ambrosimi P, Fisher P, Bird H, Aluwahlia S (1983) A children's global assessment scale (CGAS). Arch Gen Psychiatry 40:1228–1231
Steinhausen H-C (1985) Eine Skala zur Beurteilung psychisch gestörter Kinder und Jugendlicher. Z Kinder Jugendpsychiatr 13:230–240
Strauss J, Carpenter WT, Bartko J (1974) The diagnosis and understanding of schizophrenia. III. Speculation on the processes that underlie schizophrenic symptoms and signs. Schizophr Bull 1:61–69
Stutte H (1960) Kinderpsychiatrie und Jugendpsychiatrie. In: Gruhle HW, Jung R, Mayer-Gross W, Müller M (eds) Psychiatrie der Gegenwart, vol 2. Springer, Berlin Göttingen Heidelberg
Stutte H (1969) Psychosen des Kindesalters. In: Opitz H, Schmid F (eds) Neurologie-Psychologie-Psychiatrie. Springer, Berlin Heidelberg, New York, pp 908–937 (Handbuch der Kinderheilkunde, vol 8/1)

Stutte H, Dauner I (1971) Systematized delusions in early life schizophrenia. J Autism Child Schizophr 1:411–420
Süllwold L (1977) Symptome schizophrener Erkrankungen. Uncharakteristische Basisstörungen. Springer, Berlin Heidelberg New York
Von Zerssen D (1976a) Beschwerde-Liste (BL). Beltz, Weinheim
Von Zerssen D (1976b) Paranoid-Depressivitäts-Skala (PDS). Beltz, Weinheim
Walker E., Lewine RJ (1988) The positive/negative symptom distinction in schizophrenia. Validity and etiological relevance. Schizophr Res 1:315–328
Wechsler D (1964) Die Messung der Intelligenz Erwachsener. Textband zum Hamburg-Wechsler-Intelligenztest für Erwachsene (HAWIE), 3rd edn. Huber, Bern
Weiner IB (1982) Child and adolescent psychopathology. Wiley, New York
Werry JS (1979) The childhood psychoses. In: Quay HC, Werry JS (eds) Psychopathological disorders of childhood, 2nd edn. Wiley, New York

Negative Symptoms in the Long-Term Course of Childhood Schizophrenia: A Discussion Contribution

C. Eggers [1]

This short report is based on the results of a re-investigation of the long-term course of 57 cases of schizophrenic psychosis first manifested before the age of 14 years (11 patients were 10 years old or less at first manifestation and 46 patients between 11 and 14 years old). All diagnoses were made during the years 1925–1960, in each case after the first or second in-patient treatment. All patients were re-examined in personal interviews with them and their relatives 6–40 (average 16) years after first hospitalisation. The original diagnoses have been reassessed according to International Classification of Diseases (ICD) criteria (ICD 295.0–295.4). The results of the follow-up investigation were published in 1973 and 1978 (Eggers 1973, 1978). I agree with Tsuang's statement demanding caution in evaluating negative and positive symptoms retrospectively. I too am of the opinion that prospective studies are necessary. On the other hand, however, long-term follow-up studies of patients with schizophrenic psychoses at all ages are of inestimable value, and in these studies I am forced to evaluate psychopathological symptoms retrospectively.

An acute course of illness was most frequent ($n = 42$ patients, 73.7%), whereas a chronic course beginning insidiously was less often seen ($n = 15$ patients, 26.3%; see Table 1). Here, I shall try to answer the following questions:

1. Under what circumstances did negative symptoms occur?
2. What is the relationship between positive and negative features in the long-term course of childhood schizophrenia?
3. Is there any relationship between the frequency of negative symptoms and type of course (acute or chronic)?
4. Is there a relationship between the occurrence of negative symptoms and pre-morbid character traits?
5. Are there differences in the prognosis of positive as against negative pre-pubertal schizophrenia?
6. Are negative symptoms really negative?

Negative symptoms occurrred in patients in remission whose psychosis followed an acute recurring course as well as in patients with chronically deteriorating psychoses. However, the way the negative symptoms manifested

[1] Klinik für Kinder- und Jugenpsychiatrie, Universitätsklinikum, Hufelandstraße 55, W-4300 Essen, FRG

A. Marneros / N. C. Andreasen / M. T. Tsuang (Eds.)
Negative Versus Positive Schizophrenia

Table 1. Type of course in 57 patients with childhood schizophrenia (age of onset 7–14 years, mean 11.9 years)

Acute type	*n*	Chronic insidious type	*n*
One acute psychotic episode with full recovery	6	Chronic lingering course with slight amelioration	3
One acute episode, preceded by short transitory (flat) psychotic "waves" with full recovery	5	Chronic insidious course with slight deterioration	4
Frequently recurring psychotic episodes with full recovery	4	Chronic insidious course with severe deterioration	5
Frequently recurring psychotic episodes leaving a slight schizophrenic defect (relatively good social adaptation)	9	Psychotic-like change of behaviour for a period of 1 year or longer, leading to a manifest schizophrenic psychosis	3
One acute psychotic episode, leading to a severe defective state	3		
Frequently recurring episodes leading to a deep schizophrenic defect	14		
Acute-recurring onset merging into a sluggish course with continuous deterioration	1		
Total	42		15

themselves depended largely on the course of the disease: in the acute recurring type with a favourable prognosis (non-deficit type of schizophrenia) the negative symptoms were transitory and showed greater fluctuation and lack of persistence than in the chronic insidious type, in which the negative symptoms were stable and enduring. These findings are similar to those of Carpenter et al. (1988). Altogether only 5 of 15 patients with recurrent psychosis followed by full recovery had unstable negative symptoms during or after the psychotic episodes. All 5 were female. In one girl, the negative symptoms (anergia, apathy, lack of interest, coarsened affect, indifference, incongruity of emotional responsiveness, lack of contact, silly and foolish behaviour) had been so marked that sterilisation was planned – but she recovered fully, her remission remaining constant for 30 years!

Only one (female) patient of the 27 whose psychosis followed a recurrent course leading to mild or severe post-psychotic deficiencies demonstrated distinct negative symptoms resembling typical deficit symptoms (flattening of affect, incongruity of emotional responsiveness, lack of energy and interest, silly behaviour, inappropriate reactions). These occurred after her second psychotic episode and disappeared after a few weeks, leading to complete remission without noticeable signs of alteration of personality. The girl was active, went to school, played the piano and pursued intensively interests like dancing or piano lessons. However, after 1 year she had several relapses resulting in continuing hospital treatment.

Thus, only 6 of the 42 patients whose psychosis followed an acute recurring course demonstrated negative symptoms. These were on the whole fluent and non-persistent, disappearing early.

By contrast, in all 15 patients with chronic insidious psychoses (5 female, 10 male) negative symptoms were stable and endured for at least 12 months, with a maximum of 17 years (mean 8.2 years). Thus, the negative symptoms seen in acute recurring psychoses differed distinctly from those present as persistent features of chronic schizophrenic psychoses beginning at an early age (manifestation in 8 patients at age $\geqq 10$ years).

These children grew up quite unremarkably until the onset of their psychosis and then unexpectedly showed strange personality changes. These included increasing loss of contact with reality, reduced activity, diminishing of interests or narrowing of interests to those no longer appropriate to the child's age, indifference to the usual games and pursuits, disturbed motility (stereotypies, peculiar mannerisms, bizarre postures), negativism, disturbed contacts, retreat into their own autistic world and speech disturbances. Emotional changes manifested themselves as moodiness, often accompanied by anxiety, excessive distrust and affective bluntness, and included coldness and even brutality. Some children who had loved animals tortured their own pets without reason. Previously affectionate children suddenly turned unkind, cold and stubborn and no longer showed affection toward loved persons around them.

In all of the 15 patients with chronic psychoses the negative symptoms had been present from the beginning. In 9 of them the negative symptoms dominated the clinical picture for many years before positive symptoms and productive florid paranoid hallucinatory episodes became manifest, which in the patient with the longest delay happened 10 years after onset. In another patient, negative and productive symptoms were present from the beginning and persisted throughout the entire course of psychosis. Five of the 15 patients (1 female, 4 male) had exclusively negative symptoms, developing no positive symptoms such as delusions, hallucinations, positive formal thought disorder or stuporous-catatonic behaviour. Thus, in two-thirds of the 15 patients, positive symptoms and productive psychotic phenomena occurred within a negative schizophrenia, mainly later in the course of the psychosis.

As an example, I shall describe the course of psychosis in a 9-year-old boy. For 4 years this child had exclusively negative symptoms before positive, productive symptoms appeared at the age of 13 years. At the age of 9 years the following symptoms arose: increasing shyness, unmotivated running away, unmotivated damage to property, destructive behaviour, school truancy, excessive masturbation, aggressiveness, increasing isolation and emotional unresponsiveness. At 13 years he was admitted for psychiatric treatment as an in-patient. There was affective flattening and dulling; the boy was closed off and completely isolated, with poverty of speech, unchanging facial expression, a slumped posture and stiff, mannerised movements with a paucity of expressive gesture. He was subject to imperative acoustic hallucinations (voices ordering him to kill himself or abusing him) and to paranoid delusions; he carried out suicide attempts and suffered catatonic-stuporous states. The patient said, among other things, "Hold me, I can't go on; hold my head straight; my left needs splinting." He was sexually completely uninhibited, exhibited silly and foolish behaviour and was very anxious and suspicious, feeling himself to be under the influence of outside powers and reporting acoustic and olfactory hallucinations, thought blocking, thought hearing and incoherence of thought. At age 15 there was a gradual but constant improvement. The patient felt good and was active and reasonable; unlike previously, he was clean and tidy. He was able to be released from psychiatric treatment and to take an employment in a paper mill. At age 18, however, his condition deteriorated, with an increasing tendency to neglectfulness.

In only 5 of the 15 patients with chronic psychoses could a negative correlation be observed between negative and positive symptoms, and I cannot support the statement by Johnstone (1989) and Pfohl and Winokur (1982) that positive symptoms are characteristic of earlier and negative symptoms of later phases of schizophrenic psychoses. My findings, on the contrary, parallel those of Lewine et al. (1983) and Pogue-Geile and Harrow (1984), who also observed no negative correlation between positive and negative symptoms. I also agree with Lieberman et al. (this volume), who state that there is a high correlation between negative and positive symptoms before and during acute treatment but not at remission.

As we have seen, if negative symptoms are present during or between acute episodes with positive, productive symptoms, they are fluent, unstable and transient and are not associated with an unfavourable course. In such cases, negative symptoms seem to be secondary, i.e. responses by the patients to overwhelming psychotic phenomena which appear strange and stressful and provoke anxiety. It is not surprising that in the patients with acute recurring psychoses it was difficult to differentiate between negative and depressive symptoms. Similar observations have recently been reported by Kulhara et al. (1989).

By contrast, in psychoses with a chronic course, negative symptoms were much more frequent, stable and persistent and were present from the beginning. In some of these cases productive symptoms appeared after a few years, in parallel with the negative ones.

Four of the 5 cases showing exclusively negative symptoms stable over the whole period of the disease (9–17 years, mean 12.5 years), were cases of typical hebephrenia (ICD 295.1), and one was a typical schizophrenia simplex (ICD 295.0). Although the diagnosis of simple schizophrenia has disappeared from American nosology and is not included in American classification schemes

Table 2. Comparison of the pre-morbid character structures in 15 patients with negative schizophrenia and 42 patients with positive schizophrenia

Negative symptoms	Abnormal	Normal	Total
Yes	11 19.3%	4 7.0%	15 26.3%
No	19 33.3%	23 40.4%	42 73.7%
Total	30 52.6%	27 47.4%	57 100%

$\chi^2 = 3.49$; exact test according to Fisher: $P = 0.057$.

such as the Diagnostic and Statistical Manual (DSM-III), it has been retained in ICD-9 and is well-known and used in European countries. Black and Boffeli (1989) discuss the concept of schizophrenia simplex and propose operational criteria for this diagnostic category and recommend its inclusion in the DSM-IV.

The relationship between the pre-morbid level of personality adjustment and the presence of negative symptoms in the 15 patients with chronic insidious psychosis (the negative symptoms being present for at least 12 months) is shown in Table 2. The 15 patients were compared with the other patients with positive schizophrenia but without negative symptoms (36 patients) or whose negative symptoms were fluent and unstable and disappeared within a few weeks (6 patients).

Eleven of the 15 patients with a chronic insidious course and stable negative symptoms were described pre-morbidly as shy, inhibited, introverted, insecure, quiet and socially withdrawn, while the remaining were described as well adjusted. In the other group, the 42 patients with positive schizophrenia, 19 patients showed poor pre-morbid adjustment, whereas 23 were well adjusted, friendly, harmonious, self-confident and outgoing. Comparison of the pre-morbid character structure in the 15 patients with enduring negative symptoms and in the 42 patients with positive schizophrenia reveals no statistically significant difference ($\chi^2 = 3.49$), but the over-representation of pre-morbidly maladjusted personalities in the group of 15 patients with negative schizophrenia is obvious. This is in line with the findings of other authors who have reported an association between negative symptoms and poor pre-morbid adjustment (Andreasen and Olsen 1982; Buchanan et al. 1990; Kay et al. 1987; Pogue-Geile and Harrow 1984; Rohde et al., this volume).

Evaluating the prognostic character of negative symptoms in the long-term course of early-onset schizophrenia I can say that, in those 15 cases with stable and enduring negative symptoms, the negative symptoms in 13 patients were associated with a deteriorating course and a poor prognosis. Comparing the course of illness in 15 patients with negative schizophrenia and that in 42 patients with positive schizophrenia, there is a statistically significant difference in prognosis (Table 3). It appears that a significant association exists

Table 3. Comparison of the degree of remission in 15 patients with negative schizophrenia with 42 patients with positive schizophrenia

Negative symptoms	Good	Poor	Total
Yes	2 3.5%	13 22.8%	15 26.3%
No	25 43.9%	17 29.8%	42 73.7%
Total	27 47.4%	30 52.6%	57 100%

$s^2 = 9.45$, $P = 0.002$.

between negative symptoms, if they are stable (at least 12 months), and poor outcome in early-onset schizophrenic psychoses. Similar findings in adult schizophrenia have been reported by Biehl et al. (1986), Deister et al. (this volume), Kay et al. (1986), Johnstone et al. (1979) and Pogue-Geile (1989). It should, of course, be borne in mind that nearly all patients with stable negative symptoms had a poor prognosis, but this was also the case for nearly 30% of the patients with positive symptoms (see Table 3).

I have shown elsewhere that there is a significant association between pre-morbid character structure and prognosis, i.e. children who before their illness were well-adjusted, harmonious, active and well-balanced had a significantly better chance of recovery than those with maladjusted personalities, who were insecure, inhibited, shy, timid and introverted (Eggers 1973, 1978). I found a markedly increased incidence of anomalous pre-morbid features to be associated with negative symptoms. It is difficult to decide whether the poor prognosis is really attributable to the one, the other or perhaps both.

In the negative form of schizophrenia it is unclear whether pre-morbidly maladjusted children with weak ego functions may be at risk of the development of negative symptoms with an unfavourable prognosis, or whether these early anomalous features reflect nascent negative symptoms at the beginning of the psychosis.

As already stated, negative symptoms, particularly if they are present in acute recurring productive episodes with positive symptoms, can be interpreted as reactions by the patient to the overwhelming psychosis with which he or she is confronted. However, even chronically psychotic patients with a negative course and marked post-psychotic deficit symptoms showed at follow-up a degree of warm-hearted sensitivity, a need to relate and an emotional capability. Indeed, the follow-up interview showed that even if it was another form of abnormal affect that had replaced the flat affect previously observed, there was a responsive relationship with the investigator. On the basis of this experience I emphatically support the thesis of Strauss and Carpenter (1981) that "as part of understanding severe mental disorders and improving their treatment, one must use an interactive developmental model".

References

Andreasen NC, Olsen S (1982) Negative vs. positive schizophrenia: definition and validation. Arch Gen Psychiatry 30:789–794

Biehl H, Maurer K, Schubart C et al. (1986) Prediction of outcome and utilization of medical services in a prospective study of first onset schizophrenics. Eur Arch Psychiatry Neurol Sci 236:139–147

Black DW, Boffeli TJ (1989) Simple schizophrenia: past, present, and future. Am J Psychiatry 146:1267–1273

Buchanan RW, Kirkpatrick B, Heinrichs DW, Carpenter WT (1990) Clinical correlates of the deficit syndrome of schizophrenia. Am J Psychiatry 147:290–294

Carpenter WT, Heinrichs DW, Wagmann AMI (1988) Deficit and nondeficit forms of schizophrenia: the concept. Am J Psychiatry 145:578–583

Eggers C (1973) Verlaufsweisen kindlicher und präpuberaler Schizophrenien. Springer, Berlin Heidelberg New York (Monographien aus dem Gesamtgebiet der Psychiatrie)

Eggers C (1978) Course and prognosis of childhood schizophrenia. J Autism Child Schizophr 9:21–36

Johnstone EC (1989) The assessment of negative and positive features in schizophrenia. Br J Psychiatry 155:41–44

Johnstone EC, Frith CD, Gold A et al. (1979) The outcome of severe acute schizophrenic illnesses after one year. Br J Psychiatry 134:28–33

Kay SR, Opler LA, Fiszbein A (1986) Significance of positive and negative syndromes in chronic schizophrenia. Br J Psychiatry 149:439–448

Kay SR, Fiszbein A, Opler LA (1987) The positive and negative syndrome scale (PANSS) for schizophrenia. Schizophr Bull 13:261–276

Kulhara P, Avasthi A, Chadda R, Chandiramani K, Mattoo SK, Kota SK, Joseph S (1989) Negative and depressive symptoms in schizophrenia. Br J Psychiatry 154:207–211

Lewine RRJ, Fogg L, Meltzer HY (1983) Assessment of negative and positive symptoms in schizophrenia. Schizophr Bull 9:368–376

Pfohl B, Winokur G (1982) Evolution of symptoms in institutionalised hebephrenic/catatonic schizophrenics. Br J Psychiatry 141:567–572

Pogue-Geile MF (1989) The prognostic significance of negative symptoms in schizophrenia. Br J Psychiatry 155:123–127

Pogue-Geile MF, Harrow M (1984) Negative and positive symptoms in schizophrenia and depression: a follow-up. Schizophr Bull 10:371–387

Strauss JS, Carpenter WT Jr (1981) Schizophrenia. Plenum, New York

The Negative/Positive Dichotomy: Does It Make Sense from the Perspective of the Genetic Researcher?

P. McGuffin [1], I. Harvey, and M. Williams [2]

Introduction

At the present time, we cannot solve the problem of dissecting schizophrenia into its natural sub-divisions. Nonetheless, we do have the practical need of characterising the various clinical pictures that present themselves to us in this disease by terms corresponding, at least, to rather broad and crude sub-divisions. This much is possible, but not much more (Bleuler 1911).

Although tentative about how much could be achieved in sub-typing schizophrenia on the basis of clinical signs and symptoms, Bleuler had enough conviction about the probable existence of heterogeneity to subtitle his famous monograph on dementia praecox "The *Group* of Schizophrenias" (our italics). Probably the majority of biologically orientated researchers since then, impressed by the clinical variety of patients described as "schizophrenic", have followed Bleuler and attempt to seek ways in which to split the syndrome rationally. Psychiatric geneticists in particular have been on the side of the would-be splitters (even though for most practical purposes in carrying out family, twin and adoption studies, they have had to content themselves with lumping the whole syndrome together). Thus, there has been a general assumption that aetiological heterogeneity is "inherently probable" (Slater 1947). The main difficulty is that there has been no clear consensus about what is the most useful approach to clinical heterogeneity, and until recently there has been a lack of explicit and reliable ways of describing clinical sub-types.

The comparatively recent growth of interest in categorising schizophrenia on the basis of positive versus negative symptoms (Carpenter et al. 1974; Crow 1980; Andreasen 1985; Pogue-Geile and Ho 1985) is therefore an interesting phase of a much older and still unresolved debate on the unity and diversity of schizophrenia (British Medical Journal 1969). In attempting to make sense of a potential sub-typing scheme for schizophrenia in which there may be two differing but overlapping syndromes characterised by the positive or negative symptoms, the genetic researcher is faced with three problems. The first is a familiar one in all psychiatric genetic research and concerns how best to define the phenotypes. There have been several carefully considered and in some cases precisely defined accounts of what constitute negative symptoms and how

[1] Department of Psychological Medicine, University of Wales College of Medicine, Heath Park, Cardiff, CF4 4XN, United Kingdom
[2] Institute of Psychiatry, De Crespigny Park, Denmark Hill, London, United Kingdom

A. Marneros / N. C. Andreasen / M. T. Tsuang (Eds.)
Negative Versus Positive Schizophrenia

these can be elicited (Andreasen 1982; Pogue-Geile and Harrow 1985; Crow 1980, 1985), but such accounts tend to differ in detail if not in essence so that we have a number of varying definitions of the same concept. Second, rather different notions about the clinical relationship between positive and negative symptoms have been put forward (e.g. Crow 1980; Wing 1988; Murray et al. 1988), but it is unclear what implications these have for the construction of testable formal genetic models. A third and most obvious obstacle to understanding is that there is simply a lack of useful genetic data. There have been some attempts (e.g. Dworkin and Lenzenweger 1984; McGuffin et al. 1987) to reassess twin study material in the light of a possible negative/positive symptom dichotomy but as yet there are no published family, twin or adoption studies which have been "purpose-built" for this type of approach.

Elsewhere in this book, there are detailed and informed discussions of the clinical aspects of positive and negative symptoms, how such symptoms can be defined and the possible pathogenetic mechanisms. In this chapter, therefore, we will consider only briefly the problems concerning the definition of the phenotype. We will then review the previously published analyses of twin studies and will also describe new family data before going on to propose a model of transmission of positive and negative symptoms and to test this using a maximum likelihood model-fitting approach.

Negative and Positive Phenotypes

According to Berrios (1985), the idea that certain neurological symptoms due to loss of function could be classed as negative (e.g. paralysis) while others due to an excess of function could be classed as positive (e.g. muscular spasms) was put forward by Reynolds, writing in the nineteenth century. It was only later that Hughlings-Jackson proposed the more sophisticated hierarchical model in which negative symptoms are said to occur after loss of higher centre function that in turn facilitates a release of lower centres. Thus, a prerequisite for having positive symptoms which are caused by the uninhibited but otherwise normal functioning of lower centres is that there are already negative symptoms resulting from damage at a higher level. As Berrios has pointed out, the modern notion that there may be two distinct, albeit overlapping syndromes characterised by mainly positive or mainly negative symptoms is at variance with Jackson's model. In particular, Crow (1980) has suggested that a type I syndrome characterised by positive symptoms and a good response to neuroleptics may have a different aetiology to a type II syndrome which is associated with negative symptoms, cognitive impairment and cerebral ventricular enlargement on CT scan. In this formulation, negative symptoms are regarded as more-or-less permanent, and the hypothesis is of a neo-Kraepelinian type, with worsening over several years resulting in the "dementia of dementia praecox" (Johnstone et al. 1976).

A contrasting hypothesis is that of Murray et al. (1988) who view schizophrenia as a neurodevelopmental disorder. They suggest that in addition to genetic factors, early cerebral insults may have an important aetiological role. Subtle early damage may then result in negative symptoms which precede the positive ones by many years. Yet another view has been put forward by Wing (1988) who suggests that the pattern of clinical symptoms actually fluctuates considerably. Rather than there being a fixed pattern, positive or negative symptoms may predominate depending on certain environmental factors. Thus, for example, a pressure to perform at a high level in an over-stimulating environment could produce an increase in delusions and hallucinations, while under-stimulation in an impoverished milieu may lead to a predominantly negative picture.

In summary, from our perusal of the recent literature, there does not appear to be much consensus over the stability of syndromes characterised by negative or positive symptoms and still less consensus about the possible mechanisms involved in the psychogenesis or pathogenesis. This presents potential difficulties for genetic analysis which, ideally, requires phenotypes that are stable and can be unequivocally recognised in a variety of settings. Moreover, we have in our own studies noted that while some patients whose symptoms are rated on a "lifetime ever" basis appear to have only positive or type I symptoms, very few seem to show a pure form of negative symptom schizophrenia or type II syndrome (Farmer et al. 1987). Instead, most patients with negative symptoms have also at some stage had positive symptoms (this is just the opposite of what is predicted by the Jacksonian hierarchical model) and therefore have to be classified as having a "mixed" syndrome. We will therefore adopt a pragmatic solution to this problem, and for the rest of this chapter, we will assume that the most stable phenotypes are provided by a division into two broad categories: a pure positive symptom or type I syndrome and a type II/"mixed" syndrome consisting mainly of patients with a mixture of positive and negative factors plus a minority with a pure type II picture.

Twin and Family Data

At present the only published twin data derive from a "recycling" of the material from those already existing studies in which clinical written material is available in sufficient detail to allow rating of negative symptoms according to recent conventions and sub-classification according to current concepts. For example, with the author's guidance, we cast Crow's (1980) clinical criteria in an operational format and were able to show that this afforded good inter-rater reliability (Farmer et al. 1987). We then re-examined the clinical abstracts for the Maudsley Hospital schizophrenic twin series described by Gottesman and Shields (1972) and reclassified affected individuals into type I, mixed and type II categories. The results of this are summarised in Table 1 (McGuffin et al. 1987), and again as we have mentioned in connection with a different study (Farmer et al. 1987), pure type II cases proved to be rare. However, it was noteworthy that in twins who were concordant for schizophrenia, there was a tendency towards concordance for a sub-type, but the numbers involved are

Table 1. Proband-wise concordance in the Maudsley (1948–1964) Schizophrenic Twin Series (from McGuffin et al. 1987)

Subtypes of Crow (1980) concordance for	Monozygotic		Dizygotic	
	(*n*)	(%)	(*n*)	(%)
Schizophrenia, where proband is:				
Type I	8/15	53	4/21	19
Mixed type	7/11	64	0/11	0
Type II	0/0	0	0/2	0
Subtype, where both twins are diagnosed schizophrenic	11/15	73	3/4	75

small, and the degree of homotypia (or tendency for "like to go with like") was incomplete; the proportion of homotypic twins was about three-quarters in both the monozygotic (MZ) and dizygotic (DZ) samples. Regarding overall concordance for schizophrenia, there appeared to be an obvious effect due to the sub-type of the proband. Thus, the difference between MZ and DZ concordance was greater when the proband had a mixed or type II syndrome than if the proband had a type I syndrome. This could suggest that the mixed/Type II syndrome is a "more genetic" condition than type I schizophrenia, but again we cannot reach firm conclusions on the basis of the data shown in Table 1 because of the comparatively small numbers involved.

There is, however, some evidence which derives from a similar strategy of reassessing earlier twin series for the presence of negative or positive symptoms as described in case abstracts (Dworkin and Lenzenweger 1984). Using a method which is partially based on Andreasen's (1982) system for scoring negative symptoms, these authors rated 302 case histories of a total of 151 monozygotic twin pairs described in five different studies (Fischer 1973; Gottesman and Shields 1972; Kringlen 1967; Slater 1953; Tienari 1963). It was found that concordance rates in MZ twins were significantly higher when the probands had a greater number of negative symptoms (except in Kringlen 1967). Thus, the probands were divided into "high negative" and "low negative" categories, which resulted in a fairly consistent pattern. A similar effect was not observed for positive symptoms, that is, higher rates of positive symptoms in probands were not associated with higher concordances.

These authors (Dworkin et al. 1988; Lenzenweger et al. 1989) then went on to complete a series of multivariate statistical analyses of the reassessed twins. First, discriminant analyses were carried out which suggested that negative symptoms, premorbid social competence and the presence of paranoid symptoms each contributed to the ability to differentiate between concordant and discordant pairs. The authors suggested that these categories of symptoms might reflect three different functional processes involved in the development of schizophrenia (Dworkin et al. 1988). Secondly (Lenzenweger et al. 1989), a confirmatory factor analysis was carried out using the LISREL VI package (Joreskog and Sorbom 1984). Here the aim was to test three rather different theoretical models for the development of negative and positive symptoms by examining the covariance matrix based on ten groups of symptoms from ratings of 151 probands and 69 schizophrenic co-twins. The models assessed were the "bipolar" model proposed by Andreasen and Olsen (1982), in which negative and positive symptoms are considered as being at different ends of the same single dimension; Crow's "dual process" model (Crow 1980), in which positive and negative symptoms are thought of as characterising independent processes; and a severity-liability model proposed by us (Gottesman et al. 1987; McGuffin et al. 1987). The severity-liability model as reformulated by Lenzenweger et al. (1989) is like the bipolar model of Andreasen and Olson in being unidimensional but differs in that it predicts that positive and negative symptoms will both have positive loadings on the same factor, varying only in the size of the loading. The main results were that Crow's dual process model was favoured over the severity-liability model which, in turn, appeared more satisfactory than the bipolar model. However, none of the models provided a perfect fit to the data, and although their analysis represented an advance over previous attempts to use exploratory factor analytic methods in studies of positive and negative symptoms, the findings do not shed any new light specifically on the genetic aspects of negative and positive symptoms.

Indeed, although their analyses were based on twins, Lenzenweger et al. did not test any specifically genetic hypothesis, and, in particular, they tested only one aspect of the severity-liability model, that positive and negative symptoms lie on a continuum. In fact, our proposed model (McGuffin et al. 1987; Gottesman et al. 1987) is merely a particular application of a general class of models (Falconer 1965; Reich et al. 1972) in which it is assumed that liability to develop a disorder is a continuous variable that is normally distributed in the population (or can be transformed to normality) such that only those individuals whose liability at some time exceeds a certain threshold manifest the disorder. Threshold models are of particular interest in disorders which occur in two or more forms (Reich et al. 1972). It is postulated that those individuals who lie beyond the first threshold show a "broad", milder form of the disorder while those beyond a second, more extreme threshold show a "narrow", more severe form. Relatives of all affected individuals will show a mean liability which is greater than that of the general population, and thus more will lie beyond the threshold for being affected. The "isocorrelational" version of this model (Reich et al. 1979; and see below) predicts that the mean liability of relatives of "narrow" cases will be greater than that of relatives of "broad" cases (this model is illustrated in a somewhat simplified form in Fig. 1), and therefore those with the narrow form of the disorder will have more affected relatives than those with the broad form. As we have seen so far, both our re-analysis of the Gottesman and Shields twins and that of Dworkin et al. of these and other datasets suggest that probands with negative symptoms are more likely to have affected MZ co-twins than probands without such symptoms. We might therefore speculate that negative symptom or type II/"mixed" categories could be classed as "narrow" disorder lying beyond the second more extreme threshold with pure positive symptom or type I disorder

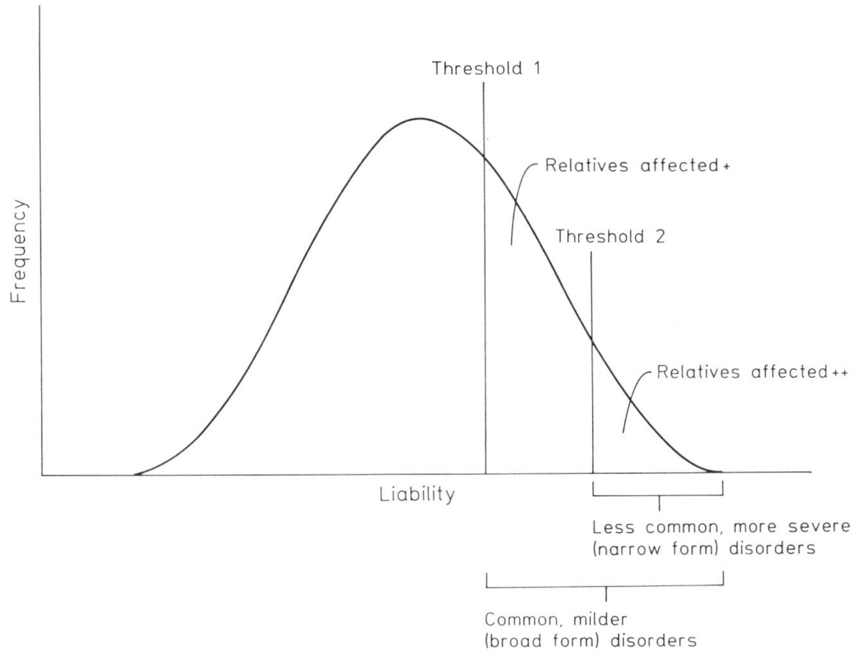

Fig. 1. The two-threshold model (see text for explanation)

being a "broad but not narrow" form lying between the first and second thresholds.

As we have noted earlier, there are little family data available to test this further. Kay et al. (1985) have briefly described a series of 101 inpatients and reported that a negative syndrome was significantly associated with a history of psychosis in first degree relatives while a positive syndrome was more closely associated with sociopathy in family members. Precisely what this means is unclear, but perhaps again it suggests that specific genetic factors for schizophrenia are most evident in patients in whom negative symptoms are prominent. We have also recently studied a consecutive series of inpatients with psychosis admitted to an acute admission ward of the King's College Hospital (Dulwich North) Psychiatry Unit in London (Harvey et al. 1990). Although not designed primarily as a family study, this investigation did yield data which have a bearing on the problem of the genetic basis of negative symptoms, and we will now therefore briefly summarise the relevant findings.

The King's College Hospital Study

The patient series has been described in detail elsewhere (Harvey et al. 1990) and consisted of 150 consecutively admitted adults who fulfilled broad but highly reliable criteria for psychosis and who were drawn from an inner city catchment area, aged 15–59 years, 70 men and 80 women. All patients were interviewed using the Present State Examination (PSE) (Wing et al. 1974), and an Operational Criteria Checklist for Psychotic Illness (OPCRIT) (McGuffin et al. 1984, 1991) was completed on the basis of both interview and case note information. Interviews with informants were carried out, the majority of whom were mothers, and a structured family history schedule was completed.

A total of 103 subjects fulfilled Research Diagnostic Criteria (RDC) (Spitzer et al. 1978) for schizophrenia or schizoaffective disorder and in further discussion are here referred to as the KCH probands. Of this group, 55 at some stage showed definite negative symptoms consisting of affective blunting, self-neglect or poverty of the content of speech as rated on the PSE and/or negative thought disorder or restricted or blunted affect as rated on the OPCRIT checklist. Some 54 of these fulfilled our operational version of Crow's (1980) criteria for mixed schizophrenia, only 1 being a pure type II case. We therefore lump the 55 together as mixed/type II probands. The remaining 48 probands showed no negative symptoms and were classified as type I.

It is well-known that a family history method, compared with a family study method in which all relatives are personally interviewed, tends to underestimate the frequency of psychopathology in relatives. This bias can be reduced by interviewing at least one informant other than the proband and by collecting the pedigree information in a systematic and structured way. Thus, using our structured family history questionnaire we obtained results fairly closely similar to the reported morbid risks for broadly defined schizophrenia in earlier studies of the relatives of schizophrenics (Gottesman and Shields 1982) and this provides some assurance as to the dependability. After applying an age correction using the shorter Weinberg method (McGuffin 1984), we obtained a morbid risk of schizophrenia or other non-affective psychosis of 5% in parents, 10.5% in siblings and 9.3% in offspring of the 103 KCH probands.

Table 2 summarises the results of splitting the relatives into those of type I and those of mixed/type II probands. As can be seen in all three categories of relatives, those of mixed/type II probands are more commonly affected than those of type I probands. In the case of siblings and offspring, the morbid risk in relatives of mixed/type II probands is double that of the relatives of type I probands. However, the differences are even more striking in parents. Thus,

Table 2. The morbid risk (MR) of schizophrenic or other non-affective psychosis in relatives of schizophrenics according to proband type

Category of relative	Proband type	Relatives at risk (BZ)	Non-affected	MR (%)
Parents	I	82	1	1.2
($n = 206$)	mixed/II	97	8	8.3
Siblings	I	110.5	7	6.3
($n = 336$)	mixed/II	109	16	14.7
Offspring	I	44	3	6.8
($n = 139$)	mixed/II	20.5	3	14.6

looking at the data in a slightly different way, 8 of 55 mixed/type II probands have an affected parent compared with 1 of 48 type I probands (since no proband has both parents affected). This difference is significant at the $P = 0.026$ level on applying Fisher's exact test.

Once again, these results are in keeping with the general hypothesis that schizophrenics with negative symptoms tend to have a more familial form of the disorder than those without such symptoms and lead us to postulate that this might be explicable in terms of a continuum of liability with multiple thresholds. Previously, because of the small sample size, we were reluctant to attempt formal testing of such a model on the re-assessed Gottesman and Shields (1972) twin data (McGuffin et al. 1987). However, having reasonably dependable family data in addition to twin data enables us to obtain a stronger purchase on the problem, and it is feasible to begin exploring the question of genetic model fitting.

Negative/Positive Symptom Schizophrenia as a Two-Threshold Trait

Knowing the proportion of affected individuals in the general population and the proportion of affected relatives of probands (and assuming that the underlying distributions are normal), we can on applying a liability/threshold model calculate the correlations in liability between pairs of relatives (Falconer 1965; Reich et al. 1972). The correlation in liability is essentially an approximation to Pearson's tetrachoric correlation coefficient. When two or more categories of disorder can be defined, the number of correlations which can be obtained between relatives increases. Thus, for a two-threshold disorder there are four possible correlations (Table 3). As we have outlined earlier, the simplest two-threshold model (Reich et al. 1972) predicts that relatives of patients with the narrow form will be more commonly affected than relatives of patients with the broad form. More particularly, if the narrow form is simply a subset of the broad form, we would expect that all of the correlations r_{11}, r_{12}, r_{21} and r_{22} would be equal. This has been called the isocorrelational model by Reich et al. (1979). An alternative hypothesis is that the narrow and broad forms do not both lie on the same continuum of liability but are in fact independent disorders so that the correlations across disorders, r_{21} and r_{12}, will be substantially lower than the correlations r_{11} and r_{22}. In extreme case when the forms are completely distinct and separate, r_{12} and r_{21} will tend to zero.

Table 3. Correlations in liability for a disorder existing in two forms, "broad" and "narrow"

		Relatives	
		broad (1)	narrow (2)
Probands	broad (1)	r_{11}	r_{12}
	narrow (2)	r_{21}	r_{22}

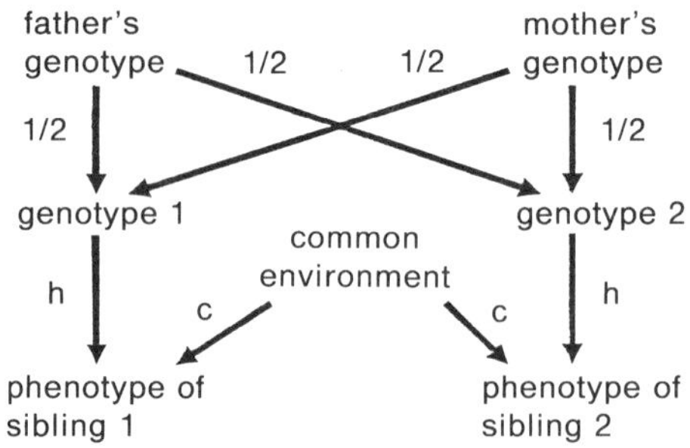

Fig. 2. Path diagram of the sources of resemblance in siblings or twins and their parents

In order to attempt to test models of this type completely, we would need to divide both probands and affected relatives into the two forms of disorder. However, quite often, as is the case with our family data described earlier, we are able to divide probands into a narrow and broad form but are only able to classify relatives as affected or unaffected. Therefore, if we consider that the narrow form is contained within the broad form, we are able to calculate the values of the two correlations r_{11} and r_{21}. Providing the sample size is large enough, this would still enable us to test whether a set of data is compatible with the hypothesis that the broad and narrow forms are on the same continuum of liability such that r_{11} equals r_{21}, as against a more general model which would suggest the broad and narrow form are separate conditions such that r_{11} is not equal to r_{21}.

In order to apply such a test we next need to consider the genetic and environmental sources of resemblance between relatives of various categories and derive expressions for the expected correlations. This can be effected by path analysis. A comparatively simple path model is shown in Fig. 2 in which there are two sources of resemblance between pairs of relatives, genes and shared (family) environment. The phenotype of sibling 1 is dependent on having genotype 1 and having a common environment which is shared with sibling 2. In addition, non-shared environment (not shown in the figure) contributes to the liability to the disorder of sibling 1 but does not have any effect on the phenotypic resemblance between sibling 1 and sibling 2. The common environment includes all of the shared experiences of sibling 1 and sibling 2 resulting from their being raised in the same family, while non-shared environment might include such social factors as attending different schools or having different circles of friends and such physical factors as trauma or exposure to certain infections.

In the model illustrated in Fig. 2 the only source of resemblance between parents and offspring is genetic such that each individual receives half of his or her genotype from the mother and half from the father. Allowing only genetic similarities between parents and offspring may of course be an over-simplification when considering a complex trait such as schizophrenia, and more complicated models (e.g. McGue et al. 1985) have been proposed which incorporate "cultural transmission" as well as genetic inheritance and allow for the possibility that there may assortative mating producing a positive correlation between the phenotypes of parents. However, it could also be argued that one should start off with a simple model with a small number of parameters and work up to more complex formulations only if this provides an unsatisfactory explanation of the data. Therefore, we will content ourselves with the simpler model here.

According to the fundamental calculus of path analysis (Li 1975), the expected correlation between variables is the sum of the permissible paths connecting them. Thus, for siblings 1 and 2 the phenotypic correlation (r_{sib}) is given by the sum of the connecting paths via the parental genotypes and the common environment. The path coefficients are standardised partial regression coefficients, and that from genotype of parent to genotype of offspring is 1/2, from genotype to phenotype is denoted by h and from common environment to phenotype by c. Thus, r_{sib} is the sum of the paths via the father's genotype, i.e. $h \times 1/2 \times 1/2 \times h$, the path via the mother's genotype, i.e. $h \times 1/2 \times 1/2 \times h$, and the path via common environment, i.e. $c \times c$. The sum is $1/4h^2 + 1/4h^2 + c^2 = 1/2h^2 + c^2$. Providing we assume that there is no greater environmental similarity between DZ twins than between full siblings, the expected correlation between DZ twins (r_{DZ}) is given by the same expression. However, if sibling 1 and 2 are MZ twins then genotypes 1 and 2 are identical so that the phenotypic correlation (r_{MZ}) is given by:

$$r_{MZ} = h^2 + c^2$$

If the path between parental genotypes and phenotypes (not shown in Fig. 1) in each case is also h, then the phenotypic correlation between probands and their offspring (r_{off}) is given by:

$$r_{off} = 1/2\ h^2$$

and similarly the expected correlation between probands and their parents (r_{par}) is given by:

$$r_{par} = 1/2\ h^2$$

Therefore, given the data for the twins shown in Table 1 and the family data summarised in Table 2, we should, provided we have estimates of population frequencies, be in a position to calculate correlations in liability for five categories of relative, r_{MZ}, r_{DZ}, r_{sib}, r_{off}, r_{par}. We could then, using a maximum likelihood method (Morton 1982) obtain the best-fit estimates of h^2 and c^2. Furthermore, if we postulate that type I and mixed/type II schizophrenia are different disorders, then we have to assume that the correlations for each of these categories of relatives vary between types and hence that the two disorders have different heritabilities and different common environmental contributions to the variance in liability. Therefore, the heritability for the broad form of the disorder (h_b^2) would differ from that of the narrow form (h_n^2) and similarly we would not expect the common environmental parameters for the broad form (c_b^2) and the narrow form (c_n^2) to be equal. However, we can postulate that the genotypes might be correlated as might the common environmental factors such that there is a genetic correlation, $r_g > 0$, and an environmental correlation, $r_e > 0$, between the two forms. Then the expected correlation between narrow-form probands and broad-form DZ co-twins or siblings becomes:

$$r_{DZ} = r_{sib} = 1/2\ h_b r_g h_n + c_b r_e c_n$$

and the corresponding expression for MZ twins becomes:

$$r_{MZ} = h_b r_g h_n + c_b r_e c_n$$

and that for parents and offspring:

$$r_{par} = r_{off} = 1/2\ h_b r_g h_n$$

The hypothesis that type I and mixed/type II syndromes are different forms of the same disorder distinguished from each other only on the basis of severity of liability can be tested by comparing the fit of a general model when $h^2 = h_b^2$ and $c_n^2 = c_b^2$ with reduced models where r_g and r_e are fixed at 1, or where both $r_g = r_e = 1$ and $h_b^2 = h_n^2 = h^2$, $c_n^2 = c_b^2 = c^2$.

This was carried out using a FORTRAN computer program, FTWIN, which calls on the GEMINI sub-routine (Lalouel et al. 1983) to maximise a likelihood function of the form:

$$\ln L = \sum_{i=1}^{N} a_i \ln(p_i) + u_i \ln(1 - p_i)$$

Where for the ith class of relatives, a_i is the number affected, u_i is the number unaffected, p_i is the predicted proportion affected, and $1 - p_i$ is the predicted proportion unaffected.

Models can be compared by carrying out a likelihood ratio test which depends on the fact that minus twice the difference in log likelihoods between two comparable models is asymptotically a χ^2 with degrees of freedom equal to the difference in the number of parameters. The results of our analyses are summarised in Table 4. We fixed the frequency of the broad form of schizophrenia at 0.86% (Gottesman and Shields 1982) and hence had seven parameters to estimate in the general model consisting of the two heritabilities (h_n^2, h_b^2), the two common environmental components (c_n^2, c_n^2), the genetic correlation (r_g), the environmental correlation (r_c) and the population frequency (Kp_n). Constraining the heritabilities and the common environmental components to be equal did not result in a significant change in the likelihood ($\chi^2 = 0.12$, 2 df, NS). Thus, an isocorrelational model in which type I and mixed/type II disorder are considered to differ only in terms of severity of liability fits just as well as a general model in which the correlations across the two types of disorder are not constrained to be equal. Hence, on grounds of parsimony, an isocorrelational model is favoured. We then went on to explore the significance of the genetic and the common environmental components. Testing an isocorrelational model in which only genetic transmission was

Table 4. Application of a two-threshold model to twin and family data

Model	Parameters							$-2\ln L$
	h_b^2	c_b^2	h_n^2	c_n^2	$K p_n$	r_g	r_e	
General (g)	0.766	0.112	0.827	0.0079	0.0062	1.0	1.0	504.312
Isocorrelational (i)	0.783	0.098	0.783 [a]	0.098 [b]	0.0049	[1.0]	[1.0]	504.437
Isocorrelational genetic (ig)	0.884	[0.0]	0.884 [a]	[0.0]	0.0048	[1.0]	[1.0]	508.043
Isocorrelational environmental (ie)	[0.0]	0.553	[0.0]	0.553 [b]	0.0055	[1.0]	[1.0]	612.381

Parameters in square brackets, e.g. [0.0], are fixed. For abbreviations, see text.
[a] h_n^2 constrained to be equal to h_b^2.
[b] c_n^2 constrained to be equal to c_b^2.
Likelihood ratios: g − i = 0.125, 1 df, *NS*
i − ig = 3.606, 1 df, $P < 0.1$
i − ie = 104.338, 1 df, $P = 0.000$.

present and in which c^2 was fixed at zero produced a fall in the likelihood which just fails to meet conventional levels of significance ($\chi^2 = 3.61$, 1 df, $P < 0.1$). On the other hand, the purely environmental model in which heritability is fixed at zero can be rejected by comparison with the isocorrelational model incorporating both genetic and environmental effects ($\chi^2 = 104.34$, 1 df, $P = 0.000$). We can conclude that a severity of liability model in which type I and mixed/type II syndromes differ only in terms of their positions on the continuum of liability provides a satisfactory explanation of the data. Furthermore, there is a highly significant genetic component to the liability but common environmental effects can be dropped from the model without any substantial or significant reduction in the likelihood.

Conclusions

Such genetic data as are available so far allow fairly limited conclusions about the negative/positive symptom dichotomy in schizophrenia. The twin data, based on a reworking of previously published studies, does not allow a clear separation of two distinct sub-types of schizophrenia. Indeed, although pure positive symptom schizophrenia appears to be common, pure negative symptom schizophrenia is rare, and most affected individuals with negative symptoms have also had positive symptoms at some stage or other in their illness. There is fairly consistent evidence from the published twin results and from our own family data that probands who have experienced negative symptoms tend to have more affected relatives than probands who have had only positive symptoms. We therefore tested a liability/threshold model in which negative or "mixed" schizophrenia was postulated to be a more severe disorder lying beyond a more extreme threshold on a liability continuum than positive symptom schizophrenia, which was postulated to be a less severe condition lying beyond a less extreme threshold. Such a model provided a satisfactory explanation of the data, providing just as good a fit as more complicated models under which the "narrow" and "broad" forms of schizophrenia were considered as separate disorders. In other words, the simple model in which negative and positive symptom forms differ only quantitatively in terms of their positions on the same continuum of liability cannot be rejected and on grounds of parsimony can be favoured over a model in which the two clinical forms are construed as separate conditions. The results therefore are reminiscent of our previous attempt at model-fitting with more traditional sub-types of schizophrenia and our findings (McGuffin et al. 1987) regarding sub-types derived from multivariate statistical analyses (Farmer et al. 1983; McGuffin et al. 1987). Here again, the findings were suggestive of quantitative rather than qualitative differences. This led us to conclude that different ways of sub-classifying schizophrenia which were based purely on signs and symptoms fail to provide a means of "carving nature at the joints" but instead may lead to various ways of slicing up a salami.

References

Andreasen NC (1982) Negative symptoms in schizophrenia: definition and reliability. Arch Gen Psychiatr 39:784–788

Andreasen NC (1985) Positive versus negative schizophrenia: a critical evaluation. Schizophr Bull 11:380–389

Andreasen NC, Olsen S (1982) Negative vs. positive schizophrenia: definition and validation. Arch Gen Psychiatr 39:784–794

Berrios GE (1985) Positive and negative symptoms and Jackson. A conceptual history. Arch Gen Psychiatr 42:95–97

Bleuler E (1911) Dementia praecox or the group of schizophrenias. (Translation) International Universities Press, New York

British Medical Journal (1969) Editorial. Unity and diversity in schizophrenia. Br Med J 4:673–674

Carpenter WT, Sacks MH, Strauss JS, Bartko JJ, Rayner J (1976) Evaluating signs and symptoms: comparison of structured interview and clinical approaches. Br J Psychiatr 128:397–403

Crow TJ (1980) Molecular pathology of schizophrenia: more than one disease process? Br Med J 280:66–68

Crow TJ (1985) The two syndrome concept: origins and current status. Schizophr Bull 11:471–486

Dworkin RH, Lenzenweger MF (1984) Symptoms and the genetics of schizophrenia: implications for diagnosis. Am J Psychiatr 141:1541–1546

Dworkin RH, Lenzenweger MF, Moldin SO, Skillings GF, Levick SE (1988) A multidimensional approach to the genetics of schizophrenia. Am J Psychiatr 145:1077–1083

Falconer DS (1965) The inheritance of liability to certain disease, estimated from the incidence among relatives. Ann Hum Genet 29:51–76

Farmer AE, McGuffin P, Spitznagel E (1983) Heterogeneity in schizophrenia: a cluster analytic approach. Psychiatries 8:1–12

Farmer AE, Jackson R, McGuffin P, Storey P (1987) Cerebral ventricular enlargement in schizophrenia: consistencies and contradictions. Br J Psychiatr 150:324–330

Fischer M (1973) Genetic and environmental factors in schizophrenia: A study of schizophrenic twins and their families. Acta Psychiatr Scand (Suppl) 49[Suppl 238]:1–158

Gottesman II, Shields J (1972) Schizophrenia and genetics: a twin study vantage point. Academic, New York

Gottesman II, Shields J (1982) Schizophrenia: the epigenetic puzzle. Cambridge University Press, Cambridge

Gottesman II, McGuffin P, Farmer AE (1987) Clinical genetics as clues to the "real" genetics of schizophrenia. (A decade of modest gains while playing for time). Schizophr Bull 13:23–48

Harvey I, Williams M, Toone BK, Lewis SW, Turner SW, McGuffin P (1990) The ventricular brain ratio (VBR) in functional psychoses: the relationship of lateral ventricular and total intracranial area. Psychol Med 20:55–62

Johnstone EC, Crow TJ, Frith CD, Husband T, Kreel L (1976) Cerebral ventricular size and cognitive impairment in chronic schizophrenia. Lancet ii:924–926

Joreskog KG, Sorbom D (1984) LISREL VI: analysis of linear structural relationship by maximum likelihood, instrumental variables and least squares methods, 3rd edn. Scientific Software, Mooresville

Kay SR, Opler LA, Fiszbein A (1985) Genetics of schizophrenia and the positive-negative dimension. Am J Psychiat 142:994–995

Kringlen E (1967) Heredity and environment in the functional psychoses: an epidemiological-clinical twin study. Heinemann, London

Lalouel JM, Rao DC, Morton NE (1983) A unified model for complex segregation analysis. Am J Hum Genet 35:816–826

Lenzenweger MF, Dworkin RH, Wethington E (1989) Models of positive and negative symptoms in schizophrenia: an empirical evaluation of latent structures. J Abnorm Psychol 98(1):62–70

Li CC (1975) Path analysis – a Primer. Boxwood, Pacific Grove, CA

McGue M, Gottesman II, Rao DC (1985) Resolving genetic models for the transmission of schizophrenia. Genet Epidemiol 2:99–110

McGuffin P (1984) Principles and methods in psychiatric genetics. In: McGuffin P, Shanks M (eds) Scientific Principles of Psychopathology. London, Grune and Stratton, pp 155–172

McGuffin P, Farmer AE, Gottesman II (1984) Twin concordance for operationally defined schizophrenia: confirmation of familiality and heritability. Arch Gen Psychiatr 41:541–545

McGuffin P, Farmer AE, Gottesman II (1987) Is there really a split in schizophrenia? The genetic evidence. Br J Psychiatr 150:581–592

McGuffin P, Sargeant M, Hett G, Tidmarsh S, Whatley S, Marchbanks RM (1990) Exclusion of a susceptibility gene from the chromosome 5q11-5q13 region. New data and reanalysis of previous reports. Am J Hum Genet 47:524–535

Morton NE (1982) Outline of genetic epidemiology. Karger, Basel

Murray RM, Lewis SW, Owen MJ, Foerster A (1988) The neurodevelopmental origins of schizophrenia. In: Bebbington P, McGuffin P (eds) Schizophrenia: The major issues. Heinemann, Oxford, pp 90–106

Pogue-Geile MF, Harrow M (1985) Negative symptoms in schizophrenia: their longitudinal course and prognostic importance. Schizophr Bull 11:427–439

Reich T, James JW, Morris CA (1972) The use of multiple thresholds in determining the mode of transmission of semi-continuous traits. Ann Hum Genet 36:163–184

Reich T, Cloninger CR, Wette R, James J (1979) The use of multiple thresholds and segregation analysis in analysing the phenotypic heterogeneity of multifactorial traits. Ann Hum Genet 42:371

Slater E (1947) Genetic causes of schizophrenic symptoms. Monatsschr Psychiatr Neurol 113:50–58

Slater E (1953) Psychotic and neurotic illness in twins. Medical Research Council Special Report Series No. 278. H. M. Stationery Office, London

Spitzer RL, Endicott J, Robins E (1978) Research Diagnostic Criteria, Instrument No. 58. New York State Psychiatric Institute, New York

Tienari P (1963) Psychiatric illness in identical twins. Acta Psychiatr Scand (Suppl) 171

Wing JK (1988) The concept of negative symptoms. Br J Psychiatr

Wing JK, Copper JE, Sartorius N (1974) The measurement and classification of psychiatric symptoms. Cambridge University Press, Cambridge

Genetic Transmission of Negative and Positive Symptoms in the Biological Relatives of Schizophrenics *

M. T. Tsuang, [1] M. W. Gilbertson, [2] and S. V. Faraone [1]

Introduction

Despite strong evidence for the role of genetics in schizophrenia, the nature of the underlying mechanisms remains elusive. Knowledge is limited regardless of recent advances in the statistical analysis of family data and the ability to detect complex segregation patterns in the pedigrees of schizophrenic probands. This has prompted the development of alternative approaches which move beyond the traditional concept of schizophrenia. In this regard, increasing interest has been devoted to the understanding of disorders or traits which may be related to schizophrenia and observed in biological relatives who do not themselves manifest a "full-blown" schizophrenic syndrome. The delineation of the so-called "spectrum disorders" such as schizotypal personality disorder is one example of this approach. It is suggested (Risch and Baron 1984; Tsuang and Faraone 1984) that such traits or disorders may prove to be manifestations of the underlying "schizophrenia gene(s)," with clinical schizophrenia being only one extreme phenotypic expression. If so, these other, more common traits may provide more sensitive indices in genetic analyses. Their identification as alternative schizophrenic phenotypes or "schizotypes" would therefore constitute a significant contribution to the understanding of the mechanisms underlying schizophrenia.

Perhaps one of the most fascinating and productive areas of interest to emerge in recent years regarding the description of the schizophrenic phenotype has been the distinction made in positive versus negative symptom complexes. The focus of this discussion will be to review the literature relevant to subthreshold pathology in first-degree relatives of schizophrenics as it applies to this distinction. More specifically, the issue will be examined as to whether negative or positive symptoms, even in the absence of clinical schizophrenia, may be regarded as relevant dimensions in the search for schizotypal markers of the schizophrenic genotype.

---

* Preparation of this article was supported in part by the Veterans Administration's Health Services Research and Development Program and National Institute of Mental Health Grants 1 R01MH41879-01 and 1 R37MH43518-01.

[1] Harvard Departments of Psychiatry and Epidemiology, Brockton/West Roxbury, VA Medical Center, 940 Belmont Street, Brockton, MA 02401, USA

[2] Highland Drive, VA Medical Center, Schizophrenia Research, Center Unit, Pittsburgh, PA 15206, USA

A. Marneros / N. C. Andreasen / M. T. Tsuang (Eds.)
Negative Versus Positive Schizophrenia

The Genetic Nature of Schizophrenia: Current Limitations and the Need to Identify Spectrum Phenotypes

Multiple research paradigms have provided evidence for a substantial genetic component in the etiology of schizophrenic disorders. The earliest and most basic observation relating to the genetic basis of schizophrenia has been provided by family aggregation studies. That is, if schizophrenia is an inherited disorder, relatives of schizophrenic patients should manifest a higher incidence of schizophrenia than is found in the general population. Both early European and contemporary studies support this familial pattern and report, for example, the risk of schizophrenia arising in the first-degree relatives of schizophrenic probands to exceed the observed rate in the general population by five to ten times (Faraone and Tsuang 1985).

Additional and stronger evidence is provided by twin studies which appear to support overwhelmingly the genetic hypothesis. All of the 11 studies reviewed by Gottesman and Shields (1982) noted that individuals who have a schizophrenic MZ twin are over four times more likely to develop schizophrenia than individuals who have a schizophrenic DZ twin. Compelling support is also supplied by adoption studies which rule out a postnatal influence (Heston 1966; Rosenthal et al. 1968, 1975; Wender et al. 1977). There appears to be little doubt, then, that genetic factors play a substantial role in the etiology of schizophrenic disorders. In reviewing this literature, Kendler (1988) reports the genetic heritability of schizophrenia (i.e., the proportion of variation attributable to genetic factors) to be rather substantial, between 60% and 70%. In contrast, it is suggested that environmental familial factors appear to account for less than 20% of the variance in the liability to schizophrenia.

Given the substantial evidence favoring the genetic hypothesis of schizophrenia, attention has more recently been directed toward the elucidation of its mode of transmission. Both quantitative modeling studies (e.g., pedigree segregation analysis) and genetic linkage analyses represent specific attempts to identify the genetic mechanism and mode of inheritance responsible for the familial distribution of schizophrenia. These investigations have centered primarily upon single gene versus polygenic inheritance models (Bassett et al. 1988; Carter and Chung 1980; Debray et al. 1978; Elston et al. 1978; Kennedy et al. 1988; Matthysse et al. 1986; McGue et al. 1983; Risch and Baron 1984; St. Clair et al. 1989; Sherrington et al. 1988; Stewart et al. 1980; Tsuang et al. 1982). Unfortunately, their results have been contradictory and have yet to produce conclusive findings.

The inconsistent results of mathematical modeling and linkage studies suggest that the genetic mechanisms underlying schizophrenia and/or its phenotypic manifestations may be heterogeneous. Of relevance to the current discussion is the concept of phenotypic heterogeneity, which suggests that a given pathogenic genotype can be expressed as one of several phenotypes. It is not uncommon for a single gene to have different phenotypic effects in different individuals; this is known as pleiotropy. Future genetic research must not only address clinical schizophrenia per se but will need to attend closely to the

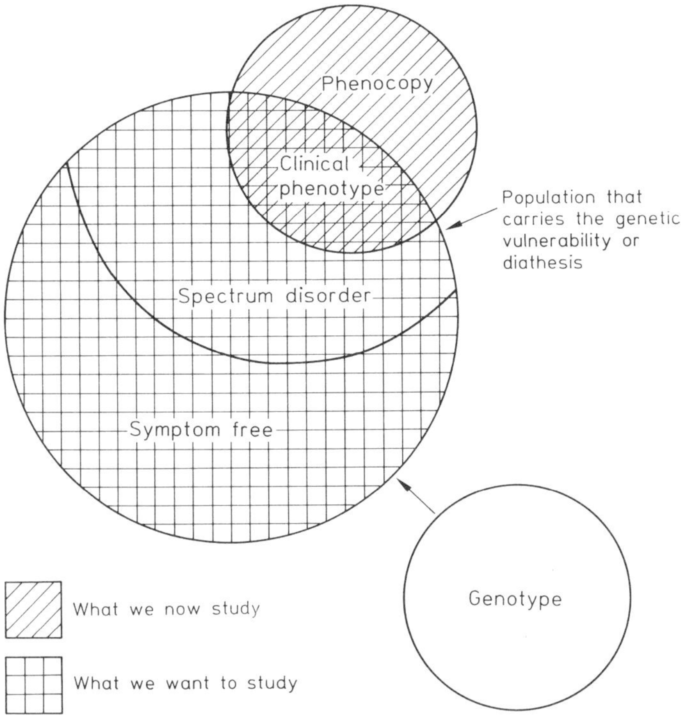

Fig. 1. Genetic and phenotypic heterogeneity model. (From Tsuang et al. (1989) "Problems of diagnosis in family studies". J Psychiat Res 21:391–395)

specification of phenotypes that may be genetically related to schizophrenia. For example, the results of Faraone and Tsuang (1988) suggest that the schizophrenia-like psychoses are related to schizophrenia. A similar relation is suggested for schizotypal personality disorder by Risch and Baron (1984).

Phenotypic heterogeneity is graphically displayed in Fig. 1. This diagram indicates that a pathogenic genotype can lead to a specific clinical phenotype (e.g., schizophrenia), a spectrum phenotype (e.g., schizotypal personality disorder), or no clinical symptomatology. Clearly, if one only studies the clinical phenotype, many genotypically abnormal individuals will be considered normal. This will make the mode of inheritance quite difficult to detect. As Fig. 1 suggests, progress in psychiatric genetics would greatly benefit from a more rigorous and comprehensive description of phenotypes related to pathogenic genotypes. Psychiatric genetics has, perhaps, reached a point at which the sophistication of available experimental tools such as molecular genetic technologies and statistical procedures has surpassed the ability to describe relevant phenotypes. It is unlikely that advances in statistical or linkage analyses per se will resolve the problems posed by phenotypic heterogeneity. Rather, what is required is the rigorous use of these technologies in populations which expand beyond the mere clinical phenotype (i.e., schizophrenic disorder) to "spectrum" phenotypes. The validation of spectrum phenotypes is relatively straightforward. The basic experimental designs of psychiatric genetics can indicate whether a specific disorder or set of clinical symptoms is more common among relatives of probands manifesting the clinical phenotype in comparison with relatives of control probands. Conceivably, the identification of individuals who carry the pathogenic genotype may extend to relatively discrete behavioral traits (e.g., individual negative and positive symptoms) which greatly broaden the boundaries of the spectrum disorder.

Kendler (1985) provides a useful analogy emphasizing the need to elucidate important symptoms of a disorder which may find genetic expression in family members and in turn provide important etiological insights (p. 549):

> Consider that the severely affected relative is an individual who has had a hemorrhagic cerebrovascular accident secondary to hypertension, and now displays severe right-sided weakness and aphasia. What kinds of signs and symptoms would we expect in his affected relatives? Rarely, he might have an affected relative with a similar condition. More frequently, his affected relatives will have hypertension only, which may present with no symptoms, or with symptoms of headache, congestive heart failure, etc. We would not expect his affected relatives to have mild right-sided weakness and mild aphasia. Using the same logic, we would not necessarily expect the deviant relatives of schizophrenic patients to display attenuated forms of all the classic symptoms of schizophrenia, such as hallucinations, delusions, formal thought disorder, and primary process thinking. ... Instead they tend to be socially withdrawn, eccentric, odd, and suspicious... it would suggest that just as the hypertensive relatives of the individual with the hemorrhagic stroke reveal to us the underlying pathology of his disorder, so the characteristic symptoms of the deviant relatives of schizophrenics tell us something important about the fundamental psychopathology underlying schizophrenia.

The purpose of the remaining discussion will be to review available literature relevant to the issue of subthreshold pathology in the family members of schizophrenics. The general hypothesis to be forwarded in the following discussions will assert that so-called negative symptoms may represent the analogue in schizophrenia of Kendler's example of "hypertension in cerebrovascular accidents." That is, negative symptomatology may represent a relevant phenotypic manifestation of the hypothesized schizophrenia genotype. If so, it may prove to be a useful construct for inclusion in segregation studies and consequently help to shed light on the mechanism of genetic transmission in schizophrenia. The review will begin with a brief discussion of the negative/positive symptom distinction and its relevance to schizophrenia. This will be followed by a historical and critical review of the "search" for subthreshold genetic traits in the biological relatives of schizophrenics and its relation to the negative-positive symptom construct.

Negative Versus Positive Symptom Distinctions in Schizophrenia

As previously suggested, the area of positive/negative symptom distinctions in schizophrenia has enjoyed renewed and vigorous interest in recent years. Positive symptoms have come to refer to such specific manifestations as paranoid delusions, auditory hallucinations, and formal thought disorder. Alternatively, negative features encompass those symptoms characterized as flat or blunted affect, apathy, loss of interest and pleasure, alogia, and social withdrawal. The purpose here is not to provide an exhaustive and critical review of the literature relevant to negative/positive symptoms in schizophrenia, as this is found elsewhere (Andreasen 1985; Pogue-Geile and Zubin 1988). However, a brief and somewhat general review will provide a context for understanding the relevance of positive/negative symptom distinctions in the examination of subthreshold pathology in family members to be discussed later.

While neither Kraepelin (1971) nor Bleuler (1950) utilized these specific terms, the salience of "positive" and "negative" symptom clusters appears at least implicit in their theoretical formulations. Interestingly, the negative symptom component seems to assume a central role in both formulations. While Kraepelin adopted an exhaustively polythetic view of dementia praecox, he seemed to recognize such features as emotional blunting to be core manifestations of the disorder. A hallmark of the Kraepelinean view, of course, was the concept of "progressive cognitive deterioration," which focused upon loss of function. This notion seems in spirit to embody the very concept of negative symptom presentation and the defect state as observed in poverty of speech, poverty of content, flat affect, apathy, etc. Bleuler was perhaps even more explicit in defining affective disturbance, autism, ambivalence, and loss of association as fundamental symptoms of schizophrenia, while relegating delusions and hallucinations to accessory symptom status. Much of what would be considered negative symptomatology in schizophrenia falls within at least a portion of Bleuler's concept of fundamental symptomatology, and as he himself notes, "In the outspoken forms of schizophrenia, the emotional deterioration stands in the forefront of the clinical picture" (Bleuler 1950, p 40).

Although references to the distinction of positive and negative symptoms in psychiatry were made by de Clearambault (1942), it was Strauss et al. (1974) who were perhaps the first to make an explicit division of schizophrenic symptoms into positive and negative categories. The evolution of this concept most probably had its origin in the work and writings of the neurologist, Hughlings-Jackson (1889), although it has been suggested that the concepts were predated by J. R. Reynolds (cf. Berrios 1985). The question as to whether positive and negative symptoms represent distinct subtypes of schizophrenia or whether one may be more fundamental to the schizophrenic process than the other has been the object of controversy in recent years. While the early Kraepelinean and Bleulerian formulations appeared to emphasize the importance of negative-based symptomatology, the past few decades have seen this view shift to a primary interest in positive symptoms as the core feature of schizophrenic illness. As suggested by Andreasen (1982), the shift of focus to delusions and hallucinations may have been precipitated by an interest in improving the reliability of psychiatric diagnosis and subsequently an enhanced concordance of diagnostic practices in the USA and Europe. Certainly the advantage of such a focus lies in its attempt to define schizophrenia on the basis of very clear-cut and reliably rated symptoms. In contrast, negative symptomatology requires the operationalizing of such vague and amorphous concepts as "blunted affect" and "avolition".

The work of Schneider (1959) and his development of "first-rank symptoms" exemplifies the positive symptom approach. Schneider's clinically derived terms include such well-known and easily defined symptoms as thought withdrawal and insertion, delusions of control, and auditory hallucinations involving two or more voices. For a time, Schneiderian first-rank symptoms were believed to represent unique and pathognomonic markers of schizophrenia, as witnessed by their incorporation into most of the major diagnostic systems, including the Present State Examination (Wing et al. 1974), the Research Diagnostic Criteria (Spitzer et al. 1978), and the Diagnostic and Statistical Manual (DSM-III; American Psychiatric Association 1980). However, while useful in the description of schizophrenia, empirical validation for the pathognomonic nature of these symptoms has been questioned (Andreasen and Akiskal 1983; Carpenter et al. 1973; Kendell et al. 1979; Koehler 1979; Mellor 1982). Both clinical and research experience have demonstrated that such positive symptoms occur with some frequency in other disorders including depression and bipolar illness and do not appear to be highly successful in predicting outcome.

Combined with the apparent failure of first-rank symptoms to become a dependable diagnostic "litmus test" for schizophrenia, two additional factors appear to have generated a renewed interest in negative symptoms and a renaissance of the original Kraepelinean and Bleulerian formulations. First is the development of rating instruments which produce a reasonably reliable documentation of negative symptomatology. Among these are the Schedule for the Assessment of Negative Symptoms (SANS; Andreasen 1984a), the Negative Symptom Rating Scale (NSRS; Iager et al. 1985), the Positive and Negative Syndrome Scale (PANSS; Kay et al. 1987), the Rating Scale for Emotional Blunting (RSEB; Abrams and Taylor 1978), and a Schedule for Affective Disorders and Schizophrenia (SADS) modification (Lewine et al. 1983). A second major factor would appear to be the much-cited recent work by Crow (1980) and the subsequently proposed delineation of schizophrenia into a type I (positive) and type II (negative) syndrome which is suggested to represent etiologically distinct subtypes. Validating data appear to support the presence of an association of negative symptoms with gross and diffuse structural atrophy of the brain while positive symptoms appear in association with dopaminergic overactivity in subcortical limbic pathways. Further elucidation of the construct (Crow 1980, 1986, 1987; Andreasen 1985; Andreasen and Olsen 1982) suggests that the positive syndrome is most commonly seen in acute, remitting schizophrenia and is characterized by a good response to neuroleptic medication and an absence of intellectual deterioration. In contrast, the negative symptom complex is most often represented in chronic course (defect state) schizophrenia and frequently presents with irreversible outcome and typically poor response to neuroleptics, although not all results have been consistent with this formulation (Breier et al. 1987; Goldberg 1985). Numerous studies have demonstrated an association between negative symptomatology and indices of cortical atrophy, ventricular enlargement, neuropsychological impairment, and intellectual deterioration (Pogue-Geile and Harrow 1985; Keefe et al. 1987; Seidman 1983; Goetz and van Kammen 1986; Kemali 1985; Kay et al. 1986).

It has been suggested that the association between negative symptoms and structural brain damage may indicate a form of schizophrenia which has a lower genetic loading owing to a potentially greater chance of environmental insult (Seidman 1983). However, preliminary data (Dworkin and Lenzenweger 1984; Kay et al. 1985) suggest that negative symptom schizophrenia may not only present clinical and outcome features which differentiate it from positive symptom schizophrenia but may also, in fact, be associated with a more salient genetic component. Dworkin and Lenzenweger (1984) have reported a higher concordance among twins in which the schizophrenic proband demonstrates a clinical picture dominated by negative symptoms, while Kay et al. (1985) presented data supporting a differentially increased incidence of psychosis in the first-degree relatives of schizophrenic probands characterized by a negative symptom complex. Neither finding is conclusive regarding genetic factors, of course, nor do they necessarily rule out other explanations such as environmental insult. Taken together, however, these reports do offer the hypothesis that negative symptomatology may define a meaningful subset of those patients labelled as schizophrenic. Furthermore, they may uniquely classify a more fundamental feature of the disorder that may be of genetic relevance and potentially observable in biological relatives. In the next section we will examine the search for observable symptoms in relatives of schizophrenic patients.

Negative/Positive Symptoms and the Search for Schizotypal Traits in the Biological Relatives of Schizophrenics

Historical Background

The search for subthreshold pathology in the family members of schizophrenics as a strategy for uncovering alternative phenotypes is neither new nor unfamiliar. Beginning even with the early works of Kraepelin and Bleuler, there has long been an interest in and acknowledgement of the "eccentric" personalities noted to exist in some biological relatives. The first detailed account was provided by Kretschmer (1970) who coined the terms "schizothyme" or "schizoid" to describe these individuals. Kretschmer emphasized the importance of poor social relations and limited affective response as features characteristic of the family members of schizophrenics. More specifically, he identified three major descriptors of the schizoid character: (1) unsociable, humorless; (2) timid, shy; (3) indifferent, dull-witted.

Kallmann (1938) identified a somewhat similar pattern which he termed "schizoid psychopath." In addition, he was perhaps one of the first to examine more systematically the frequency of such disorders in the family members of schizophrenics, as he noted that one-third of the offspring of schizophrenics displayed such schizoid disturbances. The emphasis by Kallmann in characterizing the relatives of schizophrenics appeared to center upon defects in emotional functioning, social withdrawal, and eccentric or autistic preoccupations. Prior to the development of DSM-III criteria for schizoid and schizotypal personality disorders, work by investigators examining the abnormal features aggregating in the family members of schizophrenics continued to demonstrate the salience of a "schizoid personality" characterized by social and emotional withdrawal as well as suspiciousness and interpersonal anxiety (Inouye 1970; Stephens et al. 1975). Thus, as one reviews the early familial origins of schizoid or schizotypal traits, it would appear that the negative symptom oriented features of social withdrawal, emotional constriction, and odd or eccentric rapport have most often been reported to characterize the biological relatives of schizophrenics. It is perhaps important to note that this literature has not, historically, supported the salience of subthreshold, psychotic-like, positive symptoms (e.g., thought disorder, magical thinking, illusions, and perceptual aberrations) in the family members of schizophrenics.

Current perspectives regarding familial pathology and the schizophrenia spectrum have centered upon the aggregation of DSM-III personality disorders in biological relatives. Interest has primarily been focused upon the familial prevalence of three disorders: schizotypal, schizoid, and paranoid personality disorders (PD). In simplistic terms, one might view paranoid PD as constituting a syndrome oriented toward positive symptoms (i.e., subthreshold delusional disorder), schizoid PD as constituting primarily negative-oriented symptoms (e.g., social withdrawal), and schizotypal PD as containing elements of both (e.g., magical thinking, constricted affect). It might be argued that the prevalence of these disorders may serve as crude measures of the salience of negative and positive symptoms in biological relatives. The findings are far from clear-cut, however.

Results of familial analyses of schizoid and paranoid PD have been somewhat controversial and contradictory. Baron et al. (1985) have noted an increase in paranoid PD in the relatives of schizophrenic probands (7.3%) versus control probands (2.7%). However, their results have been criticized (Rogers and Winokur 1988) on the grounds that the sample of research diagnostic criteria (RDC)-defined schizophrenic probands may have also included delusional disordered probands, therefore artificially inflating estimates of paranoid PD in relatives. It has been suggested, based on family studies (Kendler et al. 1984; Kendler and Hayes 1981; Winokur 1985), that schizophrenia and delusional disorder "breed true." More to the point, Winokur has demonstrated increased rates of paranoid traits in relatives of delusional disorder patients but not in the relatives of schizophrenics. Furthermore, Kendler et al. (1985) have shown that the rate of DSM-III paranoid PD is not increased in the relatives of schizophrenics but do demonstrate a higher rate in delusional disordered probands as compared with control probands. Currently, then, there does not appear to be strong evidence favoring paranoid PD as a clear member of the schizophrenia spectrum, although closure on this issue may be premature.

Surprisingly, schizoid PD has received relatively little interest and examination despite its apparent similarities to traits cited in the older familial literature as relevant to family member pathology in schizophrenia (e.g., social isolation, affective impoverishment). In part, this may be attributable to a historical shift in which the schizoid personality came to be interpreted in a more generalized and psychodynamic fashion, thereby losing its specific familial context with schizophrenia (Siever and Gunderson 1983). Beyond this, however, Kety et al. (1968, 1975) and the Danish adoption studies are most frequently cited as providing the evidence which potentially refutes a schizoid-schizophrenia genetic link. Given the utilization of a rather general DSM-II definition of schizoid personality disorder, it is difficult to know precisely how such individuals were judged and conceptualized. More importantly, though, Kety et al. (1975) themselves indicated the following in reference to schizoid and inadequate personalities (p. 155):

> Although our earlier studies did not develop evidence that those diagnoses per se significantly differentiated biological relatives of schizophrenics from controls (they were simply part of the spectrum which did), we are not prepared to dismiss the possibility that there is a schizoid or inadequate personality which is genetically related to schizophrenia. . . . In the present study, if we limit the examination to first-degree relatives or if we include only those inadequate or schizoid personalities where at least one rater made a stronger diagnosis, we find a significant concentration in the biological index relatives.

The preliminary findings of a more recent replication in an adoption sample (Kety 1988) indicate results similar to Kety et al.'s earlier report. The recent data, however, of Baron et al. (1985), utilizing DSM-III criteria for schizoid PD, failed to uncover statistically significant differences, although the relatives of schizophrenics did show a higher rate of schizoid PD than control relatives (1.6% versus 0%). Of interest is the fact that Baron and coworkers incorporated a "probable schizotypal PD" category which required patients to have only 2 of the necessary 4 DSM-III criteria for inclusion. Relative to family members of controls, the family members of schizophrenics demonstrated a significantly higher rate of probable schizotypal PD (12.1% versus 6.5%). Since a symptom overlap exists between the DSM-III criteria for schizotypal and schizoid PDs (e.g., affective constriction, social isolation), it is clearly possible that family members who would otherwise have been placed in schizoid PD were instead diagnosed as "probable schizotypal" PD. Finally, Kendler et al. (1984, 1985) have demonstrated an increased prevalence of a combined "schizotypal-schizoid" PD in biological relatives of schizophrenics, but unfortunately their reported results do not allow for a distinction between schizotypal and schizoid traits. Thus, as with paranoid PD, strong evidence has yet to be presented for establishing a link between schizophrenia and schizoid PD. However, closure on the genetic relatedness of schizoid PD and schizophrenia is clearly premature.

By far the most prominent portion of the schizophrenia spectrum has been attributed to schizotypal PD. The investigation of DSM-III schizotypal PD has led to numerous studies which have subsequently documented its increased prevalence in the biological relatives of chronic schizophrenic probands. These results have demonstrated consistency across family studies (Baron et al. 1983, 1985; Kendler et al. 1984), adoption studies (Gunderson et al. 1983; Kendler et al. 1981; Kety 1988), and twin studies (Siever and Gunderson 1979; Torgersen 1985). However, at least one recent study failed to find a higher rate of schizotypal PD among relatives of schizophrenic probands (Coryell and Zimmerman 1989). In general, relatively little controversy is generated by the assertion that the biological relatives of schizophrenics demonstrate subthreshold pathology in the form of schizotypal PD. The incidence of such disorders in schizophrenic families has been estimated at between 4.2% and 14.6% (Baron et al. 1985; Kendler et al. 1981, 1984, 1985). If "probable" schizotypal PD is included, estimates may run as high as 26.8% (Baron et al. 1985).

In summary, then, only schizotypal PD has received strong and consistent support in family studies as a significant non-psychotic spectrum disorder. It currently represents the best candidate for constituting a schizophrenia-related phenotype. As alluded to above, it describes a constellation of both negative and positive symptoms. It is therefore of interest ot examine more critically this concept, with the intent of identifying those specific features which may serve as optimal genetic markers.

Schizotypal Personality Disorder: Familial Versus Clinical Traditions

The following eight criteria constitute the DSM-III category of schizotypal PD:

1. Magical thinking
2. Ideas of reference
3. Social isolation
4. Recurrent illusions
5. Odd speech
6. Inadequate rapport and constricted affect
7. Suspiciousness or paranoid ideation
8. Undue social anxiety or hypersensitivity

It is obvious upon examination that positive symptoms dominate the criteria, with only nos. 3 and 6 clearly representing more negative-based symptomatology. This will become relevant to the discussion of clinical versus familial origins of the disorder. At first glance, however, the criteria certainly appear at odds with the previously reviewed familial literature regarding schizoid and schizotypal traits. As outlined earlier, this tradition has supported the presence of negative-based symptomatology in family members of schizophrenics, while DSM-III schizotypal PD, as seen in the criteria above (and as slightly modified in DSM-III-R), appears to emphasize positive-based symptoms. Several important factors are relevant to this apparent contradiction and require clarification.

The DSM-III concept of schizotypal PD has developed from a complicated history which has perhaps compromised its full utility as a descriptor of schizophrenic proband's relatives (Frances 1985; Gunderson and Siever 1985; Kendler 1985; Kety 1985; Torgerson 1985; Shields et al. 1975; Siever and Gunderson 1983). Of principle concern is its hybrid ancestry which has taken root in two somewhat disparate traditions: the familial and clinical approaches. The familial tradition has emphasized the description of traits observed in the nonpsychotic biological relatives of schizophrenic probands. Again, this literature has suggested negative-like symptoms to be salient markers. Conversely, the clinical tradition has maintained an emphasis upon the identification of patients seeking treatment who are not classically schizophrenic yet demonstrate attenuated forms of symptoms thought to be fundamental to schizophrenia. Genetic or familial association to schizophrenia is not necessarily implicit to this latter approach. Representative of such formulations are, for example, Zilboorg's (1941, 1957) "ambulatory schizophrenics" and Deutsch's (1942) "as-if personalities." Zilboorg's conceptualization, while not including florid psychotic symptoms, did emphasize disordered thinking, deviant sexuality, profound anger, lack of deep interpersonal relations, and preoccupation with fantasy. It therefore appeared to feature more positive-oriented symptomatology than the familial descriptions of schizoid or schizotypal traits.

Perhaps the most influential of the early investigators of the clinical tradition were Hoch and Polatin (1949) and their development of the diagnostic concept of "pseudoneurotic schizophrenia."In outlining its features, such symptoms as primary process thinking, brief psychotic episodes (micropsychosis), distorted self-concept and body image, deviant sexuality, and acting-out behavior were clearly emphasized. In addition, the three characteristics of pananxiety, pansexuality, and panneurosis were also deemed as central manifestations. In none of the cases reported was there a family history of schizophrenia. In many respects, Hoch et al. set the tone for the clinical tradition and in so doing created a description of schizotypal traits which was oriented toward positive symptomatology.

Of some interest within the clinical tradition are the contributions of Rado (1953) and Meehl (1962), both of whom emphasized the importance of genetics in their clinical formulations. Rado (1953) first coined the term schizotypal as shorthand for describing the schizophrenic genotype. In positing a common genetic underpinning to both schizophrenia and schizotypy, Rado outlined two fundamental abnormalities: (1) integrative pleasure deficiency or anhedonia; (2) proprioceptive disorder or a distorted body awareness. In addition, Rado viewed schizotypal patients as particularly prone to cognitive disorganization and thought disorder.

Following closely upon Rado's concepts, Meehl (1962) introduced a further elaboration of the model connecting yet a third entity, schizotaxia, to the concepts of schizophrenia and schizotypy. According to Meehl's formulation, the schizotaxon referred to core molecular features (integrative neural defect) closely tied to the genotype underlying the schizophrenic-like disorder. Contingent upon certain environmental and genetic influences, schizotaxia may manifest as either schizotypy or clinical schizophrenia. The schizotype, according to Meehl, would be apparent in particular members carrying the schizotaxic gene by virtue of subtle psychological deficits. He cited four core traits characteristic of the schizotype: (1) cognitive slippage (mild thought disorder); (2) interpersonal aversiveness; (3) anhedonia; (4) ambivalence. Of these, Meehl appeared to emphasize the importance of cognitive slippage as the most salient schizotypal marker. In general, Rado and Meehl present a picture of schizotypal traits which is consistent in many respects with the clinical tradition. Anhedonic features and interpersonal impairment, however, are characteristics shared with the more negative-oriented symptoms of the familial tradition. Symptoms and traits relevant to both the familial and clinical traditions of schizotypy research are summarized in general form in Table 1.

Interestingly, the rather different perspectives offered by both traditions have all contributed to the current definition of DSM-III schizotypal PD. Schizotypal PD as defined in DSM-III represents quite directly the distillation of work resulting from the Danish Adoption Studies (Kety et al. 1968) and subsequently that of Spitzer et al. (1979). Utilizing symptoms and variables developed in Kety et al.'s adoption studies for the identification of borderline schizophrenia and applying them in operationalized form to a mixed sample composed of biological and adoptive relatives of schizophrenics and controls, Spitzer et al. extracted the eight symptoms (listed previously) which appeared to differentiate most clearly borderline schizophrenics from controls. It is thus of interest to examine the criteria employed by these authors in identifying borderline schizophrenics. Kety et al. (1968) appeared to draw heavily upon the clinical tradition. This appears evident in the explicit reference to pseudoneurotic schizophrenia, ambulatory schizophrenia, and psychotic character (p. 352). The criteria loosely included: (1) strange and atypical mentation and speech; (2) brief episodes of cognitive distortion and micropsychosis; (3) anhedonia; (4) chaotic interpersonal and sexual adjustment (including "as-if" personality); and (5) multiple neurotic manifestations and severe widespread anxiety. The influence of Hoch and Polatin (1949) appears clear. What also seems apparent is the relative absence of negative symptomatology (impoverished affect, social isolation, inadequate rapport, etc.) which has most often been cited in the familial literature. The nature of Spitzer et al.'s approach, which relied heavily upon the Kety et al. adoption studies as its source, may have dictated that their symptom pool would be biased in the direction of positive symptomatology. Kety later asserted (1985), however, that the absence of negative symptomatology in the eight DSM-III criteria for schizotypal personality arose not from a failure to observe them in the original adoption study interviews but from a relative overemphasis on positive symptoms by Spitzer et al. (1979). It is perhaps tempting to speculate that this emphasis parallels in an analogous fashion that which had been placed upon positive symptoms in schizophrenia over the past several decades.

A second issue of concern with regard to Spitzer et al.'s use of the Danish Adoption Study data lies in the re-extraction of symptom items from the identical population onto which they were then validated. That is, utilizing

Table 1. Symptoms and traits relevant to schizophrenia

Putative schizotypal traits	Familial								Clinical					
	Kretschmer (1970)	Kallman (1938)	Inouye (1970)	Stephens et al. (1975)	Gunderson et al. (1983)	Kendler et al. (1983)	Torgersen (1985)	Silverton (1988)	Zilboorg (1941)	Hoch and Polatin (1949)	Rado (1953)	Meehl (1962)	Kety et al. (1968)	Widiger et al. (1986)
Social isolation	×	×		×	×	×	×							
Affective impoverishment (constricted, aloof)	×	×	×	×	×	×								
Odd rapport, distant (indifference, autistic)	×		×	×	×				×		×	×	×	
Hypersensitivity (fear of social rejection)	×		×											
Suspiciousness			×	×	×	×	×							×
Widespread anxiety	×			×	×						×		×	
Somatic complaints					×								×	
Anger irritability	×	×							×		×			
Anhedonia											×	×	×	
Antisocial traits (criminality)	×							×		×				
Odd speech (thought disorder)				×		×			×	×	×	×	×	
Deviant sexuality									×	×			×	
Micropsychosis (recurrent illusions)										×			×	×
Perceptual aberration (depersonalization)										×	×		×	
Magical thinking (preoccupation with fantasy)									×	×			×	×
Ambivalence												×		
Ideas of reference														×

original items and interview observations from Kety et al.'s data, Spitzer and colleagues operationalized and reapplied them to the same cases to achieve what appeared to be an impressive 86% sensitivity and 95% specificity. Unfortunately, such a methodological strategy, which may capitalize upon sample-specific factors, is not unique to Spitzer et al.'s study. One can question the interpretation of a number of studies which have attempted to apply the DSM-III criteria for schizotypal PD to the Danish adoption studies from which the criteria were developed (Kendler et al. 1981; Khouri et al. 1980). It is perhaps not surprising, then, that such studies have "validated" the schizotypal PD criteria as outlined in DSM-III. To their credit, Spitzer et al. (1979) did attempt to cross-validate the eight criteria on an additional data set [although subjects in this second data set were also diagnosed by Kety et al. (1968) with presumably similar criteria]. They found that the sensitivity of the criteria dropped to 63% and attributed this to a lowering of the threshold by Kety et al. in making borderline diagnoses in the second data set. However, such a phenomenon is well-known in cross-validation methodology. It would appear that an equally likely explanation for the drop in sensitivity is attributable to the inflated estimate of the original validation which capitalized on sample-specific variance.

Finally, and perhaps most importantly, Spitzer et al. did not specifically identify biological relatives of schizophrenics in establishing their criteria for schizotypal PD. Although 61% of those identified were indeed biological relatives of schizophrenic adoptees, the remaining individuals included both adoptive relatives and biological relatives of control adoptees. Therefore, it is not clear that the eight criteria established provide the optimal discrimination of subthreshold pathology in the biological relatives of schizophrenic probands.

Certainly, the methodological issues outlined above may provide, in part, an explanation for the discrepant relationship between DSM-III schizotypal PD and the familial tradition discussed earlier. In addition, it leads to the speculation that DSM-III schizotypal PD, despite its clear association with schizophrenia, may not optimally define the genetic schizotype. Based upon the competing clinical and familial perspectives, two types of schizotypal PD clinical pictures have been delineated: a so-called positive symptom or cognitive-perceptual one (e.g., magical thinking, recurrent illusions) and a negative symptom or social-interpersonal one (e.g., social isolation, constricted affect). As predicted by the clinical tradition literature, the positive-symptom picture has demonstrated greater diagnostic efficiency and outcome prediction in the assessment of clinical populations of schizotypal PD patients seeking treatment (Widiger et al. 1986, 1987; McGlashan 1987). Genetic associations with schizophrenia are not necessarily hypothesized to exist in this population, however. That is, these patients tend not to be the relatives of schizophrenic probands. Of interest, then, for the current discussion are the biological relatives of schizophrenic patients and whether a subset of schizotypal symptoms (e.g., negative-oriented, social-interpersonal features) may serve as an improved genetic marker.

The Search for Optimal Schizotypal Markers

To date, few studies have attempted to examine differences in the clinical and familial descriptions of schizotypy and explore what specific features may more optimally discriminate biological relatives of schizophrenic probands. There are a small number of investigations, however, which do shed light on this important question. Gunderson et al. (1983) re-examined interviews from the Danish adoption studies and, broadening the symptom base, attempted to identify particular symptoms which provided a better discrimination specifically of the relatives of schizophrenic patients. The authors found that symptoms relating to social isolation, deficient interpersonal relations, and impoverished affective experience were the best. Additionally, they discovered that positive-oriented, psychotic-like symptoms such as recurrent illusions and magical thinking were more common in individuals diagnosed with borderline PD. Hence, they strongly argued for a revision of the schizotypal PD category and proposed the following criteria (p. 21):

1. Social isolation
2. Suspicious, superficial, distant interpersonal relations
3. Odd, eccentric, "off-putting" appearance and behavior
4. Frequent somatic problems
5. Detached, constricted, flattened affect
6. Serious social dysfunction at school and work

It seems clear that the above criteria reflect a much more negative-oriented symptomatology and appear consistent with the descriptions posited by the earlier familial tradition.

A second attempt to examine specific discriminating features was undertaken by Kendler et al. (1983). Utilizing a different patient and family population (Iowa 500 study) from that of the Danish adoption studies, they divided the eight schizotypal PD criteria into negative and positive symptoms (negative = social isolation, odd speech, constricted affect, suspiciousness, and possibly social anxiety; positive = magical thinking, ideas of reference, and recurrent illusions). The authors reported four criteria, all negative, which occurred more frequently in the family members of schizophrenic probands: social isolation, constricted affect, suspiciousness, and odd speech. Again, these results appear consistent with the familial descriptions of subthreshold pathology and suggest that a subset of the current criteria for schizotypal PD may more optimally characterize these relatives.

Finally, Torgersen's (1984) recent twin study which looked at MZ and DZ twin pairs of DSM-III schizotypal PD probands found that social dysfunctional, schizoid, and milder paranoid features were observed significantly in the co-twins of schizotypal subjects. Co-twins did not display the more dramatic features of the schizotypal PD syndrome, such as mild hallucinations, perceptual distortions, depersonalization, derealization, and catastrophic anxiety. This result is in accordance with the familial tradition.

In summary, the literature to date appears to support most clearly the existence of negative symptomatology as being characteristic of the biological relatives of schizophrenic patients. It is of interest to note that such features may manifest in early childhood. Kendler et al. (1982), in an independent analysis of the Danish Adoption Study, reported that the childhood features of social withdrawal/isolation differentiate the biological relatives of schizophrenic and control adoptees. This negative-symptom-based, social-interpersonal realm may therefore best define the schizotypal traits potentially serving as a more sensitive phenotype for genetic analysis.

Preliminary Findings from the Brockton-Harvard Project

In order to examine further the relevance of negative and positive symptoms in the description of biological relatives of schizophrenics, a preliminary series of analyses were performed utilizing a subsample of family members from the authors' ongoing, large-scale Brockton-Harvard Project at the Brockton-West Roxbury VA Medical Center. First-degree relatives of schizophrenic and control probands were directly interviewed and assessed utilizing Andreasen's (1984 b) Scale for the Assessment of Positive Symptoms (SAPS) and SANS. The findings to be reported enlarge upon data previously given in the literature by adopting a prospective measurement of positive and negative symptoms observed in direct, blind interviews of relatives. Earlier studies have most often incorporated retrospective, "second-hand" data not designed to assess directly and systematically the traits in question.

Psychiatric probands were found via consecutive admissions to the inpatient and outpatient services of the Brockton VA Medical Center and interviewed utilizing Endicott and Spitzer's (1978) SADS. DSM-III-R diagnoses were assigned by a consensus panel of two psychiatrists and two psychologists, according to all information obtained from the standardized SADS interview, structured symptom data from treating clinicians, and a review of the patient's medical record. For the current study, probands were selected to represent two individual diagnostic categories: schizophrenia and mixed depressive disorder. The latter group was selected to serve as a control group and included patients who met DSM-III-R criteria for major depression or depressive disorder Not Otherwise Specified (NOS).

Several considerations led to selection of a depressive disorder control group. First, this is a class of disorders which is believed to be genetically distinct from schizophrenia. Family studies have demonstrated an apparent genetic distinction between schizophrenia and unipolar affective disorder, as observed in morbid risks for each disorder in first-degree relatives (Kendler 1985; Crow 1986). Secondly, a depressive control group offers a relevant comparison specific to negative symptoms. Much controversy has been generated regarding the presence of negative-like symptoms in depression and whether such symptoms are therefore not unique to schizophrenia (Berenbaum et al. 1987; Carpenter et al. 1985; Gibbons et al. 1985; Mayer et al. 1985). Thus, the question of the genetic specificity of negative symptoms per se can also be examined. Thirdly, the depressive group provides a better control than a simple normal group over non-specific psychiatric factors. While a normal control group may enhance the likelihood of finding differences, the use of the former increases the likelihood of uncovering genetically relevant factors and identifying differences specific to schizophrenia. Since relatives of depressive patients also cope socially, culturally, and psychologically with a psychiatrically ill proband, some degree of nongenetic factors are thereby controlled for.

A total of 58 DSM-III-R schizophrenic probands and 31 depressed control probands (21 major depression, 10 depressive disorder NOS) were included in the final sample, and an attempt was made to contact all possible first-degree relatives. Some 459 living relatives of the schizophrenic patient sample were ascertained, and it was subsequently possible to locate 70% ($n = 321$). Of this available group of family members, 135 (42%) consented to the face-to-face interview required in order to make ratings on Andreasen's SANS/SAPS instruments. A total of 164 living first-degree relatives of depressed control probands were ascertained, and 85% ($n = 139$) were located. Of the available control families, 75 relatives (54%) consented to a direct interview and were rated for the presence of negative and positive symptoms on the SANS/SAPS. Thus, a final total of 210 first-degree relatives was available for analysis.

Andreasen's SANS/SAPS instrument is intended to provide an assessment of symptomatology in the following broad domains:

Negative symptoms
1. Affective blunting or flattening
2. Alogia
3. Avolition-apathy
4. Anhedonia-asociality
5. Attention deficit.

Positive symptoms
1. Positive formal thought disorder
2. Hallucinations
3. Delusions
4. Bizarre behavior.

In order to enhance the variability of individual measures, sum scores across all individual items in each of the nine domains above were utilized as the dependent measures of interest. Table 2 lists all individual items of each of the four SAPS subscales, while Table 3 lists all items included in each of the five SANS subscales. Thus, a total of nine independent subscale scores were obtained. In each case, individual items were rated on a 0–5 point scale (absent to severe) in which a higher score value constitutes a greater pathological deficit. A total SANS score is obtained by summing all five negative symptom subscales, and a total SAPS score is obtained by summing the four positive symptom subscales. In this sample of family members, total SAPS scores ranged from 0–35, while total SANS scores had a range of 0–36.

Figures 2 and 3 graphically display the comparison of percentages of first-degree relatives in schizophrenic versus depressed pedigrees achieving total SAPS (Fig. 2) and total SANS (Fig. 3) scores above variously defined bondary scores. (Note: for simplification, the graphs extend only to a cut-off score of 12, since both groups continue to "flatten" considerably after this point and no longer provide useful information regarding differences.) As seen in Fig. 2,

Table 2. Individual Scales for the Assessment of Positive Symptoms (SAPS)

Hallucinations:	1. Auditory hallucinations	
	2. Voices commenting	
	3. Voices conversing	
	4. Somatic/tactile	
	5. Olfactory	
	6. Visual	
Delusions:	1. Persecutory	7. Reference
	2. Jealousy	8. Being controlled
	3. Guilt or sin	9. Mind reading
	4. Grandiose	10. Thought broadcast
	5. Religious	11. Thought insertion
	6. Somatic	12. Thought withdrawal
Bizarre behavior:	1. Clothing and appearance	
	2. Social and sexual behavior	
	3. Aggressive and agitated behavior	
	4. Repetitive or stereotyped behavior	
Thought disorder:	1. Derailment	5. Circumstantiality
	2. Tangentiality	6. Pressure of speech
	3. Incoherence	7. Distractible speech
	4. Illogicality	8. Clanging

All items rated on 0–5 point scale (absent → severe).

Table 3. Individual Scales for the Assessment of Negative Symptoms (SANS)

Affective flattening:	1. Unchanging facial expression
	2. Decreased spontaneous movements
	3. Paucity of expressive gestures
	4. Poor eye contact
	5. Affective nonresponsivity
	6. Lack of vocal inflections
Alogia:	1. Poverty of speech
	2. Poverty of content of speech
	3. Blocking
	4. Increased latency of response
Avolition-apathy:	1. Grooming and hygiene
	2. Impersistence at work or school
	3. Physical anergia
Anhedonia-asociality:	1. Recreational interests and activities
	2. Ability to feel intimacy and closeness
	3. Relationships with friends and peers
Attention:	1. Social inattentiveness
	2. Inattentiveness during mental status testing

All items rated on 0–5 point scale (absent → severe).

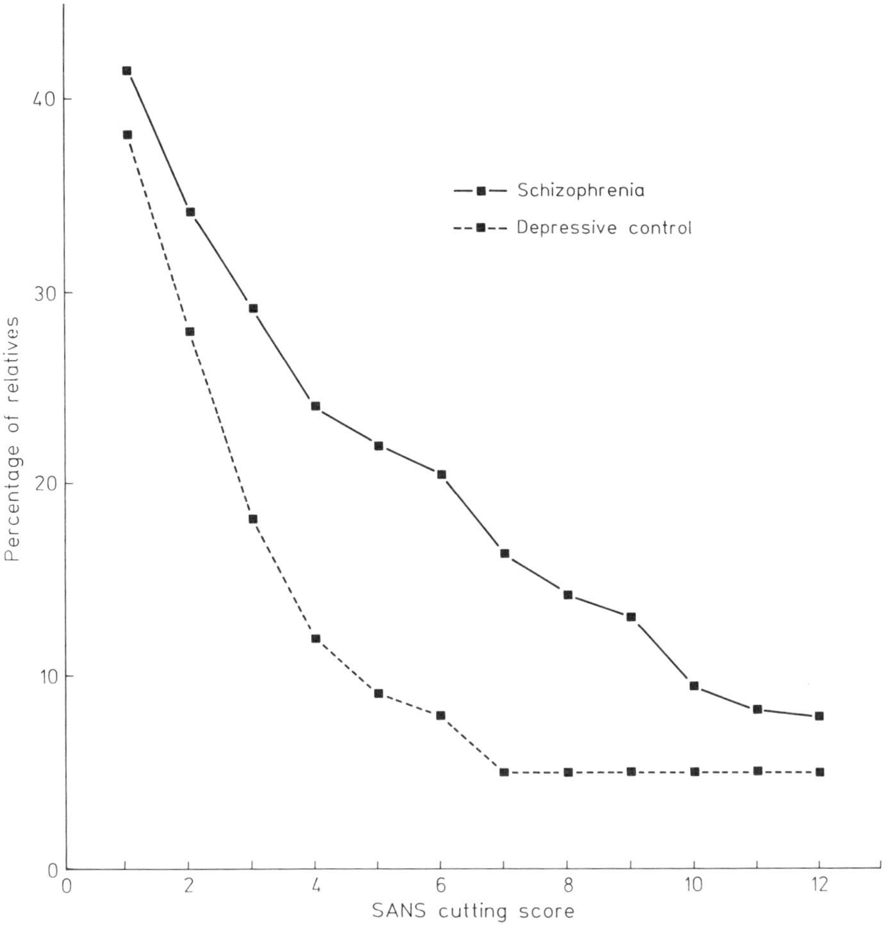

Fig. 2. Positive symptoms in first-degree relatives: Total scale for the assessment of positive symptoms (SAPS) score

family members of schizophrenics and depressed controls do not appear to differ significantly at any of the specified cut-off levels. Alternatively, in Fig. 3 it appears evident that relatives of schizophrenics do show a clearer pattern of greater overall negative symptomatology at most cut-off levels. Discrimination between groups appears to maximize at a cut-off score of 6, at which point over 20 % of relatives of schizophrenic probands are "affected" compared with only 8 % of the relatives of depressed controls. At this boundary, the total SANS score significantly discriminates the two groups of family members ($\chi^2[1] = 5.57$, $P = 0.018$). The greatest apparent level of discrimination of groups in total SAPS scores occurs at a cut-off score of 2, which is not statistically significant ($\chi^2[1] = 2.35$, $P = 0.125$).

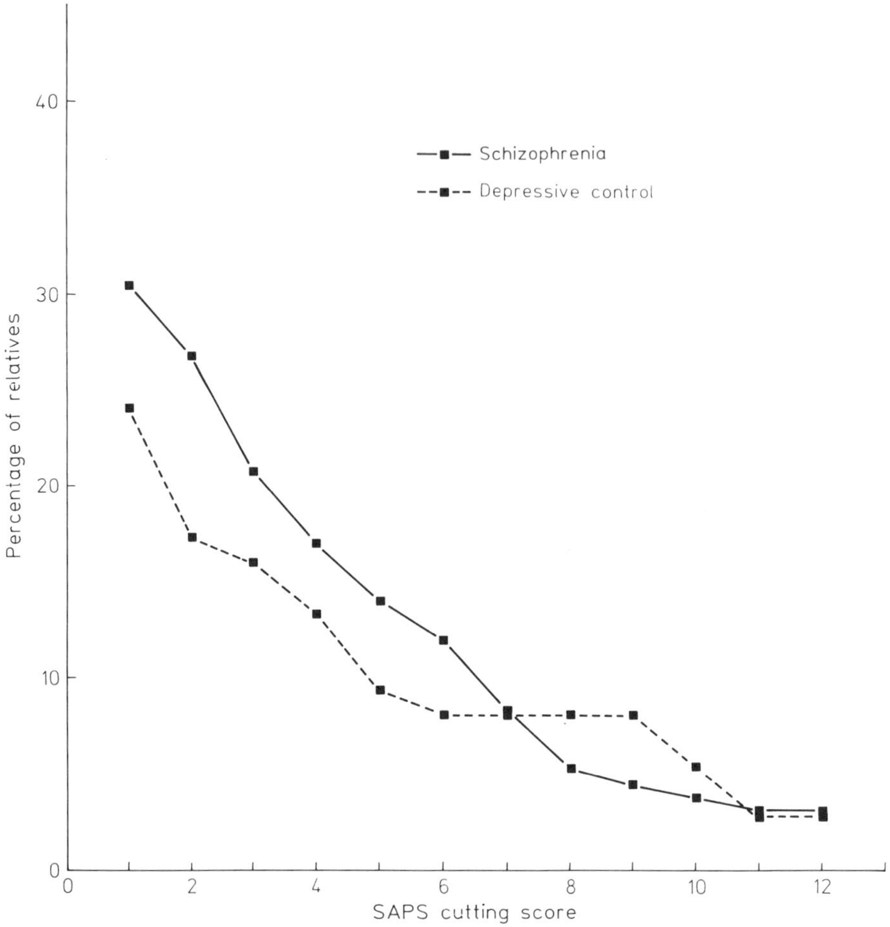

Fig. 3. Negative symptoms in first-degree relatives: total scale for the assessment of negative symptoms (SANS) score

In order to examine differences between pedigree groups more systematically and make better use of the continuous nature of individual SANS and SAPS subscale scores, a logistic regression analysis was performed to determine whether either negative or positive symptom clusters could successfully discriminate the biological relatives of schizophrenic probands from those of depressed controls. Given the highly skewed and nonnormal distribution of SANS/SAPS scores, as well as the categorical nature of their scaling, this particular analysis was employed as an appropriate nonparametric alternative to linear discriminant analysis (Press and Wilson 1978; Aldrich and Nelson 1985; Fleiss et al. 1986). The model underlying logistic regression is similar to traditional discriminant analysis except that it is a logarithmic transformation of the probability of membership in one group versus another (e.g., relative of

Table 4. Results of logistic regression analysis modeling SAPS subscales to the discrimination of schizophrenic and depressed pedigrees

Source	Estimate	Standard error	df	χ^2	Probability
Intercept	0.3960	0.1558	1	6.46	0.0110
Thought disorder	0.0663	0.0647	1	1.05	0.3059
Hallucination	−0.1735	0.1507	1	1.33	0.2494
Delusion	0.2754	0.2942	1	0.88	0.3492
Bizarre	−0.6255	0.8917	1	0.49	0.4830
Overall model likelihood ratio			23	38.8	0.0249

SAPS, Scale for the Assessment of Positive Symptoms.

schizophrenic proband versus depressed control), which is assumed to vary linearly with the set of predictors (e.g., negative and positive symptoms). Therefore, it has less restrictive assumptions regarding measurement scaling and multivariate normality.

Logistic regression was performed in the current study utilizing the CATMOD procedure of SAS (1987) which applies the statistical method of maximum likelihood estimation. Two sets of statistics will be reported. First, an overall likelihood ratio goodness-of-fit test assesses how well the specified model with all included variables fits the sample data. It is important to note, in this regard, that a significant test statistic (e.g., $P < 0.10$) demonstrates a poor fit between model and data. That is, the optimal model constructed by maximum likelihood logistic regression to discriminate schizophrenic and depressed control pedigrees on the basis of symptom scores departs significantly from the data (and therefore fails to discriminate the groups). However, a nonsignificant test statistic indicates that the specified model provides a good fit to the data and therefore successfully discriminates the two groups of family members. The second set of statistics reported are χ^2 values which provide a test for the independent significance of each of the individual discriminating variables (e.g., individual SANS and SAPS subscales) in the model. That is, are any of the subscales (flat affect, alogia, etc.) significant predictors of pedigree membership beyond their joint ability to predict membership within the overall model? In this case, a significant test statistic (in direct contrast to the interpretation of a significant test in the overall model likelihood ratio described above) indicates that the individual subscale does contribute independently to the discrimination of the two family groups.

Results of the logistic regression of positive symptoms (SAPS subscales) in the two groups are summarized in Table 4. As can be seen, the maximum likelihood analysis of variance table reveals that none of the four positive symptom measures make significant individual contributions to the overall model. More importantly, the overall goodness-of-fit statistic is significant ($P = 0.02$), which indicates that positive symptoms as measured by the overall SAPS score fail to model a discrimination between the two groups of family members.

Table 5. Results of logistic regression analysis modeling SANS subscales to the discrimination of schizophrenic and depressed pedigrees

Source	Estimate	Standard error	df	χ^2	Probability
Intercept	0.4948	0.1630	1	9.22	0.0024
Flat affect	0.1743	0.1014	1	2.95	0.0858
Alogia	−0.2113	0.1705	1	1.54	0.2152
Avolition	0.9439	0.5514	1	2.93	0.0869
Asocial	−0.1248	0.1230	1	1.03	0.3105
Attention	0.6639	0.4454	1	2.22	0.1361
Overall model likelihood ratio			51	49.26	0.5429

SANS, Scale for the Assessment of Negative Symptoms.

A similar logistic regression summary is provided for negative symptoms (SANS subscales) in Table 5. As noted, both flat affect and apathy-avolition approach significance ($P < 0.09$) in their individual contributions to the negative symptom model. Of particular note, however, is the highly nonsignificant goodness-of-fit test for the overall model ($P = 0.54$), which indicates a good fit to the data. Thus, in this preliminary set of analyses, negative symptom scores appear to model successfully a discrimination between the relatives of schizophrenic probands and depressed controls.

While preliminary in nature, these findings, which utilize a prospective measurement of positive and negative symptoms, are in accordance with the previously reviewed literature. That is, negative symptomatology appears to serve as a more powerful descriptor of the relatives of schizophrenic probands than positive symptomatology. In particular, affective flattening and apathy/avolition appear to be relevant dimensions in this description. These results are intended to highlight only a precursory examination of positive/negative symptom distinctions in biological relatives in the current Brockton-Harvard sample. In so doing, they lend strong support to the earlier theories but are not conclusive. It should be noted, for example, that Andreasen's SAPS instrument is designed for the assessment of more classic positive symptoms (e.g., full-blown delusions and hallucinations) and may therefore fail to capture adequately the more subtle positive pathology of schizotypy (e.g., magical thinking, illusory experiences). In this regard, other structured instruments or psychometric rating scales, such as Kendler et al.'s (1990) Structured Interview for Schizotypy or Eckblad and Chapman's (1983) Magical Ideation Scale may provide more sensitive indices of positive symptomatology.

Despite these caveats, such findings offer continued promise regarding the utility of negative symptomatology in the future demarcation of relevant spectrum phenotypes. The Brockton-Harvard Project will continue to assess the usefulness of these and other measures of the positive/negative symptom contrast in larger samples of family members as well as to examine their relationship to other factors such as age, gender, and the presence of axis I pathology in the relatives themselves. As findings emerge, it may be possible to build more complex multivariate models of symptom pathology in the biological relatives of schizophrenic probands. As these models are elucidated, they offer great hope in providing more sensitive spectrum phenotypes which can enhance the utility of sophisticated segregation and linkage analysis technologies. Given current indications, negative symptom features are likely to play a prominent role in this effort and ultimately in the advancement of our genetic understanding of schizophrenia.

References

Abrams R, Taylor MA (1978) A rating scale for emotional blunting. Am J Psychiatry 135:226–229

Aldrich JH, Nelson FD (1985) Linear probability, logit, and probit models. Sage, Beverly Hills

American Psychiatric Association (1980) DSM-III: Diagnostic and statistical manual of mental disorders, 3rd edn. APA, Washington

Andreasen NC (1982) Negative symptoms in schizophrenia. Arch Gen Psychiatry 39:784–788

Andreasen NC (1984a) Scale for the assessment of negative symptoms (SANS). University of Iowa, Iowa City

Andreasen NC (1984b) Scale for the assessment of positive symptoms (SAPS). University of Iowa, Iowa City

Andreasen NC (1985) Positive vs. negative schizophrenia: a critical review. Schizophr Bull 11:380–389

Andreasen NC, Akiskal HS (1983) The specificity of Bleulerian and Schneiderian symptoms: A critical reevaluation. Psychiatr Clin North Am 6:41–54

Andreasen NC, Olsen S (1982) Negative vs. positive schizophrenia. Arch Gen Psychiatry 39:789–794

Baron M, Gruen R, Asnis L, Kane J (1983) Familial relatedness of schizophrenia and schizotypal states. Am J Psychiatry 140:1437–1442

Baron M, Gruen R, Rainer JD, Kane J, Asnis L, Lord S (1985) A family study of schizophrenic and normal control probands: implications for the spectrum concept of schizophrenia. Am J Psychiatry 145:447–455

Bassett AS, Jones BD, McGillivray BC, Pantzar JT (1988) Partial trisomy of chromosome 5 cosegregating with schizophrenia. Lancet 1:799–800

Berenbaum SA, Abrams R, Rosenberg S, Taylor MA (1987) The nature of emotional blunting: a factor analytic study. Psychiatry Res 20:57–67

Berrios GE (1985) Positive and negative symptoms and Jackson: A conceptual history. Arch Gen Psychiatry 42:95–97

Bleuler E (1950) Dementia praecox or the group of schizophrenias. International Universities Press, New York (Original 1911)

Breier A, Wolkowitz OM, Doran AR, Roy A, Boronow J, Hammer DW, Pickar D (1987) Neuroleptic responsivity of negative and positive symptoms in schizophrenia. Am J Psychiatry 144:1549–1555

Carpenter WT, Strauss JS, Muleh S (1973) Are there pathognomonic symptoms in schizophrenia? Arch Gen Psychiatry 28:847–852

Carpenter WT, Heinrichs DW, Alphs LD (1985) Treatment of negative symptoms. Schizophr Bull 11:440–452

Carter CL, Chung CS (1980) Segregation analysis of schizophrenia under a mixed genetic model. Hum Hered 30:350

Coryell WH, Zimmerman M (1989) Personality disorder in families of depressed, schizophrenic, and never-ill probands. Am J Psychiatry 146:496–502

Crow TJ (1980) Molecular pathology of schizophrenia: more than one disease process? Br Med J 12:66–67
Crow TJ (1986) The continuum of psychosis and its implication for the structure of the gene. Br J Psychiatry 149:419–429
Crow TJ (1987) Two syndromes of schizophrenia as one pole of the continuum of psychosis: A concept of the nature of the pathogen and its genomic locus. In: Henn, DeLisi (eds) Neurochemistry and neuropharmacology of schizophrenia. Elsevier, Amsterdam (Handbook of schizophrenia, vol 2)
Debray Q, Caillard V, Stewart J (1978) Schizophrenia: a study of genetic models and some of their implications. Neuropsychobiology 4:217
De Clerambault G (1942) Oeuvre psychiatrique. Presses Universitaires de France, Paris
Deutsch H (1942) Some forms of emotional disturbance and their relationship to schizophrenia. Psychoanal Q 11:301–321
Dworkin RH, Lenzenweger MF (1984) Symptoms and the genetics of schizophrenia: Implications for diagnosis. Am J Psychiatry 141:1541–1546
Eckblad M, Chapman LJ (1983) Magical ideation as an indicator of schizotypy. J Consult Clin Psychol 51:215–225
Elston RC, Namboodiri KK, Spence MA, Rainer JD (1978) A genetic study of schizophrenia pedigrees: One-locus hypotheses. Neuropsychobiology 4:193
Endicott J, Spitzer RL (1978) A diagnostic interview: The schedule for affective disorders and schizoghrenia. Arch Gen Psychiatry 35:837–844
Faraone SV, Tsuang MT (1985) Quantitative models of the genetic transmission of schizophrenia. Psychol Bull 98:41–66
Faraone SV, Tsuang MT (1988) Familial links between schizophrenia and other disorders: Application of the multifactorial polygenic model. Psychiatry: Interpersonal and biological processes 51:37–47
Fleiss JL, Williams JB, Dubro AF (1986) The logistic regression analysis of psychiatric data. J Psychiatr Res 20:195–209
Frances A (1985) Validating schizotypal personality disorders: Problems with the schizophrenia connection. Schizophr Bull 11:595–597
Gibbons RD, Lewine RJ, Davis JM, Schooler NR, Cole JO (1985) An empirical test of a Kraepelinian vs. a Bleulerian view of negative symptoms. Schizophr Bull 11:390–396
Goetz KL, van Kammen DP (1986) Computerized axial tomography scans and subtypes of schizophrenia: A review of the literature. J Nerv Ment Dis 174:31–41
Goldberg SC (1985) Negative and deficit symptoms in schizophrenia respond to neuroleptics. Schizophr Bull 11:453–456
Gottesman II, Shields J (1982) Schizophrenia: the epigenetic puzzle. Cambridge University Press, New York
Gunderson JG, Siever LJ (1985) Relatedness of schizotypal to schizophrenic disorders. Schizophr Bull 11:532–537
Gunderson JG, Siever LJ, Spaulding E (1983) The search for a schizotype: Crossing the border again. Arch Gen Psychiatry 40:15–22
Heston LL (1966) Psychiatric disorders in foster home reared children of schizophrenic mothers. Br J Psychiatry 112:819–825
Hoch PH, Polatin P (1949) Pseudoneurotic forms of schizophrenia. Psychiatr Q 23:248–276
Hughlings-Jackson J (1889) On postepileptic states: a contribution to the comparative study of insanities. J Ment Sci 34:490–500
Iager A, Kirch DG, Wyatt RJ (1985) A negative symptom rating scale. Psychiatry Res 16:27–36
Inouye E (1970) Personality deviation seen in monozygotic co-twins of the index cases with classical schizophrenia. Acta Psychiatr Scand [Suppl] 219:90–96
Kallmann FJ (1938) The genetics of schizophrenia. Augustin, New York
Kay SR, Opler LA, Fiszbein A (1985) Genetics of schizophrenia and the positive-negative dimension. Am J Psychiatry 142:994–995
Kay SR, Opler LA, Fiszbein A (1986) Significance of positive and negative syndromes in chronic schizophrenia. Br J Psychiatry 149:439–448

Kay SR, Fiszbein A, Opler LA (1987) The positive and negative syndrome scale (PANSS) for schizophrenia. Schizophr Bull 13:261–276

Keefe RSE, Mohs RC, Losonczy MF, Davidson M, Silverman JM, Kendler KS, Horvath TB, Nora R, Davis KL (1987) Characteristics of very poor outcome schizophrenia. Am J Psychiatry 144:889–895

Kemali D (1985) Clinical and neuropsychological correlates of cerebral ventricular enlargement in schizophrenia. J Psychiatr Res 19:587–596

Kendell RE, Brockington IF, Leff JP (1979) Prognostic implications of six alternative definitions of schizophrenia. Arch Gen Psychiatry 36:25–31

Kendler KS (1985) Diagnostic approaches to schizotypal personality disorder: a historical perspective. Schizophr Bull 11:538–553

Kendler KS (1988) The genetics of schizophrenia: An overview. In: Tsuang MT, Simpson JC (eds) Nosology, epidemiology and genetics of schizophrenia. Elsevier, New York (Handbook of schizophrenia, vol 3)

Kendler KS, Hayes P (1981) Paranoid psychosis (delusional disorder) and schizophrenia. Arch Gen Psychiatry 38:547

Kendler KS, Gruenberg AM, Strauss JS (1981) An independent analysis of the Copenhagen sample of the Danish adoption study of schizophrenia. II. the relationship between schizotypal personality disorder and schizophrenia. Arch Gen Psychiatry 38:982–984

Kendler KS, Gruenberg AM, Strauss JS (1982) An independent analysis of the Copenhagen sample of the Danish adoption study of schizophrenia. V. The relationship between childhood social withdrawal and adult schizophrenia. Arch Gen Psychiatry 39:1257–1261

Kendler KS, Gruenberg AM, Tsuang MT (1983) The specificity of DSM-III schizotypal symptoms. Abstracts of the 135th Annual Meeting of the American Psychiatric Association. APA, Washington

Kendler KS, Masterson CC, Ungaro R, Davis KL (1984) A family history study of schizophrenia-related personality disorders. Am J Psychiatry 141:424–427

Kendler KS, Masterson CC, Davis KL (1985) Psychiatric illness in first-degree relatives of patients with paranoid psychosis, schizophrenia, and medical illness. Br J Psychiatry 147:524

Kendler KS, Lieberman JA, Walsh D (1989) The structured interview for schizotypy (SIS): A preliminary report. Schizophr Bull 15:559–591

Kennedy JL, Giuffra LA, Moises HW, Cavalli-Sforza LL, Pakstis AJ, Kidd JR, Castiglione CM, Sjorgren B, Wetterberg L, Kidd KK (1988) Evidence against linkage of schizophrenia to markers on chromosome 5 in a northern Swedish pedigree. Nature 336:167–170

Kety SS (1985) Schizotypal personality disorder: An operational definition of Bleuler's latent schizophrenia? Schizophr Bull 11:590–594

Kety SS (1988) Schizophrenic illness in the families of schizophrenic adoptees: findings from the Danish national sample. Schizophr Bull 14:217–222

Kety SS, Rosenthal D, Wender PH, Schulsinger F (1968) The types and prevalence of mental illness in the biological and adoptive families of adopted schizophrenics. In: Rosenthal D, Kety S (eds) The transmission of schizophrenia. Pergamon, New York

Kety SS, Rosenthal D, Wender PH, Schulsinger F, Jacobsen B (1975) Mental illness in the biological and adoptive families of adopted individuals who have become schizophrenic: A preliminary report based on psychiatric interviews. In: Fieve R, Rosenthal D, Brill H (eds) Genetic research in psychiatry. Johns Hopkins University Press, Baltimore

Khouri PJ, Haier RJ, Rieder RO, Rosenthal D (1980) A symptom schedule for the diagnosis of borderline schizophrenia: a first report. Br J Psychiatry 137:140–147

Koehler K (1979) First rank symptoms of schizophrenia: Questions concerning clinical boundaries. Br J Psychiatry 134:236–248

Kraepelin E (1971) Dementia praecox and paraphrenia. Krieger, New York (Original 1919)

Kretschmer E (1970) Physique and character: an investigation of the nature of constitution and of the theory of temperament. Cooper Square, New York (Original 1921)

Lewine RJ, Fogg L, Meltzer HY (1983) Assessment of negative and positive symptoms in schizophrenia. Schizophr Bull 9:368–376
Matthysse S, Holzman PS, Lange K (1986) The genetic transmission of schizophrenia: Application of Mendelian latent structure analysis to eye tracking dysfunctions in schizophrenia and affective disorder. J Psychiatr Res 20:57–65
Mayer M, Alpert M, Stastny P, Perlick D, Empfield M (1985) Multiple contributions to clinical presentation of flat affect in schizophrenia. Schizophr Bull 11:420–426
McGlashan TH (1987) Testing DSM-III symptom criteria for schizotypal and borderline personality disorders. Arch Gen Psychiatry 44:143–148
McGue M, Gottesman I, Rao DC (1983) The transmission of schizophrenia under a multifactorial threshold model. Am J Hum Genet 35:1161–1178
Meehl P (1962) Schizotaxia, schizotypy, schizophrenia. Am Psychol 17:827–838
Mellor CS (1982) The present status of first-rank symptoms. Br J Psychiatry 140:423–424
Pogue-Geile MF, Harrow M (1985) Negative symptoms in schizophrenia: Their longitudinal course and prognostic importance. Schizophr Bull 11:427–439
Pogue-Geile MF, Zubin J (1988) Negative symptomatology and schizophrenia: a conceptual and empirical review. Int J Ment Health 16:3–45
Press SJ, Wilson S (1978) Choosing between logistic regression and discriminant analysis. J Am Stat Assoc 73:699–705
Rado S (1953) Dynamics and classification of disordered behavior. Am J Psychiatry 110:406–416
Risch N, Baron M (1984) Segregation analysis of schizophrenia and related disorders. Am J Hum Gen 36:1039–1059
Rogers KL, Winokur G (1988) The genetics of schizoaffective disorder and the schizophrenia spectrum. In: Tsuang MT, Simpson JC (eds) Nosology epidemiology and genetics. Elsevier, New York (Handbook of schizophrenia, vol 3)
Rosenthal D, Wender PH, Kety SS, Schulsinger F, Welner J, Ostergaard L (1968) Schizophrenics' offspring reared in adoptive homes. In: Rosenthal D, Kety SS (eds) The transmission of schizophrenia. Pergamon, Oxford
Rosenthal D, Wender PH, Kety SS, Schulsinger F, Welner J, Rieder R (1975) Parent-child relationships and psychopathological disorder in the child. Arch Gen Psychiatry 32:466–476
SAS (1987) SAS/STAT Guide for personal computers, version 6 edition. SAS, Cary
Schneider K (1959) Clinical psychopathology. Grune and Stratton, New York
Seidman L (1983) Schizophrenia and brain dysfunction: an integration of recent neurodiagnostic findings. Psychol Bull 94:195–238
Sherrington R, Brynjolfsson J, Petrusson H, Potter M, Dudleston K, Barraclough B, Wasmuth J, Dobbs M, Gurling H (1988) Localization of a susceptibility locus for schizophrenia on chromosome 5. Nature 336:164–167
Shields J, Heston LI, Gottesman II (1975) Schizophrenia and the schizoid: The problem for genetic analysis. In: Fieve R, Rosenthal D, Brill H (eds) Genetic research in psychiatry. Johns Hopkins University Press, Baltimore
Siever LJ, Gunderson JG (1979) Genetic determinants of borderline conditions. Schizophr Bull 5:59–86
Siever LJ, Gunderson JG (1983) The search for a schizotypal personality: Historical origins and current status. Compr Psychiatry 24:199–212
Silverton L (1988) Crime and the schizophrenia spectrum: A diathesis-stress model. Acta Psychiatrica Scandinavica 78:72–81
Spitzer RL, Endicott J, Robins E (1978) Research disgnostic criteria: Rationale and reliability. Arch Gen Psychiatry 35:773–782
Spitzer RL, Endicott J, Gibbon M (1979) Crossing the border into borderline personality and borderline schizophrenia: The development of criteria. Arch Gen Psychiatry 36:17–24
St Clair D, Blackwood D, Munir W, Baillie D, Hubbard A, Wright A, Evans HJ (1989) No linkage of chromosome 5q11-q13 markers to schizophrenia in Scottish families. Nature 339:305–309

Stephens DA, Atkinson MW, Day DWK, Roth M, Garside RF (1975) Psychiatric morbidity; in parents and sibs of schizophrenics and non-schizophrenics. Br J Psychiatry 127:97–108
Stewart J, Debray Q, Caillard V (1980) Schizophrenia: The testing of genetic models of pedigree analysis. Am J Hum Genet 32:55
Strauss JS, Carpenter WT, Bartko JJ (1974) The diagnosis and understanding of schizophrenia. III. Speculations on the processes that underlie schizophrenic symptoms and signs. Schizophr Bull 1:61–69
Torgersen S (1984) Genetic and nosological aspects of schizotypal and borderline personality disorders: A twin study. Arch Gen Psychiatry 41:546–554
Torgersen S (1985) Relationship of schizotypal personality disorder to schizophrenia: Genetics. Schizophr Bull 11:554–563
Tsuang MT, Bucher KD, Fleming JA (1988) Testing the monogenic theory of schizophrenia: An application of segregation analysis to blind family study data. Br J Psychiatry 140:595–599
Wender PH, Rosenthal D, Rainer JD, Greenhill L, Sarlin MB (1977) Schizophrenics' adopting parents: Psychiatric status. Arch Gen Psychiatry 34:777
Widiger TA, Frances A, Warner L, Bluhm C (1986) Diagnostic criteria for the borderline and schizotypal personality disorders. J Abnorm Psychol 95:43–51
Widiger TA, Frances A, Trull TJ (1987) A psychometric analysis of the social-interpersonal and cognitive-perceptual items for the schizotypal personality disorder. Arch Gen Psychiatry 44:741–745
Winokur G (1985) Familial psychopathology in delusional disorder. Compr Psychiatry 26:241–248
Wing JK, Cooper JE, Sartorius N (1974) Present state examination. Cambridge University Press, London
Zilboorg G (1941) Ambulatory schizophrenias. Psychiatry 4:141–155
Zilboorg G (1957) Further observations on ambulatory schizophrenia. Am J Orthopsychiatry 27:677–682

Neuropathological and Brain Imaging Studies in Positive and Negative Schizophrenia

B. BOGERTS,[1] P. FALKAI,[1] G. DEGREEF,[2] and J. A. LIEBERMAN[2]

Introduction

Recent interest in neuroanatomical schizophrenia research has focused on three major brain regions: (1) the limbic system with its important telencephalic components comprising the medial temporal lobe structures and the cingulate gyrus; (2) the prefrontal cortex, which roughly consists of frontal cortical areas anterior to the level of the genu of the corpus callosum; and (3) the basal ganglia, most importantly the globus pallidus.

Interest in the medial temporal and related limbic structures was raised by postmortem brain studies demonstrating neuroanatomical anomalies in the hippocampus, amygdala, entorhinal cortex, and the parahippocampal and cingulate gyri in a substantial proportion of schizophrenics (Bogerts 1984; Bogerts et al. 1985; Kovelmann and Scheibel 1984; Brown et al. 1986; Falkai and Bogerts 1986; Jakob and Beckmann 1986; Benes 1987; Falkai et al. 1988a; Jeste and Lohr 1989). Prefrontal cortical dysfunction in schizophrenia has mainly been indicated by various functional brain studies such as regional cerebal blood flow studies (rCBF), positron emission tomography (PET), and single photon emission computed tomography (SPECT) (Ingvar and Franzen 1974; Buchsbaum et al. 1982, 1984; Weinberger et al. 1986; Geraud et al. 1987). Structural and functional disturbances of the globus pallidus, which is considered to be a part of the extrapyramidal and limbic system, have been reported by some postmortem and PET studies (Stevens 1982, 1986; Bogerts 1984; Bogerts et al. 1985; Early et al. 1987; Luchins et al. 1989).

Dysfunction of these three brain systems (medial temporal lobe, prefrontal cortex, pallidum) may influence the psychopathology of the disease in a different way. There is some evidence that prefrontal cortical hypofunction correlates with what are termed negative schizophrenic symptoms (such as social withdrawal, apathy, anhedonia, lack of drive and initiative), while left temporolimbic pathology may be related to positive symptoms (e.g., delusions, hallucinations, and paranoid symptoms). Some reports indicate that catatonia is associated with structural (Stevens 1986; Bogerts et al. 1986) and functional

[1] Psychiatrische Klinik, Universität Düsseldorf, Bergische Landstraße 2, W-4000 Düsseldorf, FRG
[2] Hillside Hospital, Long Island Jewish Medical Center, P.O. Box 38, Glen Oaks, NJ 11004, USA

A. Marneros / N. C. Andreasen / M. T. Tsuang (Eds.)
Negative Versus Positive Schizophrenia

(Luchins et al. 1989) disturbances of the pallidum. The present chapter gives a brief summary of brain imaging and postmortem brain studies related to positive and negative schizophrenia and displays data of our most recent computed tomography (CT) and magnetic resonance imaging (MRI) studies on this subject.

Before reviewing the literature, it should be emphasized that we regard neuroanatomical aspects as only one component of many pathophysiological and psychosocial factors which contribute to the clinical picture of schizophrenia. There are convincing arguments linking positive and negative psychotic symptoms to biochemical factors such as an imbalance of cerebral dopaminergic (Meltzer and Stahl 1976; McKenna 1987), cholinergic (Tandon and Greden 1990), and noradrenergic (D. P. van Kammen, this volume) mechanisms. Moreover, the role of psychosocial factors, e.g., stress, in precipitating acute psychotic symptoms (Zubin and Spring 1977; Curran and Cireilli 1988) and the consequences of long-term hospitalization and social deprivation for the development of syndromes similar to negative schizophrenia (see H. D. Brenner et al., this volume) are well known.

Another problem in correlating positive and negative schizophrenic symptoms with pathomorphological findings is that both types of symptoms can occur simultaneously (J. Lieberman et al., this volume) or in alternating periods (A. Marneros, this volume) in the same patient. The reported neuroanatomical changes are believed to be stable over time and not as mutable as the psychopathology. There is, however, a subgroup of patients in which negative symptoms predominate during the whole course of the disease and a larger group in which positive symptoms are most obvious; most patients can be characterized by mixed (positive and negative) symptoms. This review focuses mainly on the first two (unmixed) groups. Schizophrenic patients with mixed symptoms may have pathomorphological and pathophysiological deviations of both positive and negative schizophrenia.

Postmortem Brain Studies

After the failure of classical neuropathological schizophrenia research to convincingly demonstrate anatomical anomalies in the brains of schizophrenics, a new era of pathomorphological interest in schizophrenia started some years ago. It received strong impetus from modern neuroimaging techniques. In the last 10 years, about 20 well-controlled, quantitative morphometric (Tables 1, 2) and 7 qualitative (Table 3) postmortem brain studies have been published showing various types of pathomorphological deviation in the brains of schizophrenics. Most of these studies described anatomical anomalies in the key limbic structures of the medial temporal lobe (Tables 1, 3). Only two studies investigating the medial temporal lobe reported negative results (Christison et al. 1989; Heckers et al. 1990). The latter of these two studies was based on patients of advanced age, a fact which might explain its negative results. Some authors reported anatomical changes outside limbic structures,

Table 1. Morphometric postmortem studies in limbic structures of schizophrenics

Reference	Findings
Bogerts (1984), Bogerts et al. (1985)	Reduced volumes of hippocampus, parahippocampal gyrus, and amygdala (Vogt collection)
Kovelman and Scheibel (1984)	Disarray of hippocampal pyramidal cells
Lesch and Bogerts (1984)	Reduced thickness of diencephalic periventricular gray matter
Brown et al. (1986)	Reduced thickness of parahippocampal cortex, temporal horn enlargement
Falkai and Bogerts (1986)	Reduction of hippocampal pyramidal cells
Benes et al. (1986), Benes (1987)	Lower neuronal densities and cytoarchitectural disturbances in the cingulate gyrus
Colter et al. (1987)	Reduced parahippocampal white matter
Altshuler et al. (1987)	Correlation between hippocampal pyramidal cell disarray and severity of clinical symptoms
Falkai et al. (1988b)	Lower volume and cell densities in the entorhinal cortex
Falkai and Bogerts (1989)	Abnormal location of entorhinal pre-alpha cell clusters
Jeste and Lohr (1989)	Reduction of hippocampal volume and pyramidal cell numbers
Christison et al. (1989)	No disarray of hippocampal pyramical cells
Crow et al. (1989)	Selective left temporal horn enlargement
Bogerts et al. (1990a)	Reduced hippocampal volume (new Düsseldorf collection)
Heckers et al. (1990)	Unchanged volume of parahippocampal gyrus

e.g., in the basal ganglia, corpus callosum, and frontal cortex (Table 2). These findings were, however, less often reported than limbic system abnormalities and need confirmation by future studies.

The pathomorphological changes in schizophrenia are subtle and not comparable in magnitude to the brain tissue loss seen in the well-known degenerative brain disorders. The changes cannot be seen in all schizophrenic patients and, morphometrically, only a minority (some 20%–30%) have values below the range of matched healthy controls. These structural changes also differ from those of neurodegenerative disorders in that, at least in most patients, they are not progressive and probably were acquired very early in life (Weinberger 1987; Bogerts 1989, 1990).

Table 2. Reported neuroanatomical anomalies in other than limbic structures (morphometric studies)

Reference	Findings
Dom et al. (1981)	Reduced microneuron density in the pulvinar of catatonic patients
Nasrallah et al. (1983c)	Smaller corpus callosum in late onset vs. early onset schizophrenics
Bogerts et al. (1983)	Reduced volume of the lateral substantia nigra
Bogerts et al. (1985)	Reduced volume and cell numbers in the inner pallidal segment of catatonic patients
Benes et al. (1986)	Reduced neuronal density in the prefrontal cortex
Pakkenberg (1987)	Reduced volumes of cortical gray and white matter, increased ventricular volume
Lohr and Jeste (1988)	Reduced neuropil in the locus coeruleus

Table 3. Qualitative postmortem studies in limbic structures of schizophrenia

Reference	Findings
Nieto and Escobar (1972)	Gliosis in the hippocampus of 4 out of 10 patients
McLardy (1974)	Reduced thickness of the granule cell layer in the hippocampal formation
Averback (1981)	Cellular degeneration in the nucleus of the ansa lenticularis
Scheibel and Kovelman (1981)	Disorientation of hippocampal pyramidal cells
Stevens (1982)	Gliosis in the hippocampus and amygdala in 6 of 25 patients
Jakob and Beckmann (1986)	Cytoarchitectonic abnormalities in the rostral entorhinal region, abnormal pattern of temporal sulci

Theoretically, a broad range of schizophrenic symptoms can be explained by a temporolimbic system disorder. The limbic parts of the temporal lobe are anatomically and functionally interposed between the neocortical supramodal sensory associations and integration areas (these are mainly the prefrontal cortex, parts of the parietal and temporal neocortex) on the one hand, and the septum-hypothalamus complex on the other. All sensory information finally converges in the entorhinal cortex, hippocampus, and amygdala (Jones and Powell 1970; Mesulam 1986). These key limbic structures play an important role in what is called sensory gating, that is, the filtering out of irrelevant sensory stimuli by the neuronal comparison of present with past experience (Schmajuk 1987; Swanson 1983).

Furthermore, amygdala and hippocampus link by means of several fiber bundles, neocortical cognitive activities to the phylogenetically old basic drives and emotions which are generated in neuronal networks of the septum-hypothalamus complex (Palkovits and Zaborski 1979). Thus, in addition to disturbed sensory information processing, limbic pathology could also explain the dissociation between cognitive activities and emotional reactions to these activities, and dyscontrol syndrome of basic emotions which is frequently seen in schizophrenics (Bogerts 1985, 1989, 1990).

Limbic dysfunction causing neocortical-hypothalamic and, hence, cognitive-emotional dissociation may result in an inappropriate emotional categorization of sensory perceptions and thoughts and thus to the schizophrenic loss of reality and paranoid symptoms. Moreover, there are intensive feedback projections from the key temporolimbic structures to widespread cortical association and integration areas (Swanson and Köhler 1986). It is conceivable that dysfunction of these mesiotemporal-neocortical feedback loops, which are involved in the integration and coordination of neocortical activities (White et al. 1990), is related to schizophrenic thought disorder.

Clinicoanatomical correlations in postmortem studies are problematic and, therefore, have not been performed in most of the above-mentioned studies. Postmortem brains are usually from patients who were chronically hospitalized and had, during the long course of their disease, alternating periods of positive and negative symptoms. Most neuropathological investigations were performed on relatively old brain collections (Vogt Collection, Düsseldorf; Yakovlev Collection, Washington; Runwell Collection, UK) and, therefore, retrospective assessment of patients' psychopathology using modern rating scales was difficult. However, several of the postmortem studies reported some preliminary correlations between brain morphology and clinical symptoms. In the Vogt Collection, patients who were characterized in the extensive and well-preserved clinical records as having predominant paranoid and hallucinatory symptoms had the focus of pathology in the medial temporal lobe, whereas patients with predominant catatonic symptoms had more basal ganglia pathology (Stevens 1986; Bogerts et al. 1986).

Cytoarchitectural changes in the limbic allocortex have been reported to occur more frequently in hebephrenic than in paranoid patients (Jakob and Beckmann 1986). In a qualitative study of gliosis and cell loss, Stevens (1982) found a relationship between periventricular, limbic, or hypothalamic pathology and assaultive behavior, flat affect, catatonia, and seclusiveness; disturbances of speech were associated with pathological changes in the globus pallidum, stereotypy was associated with hypothalamic and hippocampal anomalies. Because identical sections from each of these regions were not available in every case, statistical tests of these suggestive correlations could not be performed.

Investigating morphometrically postmortem brains of schizophrenics, Pakkenberg (1987) found that patients with prevailing negative symptoms had significantly larger ventricles than patients with predominantly positive symptoms. In a comprehensive semiquantitative neuropathological study,

Bruton et al. (1990) found a significant association between both brain weight and brain length and premorbid function, namely, the poorer the function, the lighter and shorter the brain.

Additional support for the assumption that medial temporal lobe pathology can cause schizophrenia-like symptoms comes from autopsy reports of organic brain diseases mimicking schizophrenia. Viral infections with high affinity to the medial temporal lobe (e.g., herpes simplex encephalitis, rabies) often produce in the initial stages of the disease severe emotional symptoms of fear, aggression, anxiety, irritability, periods of apathy or restlessness, overattention to external stimuli, distractibility, inappropriate sexual behavior, and even paranoid symptoms and hallucinations (Greenwood et al. 1983). The same symptoms can be caused by medial temporal lobe tumors, infarctions, traumas (Mulder and Daly 1952; Davison and Bagley 1969; Malamud 1967; Hillbom 1951), and temporal lobe epilepsy (Slater et al. 1963), especially if the lesion is on the left side (Flor-Henry 1969). At least in the initial stages, such organic brain diseases are frequently misdiagnosed as schizophrenia.

Investigations of the intracerebral electrical activity of schizophrenics using intracranial electrodes (Heath 1982) demonstrated spikes in the septal region, which is closely connected with the hippocampus and amygdala. The abnormalities – not observed on surface recordings – occurred only when the patients were acutely psychotic. Violence and aggression were associated with hippocampal and amygdala discharges.

Wieser (1982) demonstrated with intracerebral electrodes in chronic epileptics that stimulation of the basal mesiotemporal structures produces complex hallucinations and delusions, which frequently have a strong emotional component. Such effects were not obtained by stimulation of other brain regions.

Flor-Henry (1969) was the first to suggest that the typical acute schizophrenic symptoms are associated with a left temporolimbic disease. He derived this assumption from laterality studies of epileptic foci in temporal lobe epileptics with various types of psychoses. Several follow-up studies investigating the laterality of the focus in psychotic temporal lobe epileptics confirmed this finding (Ounsted and Lindsley 1981; Perez et al. 1984; Sherwin 1982; Trimble 1986), while Flor-Henry's original assumption that right-sided foci can be related to affective symptoms remained more controversial. A comparable observation was made by Hillbom (1951) who reported that schizophrenia-like psychoses after brain injury occurred most frequently if the lesion was in the left temporal lobe.

CT Studies

Since the introduction of CT into psychiatry, about 80 CT studies have found structural anomalies in the brains of schizophrenics. These comprise altered tissue densities, enlargement of lateral and third ventricles, and widening of cortical sulci and fissures (Shelton and Weinberger 1986). A large number of studies found that the presence of these abnormalities is associated with various clinical symptoms, such as poor premorbid adjustment, negative or positive symptoms, poor response to neuroleptic treatment, cognitive impairment, and unfavorable outcome. A few studies found no differences between patients and controls, but these might be no more than can be expected by chance.

In a comprehensive review of the CT and MRI literature relating to positive and negative symptoms, Marks and Luchins (1990) conclude that, as of now, there is no consensus on the question of which clinical symptoms correlate with the various abnormalities seen on CT and MRI. The authors subdivided the literature in four categories:

1. Fifteen CT and two MRI studies that support a relationship of enlarged ventricles and/or cortical sulci to increased negative or decreased positive symptoms.
2. Two CT reports that find no direct relationship, but note a relationship between the neuroanatomical changes and some feature which secondarily is related to negative symptoms, such as dementia.
3. Six articles that find no relationship between the structural brain abnormalities and negative or positive symptoms.
4. Three studies that find the opposite relationship between enlarged ventricles and psychopathology, i.e., more positive or fewer negative symptoms were associated with larger ventricles.

Reviewing the neuroradiological literature up to May 1990, we came to similar conclusions. Table 4 completes the CT studies listed in the review of Marks and Luchins (1990) by adding some papers which were published later. We found 16 CT studies reporting that ventricular and/or cortical sulcal size is associated with increased negative symptoms and/or cognitive impairment, whereas 9 CT articles found that ventricular and/or cortical sulcal size is not, or is even inversely correlated with negative symptoms.

Although the statistical power of most of these studies is sufficient since large sample sizes were used (Table 4, column 2) the value of the clinical-anatomical correlations of CT studies is limited. Nearly all CT studies quantitatively assessed the lateral ventricles on one standarized horizontal level, using the ventricles to brain ratio (VBR), i.e., the area of the lateral ventricles at their maximal extent expressed as a percent of the whole brain area at this level, or qualitatively or semiquantitatively assessed the cerebral cortex as a whole. With CT, only assessments of gross anatomical structures are possible. Increased VBR or "cortical atrophy" indicates that there is a lack of tissue somewhere in the hemispheres, but does not localize it in a specific brain region. Since visualization of smaller brain structures by CT is limited because of its poor resolution and poor white-gray matter contrasts, right and left cortical, basal ganglia, or limbic areas, which are now considered to play an important role in the pathophysiology of positive and negative schizophrenic symptoms, generally have not been evaluated separately by means of CT.

Table 4. CT scan studies

I. Ventricular and/or cortical sulcal size is associated with negative symptoms or cognitive impairment (16 studies)

Reference	Patients/Controls	Associated symptom or impairment
Johnstone et al. 1976, 1978	18/ 8	Ventricle
Weinberger et al. 1980	23/20	VBR
Andreasen et al. 1982	52/47	VBR
Nasrallah et al. 1982	55/27	Cortex
Luchins et al. 1984	67/62	VBR
Pearlson et al. 1984, 1985	46/46	VBR
Kolakowska et al. 1985	77/40	VBR
Williams et al. 1985	77/40	VBR
Owens et al. 1985	112/77 (psych.)	VBR
Pandurangi et al. 1986	23/23	VBR
Ota et al. 1987	25/ 0	Ventricle/cortex
Kemali et al. 1987	50/25	VBR
Keefe et al. 1987	97/ 0	VBR
van Kammen et al. 1988	10/ 0	VBR
Moscarelli et al. 1989	19/23	VBR
Mc Carley et al. 1989	9/ 9	Silvian fissure

II. Ventricular and/or cortical sulcal size is *not or inversely* correlated with negative symptoms (9 studies)

Reference	Patients/Controls	Associated symptom in impairment
Mundt et al. 1980	68/68	3rd ventricle
Nasrallah et al. 1982, 1983a, b	55/27	VBR
Bishop et al. 1983	46/39	VBR
Losonczy et al. 1986	28/21	VBR
Farmer et al. 1987	35/ 0	VBR
Keilp et al. 1988	28/ 0	VBR
Pfefferbaum et al. 1988	45/55	Ventricle/cortex
Pearlson et al. 1989	50/87	VBR
Serban et al. 1990	31/31	Ventricle/cortex

One CT article addressing the question of right-left differences in temporal brain region deserves special attention. McCarley et al. (1989) reported that positive symptoms correlate with left silvian fissure enlargement, whereas negative symptoms correlate with right silvian fissure size. Since silvian fissure enlargement mainly indicates temporal brain tissue reduction, this finding points towards left temporal lobe dysfunction in positive schizophrenia, whereas right temporal pathology is associated with negative symptoms.

To investigate further to which extent different brain regions as visualized by CT can be related to positive and negative symptoms, we measured the CSF spaces of various brain parts of 79 female schizophrenics who, during the whole course of the disease, had predominantly positive ($n = 48$), mixed ($n = 22$), or

Table 5. New Düsseldorf CT scan study (female schizophrenics)

	Positive	Mixed	Negative
n	48	22	9
Mean age in years (Range)	37.2 (18–55)	41.8 (21–58)	36.8 (19–53)
Disease duration in years (Range)	6.0 (1–27)	6.5 (1–26)	7.5 (1–24)

negative ($n = 9$) symptoms. All patients were from the Department of Psychiatry, University of Düsseldorf. Positive and negative symptoms corresponded to those described in Type I or Type II schizophrenia (according to Crow 1980), respectively. Mean age and disease duration of the subjects are given in Table 5. In each patient, the size of all clearly visible cortical sulci at the five upper axial scans was measured planimetrically on projected enlargements ($\times 4$). The scans were provided by a Philips Tomoscan 300, the distance between the levels was 0.9 mm. In addition, the VBR, the maximal area of the temporal horn, the maximal diameter of the third ventricle, and the size of the silvian fissure on three consecutive axial levels were measured. The cortical sulci were subdivided into parasagittal, right and left frontal, and right and left parieto-occipital regions, using the central sulcus as a anatomical landmark to separate the anterior from the posterior cortical regions. For each region, the sum of all planimetrically measured cortical sulci was expressed as a percentage of the whole brain area at the VBR level, thus obtaining a sulcus to brain ratio by which magnification artifacts were eliminated. Similarly, a silvian fissure to brain ratio was calculated for each of the three temporal levels. A comprehensive description of the morphometric method, which was especially developed to measure planimetrically different regions of the external and internal CSF spaces, was published previously (Bogerts et al. 1987).

The results are shown in Tables 6 and 7. The cortical and silvian fissure values of the patients with mixed (positive and negative) symptoms closely resembled those of the positive symptom group. There were no significant differences in VBR and third ventricle between the patients with positive and those with negative symptoms. Patients with negative symptoms tended to have larger frontal and parieto-occipital cortical sulci and had significantly larger interhemispheric fissures than the patients with positive symptoms (Table 6). In the patients with negative symptoms, interhemispheric fissure enlargement was most prominent in the anterior (prefrontal) portions. Compared with the negative schizophrenics, patients with positive symptoms showed a trend towards larger silvian fissures at all three temporal levels and, more interestingly, they demonstrated a highly significant increase in size in the left temporal horn (73% larger), but no significant enlargement of the right temporal horn.

Table 6. VBR and relative size of third ventricle, frontal sulci, and interhemispheric fissure in female schizophrenics

		Positive mean	(SD)	Mixed mean	(SD)	Negative mean	(SD)	Differences (%; negative minus positive)	*p* value
VBR		8.1	(3.2)	8.1	(3.7)	8.4	(3.7)	+ 4	0.80[a]
3rd Ventrile		1.44	(0.65)	1.21	(0.6)	1.19	(0.33)	−18	0.25[a]
Frontal dorsal	L	0.53	(1.22)	0.53	(1.06)	0.97	(1.43)	+46	0.33[a]
	R	0.52	(1.23)	0.48	(1.01)	1.00	(1.37)	+48	0.23[a]
Frontal basal	L	0.82	(1.33)	0.40	(0.78)	1.00	(1.19)	+18	0.63[a]
	R	0.56	(0.93)	0.37	(0.81)	0.92	(1.22)	+40	0.32[a]
Interhemispheric fissure		0.20	(0.34)	0.27	(0.45)	0.57	(0.62)	+65	0.01
Parietooccipital dorsal	L	0.28	(0.74)	0.35	(1.04)	0.87	(0.96)	+68	0.057[a]
	R	0.21	(0.54)	0.27	(0.59)	0.72	(0.92)	+71	0.054
Parietooccipital basal	L	0.82	(1.33)	0.41	(0.78)	1.01	(1.19)	+19	0.94[a]
	R	0.57	(0.93)	0.37	(0.81)	0.93	(1.22)	+39	0.46[a]

[a] not significant.

Table 7. Relative size of silvian fissure and and temporal horn in female schizophrenics

		Positive mean	(SD)	Mixed mean	(SD)	Negative mean	(SD)	Difference (%, positive vs negative)	p value
n		48		22		9		$\frac{1}{n}$	$\frac{1}{n}$
Temporal 1	L	0.546	(0.759)	0.648	(0.741)	0.342	(0.461)	−37	0.38[a]
	R	0.447	(0.635)	0.585	(0.567)	0.232	(0.267)	−48	0.30[a]
Temporal 2	L	0.942	(0.760)	1.043	(0.852)	0.597	(0.702)	−36	0.20[a]
	R	0.800	(0.743)	0.770	(0.610)	0.360	(0.416)	−55	0.06[a]
Temporal 3	L	1.110	(0.839)	1.140	(0.744)	0.710	(0.542)	−37	0.15[a]
	R	0.970	(0.835)	0.990	(0.601)	0.500	(0.397)	−49	0.06[a]
Temporal horn	L	0.21	(0.18)	0.030	(0.025)	0.05	(0.08)	−73	0.01
	R	0.27	(0.24)	0.29	(0.026)	0.20	(0.16)	−26	0.44[a]

[a] not significant.
L, left; R, right.

Although obtained by the relative poor resolution of CT technology, the results demonstrate an association between temporal lobe pathology and positive schizophrenic symptoms. In particular, left temporolimbic pathology, as indicated by left temporal horn enlargement, was most impressively associated with positive symptoms.

MRI Studies

Because of its higher resolution, better soft tissue contrasts, and its capability of multiplanar imaging, MRI provides a more powerful tool than CT for morphometric assessment of white and gray matter structures. MRI studies in schizophrenia have been performed since 1984. While the first publications were based on small sample sizes and yielded no significant differences in ventricular size, midsagittal brain areas, and periventricular signal intensities (Smith et al. 1984; P. J. Mathew and Partain 1985; Johnstone et al. 1986), more recent studies investigated larger numbers of patients and controls and reported cerebral ventricle and/or cortical fissure enlargement (Kojima et al. 1987; Besson et al. 1987; Rossi et al. 1989; Kelsoe et al. 1988; Stratta et al. 1989; Suddath et al. 1989, 1990; Andreasen et al. 1990), altered midsagittal corpus callosum areas (Mathew et al. 1985; Nasrallah et al. 1986; Uematso and Kaiya 1988; Günther et al. 1989; Günther 1990), smaller mesiotemporal tissue or whole temporal lobe volumes (DeLisi et al. 1988; Suddath et al. 1990; Rossi et al. 1990; Johnstone et al. 1989; Bogerts et al. 1990 a), and changes in T1 and T2 relaxation times in temporal or frontal brain areas (Besson et al. 1987; Smith et al. 1987, 1988).

We found five MRI studies which correlated positive and negative symptoms with the structural findings:

1. Andreasen et al. (1986) compared on midsagittal cuts the cerebral area, the frontal lobe area, and the cranial area in 38 schizophrenics and 49 controls. There was a significant association between patients with smaller cerebral and cranial sizes and negative symptoms, but no relationship between frontal lobe size and negative symptoms. Positive symptoms did not correlate with any of these measures.
2. Kojima et al. (1987) performed linear measures of the width of the third ventricle, cellae medias, fourth ventricle, interhemispheric fissure, and silvian fissures in 29 schizophrenics and 32 healthy volunteers. Symptoms were rated using the Brief Psychiatric Rating Scale (BPRS) and the Scales for the Assessment of Negative Symptoms (SANS; Andreasen 1983). Third ventricle, interhemispheric and silvian fissures were significantly larger in the patients. Total BPRS scores and the subscores, "emotional withdrawal," "conceptual disorganization," "depressive mood," and "uncooperativeness" were increased significantly in the patients with enlarged third ventricle and silvian fissures; the same patients also showed trends towards higher subscale values on the SANS.

3. Besson et al. (1987) examined ventricular size and regional spin-lattice relaxation time (T1) changes in 23 chronic schizophrenics and 15 controls. Patients with high positive symptom scores had significantly increased T1 in the left medial temporal structures, whereas high negative schizophrenics had significant higher signal intensity in the left frontal region.
4. Applying several brain imaging procedures including MRI, Günther (1990) investigated midsagittal corpus callosum areas in 31 schizophrenics and 31 controls. Of these, 15 patients had predominantly negative symptoms (Type II schizophrenics), 16 had mainly positive symptoms (Type I patients). There were no differences between the whole schizophrenic group and the controls. However, Type I schizophrenics had significantly larger corpus callosum areas than the Type II patients.
5. In a second series, Andreasen et al. (1990) determined in 55 schizophrenic patients and 47 normal control subjects, on coronal cuts, the lateral and third ventricular volumes, and on midsagittal cuts, the cranial, cerebral, frontal lobe, thalamus, and third ventricle area. The lateral ventricular volume was found to be significantly larger in the patients. Patients with prominent negative symptoms had significantly larger ventricular size than those with mixed or positive symptoms. Andreasen's et al. (1986) earlier findings of decreased frontal, cerebral, and cranial midsagittal areas in the schizophrenic group were not replicated. No relationship between the midsagittal parameters and patients' psychopathology was observed.

Using a high resolution image acquisition system, we recently performed a detailed MRI study of clinical-anatomical correlations in schizophrenics relating different components of the ventricular system to negative and positive symptoms (Degreef et al. 1990). Thirty-nine first-episode schizophrenics (25 males, 14 females; mean age 24.1 yrs.) admitted to Hillside Hospital, a division of the Long Island Jewish Medical Center, New York, were investigated; 25 nonpatient volunteers (15 men, 10 women; mean age 28.2 years) were used as controls. To determine that the structural changes were not secondary to the treatment or the chronicity of the disease itself, MR images were obtained at the beginning of the disease, and before the patients had received substantial neuroleptic medication. Psychopathology in patients was measured prior to treatment by the SANS scale for negative symptoms and the Schedule for Affective Disorders and Schizophrenia – Psychosis and Disorganization Scale (SADS PD) for positive symptoms. By using a 40° FLASH sequence provided by a Siemens 1.0 Telsa magnetom, 63 contiguous 3.1-mm coronal slices through the whole head were obtained. Using standarized anatomical landmarks (for details, see Degreef et al. 1991), the lateral cerebral ventricles were subdivided into frontal horns, central parts (bodies), occipital horns, and anterior and posterior temporal horns. Volumes were measured with a computerized semiautomated mensuration system (Ashtari et al. 1990).

With the exception of the fourth ventricle, all components of the ventricular system were larger in the schizophrenics, the left side (difference to controls: frontal horn 35%, central part 40%, occipital horn 30%, anterior temporal horn 35%, posterior temporal horn 14%) being more affected than the right side (difference to controls: frontal horn 24%, central part 33%, occipital horn 24%, anterior temporal horn 2%, posterior temporal horn 17%). The greatest laterality effect was seen in the anterior temporal horn, which is surrounded by the hippocampus-amygdala junction (difference between groups, left: 35%, right: 2%).

The psychopathological correlates of ventricular segment volumes are shown in Table 8. The subscores "formal thought disorder" on the SADS-PD scale, and "alogia" and "avolition" on the SANS scale did not correlate with any of the ventricular segments and therefore are not shown in Table 8. As displayed in the table, the significant correlations as well as the insignificant trends were greater on the left side for all ventricular portions, except for attentional impairment, which correlated with right anterior temporal horn volume. No significant correlations with psychopathology were seen in the frontal (anterior horn), central (bodies), occipital (posterior horns), diencephalic (third ventricle), and cerebellar-brainstem parts (fourth ventricle) of the ventricular system. On the left side, however, there were trends towards correlations (r values ranged from 0.25 to 0.33) of frontal horn, body, occipital horn, whole lateral ventricle, and third ventricle size with several items from the SADS-PD or SANS scales (see Table 8).

The most consistent and highly significant correlations between positive as well as negative symptoms were seen in the anterior and posterior temporal horn. The positive symptoms correlated significantly with left posterior temporal horn enlargement. The negative symptoms correlated with right and left, anterior and posterior temporal horn enlargement. The highest and most significant correlation was seen between anhedonia and left anterior temporal horn enlargement.

This study reveals that in first episode schizophrenics there is a much higher association of a broad range of typical positive and negative schizophrenic symptoms with temporolimbic than with frontal, parieto-occipital, diencephalic and cerebellar brain anomalies. The posterior temporal horn, which was measured on the coronal sections between the levels of the mamillary bodies and pulvinar pole, is surrounded by hippocampus and white matter containing afferent and efferent fibers to the parahippocampal gyrus. The anterior temporal horn is surrounded by amygdala and anterior hippocampus, and fibers to and from the anterior temporal lobe structures. Since ventricular enlargement in many brain diseases is related to dysfunction of the surrounding brain structures, the data of this study suggest left hippocampal and parahippocampal dysfunction involvement in the pathogenesis of positive symptoms, whereas more general right and left medial temporal lobe dysfunction contributes to the development of negative symptoms.

Functional Brain Anatomy: rCBF, SPECT, PET

While most of the above-mentioned postmortem and MRI studies indicate that the focus of brain pathology in schizophrenia is the medial temporal lobe,

Table 8. Linear correlation values between ventricular volumes and psychopathology of 40 first-episode schizophrenics (from Degreef et al. 1990)

		Positive symptoms (SADS-PD)				*Negative symptoms (SANS)*		
		positive symptoms sum	paranoid symptoms	hallucinations	bizarre behavior	affective flattening	attentional disturbance	anhedonia
Whole lateral ventricle	R	0.22	0.19	0.12	0.23	0.17	0.10	0.05
	L	0.31	0.19	0.14	0.32	0.27	0.25	0.01
Frontal horn	R	0.19	0.17	0.18	0.07	0.10	0.02	−0.05
	L	0.33	0.16	0.24	0.19	0.28	0.17	−0.04
Central part	R	0.25	0.15	0.11	0.24	0.08	0.09	0.00
	L	0.31	0.13	0.06	0.37*	0.17	0.32	0.04
Occipital horn	R	0.18	0.19	0.06	0.27	0.22	0.13	−0.07
	L	0.27	0.22	0.11	0.32	0.28	0.23	0.00
Whole temporal horn	R	0.14	0.02	0.28	0.06	0.40*	0.38*	0.15
	L	0.41*	0.27	0.31	0.37*	0.51**	0.40*	0.076
Posterior temporal horn	R	0.08	0.02	0.24	0.11	0.39*	0.07	−0.08
	L	0.45**	0.33	0.41*	0.53***	0.57***	0.42*	−0.01
Anterior temporal horn	R	0.12	0.00	0.14	−0.03	0.23	0.50**	0.41*
	L	0.10	0.02	−0.01	−0.06	0.17	0.18	0.67***
3rd ventricle		0.09	−0.10	−0.05	0.19	0.34	0.15	0.21
4th ventricle		0.06	−0.10	−0.05	−0.17	0.05	−0.07	0.08

Linear correlation values r *, $p < 0.05$; **, $p < 0.01$; ***, $p < 0.001$.

functional studies of mesiotemporal structures by rCBF, PET, and SPECT are scarce. DeLisi et al. (1989) compared temporal glucose rate in PET scans of 21 off-medication schizophrenics with 19 normal controls. Patients had greater metabolic activity in the left than in the right anterior temporal lobe. The extent of this lateralisation was in proportion to the severity of psychosis (BPRS total score). Tamminga et al. (1989) studied 11 schizophrenics (11 controls) using PET; a significant reduction of cerebral activity was found only in the limbic structures of the medial temporal lobe (hippocampus, amygdala) and the cingulate gyrus. The limited number of perfusion studies in the limbic temporal lobe structures can be accounted for by the poor resolution and contrasts of these brain imaging methods in visualizing the small and irregularly shaped structures situated deeply in the medial temporal lobe.

The major focus of interest in brain perfusion studies in schizophrenia were higher neocortical regions, especially the frontal lobe. Since Ingvar and Franzen (1974) reported a relative reduction of rCBF in the frontal cortex of elder and deteriorated chronic schizophrenics, this "hypofrontality" has become a matter of controversy with further investigations using these techniques. The majority of subsequent studies investigating hemispheric blood flow at rest (on rCBF, see: Ariel et al. 1983; Kurachi et al. 1985; on PET, see: Buchsbaum et al. 1982, 1984; Farkas et al. 1984; Volkov et al. 1987; A. Wolkin et al. 1988) or after special activation tasks of prefrontal lobe functions (Weinberger et al. 1986; Sagawa et al. 1990) have confirmed the presence of a relative hypofrontality in more chronic schizophrenics. Several groups, however, have not observed hypofrontality, particularly not in acute onset, medication-free patients in whom positive symptoms usually predominate (R. J. Mathew et al. 1982, 1988; Sheppard et al. 1983; Kling et al. 1986; Gur et al. 1987a, b; Early et al. 1987). There is one study with opposite results reporting that acute psychotic patients are hyperfrontal (Szechtman et al. 1988).

Some brain perfusion studies have explicitly examined negative and positive syndromes in schizophrenia. Ingvar and Franzen (1974) found a highly significant correlation between frontal hypofunction and negative symptoms. Hoyer and Oesterreich (1975) found a positive correlation of cerebral blood flow with productive symptoms. Geraud et al. (1987) reported a frontal hypofunction in clinically remitted patients, but not during psychotic exacerbation. Similar results were obtained by Warkentin et al. (1990); in addition, the latter authors found a highly significant correlation between the fronto-occipital blood flow ratio and the degree of behavioral disturbance, indicating that the more psychotic the patients were, the more *hyperfrontal* was the blood flow distribution. Warkentin et al. (1990) suggest that the inconsistencies between studies concerning the absence or presence of hypofrontality in schizophrenia are in reality related to whether the patients were acutely psychotic or not at the time of the investigation.

In a SPECT study, Anderson et al. (1990) examined six patients with, and four patients without a history of hallucinations. A statistical evaluation of selected areas of interest (frontal, temporal, basal ganglia) to cerebellum ratios revealed no hypofrontality in any subject. Five subjects demonstrated left temporal hypoperfusion, all of these patients currently experienced auditory hallucinations. None of the nonhallucinators had temporal hypoperfusion. Assessing rCBF in comparing 17 schizophrenics with 17 controls, Risberg et al. (1990) showed that the patients studied during the exacerbated stage had normal rCBF results, while patients at remission showed a redistribution of flow with lower values in the frontal areas. The authors conclude that "hypofrontality" is dependent on the clinical state of the disease.

It is questionable whether the functional abnormalities observed in the frontal cortex by rCBF, PET, and SPECT are associated with gross structural abnormalities. In the two first planimetric MRI studies of the frontal brain of schizophrenics, reduced midsagittal (Andreasen et al. 1986) or horizontal (DeMyer et al. 1988) frontal lobe areas were described, but the differences beween patients and controls disappeared after adjustment for educational level. In four subsequent investigations of frontal lobe volumes (Kelsoe et al. 1988; Suddath et al. 1989; Suddath et al. 1990) or frontal midsagittal areas (Andreasen et al. 1990), no differences between patients and controls were detected. There is, however, one histological study of three frontal cortical areas of schizophrenics (Benes et al. 1986) reporting reduced neuronal densities and subtle cytoarchitectural changes; moreover, in our above mentioned CT study, the frontal portions of the interhemispheric fissure were significantly larger in negative schizophrenics than in the positive symptom group.

Conclusions

A considerable number of postmortem and MRI studies report anatomical anomalies in temporolimbic structures in a substantial proportion of schizophrenics. In the light of recent progress in neuroanatomy and neurophysiology of the limbic system, a broad range of schizophrenic symptoms can be explained by dysfunction of these brain regions. Direct evidence linking limbic pathology to typical schizophrenic symptoms was provided by CT, MRI, and SPECT studies analyzing, morphometrically or functionally, several brain regions including the temporolimbic areas, and relating the anatomical changes to the psychopathology. The most consistent finding is an association between left temporo-limbic pathology and positive symptoms (McCarley et al. 1989; Besson et al. 1987; Degreef et al. 1990; Anderson et al. 1990). The results are in line with laterality studies in schizophrenia-like psychoses in patients suffering from temporal lobe epilepsy or brain injuries; left temporolimbic foci or lesions in organic psychoses are more frequently associated with the typical acute schizophrenic symptoms than lesions elsewhere in the brain.

Negative symptoms cannot be localized to a specific brain region as well as positive symptoms can be, and might be related to a more diffuse brain pathology. A large number of CT studies correlated lateral ventricular size with schizophrenic psychopathology. Most of these studies found a weak relationship between ventricular enlargement and negative symptoms or cognitive impairment, whereas others found no such correlations. The inconsistent results of the VBR studies may be explained by the fact that increased lateral ventricle size cannot be related to tissue loss in a special brain region. VBR enlargement may result from frontal, parietal, or occipital brain atrophy, but not from the mesiotemporal abnormalities, which are now believed to play the crucial role in the pathophysiology of the disease. In our most recent CT and MRI studies, we found negative symptoms correlated with bilateral temporal horn (MRI study) or anterior interhemispheric fissure enlargement (CT study).

Many, but not all, brain perfusion studies of schizophrenics found a relative decrease in frontal activity as compared with posterior brain areas. This "hypofrontality" seems to be a function of the state of the disease. There are reports of a normal or even hyperfrontal blood flow distribution in acute psychotic patients, while patients at remission and chronic negative patients have hypofrontal flow patterns. Reduced activity of the frontal lobes could well explain some psychopathological aspects of negative schizophrenia. Frontal lobe syndromes caused by brain tumors, injuries, lobotomy, or Pick's disease are characterized by apathy, loss of drive, inappropriate affect, social withdrawal or disinhibition, poor judgment, and psychomotor retardation. Many of these symptoms are commonly seen in patients with negative schizophrenia. Alternatively, it is conceivable that hypofrontality could be caused by other factors such as chronic neuroleptic treatment.

The prefrontal cortex and the medial temporal lobe are closely connected by bidirectional fiber systems which mutually modulate the neuronal activity of both systems. This suggests that the state-dependent reduction in frontal neuronal activity in negative schizophrenics or increased blood flow in acute psychotic stages are results of primary structural damage in temporolimbic areas.

References

Altshuler L, Conrad A, Kovelman JA, Scheibel A (1987) Hippocampal Pyramidal Cell Orientation in Schizophrenia. Arch Gen Psychiatry 44:1094–1098

American Psychiatric Association (1980) DSM-III: diagnostic and statistical manual of mental disorders, 3rd edn. APA, Washington DC

Anderson J, Gordon E, Rennie C, Meares RA (1990) The quantification of variability in ERP's and its application to schizophrenia (abstr no 6). Second international symposium of imaging of the brain in psychiatry and related fields, 13–16 June 1990 (SPECT)

Andreasen NC (1983) Scale for the assessment for of negative symptoms (SANS). University of Iowa, Iowa City, p 17

Andreasen NC, Olsen SA, Dennert JW et al. (1982) Ventricular enlargement in schizophrenia: relationship to positive and negative symptoms. Am J Psychiatry 139:297–302

Andreasen NC, Nasrallah HA, Dunn V, Oslon SC, Grove WM, Ehrhardt JC, Coffman JA, Crosset LHW (1986) Structural abnormalities in the frontal system in schizophrenia. A magnetic resonance imaging study. Arch Gen Psychiatry 43:136–143

Andreasen NC, Ehrhardt JC, Swayze VW, Alliger RJ, Yuh WTC, Cohen G, Ziebell S (1990) Magnetic resonance imaging of the brain in schizophrenia. Arch Gen Psychiatry 47:35–44

Ariel RN, Golden CJ, Berg RA, Quaife MA, Dirksen JW, Forsell T, Wilson J, Graber B (1983) Regional cerebral blood flow in schizophrenics: test using the Xe 133 inhalation method. Arch Gen Psychiatry 40:258–263

Ashtari M, Zito JL, Gold BI, Lieberman JA, Borenstein MT, Herman PG (1990) Computerized volume mensuration of brain structure. J Invest Radiol 27(7):798–805

Averback P (1981) Structural lesions of the brain in young schizophrenics. J Can Sci Neurol 8(1):73–78

Benes FM (1987) An analysis of the arrangement of neurons in the cingulate cortex of schizophrenic patients. Arch Gen Psychiatry 44:608–616

Benes FM, Davidson B, Bird ED (1986) Quantitative cytoarchitectural studies of the cerebral cortex of schizophrenics. Arch Gen Psychiatry 43:31–35

Besson JAO, Corrigan FM, Cherryman GR et al. (1987) Nuclear magnetic brain imaging in chronic schizophrenia. Br J Psychiatry 150:161–163

Bishop RS, Golden CJ, MacInnes WD et al. (1983) The BPRS in assessing symptom correlates of cerebral ventricular enlargement in acute and chronic schizophrenia. Psychiatry Res 9:225–231

Bogerts B (1984) Zur Neuropathologie der Schizophrenien. Fortschr Neurol Psychiatr 52:428–437

Bogerts B (1985) Schizophrenien als Erkrankungen des limbischen Systems. In: Huber G (ed) Basisstadien endogener Psychosen und das Borderline-Problem. Schattauer, Stuttgart, pp 163–179

Bogerts B (1989) Limbic and paralimbic pathology in schizophrenia: Interaction with age and stress related factors. In: Schulz SC, Tamminga CA (eds) Schizophrenia: scientific progress. Oxford University Press, pp 216–227

Bogerts B (1990) The neuropathology of schizophrenia: pathophysiological and neurodevelopmental implications. In: Mednick SA, Cannon TD, Barr CE (eds) Fetal neural development and adult schizophrenia. Cambridge University Press, pp 153–173

Bogerts B, Häntsch J, Herzer M (1983) A morphometric study of the dopamine containing cell groups in the mesencephalon of normals, Parkinson patients and schizophrenics. Biol Psychiatry 18:951–960

Bogerts B, Meertz E, Schönfeld-Bausch R (1985) Basal ganglia and limbic system pathology in schizophrenia. Arch Gen Psychiatry 42:784–791

Bogerts B, Falkai P, Tutsch J (1986) Cell numbers in the pallidum and hippocampus of schizophrenics. In: Shagass C et al. (eds) Biological psychiatry. Elsevier, Amsterdam, pp 1178–1180

Bogerts B, Wurthmann C, Piroth HD (1987) Hirnsubstanzdefizit mit paralimbischem und limbischem Schwerpunkt im CT Schizophrener. Nervenarzt 58:97–106

Bogerts B, Ashtari M, Degreef G, Alvir JMJ, Bilder RM, Lieberman JA (1990a) Reduced temporal limbic structure volumes on magnetic resonance images in first episode schizophrenia. Psychiatry Res (Neuroimaging) 35:1–13

Bogerts B, Falkai P, Haupts M, Greve B, Ernst S, Tapernon-Franz U, Heinzmann U (1990b) Post-mortem volume measurements of limbic system and basal ganglia structures in chronic schizophrenia. Schizophr Res 3:285–301

Brown R, Colter N, Corsellis JAN, Crow TJ, Frith CD, Jagoe R, Johnstone EC, Marsh L (1986) Postmortem evidence of structural brain changes in schizophrenia. Differences in brain weight, temporal horn area and parahippocampal gyrus compared with affective disorder. Arch Gen Psychiatry 43:36–42

Bruton CJ, Crow TJ, Frith CD, Johnstone EC, Owens DGC, Roberts GW (1990) Schizophrenia and the brain: a prospective clinico-neuropathological study. Psychol Med 20:285–304

Buchsbaum MS, Ingvar DH, Kessler R et al. (1982) Cerebral glucography with positron tomography: use in normal subjects and in patients with schizophrenia. Arch Gen Psychiatry 39:251–259

Buchsbaum MS, DeLisi LE, Holcomb HH et al. (1984) Anteroposterior gradients in cerebral glucose use in schizophrenia and affective disorders. Arch Gen Psychiatry 41:1159–1166

Christison GW, Casanova MF, Weinberger DR, Rawlings R, Kleinman JE (1989) A quantitative investigation of hippocampal pyramidal cell size, shape and variability of orientation in schizophrenia. Arch Gen Psychiatry 46:1027–1032
Ciompi L (1980) The natural history of schizophrenia in the long term. Br J Psychiatry 136:413–420
Colter N, Battal S, Crow TJ, Johnstone EC, Brown R, Bruton C (1987) White matter reduction in the parahippocampal gyrus of patients with schizophrenia. Arch Gen Psychiatry 44:1023
Crow T (1980) Molecular pathology of schizophrenia: more than one dimension of pathology? Br Med J 280:66–68
Crow TJ, Ball J, Bloom SR, Brown R, Bruton CJ, Colter N, Frith CD, Johnstone EC, Owens DGC, Roberts GW (1989) Schizophrenia as an anomaly of development of cerebral asymmetry. Arch Gen Psychiatr 46:1145–1150
Curran JP, Cireilli VA (1988) The role psychosozial factors in the etiology, course and outcome of schizophrenia. In: Tsuang MT, Simpson JC (eds) Handbook of schizophrenia, vol 3. Elsevier, Amsterdam, pp 275–297
Davison K, Bagley CR (1969) Schizophrenia-like psychosis associated with organic disorders of the central nervous system. A review of the literature. In: Hertington RN (ed) Current problems in neuropsychiatry, pp 113–187 (Br J Psychiatry Special Publication No 4)
Degreef G, Ashtari M, Bogerts B, Bilder RM, Jody DN, Alvir JMJ, Lieberman JA (1991) Volumes of ventricular system subdivisions measured from magnetic resonance images in first episode schizophrenic patients. Arch Gen Psychiatry (in press)
DeLisi LE, Dauphinais ID, Gershon E (1988) Perinatal complications and reduced size of brain limbic structures in familial schizophrenia. Schizophr Bull 14:185–191
DeLisi LE, Buchsbaum MS, Holcomb HH et al. (1989) Increased temporal lobe glucose use in chronic schizophrenic patients. Biol Psychiatry 25:835–851
DeMyer MK, Gilmor RL, Hendrie HC, DeMyer WE, Augustyn GT, Jackson RK (1988) Magnetic resonance brain images in schizophrenic and normal subjects: influence of diagnosis and education. Schizophr Bull 14:21–32
Dom R, de Saedeler J, Bogerts B, Hopf A (1981) Quantitative cytometric analysis of basal ganglia in catatonic schizophrenics. In: Perris et al. (eds) Biological psychiatry. Elsevier, Amsterdam, pp 723–726
Early TS, Reiman EM, Raichle ME et al. (1987) Left globus pallidus abnormality in never-medicated patients with schizophrenia. Proc Natl Acad Sci USA 84:561–563
Endicott J, Spitzer RA (1978) A diagnostic interview: the schedule for affective disorders and schizophrenia. Arch Gen Psychiatry 35:837–844
Falkai P, Bogerts B (1986) Cell loss in the hippocampus of schizophrenics. Eur Arch Psychiatr Neurol Sci 236:154–161
Falkai P, Bogerts B (1989) Morphometric evidence for developmental disturbances in brains of some schizophrenics. Schizophr Res 2:99–100
Falkai P, Bogerts B, Rozumek M (1988a) Cell loss and volume reduction in the entorhinal cortex of schizophrenics. Biol Psychiatry 24:515–521
Falkai P, Bogerts B, Roberts GW, Crow TJ (1988b) Measurement of the alpha-cell-migration in the entorhinal region: a marker for developmental disturbances in schizophrenia? Schizophr Res 1:157–158
Farkas T, Wolf AP, Jaeger J et al. (1984) Regional brain glucose metabolism in chronic schizophrenia: a positron emission transaxial tomographic study. Arch Gen Psychiatry 41:293–300
Farmer A, Jackson R, McGuffin P, Storey P (1987) Cerebral ventricular enlargement in chronic schizophrenia: consistencies and contradictions. Br J Psychiatry 150:324–330
Flor-Henry P (1969) Psychosis and temporal lobe epilepsy: a controlled investigation. Epilepsia 10:363–395
Geraud G, Arne-Bes MC, Guell A, Bes A (1987) Reversibility of hemodynamic hypofrontality in schizophrenia. J Cereb Blood Flow Metab 7:9–12
Greenwood R, Bhalla A, Gordon A, Roberts J (1983) Behaviour disturbances during recovery from herpes simplex encephalitis. J Neurol Neurosurg Psychiatry 46:809–817

Günther W (1990) Hirnfunktionsstörungen und Corpus-callosum Befunde bei Schizophrenen, gemessen mit EEG-Mapping, regionaler Hirndurchblutung und Kernspintomographie. In: Heinrich K, Bogerts B (eds) Pathophysiologische und pathomorphologische Aspekte bei schizophrenen Psychosesn. Schattauer, Stuttgart, pp 97–113

Günther W, Moser E, Petsch R, Brodie JD, Steinberg R, Streck P (1989) Pathological cerebral blood flow and corpus callosum abnormalities in schizophrenia: relations to EEG mapping and Pet data. Psychiatry Res 29:453–455

Gur RE, Resnick SM, Alavi A et al. (1987a) Regional brain function in schizophrenia. I. A positron emission tomography study. Arch Gen Psychiatry 44:119–125

Gur RE, Resnick SM, Gur RC et al. (1987b) Regional brain function in schizophrenia. II. Repeated evaluation with positron emission tomography. Arch Gen Psychiatry 44:126–129

Heath RG (1982) Psychosis and epilepsy: similarities and differences in the anatomic-physiologic substrate. In: Koella WP, Trimble MR (eds) Temporal lobe epilepsy, mania and schizophrenia and the limbic system. Karger, Basel, pp 106–116

Heckers S, Heinsen H, Heinsen Y, Beckmann H (1990) Morphometry of the parahippocampal gyrus in schizophrenics and controls. Some anatomical considerations. J Neural Transm 80:151–155

Hillbom E (1951) Schizophrenia-like psychoses after brain trauma. Acta Psychiatr Neurol Scand 60:36–47

Hoyer S, Oestreich K (1975) Blood flow and oxidative metabolism of the brain in patients with schizophrenia. Psychiatr Clin 8:304–313

Ingvar DH, Franzen G (1974) Abnormalities of cerebral blood flow distribution in patients with chronic schizophrenia. Acta Psychiatr Scand 50:425–462

Jakob J, Beckmann H (1986) Prenatal developmental disturbances in the limbic allocortex in schizophrenics. J Neural Transm 65:303–326

Jeste DV, Lohr JB (1989) Hippocampal pathologic findings in schizophrenia. Arch Gen Psychiatry 46:1019–1024

Johnstone EC, Crow TJ, Frith CD et al. (1976) Cerebral ventricular size and cognitive impairment in chronic schizophrenia. Lancet ii:924–926

Johnstone EC, Crow TJ, Frith C, Stevens M, Kreel S, Husband J (1978) The dementia of dementia praecox. Acta Psychiatr Scand 57:305–324

Johnstone EC, Crow TJ, MacMillan JF et al. (1986) A magnetic resonance study of early schizophrenia. J Neurol Neurosurg Psychiatry 49:317–321

Johnstone EC, Owens DGC, Crow TJ, Frith CD, Alexandropolis K, Bydder G, Colter N (1989) Temporal lobe structure as determined by nuclear magnetic resonance in schizophrenia and bipolar affective disorder. J Neurol Neurosurg Psychiatry 52:736–741

Jones EG, Powell TPS (1970) An anatomical study of converging sensory pathways within the cerebral cortex of the monkey. Brain 93:793–820

Keefe RSE, Mohs RC, Losonczy MF et al. (1987) Characteristics of very poor outcome schizophrenia 144:889–894

Keilp JG, Sweeney JA, Jacobsen P et al. (1988) Cognitive impairment in schizophrenia: specific relation to ventricular size and negative symptomatology. Biol Psychiatry 24:47–55

Kelsoe JR Jr, Cadet JL, Pickar D, Weinberger DR (1988) Quantitative neuroanatomy in schizophrenia: a controlled magnetic resonance imaging study. Arch Gen Psychiatry 45:533–541

Kemali D, Maj M, Galderisi S (1987) Clinical, biological, and neuropsychological features associated with lateral ventricular enlargement in DSM-III schizophrenic disorder. Psychiatry Res 21:137–149

Kling AS, Metter EJ, Riege WH et al. (1986) Comparison of PET measurement of local brain glucose metabolism and CAT measurement of brain atrophy in chronic schizophrenia and depression. Am J Psychiatry 143:175–180

Kojima H, Yamada S, Nakamura J et al. (1987) Morphological changes of the brain in chronic schizophrenia. In: Takahashi R et al. (eds) Cerebral dynamics, laterality and psychopathology. Elsevier, Amsterdam

Kolakowska T, Williams AO, Ardern M et al. (1985) Schizophrenia with good and poor outcome. I. Early clinical features, response to neuroleptics and signs of organic dysfunction. Br J Psychiatry 146:229–246
Kovelman JA, Scheibel AB (1984) A neurohistological correlate of schizophrenia. Biol Psychiatry 19:1601–1621
Kurachi M, Kobayashi K, Matsubara R, Hiramatsu H, Yamaguchi N, Matsuda H, Maeda T, Hisada K (1985) Regional blood flow in schizophrenic disorders. Eur Neurol 24:176–181
Lesch A, Bogerts B (1984) The diencephalon in schizophrenia: evidence for reduced thickness of the periventricular grey matter. Eur Arch Psychiatr Neurol Sci 234:212–219
Lohr JB, Jeste DV (1988) Locus ceruleus morphometry in aging and schizophrenia. Acta Psychiatr Scand 77:689–697
Losonczy MF, Song IS, Mohs RC et al. (1986) Correlates of lateral ventricular size in chronic schizophrenia. I. Behavioral and treatment response measures. Am J Psychiatry 143:976–981
Luchins D, Lewine R, Meltzer H (1984) Lateral ventricular size, psychopathology and medication response in the psychoses. Biol Psychiatry 19:29–44
Luchins DL, Metz JT, Marks RC, Cooper MD (1989) Basal ganglia glucose metabolism asymmetry during a catatonic episode. Biol Psychiatry 26:725–728
Malamud M (1967) Psychiatric disorder with intracranial tumors of the limbic system. Arch Neurol 17:113–123
Marks RC, Luchins DJ (1990) Relationship between brain imaging findings in schizophrenia and psychopathology. In: Andreasen NC (ed) Schizophrenia: positive and negative symptoms and syndromes. Karger, Basel, pp 89–123
Mathew PJ, Partain CL (1985) Midsagittal sections of the cerebellar vermis and fourth ventricle obtained with magnetic resonance imaging in schizophrenic patients. Am J Psychiatry 142(8):970–971
Mathew PJ, Partain CL, Prakash R, Kulkarni MV, Logan TP, Wilson WH (1985) A study of the septum pellucidum and corpus callosum in schizophrenia with MR imaging. Acta Psychiatr Scand 72(5):414–421
Mathew RJ, Barr DL, Weinman ML, Barr DL (1982) Regional blood flow in schizophrenia. Arch Gen Psychiatry 39:1121–1124
Mathew RJ, Wilson WH, Tant SR, Robinson L, Prakash R (1988) Abnormal resting regional blood flow patterns and their correlates in schizophrenia. Arch Gen Psychiatry 45:542–549
McCarley RW, Faux SF, Shenton M, LeMay M, Cane M, Ballinger R, Duffy PH (1989) CT abnormalities in schizophrenia. A preliminary study of their correlations with P300/P200. Electrophysiological features and positive/negative symptoms. Arch Gen Psychiatry 46:698–708
McKenna PJ (1987) Pathology, phenomenology and the dopamine hypothesis of schizophrenia. Br J Psychiatry 151:288–301
McLardy T (1974) Hippocampal zinc and structural deficits in brains from chronic alcoholics and some schizophrenics. J Orthomol Psychiatry 4:32–36
Meltzer HY, Stahl SM (1976) The dopamine hypothesis of schizophrenia: a review. Schizophr Bull 2:19–76
Mesulam MM (1986) Patterns in behavioral neuroanatomy: association areas, the limbic system, and hemispheric specialization. In: Mesulam MM (ed) Principles of behavioral neurology. Davis, Philadelphia, pp 1–70
Moscarelli M, Cesana BM, Ciussani S et al. (1989) Ventricle-brain ratio and alogia in 19 young patients with chronic negative and positive schizophrenia. Am J Psychiatry 146:257–258
Mulder DW, Daly D (1952) Psychiatric symptoms associated with lesions of the temporal lobe. JAMA 150:173–176
Mundt CH, Radü W, Glück E (1980) Computertomographische Untersuchungen der Liquorräume an chronisch schizophrenen Patienten. Nervenarzt 51:743–748

Nasrallah HA, Jacoby CG, McCalley-Whitters M, Kuperman S (1982) Cerebral ventricular enlargement in subtypes of chronic schizophrenia. Arch Gen Psychiatry 39:774–777
Nasrallah HA, Kuperman S, Jacoby CG et al. (1983a) Clinical correlates of sulcal widening in chronic schizophrenia. Psychiatry Res 10:237–242
Nasrallah HA, Kuperman S, Hamra B, McCalley-Whitters M (1983b) Clinical differences between schizophrenic patients with and without large cerebral ventricles. J Clin Psychiatry 44:407–409
Nasrallah HA, McCalley-Whitters M, Rauscher FP et al. (1983c) A histological study of the corpus callosum in chronic schizophrenia. Psychiatry Res 8:151–160
Nasrallah HA, Andreasen NC, Coffman JA, Olson SC, Dunn VD, Ehrhardt JC, Chapman SM (1986) A controlled magnetic resonance imaging study of corpus callosum thickness in schizophrenia. Biol Psychiatry 21:274–282
Nieto D, Escobar A (1972) Major psychoses. In: Minkler J (ed) Pathology of the nervous system. McGraw-Hill, New York, pp 2654–2665
Ota T, Maeshiro H, Ishido H et al. (1987) Treatment-resistant chronic psychopathology and CT scans in schizophrenia. Acta Psychiatr Scand 75:415–427
Ounsted C, Lindsley J (1981) The long-term outcome of temporal lobe epilepsy in childhood. In: Reynolds EH, Trimble MR (eds) Epilepsy and psychiatry. Churchill Livingstone, Edinburgh, pp 185–215
Owens D, Johnstone E, Crow T et al. (1985) Lateral ventricular size in schizophrenia: relationship to the disease process and its clinical manifestations. Psychol Med 15:27–41
Pakkenberg B (1987) Post-mortem study of chronic schizophrenic brains. Br J Psychiatry 151:744–752
Palkovits M, Zaborski L (1979) Neural connections of the hypothalamus. In: Morgane PJ (ed) Anatomy of the hypothalamus. Decker, New York, pp 379–509
Pandurangi A, Dewan M, Boucher M et al. (1986) A comprehensive study of chronic schizophrenic patients. II. Biological, neuropsychological, and clinical correlates of CT abnormality. Acta Psychiatr Scand 73:161–171
Pearlson G, Garbacz D, Breakey W et al. (1984) Lateral ventricular enlargement associated with persistent unemployment and negative symptoms in both schizophrenia and bipolar disorder. Psychiatry Res 12:1–9
Pearlson GD, Garbacz DJ, Moberg PJ et al. (1985) Symptomatic familial, perinatal, and social correlates of computerized axial tomography (CAT) changes in schizophrenics and bipolars. J Nerv Ment Dis 173:42–50
Pearlson GD, Kim WS, Kubos KL, Moberg PJ, Jayaram G, Bascom MJ, Chase GA, Goldfinger AD, Tune LE (1989) Ventricle-brain ratio, computed tomographic density and brain area in 50 schizophrenics. Arch Gen Psychiatry 46:690–697
Perez MM, Trimble MR, Reider I, Murray M (1984) Epileptic psychosis, a further evaluation of PSE profiles. Br J Psychiatry 146:155–163
Pfefferbaum A, Zipursky RB, Lim KO et al. (1988) Computed tomographic evidence for generalized sulcal and ventricular enlargement in schizophrenia. Arch Gen Psychiatry 45:633–640
Risberg J, Warkentin S, Graae E, Nilsson A, Franzen G (1990) Regional cerebral blood flow in schizophrenia. Second International Symposium Imaging of the Brain in Psychiatry and Related Fields, 13–16 June 1990 (abstr no 90)
Rossi A, Stratta P, Gallucci M, Passarellio R, Cassachia M (1989) Quantification of corpus callosum and ventricles in schizophrenia with nuclear magnetic resonance imaging: a pilot study. Am J Psychiatry 146:99–101
Rossi A, Stratta P, D'Albenzio L, Tartaro A, Schiazza G, di Michele V, Bolino F, Casacchia M (1990) Reduced temporal lobe areas in schizophrenia: preliminary evidences from a controlled multiplanar magnetic resonance imaging study. Biol Psychiatry 27:61–68
Sagawa K, Kawakatsu S, Shibuya I et al. (1990) Correlation of regional cerebral blood flow with performance on neuropsychological tests in schizophrenic patients. Schizophrenia Res 3:241–246

Scheibel AB, Kovelman JA (1981) disorientation of the hippocampal pyramidal cells and its processes in the schizoprenic patient. Biol Psychiatry 16:101–102
Schmajuk NA (1987) Animal models for schizophrenia: the hippocampally lesioned animal. Schizophr Bull 13(2):317–327
Serban G, George A, Siegel S, DeLeon M, Gaffney M (1990) Computed tomography scans and negative symptoms in schizophrenia: chronic schizophrenics with negative symptoms and nonenlarged lateral ventricles. Acta Psychiatr Scand 81:441–447
Shelton RC, Weinberger DR (1986) X-ray computerized tomography studies in schizophrenia: a review and synthesis. In: Nasrallah HA, Weinberger DR (eds) The neurology of schizophrenia. Elsevier, New York, pp 207–250
Sheppard G, Gruzelier J, Manchanda R, Hirsch SR (1983) 15-0 Positron emission tomographic scanning in predominantly never treated acute schizophrenic patients. Lancet ii:1448–1452
Sherwin I (1982) The effect of the location of an epileptogenic lesion on the occurrence of psychosis in epilepsy. In: Koella W, Trimble MR (eds) Temporal lobe epilepsy, mania and schizophrenia and the limbic system. Karger, Basel, pp 81–97
Salter E, Beard AW, Glithero E (1963) The schizophrenia-like psychosis of epilepsy. Br J Psychiatry 109:95–150
Smith RC, Calderon M, Ravichandran GK, Largen J, Vroulis G, Shvartsburd A, Gordon J, Schoolar JC (1984) Nuclear magnetic resonance in schizophrenia: a preliminary study. Psychiatry Res 12(2):137–147
Smith RC, Baumgartner R, Calderon M (1987) Magnetic resonance imaging studies of the brains of schizophrenic patients. Psychiatry Res 20(1):33–46
Stevens JR (1982) Neuropathology of schizophrenia. Arch Gen Psychiatry 39:1131–1139
Stevens JR (1986) Clinicopathological correlations in schizophrenia. Arch Gen Psychiatry 43:715–716
Stratta P, Rossi A, Gallucci M, Amicarelli I, Passariello R, Casacchia M (1989) Hemispheric asymmetries and schizophrenia: a preliminary magnetic resonance imaging study. Biol Psychiatry 25:275–284
Suddath RL, Casanova FMF, Goldberg TE, Daniel DG, Kelsoe J, Weinberger DR (1989a) Temporal lobe pathology in schizophrenia: a quantitative magnetic resonance imaging study. Am J Psychiatry 146:464–472
Suddath RL, Christison GW, Torrey EF, Casanova MF, Weinberger DR (1990) Anatomical abnormalities in the brains of monozygotic twins discordant for schizophrenia. N Engl J Med 322(12):62–67
Swanson LW (1983) The hippocampus and the concept of limbic system. In: Seifert W (ed) Neurobiology of the hippocampus. Academic, London, pp 3–19
Swanson LW, Köhler C (1986) Anatomical evidence for direct projections from the entorhinal area to the entire cortical mantle in the rat. J Neurosci 6:3010–3023
Szechtman H, Nahmias C, Garnett S et al. (1988) Effect of neuroleptics on altered cerebral glucose metabolism in schizophrenia. Arch Gen Psychiatry 45:523–532
Tamminga CA, Thaker GK, Alphs LD, Chase TN (1989) Limbic system: localization of PCP drug action in rat and schizophrenic manifestions in humans. In: Schulz SW, Tamminga CA (eds) Schizophrenia: scientific progress. Oxford University Press, 162–172
Tandon R, Greden JF (1990) Cholinergic hyperactivity and negative schizophrenic symptoms. Arch Gen Psychiatry 46:745–753
Trimble MR (1986) Pet in epilepsy. In: Trimble MR, Bolwig T (eds) Aspects of epilepsy and psychiatry. Wiley, Chichester, pp 147–160
Uematso M, Kaiya H (1988) The morphology of the corpus callosum in schizophrenia: an MRI study. Schizophr Res 1:391–398
Van Kammen DP, Van Kammen WB, Peters J et al. (1988) Decreased slow-wave sleep and enlarged ventricles in schizophrenia. Neuropsychopharmacology 1:265–271
Warkentin S, Nilsson A, Risberg J et al. (1990) Regional cerebral blood flow in schizophrenia: repeated studies during a psychotic episode. Psychiatry Res (Neuroimaging) 35:27–38

Weinberger DR (1987) Implications of normal brain development for the pathogenesis of schizophrenia. Arch Gen Psychiatry 44:660–669
Weinberger DR, Cannon-Spoor E, Potkin SG, Wyatt RJ (1980) Poor premorbid adjustment and CT scan abnormalities in chronic schizophrenia. Am J Psychiatry 137:1410–1413
Weinberger DR, Berman KF, Zec RF (1986) Physiological dysfunction of dorsolateral prefrontal cortex in schizophrenia. I. regional cerebral blood flow (RCBF) evidence. Arch Gen Psychiatry 43:114–125
Wieser HG (1982) Zur Frage der lokalisatorischen Bedeutung epileptischer Halluzinationen. In: Karbowski K (ed) Halluzinationen bei Epilepsien und ihre Differentialdiagnose. Huber, Bern, pp 67–92
Williams AO, Reveley MA, Kolakowska T (1985b) Schizophrenia with good and poor outcome. II. Cerebral ventricular size and its clinical significance. Br J Psychiatry 146:239–246
White TD, Tan AM, Finch DM (1991) Functional reciprocal connections of the rat entorhinal cortex and subicular complex with the medial frontal cortex: an in vivo intracellular study. Brain Res (in press)
Wolkin JA, Jaeger J, Brodie JD et al. (1988) Low frontal glucose utilisation in chronic schizophrenia: a replication study. Am J Psychiatry 145:251–253
Wolkin JA, Jaeger J, Brodie JD et al. (1985) Persistence of cerebral metabolic abnormalities in chronic schizophrenia as determined by positron emission tomography. Am J Psychiatry 142:564–571
Zubin J, Spring B (1977) Vunerability – a new view of schizophrenia. J Abnorm Psychol 86:103–126

Explorations of Dopamine and Noradrenaline Activity and Negative Symptoms in Schizophrenia: Concepts and Controversies

D. P. VAN KAMMEN, A. MOUTON, M. KELLEY, W. BREEDING, and J. PETERS [1]

Introduction

Attempts to understand the pathophysiology of negative symptoms took off when Crow (1980a, b) described the Type I and II syndromes of schizophrenia. He proposed that the Type II form was irreversible and nondopaminergic, consisting of negative symptoms, brain atrophy, poor drug response, and outcome; Type I was the reverse, i.e., positive symptoms, absence of brain atrophy (normal ventricle brain ratio, VBR), and excellent antipsychotic drug response, and consisted of a hyperdopaminergic disorder. Mackay (1980) challenged this concept and hypothesized that Type II schizophrenia was a hypodopaminergic, Kraepelinian form of schizophrenia.

The Type I/Type II conceptualization has been of tremendous heuristic value for the study of negative symptoms. This division has led investigators to define negative symptoms as a component of an irreversible deficit syndrome (Carpenter et al. 1988; Andreasen 1982; Crow 1980a, b) with large VBRs (Andreasen et al. 1982; Crow 1980a, b). Others have focussed on potential lesions in the prefrontal cortex (Weinberger 1987; Levin 1984; van Kammen et al. 1983; Rieder et al. 1979). On the other hand, negative symptoms have been described as a part of the basic symptomatology of schizophrenia (Gross 1989) or changing with clinical state (Goldberg 1985). Unfortunately, only a small fraction of patient meets all the criteria of the pure Type I or II syndrome. There is also no evidence that the distribution of VBR sizes in schizophrenia is bimodal (Harvey et al. 1990). Furthermore, it has become clear that the more components of the Type II syndrome are present, the more severe or more deteriorated, chronic, or nonremitting is the patient (Keefe et al. 1987).

The dopamine (DA) system is primarily involved in two behavioral classes (Miller et al. 1990); it can generally activate performance, and it can also act as an internal reward signal, particularly for motivating future behaviors. Miller et al. (1990) extensively reviewed the relationship between DA and these behaviors; they proposed that D_1-receptors mediate the reward function, and D_2-receptors are the main mediators of the performance function. Impairment of the DA system may then lead to anhedonia, lack of drive or motivation, lack

[1] Western Psychiatric Institute and Clinic, University of Pittsburgh Medical School, and the Department of Veterans Affairs Medical Center, Highland Drive, Pittsburgh, PA 15213, USA

A. Marneros / N. C. Andreasen / M. T. Tsuang (Eds.)
Negative Versus Positive Schizophrenia

of self-care, poverty of speech, and other negative symptoms. If lesions to the prefrontal cortical DA projection fields, like those in Parkinson's disease, are associated with negative symptoms (Levin 1984), and if a relationship between cortical atrophy and decreased cerebralspinal fluid (CSF) homovanillic acid (HVA), the major DA metabolite, exists (van Kammen et al. 1986), then negative symptoms should be present in patients with low CSF HVA.

Although DA has been recognized as the major neurotransmitter in the reward pathway (Wise 1988), noradrenaline (NA) plays a role in the reward functions of the brain as well (Bird and Kornetsky 1990). Consistent with the chronic deterioration observed in some patients (Miller 1989), Stein and Wise (1971) hypothesized that a progressive loss of noradrenergic neurons in the reward pathway caused by endogeneous neurotoxins such as 6-hydroxy-dopamine, 6-OHDA, could lead to the development of negative symptoms. Recently, Yamamoto et al. (1990) showed that 6-OHDA can induce skin conductance patterns in animals reminiscent of those found in schizophrenic patients. 6-OHDA also has a physiological role in the brain as a redox cofactor in serum amina oxidase (Janes et al. 1990). The potential role of other catecholamine-related neurotoxins, such as free radicals, needs to be examined in the deficit syndrome as well. If neurotoxins can lead to schizophrenia, we may need to differentiate between neurodevelopmental (Weinberger 1987) and neurodegenerative aspects (Miller 1989) of schizophrenia. Crow (1980a, b) claimed that negative symptoms were caused by a nondopaminergic disturbance, in contrast to a hyperdopaminergic state leading to positive symptoms, whereas Mackay (1980) postulated a hypodopaminergic condition to be associated with the more severe, chronic forms of the illness.

In the course of the debate as to whether negative symptoms are irreversible (Carpenter et al. 1988; Crow 1980a, b; Weinberger 1987) or not (Goldberg 1985), it has become clear that negative symptoms can fluctuate independently from positive symptoms (Guelfi et al. 1989; Johnstone et al. 1986; Shepherd et al. 1989), increase with psychotic exacerbation (van Kammen et al. 1990; Rosen et al. 1984), correlate with positive symptoms (Tandon et al. 1990; von Kammen et al. 1989a, 1990; Rosen et al. 1984), and change over time more than positive symptoms in patients with residual symptoms (Johnstone et al. 1986). They also can respond to neuroleptic treatment (Goldberg et al. 1967; Rosen et al. 1984; Breier et al. 1987; van Kammen et al. 1987; Tandon et al. 1990). Unless we differentiate these various negative symptoms, controversies about the nature of negative symptoms will remain.

Increased and Decreased Dopamine Activity in Schizophrenia

The original DA hypothesis of schizophrenia (Randrup and Munkvad 1974; Snyder 1976; Carlsson 1978) postulated that increased DA release or DA receptor supersensitivity leads to psychosis or positive symptoms. This formulation was based upon the pharmacological evidence that antipsychotic drugs blocked DA receptors, that amphetamine psychosis resembled schizophrenia, and that DA-releasing agents worsened schizophrenic symptomatology. These observations predicted that increased DA activity would be present during psychotic relapse or when psychotic symptoms are increased (Bowers 1974). On the other hand, amphetamine can also improve schizophrenic symptoms or leave them unchanged (for review see Angrist and van Kammen 1984; van Kammen et al. 1982a; Angrist et al. 1982).

There are also many reports that DA activity actually decreases in schizophrenia (Wyatt 1986; Karoum et al. 1987; Friedhoff 1988; Bowers and Study 1979; Meltzer 1984). Decreased CSF, plasma, or urinary HVA is associated with remission (Post et al. 1975), chronicity (Bowers and Rozitis 1974; Karoum et al. 1987), and poor drug response (Chang et al. 1990; Bowers et al. 1986; van Putten et al. 1989). CSF HVA is also decreased in patients with evidence of structural brain abnormalities such as cortical atrophy or enlarged ventricles (van Kammen et al. 1983, 1986; Nybäck et al. 1983; Jennings et al. 1985; Houston et al. 1986; Lozoncsy et al. 1986; Doran et al. 1987). Growth hormone response to apomorphine, as a measure of DA receptor sensitivity, is lower in patients with a longer duration of illness (Meltzer et al. 1984), poor premorbid functioning (Malas et al. 1983), and increased negative symptoms (Ferrier et al. 1984). In summary, decreased DA turnover and activity are associated with the severe, stable, chronic, and poor prognosis forms of schizophrenia.

In addition to the reports of increased and decreased CSF HVA or DA turnover, there are reports that CSF HVA concentration is not different in drug-free schizophrenic probands. We suggest that this lack of a difference is observed when a mixed group of schizophrenic patients with varying clinical characteristics are studied together. For instance, Nybäck et al. (1983) reported that VBRs were significantly different from that of normal controls but the CSF HVA level was not. More importantly, they found that the CSF HVA concentration correlated significantly with VBRs only in the schizophrenic patients. This relationship suggests that the so-called "nonspecific" structural brain abnormalities on computed tomography (CT) scans can be specific for schizophrenia. With more focussed examinations of these structural abnormalities with magnetic resonance imaging (MRI) (Bogerts et al. 1990), we may better able to discriminate between changes that are schizophrenia-specific and those that are not. We will not review the proposed etiologies of structural brain abnormalities and decreased DA turnover in schizophrenia, as they have recently been reviewed elsewhere (van Kammen and Kelley 1991).

Dopamine and Nonadrenaline Activity Are Both Involved in Schizophrenia

Similar to increased DA activity, increased NA activity has been related to increased psychotic symptoms (Linnoila et al. 1983). Other relapse-related symptoms, such as paranoia, anxiety, and decreased sleep, even during the prerelapse state, have been linked with hyperadrenergic activity (van Kammen and Antelman 1984; Hornykiewicz 1982; Lake et al. 1980). Plasma HVA and 3-methoxy-4-hydroxyphenylglycol (MHPG) (the main metabolites of DA and NA, respectively) levels correlate significantly with each other (van Kammen and Yao 1990, unpublished data; Chang et al. 1990; Bowers 1988), as do plasma DA and NA levels (Bondy et al. 1984) and CSF NA and DA or $DASO_4$ levels (van Kammen and Antelman 1984). Patients on chronic antipsychotic drug treatment, which decreases both DA and NA turnover, are at risk for developing symptoms that resemble negative symptoms (see Bird and Kornetsky 1990).

Acute D-amphetamine administration, which releases and blocks uptake of both DA and NA, increases emotional tone, motivation, and motor behaviors and can decrease negative symptoms (van Kammen et al. 1982a; Angrist et al. 1981). Chronic high-dose administration of D-amphetamine can lead to both a hallucinatory delusional syndrome and to negative symptoms, including flat affect, emotional withdrawal, and poverty of content of speech (Tatetsu 1963; Angrist et al. 1981; Ellinwood 1967, 1972; Connell 1958). Variability in psychotic symptom response may be explained by the changing baseline relationships between pre- and postsynaptic DA receptor activity, as well as competitive interactions between D-amphetamine's differential effects on the cell body, axons, and terminals (Groves et al. 1988; van Kammen et al. 1982a).

Evidence is accumulating that the NA and DA systems communicate with each other, despite being separate neuronal systems. NA regulates the output of target neurons (Foote et al. 1983), including DA. The two systems interact in the substantia nigra, either directly or indirectly through the serotonin system (Grenhoff and Svensson 1988; Bunney and DeRiemer 1982), in the locus coeruleus (Ornstein et al. 1987), in the prefrontal cortex (Hervé and Le Moal 1988; Goldman-Rakic 1987), and in subcortical structures (Swerdlow and Koob 1989; Hornykiewicz 1982). NA might interact with D_2- (Swerdlow and Koob 1989) or D_1-receptors (van der Heyden et al. 1986), presumably through an α_2-receptor. The α_1- and α_2-receptors may modulate D_2- (Delini and Hunn 1990; Reubenstein et al. 1989; Dickinson et al. 1988) and D_1-receptor activity (Tassin 1989, personal communication). β-receptor stimulation may affect DA release (Reisine et al. 1981; Langer 1981). DA denervation supersensitivity will not be observed in the cortex unless the NA system input into the cortex is at least partially intact (Glowinski et al. 1988). Because of this modulation of DA activity, NA should be considered in the final analysis of negative symptoms (Table 1).

Besides affecting the DA, serotonin, and other neuronal systems, it is likely that NA interacts with glial cells (Stone and Ariano 1990). Adrenergic stimulation leads to glycogenolysis which provides neighboring cells with ATP, glucose, and other metabolic substances. These mechanisms may support the energy demands of neighboring neurons. Decreased NA activity may then lead to insufficient metabolic support for neuronal metabolic demands and could be seen as the cause of hypofrontality (Warkentin et al. 1990; van Kammen and Antelman 1984) associated with clinically stable or remitted conditions. Furthermore, stimulation of α_1- and β-receptors on glial cells alters neuronal activity, presumably through releasing neurotrophic substances as well (for review, see Stone and Ariano 1990).

Table 1. Proposed model of how noradrenaline (NA) affects schizophrenic psychopathology, course, drug response, and outcome. In acutely psychotic patients the range of DA and NA release is increased. NA enhances DA effects on behavior. Increased release of DA and NA is associated with increased symptomatology (model A). In chronic patients, overall DA release is decreased, and the system is less responsive to stimuli that increase release. Increases in NA lead to changes in DA transmission

Model A (acute patients)

↑ NA and ↑ during relapse ⟶ ↑ psychosis

Model B (chronic patients)

↑ NA	Facilitates / Stimulates	D_1/D_2 receptors, α and β-receptors	↓ DA release (presynaptic); ↑ DA receptor stimulation (postsynaptic)	a) normalization; b) ↑ psychosis; c) ↑ negative symptoms

In this chapter, we describe some of the biochemical and pharmacological studies from our group relevant to the negative symptom syndrome in schizophrenia, which may help to explain some of the apparent paradoxes in the literature. These studies highlight in particular some of the problems of the concept of irreversibility of negative symptoms. While all four studies deal with pharmacological and biochemical explorations of the state-dependent influences upon negative symptoms, study IV focuses on the more stable characteristics of negative symptoms. We review the evidence that decreased DA and NA activities relate to negative symptoms, particularly in patients with residual symptomatology, and that increased NA activity leads to increased negative symptoms during psychotic relapse, through inhibiting DA release in the appropriate cortical areas. We hypothesize that psychotic relapse occurs through noradrenergic enhancement of residual psychotic symptoms and certain postsynaptic receptors in chronic patients (amygdala?). The relationship between negative symptoms and structural brain abnormalities, which are associated with decreased catecholamine activity, suggests that decreased DA and NA concentrations are linked to negative symptoms. We will show that the relationship between negative symptoms and catecholamine activity depends on the course and clinical state characteristics of the study sample. Other potential mediators of negative symptoms, such as acetylcholine (Tandon and Greden 1989), somatostatin and cholecystokinin (CCK; Ferrier et al. 1983), neuropeptide Y (Peters et al. 1990), γ-aminobutyric acid (GABA; van Kammen et al. 1982c), or serotonin (for review, see van Kammen and Gelernter 1987), will not be discussed here.

The methodology of the four studies to be discussed will not be extensively described, as all have been previously published. All patients were physically healthy and had a DSM-III or DSM-III R diagnosis of schizophrenia. Informed consent was obtained according to the guidelines of the Department of Health and Human Services. Subjects were rated daily by the blind nursing staff and weekly by the blind therapists with the Bunney-Hamburg global rating scale for psychosis (Bunney and Hamburg 1963). The Brief Psychiatric Rating Scale (BPRS) was also used weekly and, in the infusion studies, before and after the infusion. Negative symptoms were rated with the withdrawal/retardation factor of the BPRS, consisting of the emotional withdrawal, motor retardation, and blunted affect items, as well as the Scale for the Assessment of Negative Symptoms (SANS) (Andreasen 1982). Patients received lumbar punctures between 7:30 and 8:30 a.m. in lateral decubitus position. The procedure and the CSF methodology have been described elsewhere (van Kammen and Sternberg 1980; van Kammen et al. 1989a). Patients were considered to be drug-free after at least 2 weeks without medication. Patients of studies I–III were inpatients at the National Institute of Mental Health Schizophrenia Research Unit at the Clinical Center, National Institutes of Health, Bethesda, Maryland, USA. They ranged in age from 18 to 35 years (mean 24 years). The patients of study IV were admitted to the Schizophrenia Research Unit of the Highland Drive Veterans Administration Medical Center, Pittsburgh, Pennsylvania, USA, and were significantly older (mean 35 years, range 20–50 years).

Study I

Amphetamine Diminishes Negative Symptoms in Schizophrenia

Methods

Thirty schizophrenic patients (17 males and 13 females) with a mean age of 24 years received two infusions of 20 mg D-amphetamine, once after receiving blind placebo capsules for 33 ± 1 days and once after subsequently being treated with pimozide (mean $\pm$ SD: 8 ± 1 mg/day) for a mean of 37 ± 2 days. In the first phase, patients received either 20 mg of D-amphetamine or a saline placebo infusion; 3–5 days later the alternate infusate was given. During the second phase, the placebo infusion was omitted (van Kammen and Boronow 1988).

Results

Drug-Free Condition. After subtracting the placebo response from the amphetamine response, negative symptoms improved significantly following D-amphetamine administration under both the drug-free and pimozide conditions. During the placebo pretreatment, 20 out of 30 patients improved in blunted affect and 6 worsened, while 23/30 scored better and 6/30 worse in the withdrawal/retardation factor. Pimozide had no consistent effect on the BPRS

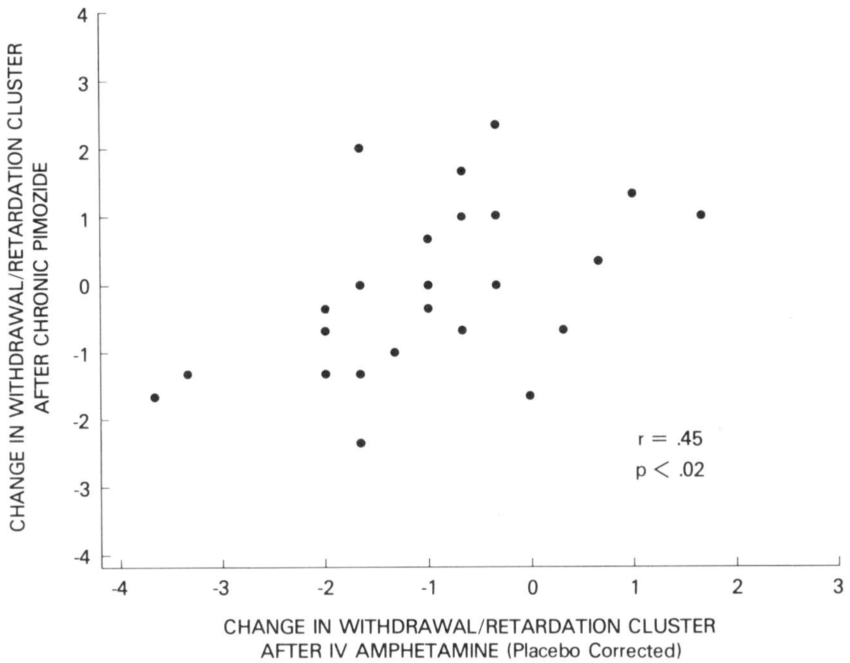

Fig. 1. Improvement of negative symptoms due to amphetamine correlates with improvement in negative symptoms due to pimozide

negative symptoms, although the 8 patients who showed overall improvement with D-amphetamine were distinguished in that pimozide attenuated significantly to the responsiveness of their negative symptoms to D-amphetamine, i.e., they were the only patients who showed the expected blockade of the amphetamine effects on the withdrawal/retardation factor.

Pimozide Effects on the Preinfusion Condition. The 8 patients who globally improved in psychosis with D-amphetamine showed a drop in their withdrawal/retardation cluster while on pimozide. Those subjects whose negative symptoms improved on amphetamine tended to be the same patients whose negative symptoms ultimately improved with pimozide treatment ($r = 0.45$, $P = 0.02$) (Fig. 1).

Negative Symptoms and Depression. Although the withdrawal/retardation cluster is distinct from the depression item and the anxiety/depression cluster of the BPRS, negative symptoms and depressive symptomatology do sometimes overlap. Nevertheless, individual depression item ratings done prior to the amphetamine infusion correlated significantly with the negative symptom cluster ($r = 0.73$, $P < 0.001$) (Fig. 2), which could mean that the raters were not discriminating negative and depressive symptomatology. After the amphetamine infusion, however, the changes in the negative and depressed

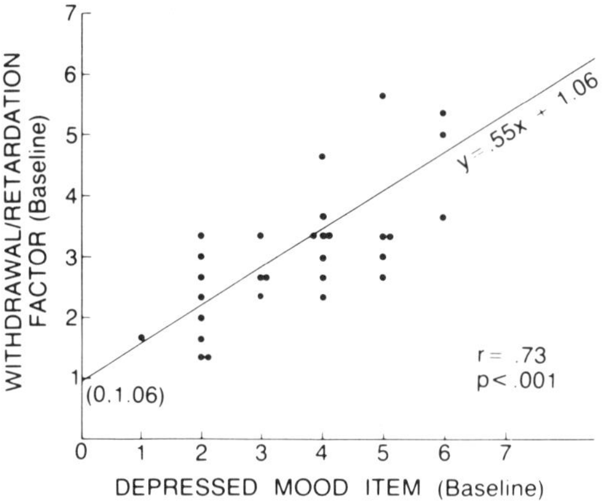

Fig. 2. Correlation of individual depression item ratings with negative symptoms cluster prior to amphetamine infusion

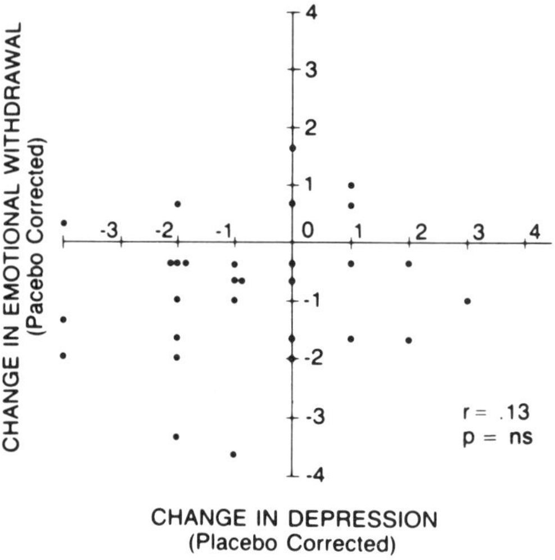

Fig. 3. Change in depressed mood does not correlate with change in withdrawal/retardation factor after amphetamine infusion

symptoms were unrelated ($r = 0.13$, $P = \text{NS}$) (Fig. 3). Only in the 8 patients who improved in psychosis did both negative and depressed symptoms improve.

Comments

D-Amphetamine has been reported to improve, worsen, and leave negative symptoms unchanged (for review see Angrist and van Kammen 1984). The data from this study (van Kammen and Boronow 1988) suggested that the response of negative symptoms to D-amphetamine, similar to positive symptoms, depends on the clinical state of the patient (van Kammen et al. 1982a, b).

Study II

Pimozide Treatment Decreases Negative Symptoms in Schizophrenia: Are Negative Symptoms State Dependent?

Methods

Twelve DSM-III diagnosed schizophrenic patients were drug-free for at least 3 weeks before being placed on double-blind pimozide treatment (6–20 mg/day, mean daily dose 15.2 mg/day). Patients were divided into pimozide improvers and nonimprovers depending on whether they showed improvement in the weekly Bunney-Hamburg global psychosis ratings of 2 points during the 5th week compared with the week prior to initiating pimozide treatment (van Kammen et al. 1987).

Results

In the pimozide responders both the thought disorder ($P < 0.03$) and the withdrawal retardation cluster ($P < 0.04$) improved. Further, in this sample patients who had hallucinations, delusions, and disorganized speech improved during pimozide treatment and also became less withdrawn and emotionally flat and had less motor retardation. Similarly, patients whose positive symptoms persisted remained as plagued with negative symptomatology as they were prior to pimozide treatment. Patients whose positive symptoms worsened during treatment tended to experience an increase in their negative symptoms as well. The patients who improved were similar in their pretreatment global psychosis and BPRS cluster scores, except for the withdrawal/retardation cluster, which was higher. Changes in the thought disorder cluster correlated with the individual negative symptom item changes: emotional withdrawal, $r = 0.61$, $P < 0.03$; motor retardation, $r = 0.60$, $P < 0.04$; and blunted affect, $r = 0.57$, $P < 0.05$.

Comments

In this particular patient sample, negative symptoms improved along with positive ones. We propose that drug-responsive and drug-nonresponsive negative symptoms have a different pathophysiology. Dinan and Aston-Jones (1985) reported that chronic haloperidol treatment decreased the firing rate of certain NA cells in the locus coeruleus, which is consistent with our earlier observation that the CSF NA decreased with pimozide treatment parallel with clinical improvement. Pimozide has been reported to be particularly effective with negative symptoms (Pinder et al. 1976).

Study III

Decreased Dopamine Metabolism in Patients with Cortical Atrophy

Methods

We examined global sulcal widening (GSW) in 31 male and 25 female drug-free schizophrenic patients who also received a lumbar puncture. CSF HVA, DOPAC, and $DASO_4$ levels were measured (van Kammen et al. 1986).

Results

Patients with GSW had significantly lower CSF HVA (188 ± 61.8 vs. 107 ± 46.4 pmol/ml, $P < 0.001$), DOPAC (2.5 ± 1.02 vs. 1.7 ± 0.67 pmol/ml, $P < 0.03$), and conjugated DOPAC (4.5 ± 3.10 vs 2.6 ± 1.73 pmol/ml, NS), but higher $DASO_4$ (3.9 ± 3.21 vs. 6.1 ± 4.80, $n = 33$, $P < 0.08$) levels than patients without GSW. Correlations were significant between GSW and HVA ($r = -0.46$; $n = 50$; $P = 0.0001$), DOPAC ($r = -0.37$; $n = 33$; $P = 0.01$), conjugated DOPAC ($r = -0.30$; $n = 31$; $P < 0.04$), and $DASO_4$ ($r = 0.24$; $n = 33$; $P = 0.08$).

In patients without GSW, the CSF HVA level correlated significantly with the withdrawal/retardation cluster of the BPRS ($r = -0.33$, $n = 32$, $P = 0.03$) and positively with the unusual thought content ($r = 0.35$, $n = 31$, $P < 0.03$). When we performed a mean split on the total DA utilization (CSF HVA + DOPAC + conjugated DOPAC/$DASO_4$) in this group, we found that patients with a low DA utilization had significantly higher ratings of blunted affect (2.8 ± 0.83 vs. 1.8 ± 1.22, $P < 0.05$) and the withdrawal retardation cluster (2.7 ± 1.13 vs. 1.7 ± 0.8, $P < 0.05$).

Study IV

Cerebrospinal Fluid Noradrenaline Level Correlates Positively in Drug-Free Relapsed Patients and Negatively in Drug-Free Stable Patients with Negative Symptoms

Methods

A total of 32 male DSM-III R diagnosed schizophrenic patients (mean age 34 ± 7.6 years) treated with oral maintenance haloperidol (mean dose 12 mg/day) participated after signing informed consent forms. CSF NA, 3-methoxy-4-hydroxyphenylglycol (MHPG), and HVA levels were determined with high-performance liquid chromatography (HPLC) (van Kammen et al. 1989a, 1990). After discontinuation of haloperidol, patients were placed on placebo for up to 6 weeks. Relapse was determined by an increase of 3 points in a 3-day mean of the Bunney-Hamburg psychosis ratings. Lumbar punctures were performed at the time of relapse ($n = 14$, 22 ± 11 days drug-free) or after 6 weeks of placebo in patients who did not relapse ($n = 18$, 45 ± 8 days) (van Kammen et al. 1989a).

Results

CSF NA was significantly higher in the haloperidol-treated patients who relapsed subsequent to haloperidol withdrawal (0.79 ± 0.356 vs. 0.52 ± 0.348 nmol/ml; $P = 0.04$, two-tailed). None of the CSF monoamine metabolites were distinguished between the two groups while on haloperidol. In the entire drug-free group, positive correlations of CSF NA and MHPG with negative ($r = 0.50$, $P = 0.006$; $r = 0.41$, $P = 0.024$, respectively) and positive symptoms ($r = 0.56$, $P = 0.001$; $r = 0.50$, $P = 0.005$, respectively) were observed. CSF NA and MHPG were significantly higher in the drug-free relapsers than in the nonrelapsers. CSF HVA was not significantly different between groups and did not change significantly following drug withdrawal in the total group of chronic schizophrenic patients. SANS ratings correlated significantly with psychosis scores ($r = 0.69$, $P < 0.0001$). In the drug-free patients, the correlations of CSF NA and MHPG with negative symptoms remained positive in the relapsers but became negative but nonsignificant in the drug-free, stable patients (Table 2).

Table 2. Two-tailed correlation coefficients for negative symptoms and psychosis rating before lumbar puncture (Bunney and Hamburg, 1963) in patients treated with haloperidol

	Relapsers		Nonrelapsers	
	NA	MHPG	NA	MHPG
Affective flattening	$r = 0.41$ NS	0.37 NS	$r = -0.08$ NS	0.15 NS
Alogia	$r = 0.50$ $P = 0.076$	0.43 NS	$r = -0.25$ NS	−0.31 NS
Avolition-apathy	$r = 0.40$ NS	0.28 NS	$r = -0.41$ NS	−0.39 NS
Anhedonia-asociality	$r = 0.52$ $P = 0.068$	0.70 0.012	$r = -0.06$ NS	−0.28 NS
Attentional impairment	$r = 0.60$ $P = 0.031$	0.62 0.030	$r = -0.12$ NS	−0.23 NS
Total score	$r = 0.54$ $P = 0.059$	0.52 0.085	$r = -0.24$ NS	−0.28 NS
Psychosis	$r = 0.57$ $P = 0.040$	0.73 0.008	$r = 0.06$ NS	0.01 NS

NA = noradrenaline.

Comments

The increases in CSF NA and MHPG levels in the relapsers suggested that positive and negative symptoms may be increased through the same mechanisms, i.e., elevated NA turnover. This observation may explain why Sternberg et al. (1981) did not observe a relationship between CSF NA and psychosis in their drug-free patients, whose clinical state was not well-defined. Based upon the elevated CSF NA levels prior to haloperidol withdrawal and the subsequent relapse, and the further significant decline in CSF NA in the nonrelapsers following haloperidol withdrawal, we propose that NA activity is relatively increased as a prodrome of psychotic relapse and that clinical stability is associated with normal or decreased CSF NA levels. In this sample the CSF HVA concentration did not correlate significantly with negative or positive symptoms. Conceivably, adrenergic receptor stimulation may have led to decreases in DA release (Reisine et al. 1981; Langer 1981; van der Heyden et al. 1986; Delini and Hunn 1990) with (i.e., relapsers) and without (i.e., nonrelapsers) postsynaptic DA-receptor activation in these patients. In other words, increased NA levels can lead to a relapse in schizophrenia if there is already a DA disturbance.

Discussion

The presented studies support both a role of decreased DA function and the concept of multiple pathophysiologies of negative symptoms. Studies of the relapse process (Docherty et al. 1978; Herz and Melville 1980; Szymanski et al. 1983) suggest that negative symptoms may emerge or worsen as prodromal symptoms to a psychotic episode (Table 3), remain as residual symptoms following resolution of the psychotic exacerbation (Miller 1989; Docherty et al. 1978), or be a part of the basic disturbance (Gross 1989). In some cases, negative symptoms may also be present prior to the development of psychotic symptoms. Carpenter et al. (1988) suggested that negative symptoms should be divided into primary (deficit syndrome) and secondary (with psychotic symptoms or neuroleptic treatment), whereas van Kammen and coworkers proposed a division into drug-responsive, drug-nonresponsive or residual, and drug-induced symptoms (van Kammen et al. 1987, 1989 a, 1990; van Kammen and Boronow 1988). These studies indicate that negative symptoms can fluctuate and respond to pharmacological interventions, in other words are *state-dependent*. Residual symptoms or the severity of negative symptoms, however, do relate to presumed trait measures such as GSW and VBR, premorbid functioning, and decreased slow-wave sleep. In other words, they are also *state-independent*. Whether negative symptoms correlate with state-dependent or -independent biochemical or other measures seems to depend on the major clinical state of the patient sample. The variable relationships of negative symptoms with CSF NA and MHPG emphasize the need to define the clinical state of the patients being studied (van Kammen et al. 1985). We suggest

Table 3.

Staging		Symptoms
Equilibrium		Normal optimal functioning; spacing of demands; appropriate relating and performing
Overextension		Subject feels "stressed out", "too much going on" at any one time, difficulty in dealing with information overload; strange bodily sensations; energy level not up to demand
Withdrawal		Depressive symptoms; negative symptoms; definite lack of energy; decreased motivation; decreased volition; negativism; emotional withdrawal; motor retardation
Prepsychotic/hypomanic	*A*	Increased energy level; increased motivation; feels "better than ever"; sexually preoccupied; new initiatives; * therapist may join with patient in believing that the illness is permanently under control
	B	Decreased sleep or lack of sleep; angry, hostile, loosening of associations; increased or reoccurrence of psychotic symptoms
Psychotic episode	*A*	Increased and fleeting delusions; increased hallucinations; confused, disorganized speech; incoherent, schizophasia; ambivalent; negativistic, angry, hostile
	B	Crystallized delusions, ongoing hallucinations; deterioration in self-care and average daily activities
Psychotic stabilization		More stable clinical picture; residual symptoms of varying intensity; crystallized delusions

that structural brain abnormalities should not be equated with the deficit syndrome (which is a behavioral syndrome) per se. It is conceivable, however, that the deficit syndrome is more likely to be observed in its pure form in clinically stable patients with such structural brain abnormalities. These differential interactions between negative symptoms, clinical state, neuroleptic status, and CSF monoamine metabolites may explain some of the discrepancies observed in the literature.

Decreased Cerebrospinal Fluid Homovanillic Acid Level and Negative Symptoms

Our data indicate that decreased DA turnover in clinically stable patients is associated with negative symptoms, albeit in a complex way. Several groups, whom we expect to have studied mainly clinically stable, drug-free patients, related anergia or other negative symptoms to decreased CSF or urinary HVA (Beckmann et al. 1983; Lindström 1985; Friedhoff 1988; Wyatt 1986; Meltzer 1984; Alpert et al. 1978). Although study III indicated that decreased CSF HVA was associated with negative symptoms in patients with normal CT scan readings, in study IV no such relationship was observed in the drug-free patients. Both age and chronicity may have played a role in study IV. Several groups were unable to find a clear positive relationship between negative symptoms and ventricular enlargement or cortical atrophy (Andreasen et al. 1982; Bishop et al. 1983; Luchins et al. 1984; Ota et al. 1987; Miller 1989), while others did (Kemali et al. 1986; Pandurangi et al. 1988; Takahashi et al. 1981). This means that (a) structural brain abnormalities are not the sole contributors to decreased DA activity or negative symptoms and (b) that negative symptoms can be state-dependent. When so many clinical descriptors, as discussed in the Introduction, are associated with decreased CSF HVA, it becomes important to know how they are distributed in a given study sample.

State-dependent changes in the underlying biochemistry (van Kammen et al. 1985) may explain these inconsistent findings. Even though cortical atrophy and enlarged VBRs tend to be associated with a decreased catecholamine turnover (van Kammen et al. 1983, 1986; Nybäck et al. 1983), DA and NA levels can still fluctuate with clinical state (van Kammen et al. 1985). Decreased DA and NA turnover, regardless of evidence of structural brain abnormalities, seem to be associated with negative symptoms in the residual state of chronic schizophrenic patients. It is therefore of interest that Warkentin et al. (1990) observed that the hypofrontality observed with cerebral blood flow measures was a function of the patient's clinical state. Regional cerebral blood flow reflects metabolic activity. Conceivably, it is under monoaminergic influence (Edvinsson and Owman 1974).

Variable Dopamine Activity in The Brain

The internal dynamics of DA in the brain are complex. Decreased DA activity in the prefrontal cortex leads to increased DA activity in the nucleus accumbens (Glowinski et al. 1988; Pycock et al. 1980) or corpus striatum (Carter and Pycock 1980). Through the work of Glowinski and Pycock and associates and that of Goldman-Rakic (1987), who reported cortico-cortical connections, the simultaneous presence of increased and decreased catecholamine activity in different parts of the brain might become understandable. These topically different activities of DA suggest that the normal adaptive ability of the cortex is impaired in schizophrenia. CSF HVA may reflect the total HVA production in the brain, irrespective of where it came from and how much was removed on the way to the lumbar region. CSF HVA may, however, provide more information about cortical DA than of striatal DA turnover (Elsworth et al. 1987). The association of decreased CSF HVA levels, cortical lesions, and negative symptoms is consistent with the work of Wyatt et al. (1989), who observed a loss of cortical DA terminals and "negative symptoms" in rats treated with cocaine. Plasma HVA has sometimes been found to be more informative than CSF HVA. This may be because of the effects of the gradient on lumbar CSF HVA, or that the central autonomic nervous system affects peripheral DA turnover, or vice versa. It is conceivable that the peripheral autonomic nervous system modulates the central nervous system (CNS) DA activity in schizophrenia, comparable to but not similar to the regulation of the locus coeruleus by the autonomic nervous system (Svensson 1987).

Increased and Decreased Noradrenaline Activity and Negative Symptoms

We interpreted the data of study IV to indicate that the increase in CSF NA preceded relapse and led to symptom aggravation, regardless of whether the symptoms were positive or negative. This increase in "gain" with increased NA levels is consistent with the proposed role of the locus coeruleus in the brain: increasing the output of target neurons (Foote et al. 1983). Many patients report decreases in intensity of voices or decreased preoccupation with hallucinations and delusions with improvement or increases in symptom intensity with worsening as if the "gain" is turned up. Furthermore, following depletion of DA, NA stimulates behavioral activation in the nucleus accumbens (Swerdlow and Koob 1989). These observations are consistent with our hypothesis that increased NA is necessary for the DA disorder to be expressed, even in the presence of low or normal HVA levels (D_2-receptor supersensitivity?) (van Kammen et al. 1990).

Inversely, in the residual state, decreased NA turnover may lead to decreased emotions, motivation, and energy, i.e., negative symptoms. This mutual relationship suggests that negative symptoms should fluctuate or sometimes disappear prior to relapse. In other words, they can be both state-dependent and -independent. This has indeed been observed (Johnstone et al. 1986; Herz and Melville 1980; Szymanski et al. 1983; van Kammen et al. 1975, unpublished observations). This may also explain why Angrist et al. (1980) reported that D-amphetamine did not change or even worsened negative symptoms in chronic schizophrenic inpatients, but in an outpatient group they (Angrist et al. 1982) observed an improvement in negative symptoms. Not only do depression and negative symptoms have some aspects in common, CSF NA can also be increased and CSF HVA concentration decreased in some depressed patients (Post et al. 1981; Jimerson et al. 1984). Study I indicates, however, that under amphetamine stimulation, negative and depressive symptomatology seem to be separable.

Noradrenergic input that is at least partially intact is required for the development of D_1 denervation supersensitivity (Glowinski et al. 1988). Lesions in the primary sulcus area (i.e., the prefrontal cortex) in nonhuman primates can lead to problems with working memory which can be restored by clonidine (Goldman-Rakic 1987). Consistent with this NA-DA connection, Fields et al. (1988) reported that treatment with the α_2-receptor agonist clonidine has improved memory in schizophrenic patients, regardless of changes in clinical state. Clonidine decreased CSF MHPG, and increased CSF HVA (van Kammen et al. 1989b); so, even though the lesion is hypothesized to be in a major DA projection field, stimulation of α_2-receptors will affect behaviors associated with this cortical area. van Kammen et al. (1989b) observed antipsychotic and antinegative symptom effects with clonidine treatment in patients with increased or normal α_2-receptor function. The above-reviewed relationship between the DA and the NA systems supports further the interpretations that both DA and NA are decreased in the deficit or residual syndrome. Optimal integration of inputs from the projections to other cortical areas and the amygdala are required for the individual to behave "normally."

Lohr and Jeste (1988) reported a decrease in cell volume in DSM-III schizophrenic patients, and Gay et al. (1989) reported increased dopamine β-hydroxylase (DBH) activity in the locus coeruleus area in postmortem brains of paranoid schizophrenic patients. Lesions in the locus coeruleus can lead to both increases and decreases of certain components of the NA metabolism. Nonnoradrenergic cell loss may lead to increased NA activity if inhibitory inputs are removed or to increased brain stem DBH levels because of a relative increase in DBH per mg protein. Although paranoid schizophrenia has been associated with decreased plasma DBH activity, there are also reports of increased CSF (Lake et al. 1980) and postmortem brain NA (Farley et al. 1978) in paranoid schizophrenic patients. Thus, it is conceivable but still unproven that the proposed dysregulation of NA activity is due to cell loss in the locus coeruleus.

Wing (1989) pointed out that there seems to be at least two environmental processes that may interact with biological vulnerability. Under conditions of social overstimulation (increased NA or DA turnover?) psychotic decompensation may occur, whereas with social deprivation symptoms such as passivity, social withdrawal and lack of initiative tend to increase (decreased DA and NA turnover?) (Wing 1989). Negative symptoms can be a defense; if they reflect a *less responsive* DA and NA system, they may also be associated with a decreased risk of relapse. On the other hand, negative symptoms under stimulus overload conditions may be a precursor to developing florid symptomatology, when associated with increased DA activity in the amygdala (van Kammen and Kelley 1991). This formulation suggests that only under optimal stimulus conditions will patients reach their optimal functioning.

Neuroleptic Treatment and Negative Symptoms

In general, negative symptoms seem to be mostly resistant to antipsychotic drug treatment. Reports, however, indicate that negative symptoms both respond (Goldberg 1985; van Kammen et al. 1987; Tandon et al. 1990; Rosen et al. 1984) and do not respond (Crow 1980a, b; Carpenter et al. 1988) to neuroleptics. In patients with residual negative symptoms who are optimally treated with neuroleptics, the deficit syndrome may be observed. On the other hand, patients who responded well to pimozide had higher pretreatment negative symptoms than those who did not respond (van Kammen et al. 1987) and showed a stronger decline in CSF NA with pimozide treatment (Sternberg et al. 1981). Patients with lower plasma HVA and MHPG tend to respond later or more poorly to neuroleptics (Chang et al. 1990; Bowers et al. 1986; Bowers 1988; van Putten et al. 1989; Garver et al. 1990).

Just as neuroleptics can induce or maintain residual positive symptoms (van Kammen et al. 1990; Marder et al. 1979; van Putten et al. 1974), negative symptoms can be drug-induced as well. Antipsychotic drugs may induce or worsen negative symptoms (Lehman and Hanrahan 1954) through decreased

DA transmission (Bird and Kornetsky 1990). That this effect is not constant but also under state-dependent control is shown in study IV. In the nonrelapsers, haloperidol withdrawal was associated with significant improvement in the withdrawal/retardation cluster of the BPRS but not in the SANS scores. There is recent evidence that clozapine may improve negative symptoms more than the traditional antipsychotic drugs that show extrapyramidal side effects. The lack of change in the nigrostriatal pathway with clozapine suggests that the residual negative symptoms on haloperidol may be, at least in part, secondary to parkinsonian side effects and as such could be drug-induced. That clonidine has a therapeutic effect on akathisia supports the possibility of treating *drug-induced* negative symptoms with clonidine. It is important that we make this differentiation among negative symptoms (Carpenter et al. 1988; van Kammen et al. 1987), because most negative symptom studies will be performed in medicated patients.

Conclusions

The insufficiency or low energy states in schizophrenia that among others Kraepelin (1893) and Berze (1914) described, e.g., anergia, passivity, and neurasthenia, may be explained by decreased NA and cortical DA activity. The proposed state-dependent changes in DA and NA turnover related to psychotic relapse (van Kammen et al. 1982a, b, 1985, 1987) can now also be extended to the regulation of negative symptoms. The interactions between NA and DA (Table 1) as well as the differential DA activity (depending on brain area and clinical state) may help us to understand the observations of too much and too little DA and NA in schizophrenia.

Our inability to diagnose different negative symptoms has led to contradictory findings and has hampered our attempts to validate the concept biochemically. Similarly, attempts to validate different subtypes of schizophrenia have not consistently been successful. The data indicate that the different clinical components that make up the Type II syndrome are usually not present all at the same time; each of these characteristics describes only partially overlapping groups. This syndrome reflects several clinical dimensions of severity rather than a distinct and separate clinical entity or category.

We have previously proposed a standardization of reporting clinical, demographic, and procedural data in CSF studies of schizophrenic patients (van Kammen and Sternberg 1980). We now propose to define schizophrenic patients in biological studies – when possible – as having a progressive or intermittent disorder, with residual symptoms or being fully remitted, clinically stable, subacute, or relapsed, with or without negative symptoms. In addition, we suggest that negative symptoms should be labeled drug-nonresponsive or residual, drug-responsive, and drug-induced (Table 4). Another way would be primary and secondary symptoms as proposed by Carpenter et al. (1988). This categorization is not always easily done in cross-sectional study designs. It requires that the investigator know his patients clinically for at least several

Table 4. Proposed categorization of negative symptoms with dopamine (DA), noradrenaline (NA), and homovanillic (HVA) activities for future research

Drug responsive	↑ or =	HVA
	↑	DA receptors
	↑	NA
Drug induced	↓ or ↑	HVA
	↓	DA receptors
	?	NA
Drug nonresponsive (residual/deficit)	↓	HVA
	↓	DA receptors
	(↓	NA)

months. It is important to note that these categories are not mutually exclusive; further studies will have to determine whether defining the negative symptoms with a more process-oriented approach is indeed meaningful in biochemical and pharmacological studies. We expect that through more practical guidelines for diagnosis and clinical descriptions, the concept of negative symptoms can be biologically validated and its etiology revealed.

Acknowledgements. We wish to thank the patients and nursing staff under Sylvia Beal, RN, of the National Institute of Mental Health (NIMH) Clinical Research Unit 4E in the Clinical Center NIH, Bethesda, MD, and the patients and nursing staff under Doris McAdam, RN, of the Schizophrenia Research Unit of the Highland Drive VA MC, Pittsburgh, PA. Without their collaboration, participation, and support, we could not have done the necessary drug-free studies that have led to our present formulation of the role of DA and NA in negative schizophrenia. Funding for this paper was provided to Dr. van Kammen in part by the Highland Drive DVAMC, DVA merit review funding and NIMH grant RO1MH44841-01.

References

Alpert M, Friedhoff AJ, Marcos LR, Diamond F (1978) Paradoxical reaction to L-Dopa in schizophrenic patients. Am J Psychiatry 135:1329–1332

Andreasen NC (1982) Negative symptoms in schizophrenia: definition and reliability. Arch Gen Psychiatry 39:7

Andreasen NC, Smith MR, Jacoby CG, Dennert JW, Olsen SA (1982) Ventricular enlargement in schizophrenia: definition and prevalence. Am J Psychiatry 139:292–298

Angrist B, van Kammen DP (1984) CNS stimulants as tools in the study of schizophrenia. Trends Neurosci 7:388–390

Angrist B, Rotrosen J, Gershon S (1980) Responses to apomorphine, amphetamine, and neuroleptics in schizophrenic subjects. Psychopharmacology (Berlin) 67:31–38

Angrist B, Burrows GD, Lader M, Lingjaerde O, Sedvall G, Wheatly D (1981) Relationships between responses to dopamine agonists: psychopathology, neuroleptic treatment response, and need for neurleptic maintenance in schizophrenic subjects. In: Angrist B,

Peselow E, Rotrosen J, Gershon S (eds) Recent advances in neuropsychopharmacology. Pergamon, Oxford, pp 49–54

Angrist B, Peselow E, Rubinstein M, Corwin J, Rotrosen J (1982) Partial improvement in negative schizophrenic symptoms after amphetamine. Psychopharmacology (Berlin) 78:128–130

Beckmann H, Waldmeier P, Lauber J, Gattaz WF (1983) Phenylethylamine and monamine metabolites in CSF of schizophrenics: effects of neuroleptic treatment. J Neurol Transm 57:103–110

Berze J (1914) Die primäre Insuffizienz der psychischen Aktivität. Deuticke, Leipzig

Bird M, Kornetsky C (1990) Dissociation of the attentional and motivational effects of pimozide on the threshold for rewarding brain stimulation. Neuropsychopharmacology 3:33–40

Bishop RJ, Golden CJ, McInnes WD, Chu C-C, Ruedrich SL, Wilson J (1983) The BPRS in assessing symptom correlates of cerebral enlargement in acute and chronic schizophrenia. Psychiatry Res 9:225–231

Bogerts B, Ashtari M, Degreef G, Alvir JMJ, Bilder RM, Lieberman JA (1990) Reduced temporal limbic structure volumes on magnetic resonance images in first episode schizophrenia. Psychiatry Res 35:1–13

Bondy B, Ackenheil M, Birzle W, Elbers R, Frohler M (1984) Catecholamines and their receptors in blood: evidence for alterations in schizophrenia. Biol Psychiatry 19:1377–1393

Bowers MB (1974) Central dopamine turnover in schizophrenic syndromes. Arch Gen Psychiatry 31:50–54

Bowers MB Jr (1988) Plasma monoamine metabolites in psychotic disorders. Arch Gen Psychiatry 45:564–567

Bowers MB, Rozitis A (1974) Regional differences in homovanillic acid concentrations after acute and chronic administration of antipsychotic drugs. J Pharmacol 26:743–745

Bowers MB, Study RE (1979) Cerebrospinal fluid cyclic amp and acid monoamine metabolites following probenecid: studies in psychiatric patients. Psychopharmacology (Berlin) 62:17–22

Bowers MB, Swigar E, Jatlow PI, Hoffman F, Giocoechea N (1986) Early neuroleptic response in psychotic men and women: correlation with plasma HVA and MHPG. Comp Psychiatry 27:181–185

Breier A, Wolkowitz OM, Doran AR, Roy A, Boronow J, Hommer DW, Pickar D (1987) Neuroleptic responsivity of negative and positive symptoms in schizophrenia. Am J Psychiatry 144:1549–1555

Bunney BS, DeRiemer S (1982) Effect of clonidine on dopaminergic neuron activity in the substantia nigra: possible indirect mediation by noradrenergic regulation of the serotonergic raphi system. Adv Neurol 35:99–104

Bunney WE Jr, Hamburg DA (1963) Methods for reliable longitudinal observation of behavior. Arch Gen Psychiatry 9:280–294

Carlsson A (1978) Does dopamine have a role in schizophrenia? Biol Psychiatry 13:3–21

Carpenter WT, Heinrichs DW, Wagman AMI (1988) Deficit and nondeficit forms of schizophrenia: the concept. Am J Psychiatry 145:578–583

Carter CJ, Pycock CJ (1980) Behavioural and biochemical effects of dopamine and noradrenaline depletion within the medial prefrontal cortex of the rat. Brain Res 192:163–176

Chang W-H, Chen T-Y, Lin S-K, Lung F-W, Lin W-L, Hu W-H, Yeh E-K (1990) Plasma catecholamine metabolites in schizophrenics: Evidence for the two type concept. Biol Psychiatry 27:510–518

Connell PH (1958) Amphetamine psychosis. Chapman and Hall, London (Maudsley monograph, no 5)

Crow TJ (1980a) Molecular pathology of schizophrenia: more than one disease process? Br Med J 280:66–68

Crow TJ (1980b) Positive and negative schizophrenic symptoms and the role of dopamine. Br J Psychiatry 137:383–386

Deline A, Hunn C (1990) Effects of single and repeated treatment with antidepressants on apomorphine-induced yawning in the rat: the implications of α_1 adrenergic mechanisms in the D_2 receptor function. Psychopharmacology (Berlin) 101:62–66

Dickinson SL, Gadie B, Tulloch IF (1988) Alpha, and alpha$_2$ adrenoreceptor antagonists differentially influence locomotor and stereotyped behavior induced by d-amphetamine and apomorphine in the rat. Psychopharmacology (Berlin) 96:521–527

Dinan TG, Aston-Jones G (1985) Chronic haloperidol inactivates brain noradrenergic neurons. Brain Res 325:385–388

Docherty JP, van Kammen DP, Siris SG, Marder SR (1978) Stages of onset of schizophrenic psychosis. Am J Psychiatry 135:420–426

Doran AR, Boronow J, Weinberger DR, Wolkowitz OM, Breier A, Pickar D (1987) Structural brain pathology in schizophrenia revisited-prefrontal cortex pathology is inversely correlated with cerebrospinal fluid levels of homovanillic acid. Neuropsychopharmacology 1:25–32

Edvinsson L, Owman C (1974) Pharmacological characterization of alpha and beta receptors mediating the vasomotor responses of cerebral arteries in vitro. Circ Res 35:853–849

Ellinwood EH Jr (1967) Amphetamine psychosis: a description of the individuals and process. J Nerv Ment Dis 144:273–283

Ellinwood EH Jr (1972) Amphetamine psychosis: individuals, settings and sequences. In: Ellinwood EH Jr, Cohen S (eds) Current concepts on amphetamine abuse. US Department of Health, Education and Welfare, Washington (Publication 72-9085)

Elsworth JD, Leahy DJ, Roth RH, Redmond DE (1987) Homovanillic acid concentrations in brain, CSF and plasma as indicators of central dopamine function in primates. J Neural Transm 68:51–62

Farley IJ, Price KS, McCullough E, Deck JH, Hordynski W, Hornykiewicz O (1978) Norepinephrine in chronic paranoid schizophrenia: above-normal levels in limbic forebrain. Science 200:456–458

Feinberg I, Braun M, Koresko RL, Gottlieb F (1969) Stage 4 sleep in schizophrenia. Arch Gen Psychiatry 21:262–266

Ferrier IN, Roberts GW, Crow TJ, Johnstone EC, Owens DGC, Lee YC, O'Shaughnessy D, Adrian TE, Polak JM, Bloom SR (1983) Reduced cholecystokinin-like and somatostatin-like immunoreactivity in limbic lobe is associated with negative symptoms in schizophrenia. Life Sci 33:475–482

Ferrier IN, Johnstone EC, Crow TJ (1984) Hormonal effects of apomorphine in schizophrenia. Br J Psychiatry 144:349–357

Fields RB, van Kammen DP, Peters JL, Rosen J, van Kammen WB, Nugent A, Stipetic M, Linnoila M (1988) Clonidine improves memory function in schizophrenia independently from change in psychosis. Schizophr Res 1:417–423

Foote SL, Bloom FE, Aston-Jones G (1983) Nucleus locus coeruleus: new evidence of anatomical and physiological specificity. Physiol Rev 63:844–914

Friedhoff AJ (1988) Dopamine as a mediator of a central stabilizing system. Neuropsychopharmacology 1:189–191

Ganguli R, Reynolds CF III, Kupfer DJ (1987) Electroencephalographic sleep in young, never-medicated schizophrenics. Arch Gen Psychiatry 44:36–44

Garver DL, Yao J, van Kammen DP (1990) Dopamine, HVA and early neuroleptic response. Proc Am Psychiatr Assoc 143:247

Gay N, Cottreaux JA, Denoroy L, Tomassi M, Kopp N (1989) Possible increase of dopamine-beta-hydroxylase activity in the locus coeruleus of paranoid schizophrenic patients: a preliminary postmortem study. Psychiatry Res 27:31–38

Glowinski J, Hervé D, Tassin JP (1988) Heterologous regulation of receptors on target cells of dopamine neurons in the prefrontal cortex, nucleus accumbens and striatum. Ann NY Acad Sci 137:112–123

Goldberg SC (1985) Negative and deficit symptoms in schizophrenia do respond to neuroleptics. Schizophr Bull 11:453–456

Goldberg SC, Schooler NR, Mattson N (1967) Paranoid and withdrawal symptoms in schizophrenia: differential symptom reduction over time. J Nerv Ment Dis 145:158–162

Goldman-Rakic PS (1987) Circuitry of primate prefrontal cortex and regulation of behavior by representational memory. In: Plum E (ed) Higher functions of the brain. Handbook of physiology, the nervous system, Sect. 1, vol 5. American Physiological Society, Bethesda, pp 373–417

Grenhoff J, Svensson TH (1988) Clonidine regularizes substantia nigra dopamine cell firing. Life Sci 42:2003–2009

Gross G (1989) The "basic" symptoms of schizophrenia. Br J Psychiatry [Suppl 7] 177:21–25

Groves P, Ryan L, Diana M, Gariano R (1988) Neurophysiological consequences of amphetamine administration. Natl Inst Drug Abuse Monogr Ser 90:213–222

Guelfi GP, Faustman WO, Csernansky JG (1989) Independence of positive and negative symptoms in a population of schizophrenic patients. j Nerv Ment Dis 177:285–290

Harvey I, McGuffin P, Williams M, Toone BK (1990) The ventricle-brain ratio (VBR) in functional psychoses: an admixture analysis. Psychiatry Res 35:61–69

Hervé S, Le Moal M (1988) Mesencephalic dopaminergic neurons: role in the general economy of the brain. Ann NY Acad Sci 537:235–253

Herz MI, Melville C (1980) Relapse in schizophrenia. Am J Psychiatry 137:801–805

Hornykiewicz O (1982) Brain catecholamine in schizophrenia – a good case for noradrenaline. Nature 299:484–486

Houston JP, Mass JW, Bowden CL, Contreras SA, McIntyre KL, Javors MA (1986) Cerebrospinal fluid HVA, central brain atrophy, and clinical state in schizophrenia. Psychiatry Res 19:207–214

Janes SM, Mu D, Wemmer D, Smith AJ, Kaur S, Maltby D, Burlingame AL, Klinmans J (1990) A new redox cofactor in eukaryotic enzymes: 6-hydroxydopamine at the active site of bovine serum amine oxidase. Science 248:981–987

Jennings WS, Schulz SC, Narasimhachari N, Hamer RM, Friedel RO (1985) Brain ventricular size and CSF monoamine metabolites in an adolescent inpatient population. Psychiatry Res 16:87–94

Jimerson DC, Rubinow DR, Ballenger JC, Post RM, Kopin IJ (1984) Cerebrospinal fluid norepinephrine metabolites in depressed patients: new methodologies. In: Usdin E, Carlsson A, Dahlstrom A, Engel J (eds) Catecholamines. Neuropharmacology and central nervous system – therapeutic aspects. Liss, New York, pp 123–129

Johnstone E, Owens D, Frith C, Crow T (1986) The relative stability of positive and negative feature in chronic schizophrenia. Br J Psychiatry 150:60–64

Karoum F, Karson CN, Bigelow LB, Lawson WB, Wyatt RJ (1987) Preliminary evidence of reduced combined output of dopamine and its metabolites in chronic schizophrenia. Arch Gen Psychiatry 44:604–607

Keefe RSE, Mohs RC, Losonczy MF, Davidson M, Silverman JM, Kendler KS, Horvath TB, Nora R, Davis KL (1987) Characteristics of very poor outcome schizophrenia. Am J Psychiatry 144:889–895

Kemali D, Maj M, Galderisi S, Salvati A, Starace F, Valente A, Pirozzi R (1986) Clinical, biological, and neuropsychological features associated with lateral ventricular enlargement in DSM-III schizophrenic disorder. Psychiatry Res 21:137–149

Kraepelin E (1893) Psychiatrie: ein kurzes Lehrbuch für Studierende und Ärzte. Abel, Leipzig

Lake CR, Sternberg DE, van Kammen DP, Ballenger JC, Ziegler MG, Post RM, Kopin IJ, Bunney WE Jr (1980) Schizophrenia: elevated cerebrospinal fluid norepinephrine. Science 207:331–333

Langer AZ (1981) Presynaptic regulation of the release of catecholamines. Pharmacol Rev 32:337–362

Lehman HE, Hanrahan GE (1954) Chlorpromazine, a new inhibiting agent for psychomotor excitement and manic states. AMA Arch Neurol Psychiatry 71:227–237

Levins S (1984) Frontal lobe dysfunctions in schizophrenia. II. Impairments of psychological and brain functions. J Psychiatr Res 18:57–72

Lindström LH (1985) Low HVA and normal 5-HIAA CSF levels in drug free schizophrenic patients compared to healthy volunteers: correlations to symptomatology and family history. Psychiatry Res 14:265–273

Linnoila M, Ninan PT, Scheinin M, Waters RN, Chang WH, Bartko J, van Kammen DP (1983) Reliability of norepinephrine and major monoamine metabolite measurements in CSF of schizophrenic patients. Arch Gen Psychiatry 40:1290–1294
Lohr JB, Jeste DV (1988) Locus coeruleus morphometry in aging and schizophrenia. Acta Psychiatr Scand 77:689–697
Losonczy MF, Song IS, Mohs RC, Mathé AA, Davidson M, Davis BM, Davis KL (1986) Correlates of lateral ventricular size in chronic schizophrenia. II. Biological measures. Am J Psychiatry 143:1113–1118
Luchins DJ, Lewine RRJ, Meltzer HY (1984) Lateral ventricular size, psychopathology, and medication response in the psychoses. Biol Psychiatry 19:29–44
Mackay AVP (1980) Positive and negative schizophrenic symptoms and the role of dopamine. Br J Psychiatry 137:379–383
Malas KL, van Kammen DP, Defraites EA, Brown GM, Gold PW (1983) Platelet monoamine oxidase and the growth hormone response to apomorphine in schizophrenia. Biol Psychiatry 18:255–259
Marder SP, van Kammen DP, Bunney WE Jr (1979) Prediction drug-free improvement from schizophrenic psychosis. Arch Gen Psychiatry 36:1080–1085
Meltzer H (1984) Dopamine and negative symptoms in schizophrenia: critique of the type I–II hypotheses. In: Alpert M (ed) Controversies in schizophrenia: changes and consistencies. Guilford, New York, pp 110–144
Meltzer HY, Kolakowska T, Fang VS, Fogg L, Robertson A, Lewine R, Strahilevitz M, Busch D (1984) Growth hormone and prolactin response to apomorphine in schizophrenia and the major affective disorders. Arch Gen Psychiatry 41:512–519
Miller R (1989) Schizophrenia as a progressive disorder: relations to EEG, CT, neuropathological and other evidence. Prog Neurobiol 33:17–44
Miller R, Wickens JR, Beninger RJ (1990) Dopamine D-1 and D-2 receptors in relationship to reward and performance; a case for the D-1 receptor for the primary site of the therapeutic action of neuroleptic drugs. Prog Neurobiol 34:143–183
Nybäck H, Berggren BM, Hindmarsh T (1983) Cerebroventricular size and cerebrospinal fluid monamine metabolites in schizophrenic patients and healthy volunteers. Psychiatry Res 9:301–308
Ornstein K, Milon H, McRae-Degueurce A, Alvarez C, Berger B, Wurzner HP (1987) Biochemical and radioautographic evidence for dopaminergic afferents of the locus coeruleus originating in the ventral tegmental area. J Neurol Transm 70:183–191
Ota T, Maeshiro H, Ishido H, Shimizu Y, Uchida R, Toyoshima H, Takazawa A, Motomura H, Noguchi T (1987) Treatment resistant chronic psychopathology and CT scans in schizophrenia. Acta Psychiatr Scand 75:415–427
Pandurangi AK, Bilder RM, Rieder RO, Mukherjee S, Hamer RM (1988) Schizophrenic symptoms and deterioration – relation to computed tomographic findings. J Nerv Ment Dis 176:200–206
Peters J, van Kammen DP, Gelernter J, Yao J, Shaw D (1990) Neuropeptide Y like immunoreactivity in schizophrenia: relationships with clinical measures. Schizophr Res 3: 287–294
Pinder RM, Brogden RN, Sawyer PR, Spencer R, Avery GS (1976) Pimozide: a review of its pharmacological properties and therapeutic uses in psychiatry. Drugs 12:1–40
Post RM, Fink E, Carpenter WT, Goodwin FK (1975) Cerebrospinal fluid amine metabolites in acute schizophrenia. Arch Gen Psychiatry 32:1063–1069
Post RM, Bunney WE Jr, van Kammen DP, Ballenger JC, Lake CR, Lerner P, Sternberg DE, Uhde PW, Goodwin FK (1981) Cerebrospinal fluid norepinephrine and dopamine-beta-hydroxylase in affective illness and schizophrenia. In: Angrist B, Burrows GD, Lader M, Lingjaerde O, Sedvall G, Wheatley D (eds) Recent advances in neuropsychopharmacology. Pergamon, New York, pp 283–288
Pycock CJ, Kerwin RW, Carter CJ (1980) Effect of cortical dopamine terminals on subcortical dopamine in rats. Nature 286:74–77
Randrup A, Munkvad I (1974) Pharmacology and physiology of stereotyped behavior. J Psychiatr Res 11:1–10

Reisine TD, Chesselet MF, Lubetzki C, Cheramy A, Glowinski J (1981) Striatal β-adrenergic receptors regulate dopamine release. Soc Neurosci Abstr 8:526

Reubenstein M, Schinder AF, Gershanik O, Stefano FJE (1989) Positive interaction between alpha-1 adrenergic and dopamine-2 receptors in locomotor activity of normo and supersensitive mice. Life Sci 44:337–346

Rieder RO, Donnelly EF, Herdt JR, Waldman IN (1979) Sulcal prominence in young chronic schizophrenic patients: CT scan findings associated with impairment on neuropsychological tests. Psychiatry Res 1:1–8

Rosen WG, Mohs RC, Johns CA, Small NS, Kendler KS, Horvath TB, Davis KL (1984) Positive and negative symptoms in schizophrenia. Psychiatry Res 13:277–284

Shepherd M, Watt D, Falloon I, Smeeton N (1989) The natural history of schizophrenia: a five year follow-up study of outcome and prediction in a representative sample of schizophrenics. Psychol Med [Suppl] 15

Snyder SH (1976) The dopamine hypothesis of schizophrenia: focus on the dopamine receptor. Am J Psychiatry 33:197–202

Stein L, Wise CD (1971) Possible etiology of schizophrenia: progressive damage to the noradrenergic reward system by 5-hydroxydopamine. Science 171:1032–1036

Sternberg DE, van Kammen DP, Lake CR, Ballenger JC, Marder SR, Bunney WE Jr (1981) The effect of pimozide on CSF norepinephrine in schizophrenia. Am J Psychiatry 138:1045–1051

Stone EA, Ariano M (1990) Are glial cells targets of the central noradrenergic system? A review of the evidence. Brain Res Rev 14:297–309

Svensson TH (1987) Peripheral, autonomic regulation of locus coeruleus noradrenergic neurons in the brain: putative implications for psychiatry and psychopharmacology. Psychopharmacology (Berlin) 92:1–7

Swerdlow NR, Koob GF (1989) Norepinephrine stimulates behavioral activation in rats following depletion of nucleus accumbens dopamine. Pharmacol Biochem Behav 33:595–599

Szymanski HV, Simon JC, Gutterman N (1983) Recovery from schizophrenic psychosis. Am J Psychiatry 140:335–338

Takahashi R, Inaba Y, Inanaga K, Kato N, Kumashiro H, Nishimura T, Okuma T, Otsuki S, Sakai T, Sato T, Shimazono Y (1981) CT scanning and the investigation of schizophrenia. In: Perris C, Struwe G, Jansson B (eds) Biological psychiatry. Elsevier/North-Holland, Amsterdam, pp 259–268

Tandon R, Greden JF (1989) Cholinergic hyperactivity and negative schizophrenic symptoms. A model of cholinergic/dopaminergic interactions in schizophrenia. Arch Gen Psychiatry 46:745–753

Tandon R, Goldman RS, Goodson JA, Greden JF (1990) Mutability and relationship between positive and negative symptoms during neuroleptic treatment in schizophrenia. Biol Psychiatry 27:1323–1326

Tatetsu S (1963) Methamphetamine psychosis. Folia Psychiatr Neurol Jpn [Suppl] 7:377–380

van der Heyden P, Ebinger G, Kanarek L (1986) Vauquelin, epinephrine and norepinephrine stimulation of adenylate cyclase in bovine retina homogenate: evidence for interaction with the D_1 receptor. Life Sci 38:1221–1228

van Kammen DP, Antelman S (1984) Impairment of noradrenergic transmission in schizophrenia? A minireview. Life Sci 34:1403–1413

van Kammen DP, Boronow J (1988) Dextro-amphetamine diminishes negative symptoms in schizophrenia. Int J Clin Psychopharmacol 3:111–121

van Kammen DP, Gelernter JA (1987) Biochemical instability in schizophrenia. II. The serotonin and gamma-aminobutyric acid systems. In: Meltzer HY (ed) Psychopharmacology: the third generation of progress. Raven, New York, pp 753–758

van Kammen DP, Kelley M (1991) Dopamine and norepinephrine activity in schizophrenia. Schizophr Res 4:173–191

van Kammen DP, Sternberg DE (1980) CSF studies in schizophrenia. In: Wood JH (ed) Neurobiology of cerebrospinal fluid, vol 1. Plenum, New York, pp 719–742

van Kammen DP, Bunney WE Jr, Docherty JP, Marder SR, Ebert MH, Rosenblatt JE, Rayner JN (1982a) D-amphetamine-induced heterogeneous changes in psychotic behavior in schizophrenia. Am J Psychiatry 139:991–997
van Kammen DP, Docherty JP, Marder SR, Schulz SC, Dalton L, Bunney WE Jr (1982b) Antipsychotic effects of pimozide in schizophrenia. Arch Gen Psychiatry 39:261–266
van Kammen DP, Sternberg DE, Hare TA, Waters R, Bunney WE Jr (1982c) CSF levels of gamma-aminobutyric acid in schizophrenia. Arch Gen Psychiatry 39:91–97
van Kammen DP, Mann LS, Sternberg DE, Scheinin M, Ninan PT, Marder SR, van Kammen WB, Rieder RO, Linnoila M (1983) Dopamine-beta-hydroxylase activity and homovanillic acid in spinal fluid of schizophrenics with brain atrophy. Science 220:974–977
van Kammen DP, Rosen J, Peters J, Fields R, van Kammen WB (1985) Are there state-dependent markers in schizophrenia? Psychopharmacol Bull 21:497–502
van Kammen DP, van Kammen WB, Mann LS, Seppala T, Linnoila M (1986) Dopamine metabolism in the cerebrospinal fluid of drug-free schizophrenic patients with and without cortical atrophy. Arch Gen Psychiatry 43:978–983
van Kammen DP, Hommer DW, Malas KL (1987) Effect of pimozide on positive and negative symptoms in schizophrenic patients: are negative symptoms state dependent? Neuropsychobiology 18:113–117
van Kammen DP, Peters J, van Kammen WB, Nugent A, Goetz KL, Yao J, Linnoila M (1989a) CSF norepinephrine in schizophrenia is elevated prior to relapse after haloperidol withdrawal. Biol Psychiatry 26:176–188
van Kammen DP, Peters JL, Rosen J, van Kammen WB, McAdam D, Linnoila M (1989b) Clonidine treatment in schizophrenia: can we predict treatment response? Psychiatry Res 27:297–311
van Kammen DP, Peters J, Yao J, van Kammen WB, Neylan T, Shaw D, Linnoila M (1990) Norepinephrine in acute exacerbations of chronic schizophrenia: negative symptoms revisited. Arch Gen Psychiatry 47:161–168
van Putten T, Mutalipassi LR, Malkin MD (1974) Phenothiazine-induced decompensation. Arch Gen Psychiatry 30:102–105
van Putten T, Marder SR, Aravagiri M, Chabert N, Mintz J (1989) Plasma homovanillic acid as a predictor of response to fluphenazine treatment. Psychopharmacol Bull 1:89–91
Warkentin S, Nilsson A, Risberg J, Karlson S, Flekköy K, Franzén G, Gustafson L, Rodriguez G (1990) Regional cerebral blood flow in schizophrenia: repeated studies during a psychotic episode. Psychiatry Res 35:27–38
Weinberger DR (1987) Implications of normal brain development for the pathogenesis of schizophrenia. Arch Gen Psychiatry 44:660–669
Wing JK (1989) The concept of negative symptoms. Br J Psychiatry [Suppl 7] 155:10–14
Wise RA (1988) Psychomotor stimulant properties of addictive drugs. Ann NY Acad Sci 537:228–234
Wyatt RJ (1986) The dopamine hypothesis: variations on a theme. II. Psychopharmacol Bull 22:923–927
Wyatt RJ, Fawcett R, Kirch D (1989) A possible animal model of defect state schizophrenia. In: Schulz SC, Tamminga CA (eds) Schizophrenia: scientific progress. Oxford University Press, New York, pp 184–189
Yamamoto K-i, Arai H, Nakayama S (1990) Skin conductance response after 6-hydroxydopamine lesion of central noradrenaline system. Biol Psychiatry, 27/28:151–160

Typical Neuroleptics in the Treatment of Positive and Negative Symptoms

H.-J. Möller [1]

Efficacy in Positive Symptoms

There is broad evidence, derived from placebo-controlled clinical studies and daily clinical practice, that neuroleptics are able to reduce positive symptoms of schizophrenia under acute and long-term conditions and prevent relapses of acute schizophrenic psychoses. To demonstrate the efficacy of neuroleptics in the treatment of acute, productive schizophrenic psychoses the results of the famous phenothiazine study carried out by the National Institute of Mental Health (NIMH) collaborative group (Cole et al. 1964, 1966) are presented in Fig. 1. After 6 weeks of treatment, about 70% of the patients were rated as much improved, most of them with a very good or good outcome. In the placebo group only about 20% demonstrated much improvement while almost 50% showed clinical deterioration. The results of this and many similar investigations supported the hypothesis, offered by Delay and Deniker (1952), that chlorpromazine and similar phenothiazines are able to reduce or to suppress productive symptoms of schizophrenia. After the development of haloperidol and other substances of the butyrophenone group by Janssen, the hypothesis was extended to embrace this pharmacological group.

The antipsychotic effect of the neuroleptics is very impressive and can be observed for all kinds of neuroleptics and in nearly all trials, whether sophisticated in design or not. Using standardized rating procedures, it has been clearly demonstrated that these drugs are not only sedative or anxiolytic and, in consequence of this, antipsychotic, but truly antipsychotic in the sense of reducing productive symptoms of schizophrenic psychoses. The analysis of the subscores of the applied scales, for example the Brief Psychiatric Rating Scale (BPRS), showed this in a convincing manner (Fig. 2). In the early development of neuroleptics and in their clinical evaluation over a long period, the emphasis was on the alleviation of positive symptoms, and the clinical opinion was widespread that negative symptoms of schizophrenia, e.g., flat affect, withdrawal, loss of motivation, and apathy, are less likely to respond to the antipsychotic drugs. It might be that this opinion was generated by the overwhelming effect of the neuroleptics on productive symptoms which was observable not only in clinical trials but also in everyday psychiatric practice.

[1] Psychiatrische Klinik und Poliklinik der Universität Bonn, Sigmund-Freud-Straße 25, W-5300 Bonn 1 (Venusberg), FRG

A. Marneros / N. C. Andreasen / M. T. Tsuang (Eds.)
Negative Versus Positive Schizophrenia

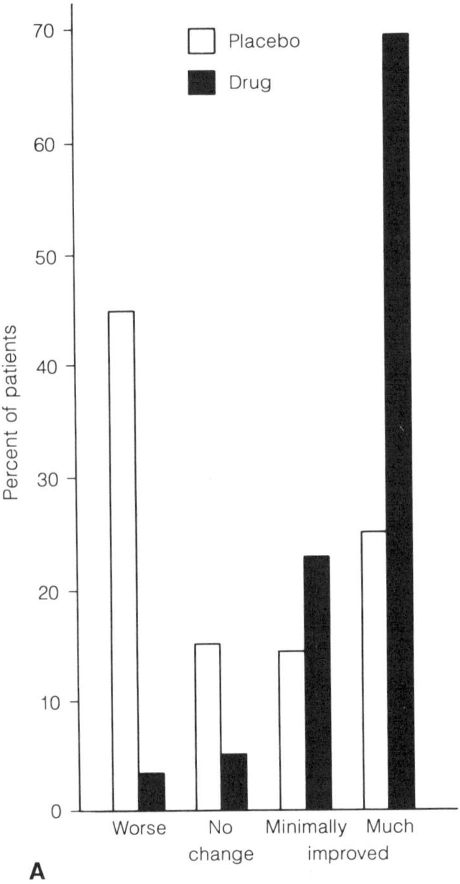

Fig. 1. Results of the treatment of schizophrenic patients with antipsychotic drugs or placebo (Cole et al. 1964, 1966)

The antipsychotic effect is usually prompt in onset under acute treatment conditions, and an impressive amelioration can be observed during the first 4–6 weeks. Whether there might be a delay between sedation at the first stage of medication and a "true" antipsychotic effect is difficult to decide because of methodological problems, but the opinion that a real antipsychotic effect appears even in the first days of treatment is becoming increasingly widespread. Several authors have even described that a prediction of the later outcome can be based on this early response (Möller et al. 1985; Nedopil and Rüther 1981; Woggon 1983).

Mode of Action

Many biological studies were performed to find out the mode of action of neuroleptics. From animal pharmacology it was concluded that all neurolep-

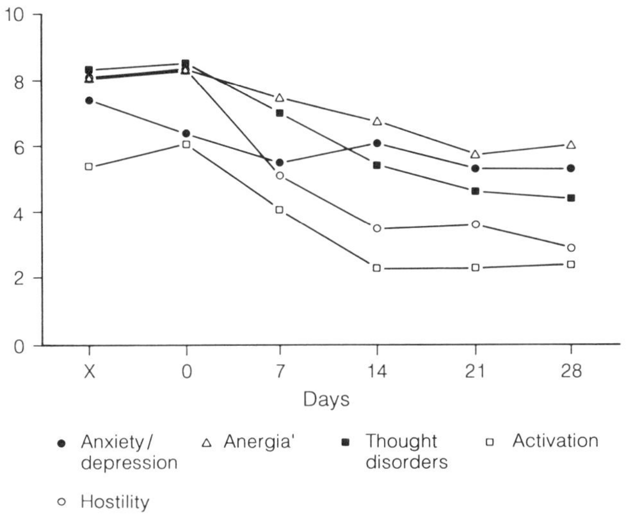

Fig. 2. Means of the BPRS subscores of 16 patients with an acute schizophrenic psychosis which demonstrate the antipsychotic efficacy of a new neuroleptic compound: savoxepine (Möller et al. 1989)

tics are antidopaminergic drugs and that the antipsychotic effect might be based on this influence on the dopaminergic system. In line with this theory, a dopamine hypothesis of schizophrenia was postulated, which explained the symptoms produced in schizophrenia by an overfunction of the dopaminergic system (Carlsson 1978). With respect to the topological distribution of dopamine receptors in the brain, the mesolimbic system was postulated as the locus of schizophrenic psychoses and of the antipsychotic action of neuroleptic drugs. The action of neuroleptics in the other dopaminergic systems such as the nigrostriatal and tuberoinfundibular systems were related to some of the side effects typically seen with neuroleptics, e.g., extrapyramidal motor disturbances, the increase in prolactin levels, and the consequences of the latter for sexual dysfunctions.

An intensive discussion tried to clarify whether the acute antidopaminergic effect of the neuroleptics or the following regulative adaptations at the dopaminergic synapsis were the biological basis for the antipsychotic activity (Müller 1987). It was also discussed whether only antidopaminergic mechanisms were related to the antipsychotic effects of neuroleptics or whether other, e.g., antiadrenergic, mechanisms (Ackenheil et al. 1978) might also be involved. As a result of receptor-binding studies, it was proven that the capacity to block the postsynaptic D_2 receptor was closely correlated with the antipsychotic potency of the different neuroleptics (Richelson 1984) (Fig. 3). A recent hypothesis that a well-balanced relation of D_2 and D_1 blockade (Wiesel et al. 1990) seems to guarantee good antipsychotic efficacy and good tolerability must be further tested.

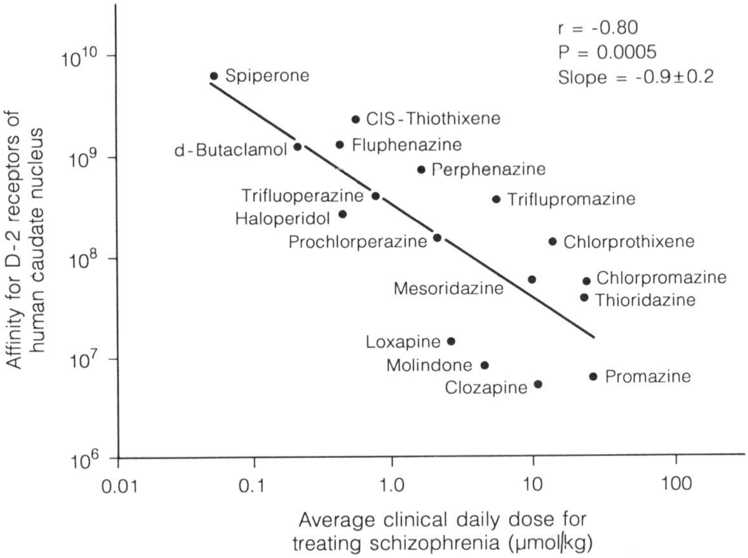

Fig. 3. Relationship between neuroleptic affinities for the dopamine (D_2) receptor of human brain caudate nucleus and average daily dose for treating schizophrenia (Richelson 1984). The equation for this regression is $y = 8.5 + 9.2\times$ ($r = -0.80$; $p = 0.0005$)

With the development of a newer generation of neuroleptics the serotonin system was also included in the theory of antipsychotic mechanisms (Gelders 1990; Niemegeers et al. 1990). To reduce extrapyramidal side effects attempts were made to develop neuroleptics which acted preferentially in the dopaminergic structures of the limbic system (Bischoff et al. 1985). Clozapine was the first so-called atypical neuroleptic. The term "atypical" was chosen to express that such a neuroleptic has a good antipsychotic effect without relevant extrapyramidal side effects.

Acute neuroleptic treatment correlates with changes in some biochemical blood and cerebrospinal fluid parameters in humans. This may be taken as an indication that transmitter or receptor processes are involved in the therapeutic action (Rüther and Müller-Spahn 1987; Rüther 1986); for example, the prolactin increase demonstrates the antidopaminergic effects of neuroleptics (Möller et al. 1981) (Fig. 4).

Clinical Profile

The classical neuroleptics are usually classified as low-potent and high-potent neuroleptics. This classification should not be misinterpreted in the sense that the high-potent neuroleptics are more effective in the treatment of schizophrenic psychoses. In general, each neuroleptic can treat the positive symptoms of schizophrenic psychoses sufficiently. The difference between high- and low-

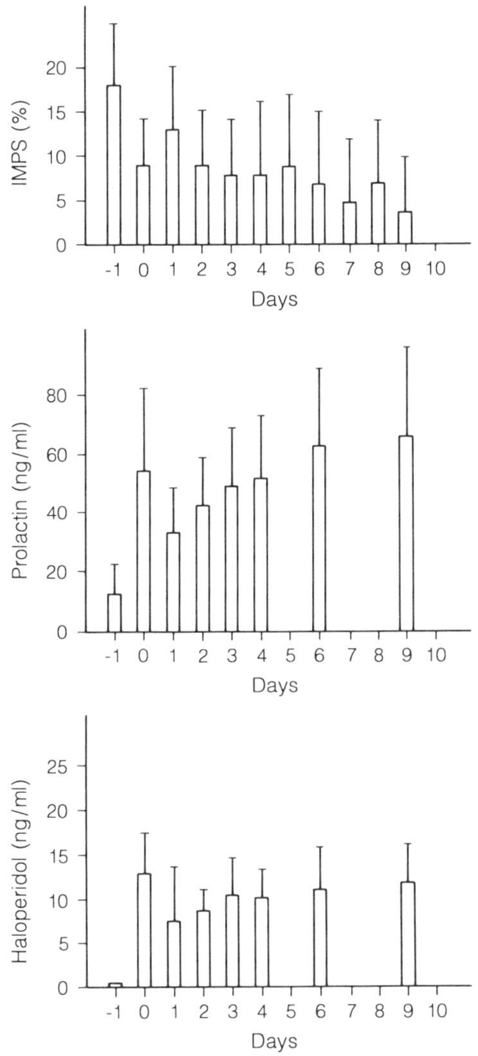

Fig. 4. Antidopaminergic effect of neuroleptic treatment demonstrated by the mean values (with standard deviations) of the plasma levels of prolactin during a 9-day treatment ($n = 29$). The productive psychotic symptoms were rated using a seven-factor score of the IMPS (Möller et al. 1981)

potent drugs is only the dosage. High-potent neuroleptics are efficacious even in small dosages, while a higher amount of low-potent neuroleptics is needed for adequate antipsychotic treatment (Table 1). Nevertheless, such a high dosage of low-potent neuroleptics can be problematic because of sedative or cardiovascular-depressive side effects. Therefore, a change to high-potent neuroleptics (e.g., most of the butyrophenones) might be necessary. In

Table 1. Antipsychotic dose equivalence of some neuroleptics related to 100 mg chlorpromazine (Davis 1974)

Generic name (brand name)	Dose ratio equivalent to 100 mg chlorpromazine (ratio S.E.M.[a])	Oral dose[b] (mg/kg)	Parenteral dose (mg/kg)
Chlorpromazine (Thorazine)	100	3.4952	1.1650
Triflupromazine (Vesprin)	28.4 ± 1.8	0.9904	0.3301
Thioridazine (Mellaril)	95.3 ± 8.2	3.3333	1.1111
Prochlorperazine (Compazine)	14.3 ± 1.7	0.5000	0.1666
Perphenazine (Trilafon)	8.9 ± 0.6	0.3100	0.1033
Fluphenazine (Prolixin)	1.2 ± 0.1	0.0419	0.0139
Trifluoperazine (Stelazine)	2.8 ± 0.4	0.0980	0.0326
Acetophenazine (Tindal)	23.5 ± 1.5	0.8190	0.2730
Carphenazine (Prokstazine)	24.3 ± 2.7	0.8380	0.2793
Butaperazine (Repoise)	8.9 ± 1.1	0.3095	0.1031
Mesoridazine (Serentil)	55.3 ± 8.3	1.93333	0.6444
Piperacetazine (Quide)	10.5	0.3671	0.1223
Haloperidol (Haldol)	1.6 ± 0.4	0.0545	0.0181
Chlorprothixene (Taractan)	43.9 ± 13.9	1.5333	0.5111
Thiothixene (Navane)	5.2 ± 1.3	0.1809	0.0603

[a] Standard error of the mean.
[b] One-third the average daily dose in a 70-kg "person".

contrast, a change from high-potent to low-potent neuroleptics may be preferable when extrapyramidal side effects are too pronounced.

This leads to the general question of the clinical profile of different neuroleptics. Hitherto, the discussion has not been totally conclusive whether certain drugs might have a special clinical profile. The assumption of specific clinical profiles was based, among other things, on the different pharmacological profiles of different neuroleptics (Fig. 5). The hypothesis of specific clinical profiles was visualized for example, using the star profiles of Liège (Bobon et al. 1972; Bobon 1990) (Fig. 6).

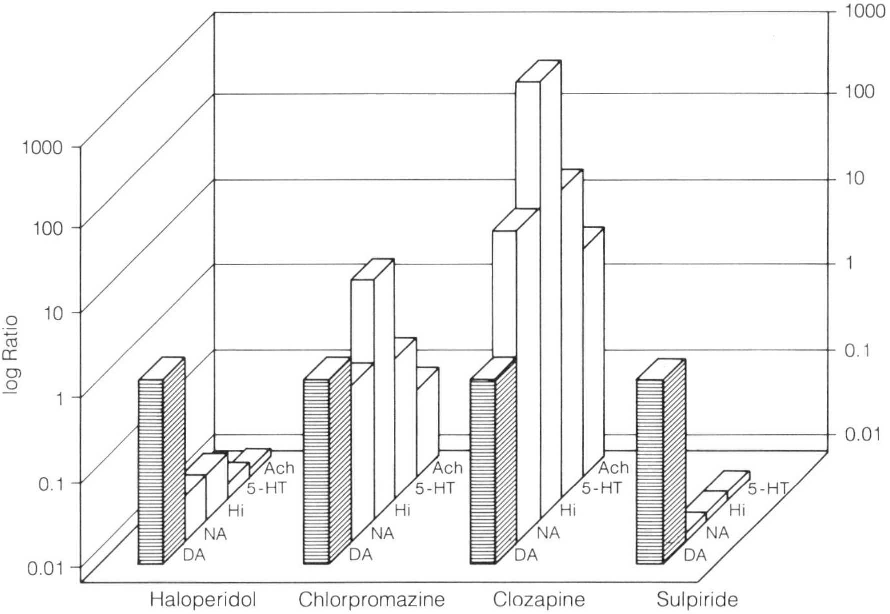

Fig. 5. Receptor-affinity profiles of four neuroleptics, related to an equivalence dose with regard to the antidopaminergic effect (Delini-Stula 1986)

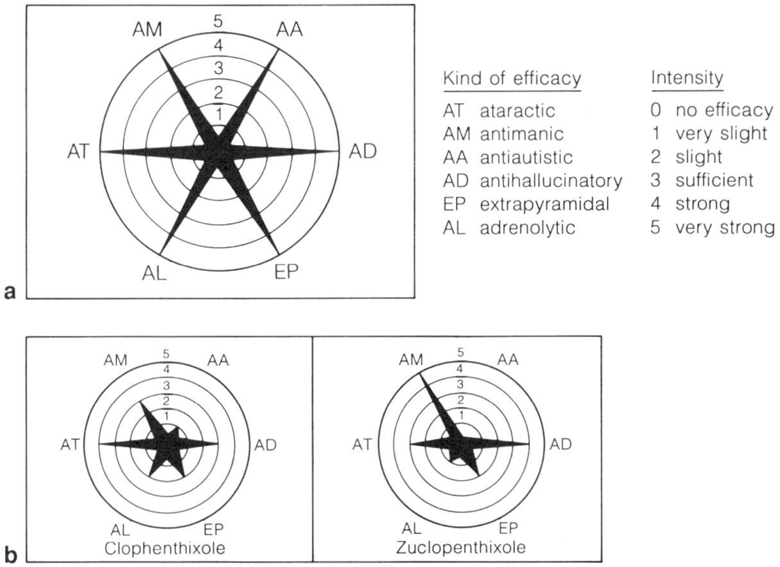

Fig. 6. a The "Liège star" for demonstration of the clinical-pharmacological action profiles of the neuroleptics (Bobon 1990). **b** Action profiles of clophenthixole and zuclopenthixole (Bobon 1990)

General opinion seems to be tending increasingly towards the hypothesis that there is no special clinical profile of certain neuroleptics with respect to antipsychotic properties (Davis and Garver 1978; Möller 1987a) and that neuroleptic drugs differ only in their sedation and extrapyramidal side effects. Other authors, however, underline that certain neuroleptics demonstrate special antiautistic, stimulating, or antidepressive properties (Sieberns 1986; de Buck 1974; Tegeler 1981). The discussion of the special profile of neuroleptics leads to the question whether neuroleptics are effective for negative symptoms of schizophrenia, a topic which is discussed elsewhere in detail (see Meltzer, this volume). In general, it can be only stated that findings concerning a special profile of certain classical neuroleptics are totally inconsistent in the literature and were merely replicated. Some authors tried to explain the inconsistency of such descriptions by different dosages (Gardos and Cole 1973; Lehmann et al. 1980; Tansella and Balestrieri 1976), tending to the position that certain effects can only be induced by certain dosages, e.g., an antidepressive effect of neuroleptics only by low dosages of neuroleptics.

Relevance of Dose and Plasma Level

Based on two meta-analyses of clinical studies on neuroleptics (Davis et al. 1980; Baldessarini et al. 1988), a dosage equivalent to 500–1000 mg chlorpromazine per day was described as sufficient to control the productive symptoms of an acute schizophrenic psychosis. This corresponds to the results of positron emission tomography (PET) dopamine receptor-binding studies which demonstrated that the receptor occupancy is nearly complete in such a dosage range (Table 2). However, in clinical practice higher dosages are in widespread use (Haag et al. 1987) (Fig. 7), perhaps indicating that, besides the antidopaminergic effect, clinicians utilize other "nonspecific" mechanisms of neuroleptics, e.g., antinoradrenergic or antiserotonergic properties (Fig. 8). Also there seems to be a subgroup of patients who are resistant to neuroleptic treatment in the usual dose range, but who profit from a higher dosage. Perhaps these are patients with an atypical pharmacokinetic situation, e.g., reduced absorption or intensified metabolism (Breyer-Pfaff 1987).

Although a certain dosage range seems to exist for an adequate antipsychotic treatment, a clear-cut relationship between plasma level and the clinical efficacy of neuroleptics has not yet been proven. This might have to do with the complicated metabolism of phenothiazines and with the high variability of the relationship between the dose and plasma levels of neuroleptics (Fig. 9). Nevertheless, there is some evidence of a relationship between plasma level and clinical efficacy for haloperidol (Breyer-Pfaff 1987) (Fig. 10).

Poor or nonresponse to neuroleptics occurs in about 20% of patients undergoing a first course of neuroleptic treatment. Several predictors of nonresponse have been described, but there is still much inconsistency in this field (Woggon 1983; Möller et al. 1985). The correlations of predictors and efficacy to neuroleptic treatment are quite low and do not provide the basis for

Table 2. D_2 receptor occupancy in schizophrenic patients with neuroleptic monotherapy (Wiesel et al. 1990)

Drug	Daily dose (mg)	Receptor occupancy (%)
Phenothiazine		
Chlorpromazine	200	80
Thioridazine	300	75
Trifluperazine	10	80
Perphenazine	8	79
Perphenazine	60	88 (EPS)
Thioxanthene		
Flupentixole	10	74
Butyrophenone		
Haloperidol	12[a]	86 (EPS)
Haloperidol	8[a]	84
Haloperidol	6	85 (EPS)
Haloperidol	6	89 (EPS)
Haloperidol	4	81 (EPS)
Melperone	300	74
Melperone	250	71
Diphenylbutylpiperidine		
Pimozide	8	77 (EPS)
Benzamide		
Sulpiride	800	82
Sulpiride	800	73
Sulpiride	800	68
Raclopride	8	72
Raclopride	6	65
Dibenzodiazepine		
Clozapine	600	65
Clozapine	300	40

EPS, extrapyramidal side effects.
[a] Same patient; because of extrapyramidal side-effects the dosage of 10 mg/day was reduced to 8 mg/day, after which they disappeared.

individual prognosis, but only for group-statistical differentiation. In the case of nonresponse, the dosage of the neuroleptic should be increased, and, in the case of nonsuccess, parenteral administration of the drug under the hypothesis of an increased first-pass metabolism or a switch to another drug with different pharmacological profile can lead to a satisfying therapeutic result (Hansen and Larsen 1985). A generally applied course of high-dosage treatment, which was recommended some years ago, does not lead to better therapeutic results. A course of high-dosage therapy with tenfold or even higher amounts should only be applied as ultima ratio in severe cases of nonresponse (Aubree and Lader 1980).

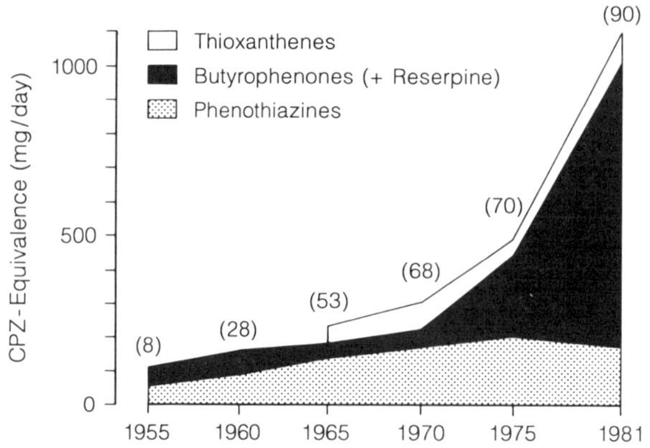

Fig. 7. Average neuroleptic dose/day (*CPZ-Equ.*, chlorpromazine equivalence) in the years 1954–1981. Numbers in parentheses are the number of patients. Only those patients who were treated in the relevant year with neuroleptics are taken into account. (Haag et al. 1987)

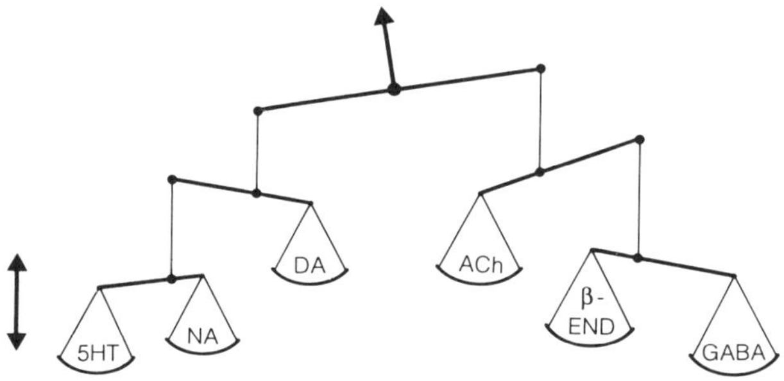

Fig. 8. "Balance" model of different transmitters/modulators (Fritze 1989)

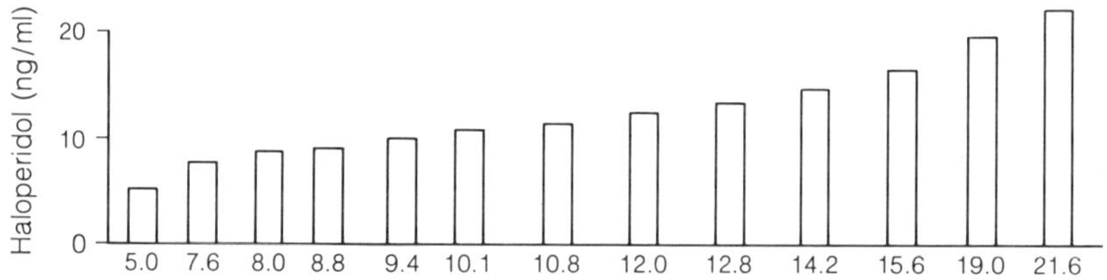

Fig. 9. Demonstration of the variability of plasma levels at the 10th day of neuroleptic treatment (oral application of 24 mg haloperidol/day; $n = 13$) (Möller and Kissling 1987)

The Problems of Negative Symptoms

When the problems of the treatment of positive symptoms had been solved more or less sufficiently, negative symptoms were defined increasingly as a focus of interest for the drug therapy of schizophrenia, especially as a primary

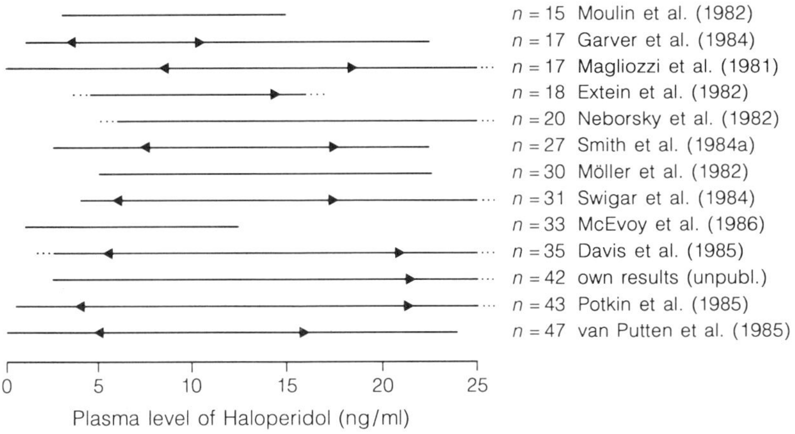

Fig. 10. Overview of concentrations of plasma levels in different publications (Breyer-Pfaff 1987). ——, total plasma level range of the patients; ...——..., not the total range is delineated; —‹— and —›—, bottom and top level of the therapeutic favorable range

goal in the development of new drugs (Meltzer and Zureick 1989). At the same time, intensified research activities were started to describe biological correlates of negative symptoms such as cortical or ventricular atrophy (Crow 1980; Andreasen et al. 1982), reduced dopamine turnover (Van Kammen et al. 1986; Lindström 1985; Nybäck et al. 1983), and disturbances of the noradrenergic and/or serotonergic transmission (Bleich et al. 1988).

A central problem of this scientific approach is that the terms "negative symptoms" or "minus symptoms" are not well defined. In addition, different authors use different concepts for the type and number of symptoms implicated (Helmchen 1988; Rösler and Hengesch 1990). According to Sommers' review, the main negative symptoms concern affect, arousal, cognition, and social functioning (Sommers 1985) and are reflected, for example, by blunted affect, apathy, attentional deficit, poverty of thought or speech, and social withdrawal. Some of these symptoms are elements of the deficit syndrome already described by Bleuler (1911) as "core symptoms" of schizophrenia, or by Huber (1957) as "basic symptoms" of schizophrenia. While some authors support a broad concept of negative symptoms (Gibbons et al. 1985; Meltzer and Zureick 1989), others prefer a narrow concept (Strauss et al. 1974; Wing 1978; or Crow, 1985, who only included flat affect and poverty of speech). The discrepancies particularly concern symptoms such as incoherence, loosening of associations, and thought blocking, which are interpreted either as negative or positive symptoms.

The concept of negative symptoms has been refined through factor-analytic studies to better determine whether they are unitary in nature, and the relationship between negative and positive symptoms, i.e., whether they are independent (Lewine et al. 1983) or part of a single dimension, as suggested by Andreasen (1982). When a broad concept of negative symptoms and in

Table 3. Correlation matrix for the Brief Psychiatric Rating Scale, the Association for Methodology and Documentation in Psychiatry system, and the Scale for the Assessment of Negative Symptoms (Zinner et al. 1990)[a]

	BPRS-ANER	AMDP-APA	AMDP-PSYORG
AMDP			
APA	0.795		
PSYORG	0.481	0.614	
SANS			
Affective flattening	0.798	0.820	0.662
Alogia	0.650	0.694	0.539
Avolition	0.499	0.521	0.388 *
Anhedonia	0.675	0.729	0.593
Attention impairment	0.464	0.422	0.525
Composite score	0.778	0.810	0.670
Summary score	0.768	0.816	0.672

[a] All $p < 0.001$ (apart from $^{*}p < 0.01$).

BPRS, Brief Psychiatric Rating Scale; AMDP, Association for Methodology and Documentation in Psychiatry; SANS, Scale for the Assesssment of Negative Symptoms; ANER, anergy; APA, apathy; PSYORG, psychoorganic syndrome.

consequence a large number of symptoms has been evaluated, nearly all factor-analytic studies have identified two or three dimensions of negative symptoms (Gibbons et al. 1985; Liddle 1987; Meltzer and Zureick 1989). For example, Meltzer and Zureick (1989) described three factors: cognitive impairment/inappropriate affect, anhedonia/anergia, retardation/flat affect. The development of special scales like the Scale for the Assessment of Negative Symptoms (SANS) or the Positive and Negative Syndrome Scale (PANSS) was an important step for a better methodological basis for research in this field, but it should be carefully taken into account that there are relevant differences between these scales, not so much with respect to the general psychopathological areas being covered, but more regarding the selection of items (Zinner et al. 1990). Such discrepancies become still more important if the apathy/anergia/retardation subscales of rating scales commonly used to assess psychotic patients, e.g., the Brief Psychiatric Rating Scale (BPRS), the Inpatient Multidimensional Psychiatric Scale (IMPS), and the rating scale of the Association for Methodology and Documentation in Psychiatry (AMDP) are used to determine negative symptoms (Tables 3, 4).

The lack of homogeneity in the definition and measurement of negative symptoms has potentially important clinical implications. Perhaps some of the inconsistencies in research results can be explained by this fact.

> "Different types of negative symptoms may appear at different stages of schizophrenia or may respond differentially to pharmacological or psychosocial treatments"

(Meltzer and Zureick 1989). In this context the differentiation between primary and secondary negative symptoms, as proposed by Carpenter et al. (1985), seems of great relevance. While primary negative symptoms are the conse-

Table 4. Inclusion of psychic functions in observer rating scales for assessment of schizophrenic minus symptoms (Zinner et al. 1990)

Scale	AMDP APA	IMPS RTD	BPRS ANER	PANSS MINUS	SANS	INSKA	BSABS
Items	8	9	4	7	25	60	98
Affect	○	○	○	○	○	○	○
Impulsion, Psychomotility	○	○	○	○	○	○	○
Social activities	○		○	○	○	○	○
Speech		○		○	○	○	○
Thinking	○			○		○	○
Attention, Perception (also Orientation and Memory)		○	○		○		○

AMDP, Association for Methodology and Documentation in Psychiatry; APA, apathy; IMPS, Inpatient Multidimensional Psychiatric Scale; RTD, Retardation; BPRS, Brief Psychiatric Rating Scale; ANER, anergy; PANSS, Positive and negative Syndrome Scale; SANS, Scale for Assessment of Negative Symptoms; INSKA, Intentionalitätsskala (intentionality scale); BSABS, Bonn Scale for the Assessment of Basic Symptoms.

Table 5. Occurrence of negative symptoms (Angst et al. 1989)

1. In the course of schizophrenia

   Prepsychotic period (Conrad 1958; Huber 1957)

   Productive psychotic period
     Mixture of positive and negative symptoms
     Negative symptoms may be hidden

   Postpsychotic period
     Residuum or defect with or without positive symptoms
     "Postpsychotic depression", endogenous or reactive (Mayer-Gross 1920)
     Postremissive exhaustion (Heinrich 1967)

2. Of other origin

   Depression and schizoaffective psychoses
   Drug-induced depression
   Neuroses and personality disorders
   Mild organic brain syndromes
   Drug-induced Parkinson syndromes
   Institutionalization

quence of a morbogenic deficit state (e.g., in the sense of type II schizophrenia of Crow, 1980), secondary negative symptoms are the consequence of:

1. Positive symptoms (e.g., social withdrawal because of paranoid ideas).
2. Extrapyramidal side effects (e.g., motor retardation as an indicator of akinesia).
3. Depressive symptoms (e.g., postpsychotic or pharmacogenic depression).
4. Social understimulation (e.g., hospitalism).

According to this theory, the treatment of negative symptoms has to be differentiated according to the different causes. In a similar direction, Angst et al. (1989) underline the diagnostic unspecifity of negative symptoms, and have listed different kinds of negative symptoms in the course of schizophrenia (Table 5). When studying the effect of neuroleptics on negative symptoms, one should, therefore, specify the stage of psychosis in which the trial is carried out.

In contrast to the concept of a type I and a type II schizophrenia (Crow 1980), which postulates the stability of a type of schizophrenia with positive symptoms and a type with negative symptoms and explains this by different biological causes, most other authors stressed the point that negative and positive symptoms can be combined cross-sectionally or longitudinally (Deister et al. 1990).

In chronic cases, negative symptoms tend to have more stability (Kay and Opler 1987). This led Angst et al. (1989) to assume that drug effects may be better in the early stage of the disorder. However, with respect to research on drug effects, it has to be considered that, especially in the early stage of schizophrenia, investigation into neuroleptic treatment of negative symptoms is complicated much more by the instability of the syndrome and by the heterogeneity of causes than in later stages of schizophrenia. Also the question has to be answered whether the negative symptoms of the early stage of schizophrenia, in which negative symptoms mostly accompany positive symptoms and have a high chance of disappearing with them, or the negative symptoms of the chronic deficit state are a greater therapeutic problem.

If one is aware of these principal difficulties and if one also takes into account the fact that earlier clinical studies on the typical (classical) neuroleptics focused mainly on positive symptoms, it is not surprising that our knowledge of neuroleptic effects in this field is quite limited and controversial. For example, Crow (1980) proposed that negative symptoms are largely unresponsive to a neuroleptic treatment because they are, in his view, manifestations of irreversible structural changes in the central nervous system. Some years later Meltzer and Zureick (1989) came to the conclusion that there is considerable empirical evidence for the proposition that negative symptoms, while not as responsive to neuroleptic treatment as positive symptoms, do diminish during the course of treatment with neuroleptic drugs and may worsen in the absence of such treatment. They concluded from their recent study:

"We have now found that typical neuroleptics produce as much improvement in cognitive impairment/inappropriate affect as in positive symptoms. Significant improvement was also noted in anhedonia/anergia and retardation/flat affect but to a much lesser extent. ... Improvement in negative symptoms was present even after controlling for improvement in positive symptoms"

(Meltzer and Zureick 1989, p. 71). It should however, be questioned in advance whether Crow on the one hand and Meltzer and Zureick on the other have different kinds of negative symptoms in mind. Apparently Crow thinks about negative symptoms in a chronic deficit state, whereas Meltzer and Zureick, like other authors, investigated negative symptoms in less chronic cases, mostly in patients suffering from more or less acute psychotic episodes with productive and negative symptoms. It seems to be an unsolved problem whether the reduction of negative symptoms accompanying positive symptoms is the same as the reduction of negative symptoms in a deficit state.

A problem in the interpretation of rating scale data from studies in this field is that negative symptoms scores correlate positively with the drug-induced Parkinson syndrome (Hoffman et al. 1987; Prosser et al. 1987). Furthermore, there is a correlation between negative symptoms and hyperkinetic neurological symptoms such as akathisia and dyskinesia (Barnes and Braude 1985; Waddington et al. 1985). One could, therefore, conclude that drugs without extrapyramidal side effects in general may be advantageous in treating negative symptoms (Woggon 1990). Similarly, the differentiation between depression and negative symptoms is nearly impossible on the basis of rating scales (Maier et al. 1990), and therapeutic effects on depressive symptoms might be misinterpreted as successful treatment of negative symptoms and vice versa (Möller 1987b). Other authors have even described that neuroleptics may induce depressive or apathetic symptoms in schizophrenic patients, a position which is not commonly accepted (see the review by Möller and Von Zerssen 1986).

Efficacy in Negative Symptoms

In the following summary of some data on typical neuroleptics demonstrating a therapeutic effect on negative symptoms, it should be taken into account that these data are not totally conclusive, especially because of semantic problems with respect to the definition of negative symptoms and their differentiation from depression and akinesia, and the distinction between primary and secondary negative symptoms.

In his review, Goldberg (1985) cited five large placebo-controlled studies to demonstrate that, contrary to the contention of Johnstone et al. (1976) and Crow (1980), negative and/or deficit symptoms in schizophrenia do indeed respond to neuroleptic treatment. He described, for example, the NIMH collaborative group studies on phenothiazines, where highly significant drug-placebo-differences were shown in a variety of "positive, negative and deficit schizophrenic symptoms". Included in the latter two categories are: indifference to environment or apathy, hebephrenic symptoms or inappropriate affect, slowed speech and movements, poor social participation, and poor self-care and confusion. According to his review, the greater drug effects were shown in "negative" symptoms like hebephrenic symptoms, poor social participation, confusion, and poor self-care rather than positive symptoms. He differentiated this vote, however, by stating that, without subtracting the placebo effect under the drug condition, the negative or deficit symptoms do not change as much as the positive symptoms (Tables 6, 7). Goldberg (1985) also quoted the review by Cole et al. (1966) as a proof of his hypothesis. In this summary of other controlled studies on phenothiazines too, similar results were found. Two of the studies demonstrated a reduction in blunted affect and indifference. Four of the studies showed an effect on withdrawal/retardation, and four of the studies showed a drug effect on autistic behavior and mannerisms. Several problems of interpreting such data that have been already discussed have to be taken into account. For example, it has to be stated that all these studies were performed in acute schizophrenic patients, and the definition of negative symptoms is very broad when hebephrenic symptoms, confusion, and mannerisms are included in this concept.

In our own investigations in large samples of schizophrenic inpatients treated under routine care conditions, mostly with haloperidol as treatment of first choice, we found that not only productive symptoms, but also symptoms of the depressive-apathic spectrum were reduced between admission and discharge (Möller and Von Zerssen 1981, 1982, 1986) (Fig. 11). At least the IMPS factor "retardation and apathy", correlating almost exactly with the global score of so-called negative symptoms scales (see above), can be interpreted as an indicator of negative symptoms, thus apparently treatment with haloperidol seems to have a therapeutic effect on negative symptoms.

With respect to the butyrophenones, different groups have reported therapeutic effects of pimozide on negative symptoms (Pinder et al. 1976;

Table 6. Greater reduction of negative and/or deficit symptoms under drug than placebo (Goldberg 1985)

	Placebo pre/post change standard scores	Drug pre/post change standard scores	*P*
Indifference to environment ($n = 214$)	0.353	1.234	< 0.01
Slowed speech and movements ($n = 245$)	0.114	0.849	< 0.01
Social participation vs withdrawal ($n = 302$)	0.788	1.776	< 0.01
Hebephrenic symptoms ($n = 150$)	0.247	1.437	< 0.01
Confusion ($n = 276$)	0.620	1.600	< 0.01
Poor self-care ($n = 224$)	0.349	1.283	< 0.01

Table 7. Greater development of negative and/or deficit symptoms under placebo than drug among initially asymptomatic patients (Goldberg 1985)

	Placebo pre/post	Drug pre/post	*p*
Poor self-care ($n = 94$)	– 0.656	– 0.192	< 0.05
Slowed speech and movements ($n = 80$)	– 1.087	– 0.257	< 0.01
Hebephrenic symptoms ($n = 175$)	– 0.865	– 0.204	< 0.01
Indifference to environment ($n = 111$)	– 1.261	– 0.572	< 0.01

Fallon et al. 1978; Wilson et al. 1982; Feinberg et al. 1988; Van Kammen et al. 1987); this is explained, among other things, by the lack of a noradrenergic receptor blockade. The blockade of noradrenergic receptors induces sedation and an unfavorable influence of the central noradrenergic reward system, which could cause negative symptoms. In addition to this special pharmacological profile of pimozide, the importance of a low-dose therapy has been stressed (Niemegeers 1988) and explained by several biochemical hypotheses. Only low-dose therapy with pimozide seems to have an activating effect. The study by Feinberg et al. (1988) was uncontrolled, the study by Falloon et al. (1978) was a control-group study versus fluphenazine, and the study by Wilson et al. (1982) was a control-group study versus chlorpromazine. These control-group studies raise the question whether pimozide really has an effect on negative

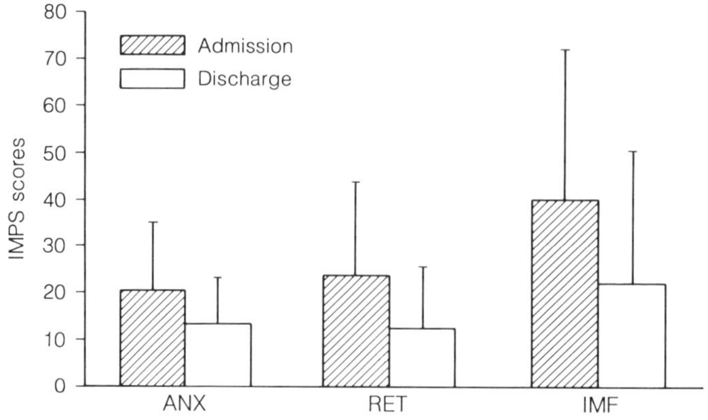

Fig. 11. Comparison of the mean values (with standard deviations) of the IMPS factor "anxious depression" (ANX), "retardation and apathy" (RET) and "impaired functioning" (IMF) at admission and discharge ($n = 280$) (Möller and Von Zerssen 1981)

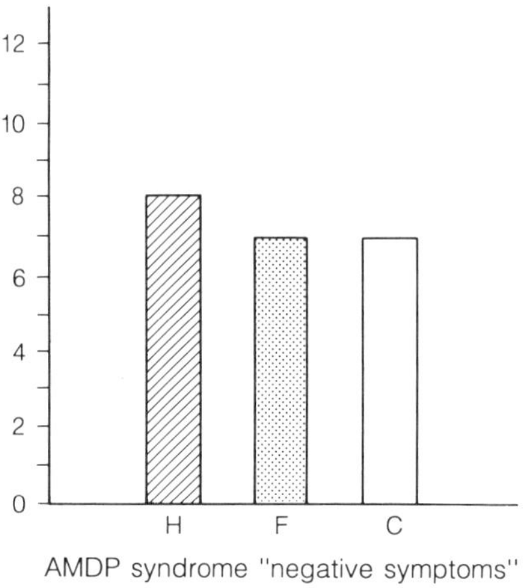

Fig. 12. Changes in negative symptoms under treatment with haloperidol (*H*), fluperlapine (*F*) or clozapine (*C*) (Angst et al. 1989)

symptoms or is only favorable insofar as it does not induce as much sedation, apathy, or akinesia as chlorpromazine or fluphenazine. The equivalence dosage used in these trials might also be relevant to the results. In the placebo-controlled study by Van Kammen et al. (1987), the neuroleptic treatment did not exert a differential effect on the positive and negative symptoms of schizophrenia (both groups of symptoms responded). Changes in the positive and negative symptoms of schizophrenia were directly related (Van Kammen

"Thus, patients whose hallucinations, delusions and disorganized speech improved during neuroleptic treatment also became less withdrawn, emotionally flat and motorically slowed"

et al. 1987, p. 115). This statement makes it clear that apparently only secondary negative symptoms in the sense of Carpenter were responsive.

In their meta-analysis, Angst and Woggon (Angst et al. 1989; Woggon 1990) compared the results of some of their own studies with haloperidol, fluperlapine, and clozapine to find out whether one or all of these drugs had a special effect on negative symptoms. The first two groups studied came from a multicenter double-blind trial (Woggon et al. 1986), the latter from five different trials on clozapine carried out in Zurich, two of them with a double-blind design. In each group 90 patients could be included in the meta-analysis. For the analysis of the data, 14 scores of the AMDP system and a new ad hoc scale for negative symptoms (NAMDP) derived from the AMDP system were used. The authors analyzed the three samples separately, i.e., patients treated with haloperidol, fluperlapine, or clozapine, respectively. Each sample comprised 90 patients in order to determine changes of the syndrome scores during treatment. The improvement of the NAMDP score was visualized by so-called scatter plots, in which values of the first measurement and those of the second measurement (20 days later) were plotted against each other. A clear and almost identical reduction of NAMDP score values showed up in all three samples. This reduction was satisfactorily homogeneous within the population as indicated by correlation coefficients between the two measurements of 0.68 (fluperlapine), 0.73 (haloperidol), and 0.72 (clozapine). Contrary to expectations, no significant differences between the three drugs could be revealed with respect to changes in the negative symptoms score of the AMDP (NAMDP) (Fig. 12).

Other studies have tried to demonstrate that especially the so-called atypical neuroleptics such as clozapine have a special therapeutic profile concerning negative symptoms. A special chapter in this book (Meltzer) is devoted to this issue.

Summary

In summary, there seems to be some evidence that typical neuroleptics can reduce negative symptoms, but, because most of these trials were performed during acute exacerbations of schizophrenic psychoses, the question arises whether only negative symptoms secondary to productive symptoms might be concerned. Because of the heterogeneity of the etiology of negative symptoms, such data cannot be interpreted in the sense that negative symptoms of a chronic deficit state of schizophrenia are sensitive to typical neuroleptics. This has to be tested in chronic schizophrenic patients who are themselves suffering from a deficit state. Observations that in maintenance studies one neuroleptic is associated with fewer negative symptoms than another cannot be accepted as a definitive proof of reduction of negative symptoms. As an alternative hypothesis, the possibility that one drug induces more depression, akinesia, or sedation etc., than another must be considered seriously. Only a placebo-controlled trial can solve such problems of interpretation, but, even under such conditions, one must carefully differentiate between an antidepressant effect – many neuroleptics are said to have antidepressant effects, especially in lower dosages – and a real effect on negative symptoms.

When a neuroleptic is described as efficacious towards negative symptoms, most clinicians think that they are helpful in reducing the negative symptoms in a deficit state. In many cases of traditional or more recently developed neuroleptics, the expectation that the drug can reduce negative symptoms in a deficit state has not been fulfilled in everyday clinical practice, although the drugs seemed to have this therapeutic profile in scientific studies. This discrepancy between research results and clinical practice might be explained by methodological problems which still exist in this field. From my viewpoint, particularly the chronic and stable negative symptoms of patients with a deficit state of schizophrenia should be taken as target symptoms for such clinical studies and not primarily the negative symptoms during an acute episode of schizophrenia, which must mostly be considered as secondary to productive symptoms and which seems to disappear under neuroleptic treatment of any kind when the productive symptoms are effectively treated. The negative symptoms which accompany acute productive symptoms do not seem to be such a problem of treatment as the chronic negative symptoms of a deficit state.

References

Ackenheil M, Hippius H, Matussek N (1978) Ergebnisse der biochemischen Forschung auf dem Schizophrenie-Gebiet. Nervenarzt 49:634–649

Andreasen NC (1982) Negative symptoms in schizophrenia: definition and reliability. Arch Gen Psychiatry 39:784–788

Andreasen NC, Smith MR, Jacoby CG, Dennert JW, Olsen SA (1982) Ventricular enlargement in schizophrenia: definition and prevalence. Am J Psychiatry 139:292–296

Angst J, Stassen HH, Woggon B (1989) Effect of neuroleptics on positive and negative symptoms and the deficit state. Psychopharmacology 99:41–46

Aubree JC, Lader MH (1980) High and very high dosage of antipsychotics. A critical review. J Clin Psychiatry 41:341–350

Baldessarini RJ, Cohen BM, Teicher MH (1988) Significance of neuroleptic dose and plasma level in the pharmacological treatment of psychoses. Arch Gen Psychiatry 45:79–91

Barnes TR, Braude WM (1985) Akathisia variants and tardive dyskinesia. Arch Gen Psychiatry 42:874–878

Bischoff S, Delini-Stula A, Maitre L (1985) Blockade der Dopamin-Rezeptoren im Hippokampus als Indikator antipsychotischer Wirksamkeit: Korrelationen zwischen neurochemischen und psycho-pharmakologischen Wirkungen von Neuroleptika. In: Pflug B, Foerster K, Straube E (eds) Perspektiven der Schizophrenie-Forschung. Fischer, Stuttgart, pp 87–103

Bleich A, Brown SL, Kahn R, Van Praag HM (1988) The role of serotonin in schizophrenia. Schizophr Bull 14:297–315

Bleuler E (1911) Dementia praecox oder Gruppe der Schizophrenien. In: Aschaffenburg G (ed) Handbuch der Psychiatrie, Deuticke, Leipzig (part 4/I) pp 1–420

Bobon D (1990) Klinische Wirkungsprofile der Thioxanthene. In: Müller-Oerlinghausen B, Möller HJ, Rüther E (eds) Thioxanthene in der neuroleptischen Behandlung. Springer, Berlin Heidelberg New York, pp 55–58

Bobon J, Bobon D, Pinchard A, Collard J, Ban TA, de Buch R, Hippius H, Lambert PA, Vinar O (1972) A new comparative physiognomy of neuroleptics: a collaborative clinical report. Acta Psychiatr Belg 72:542–554

Breyer-Pfaff U (1987) Klinische Pharmakokinetik der Neuroleptika: Ergebnisse und Probleme. In: Pichot P, Möller HJ (eds) Neuroleptika. Rückschau 1952–1986. Künftige Entwicklungen. Springer, Berlin Heidelberg New York, pp 37–46
Buck R de (1974) Antiautistic effect of flupentixol. In: Bobon P, Gottfries CG (eds) Clinical physiognomy of thioxanthenes. Acta Psychiatr Belg 74:441–568
Carlsson A (1978) Does dopamine have a role in schizophrenia? Biol Psychiatry 13:3–21
Carpenter WT, Heinrichs DW, Alphs LD (1985) Treatment of negative symptoms. Schizophr Bull 11:440–452
Cole JO, Goldberg SC, Klerman GL (1964) Phenothiazine treatment in acute schizophrenia. Arch Gen Psychiatry 10:246–261
Cole JO, Goldberg SC, Davis JM (1966) Drugs in the treatment of psychosis: controlled studies. In: Solomon P (ed) Psychiatric drugs. Grune and Stratton, New York, pp 153–180
Conrad K (1958) Die beginnende Schizophrenie. Thieme, Stuttgart
Crow TJ (1980) Molecular pathology of schizophrenia: more than one disease process? Br Med J 280:66–68
Crow TJ (1985) The two-syndrome concept: origins and current status. Schizophr Bull 11:471–486
Davis JM (1974) Dose equivalence of antipsychotic drugs. J Psychiatr Res 11:65–69
Davis JM, Garver DL (1978) Neuroleptics: clinical use in psychiatry. In: Iversen LL, Iversen SD, Snyder SH (eds) Handbook of psychopharmacology, vol. 10. Plenum Press, New York
Davis JM, Schaffer CB, Killian GA, Kinard C, Chan C (1980) Important issues in the drug treatment of schizophrenia. Schizophr Bull 6:70–87
Deister A, Marneros A, Rohde A (1990) Zur Stabilität negativer und positiver Syndromatik. In: Möller HJ, Pelzer E (eds) Neuere Ansätze zur Diagnostik und Therapie schizophrener Minussymptomatik. Springer, Berlin Heidelberg New York, pp 25–34
Delay J, Deniker P (1952) 38 cas des psychoses traités par la cure prolongée et continué de 4568 RP. Ann Med Psychol 110:364
Delini-Stula A (1986) Neuroanatomical, neuropharmacological and neurobiochemical target systems for antipsychotic activity of neuroleptics. Pharmacopsychiatry 19:134–139
Falloon F, Watt DC, Shepherd M (1978) The social outcome of patients in a trial of long-term continuation therapy in schizophrenia: pimozide vs fluphenazine. Psychol Med 8:265–274
Feinberg S, Kay S, Elijovich L, Fiszbein A, Opler L (1988) Pimozide treatment of the negative schizophrenic syndrome: an open trial. J Clin Psychiatry 49:235–241
Fritze J (1989) Einführung in die biologische Psychiatrie. Fischer, Stuttgart New York
Gardos G, Cole JO (1973) The importance of dosage in antipsychotic drug administration – a review of dose response studies. Psychopharmacologia 29:221–230
Gelders Y (1990) Die Bedeutung des 5-HT-2-Rezeptor-Antagonismus für die Bedeutung der Schizophrenie, unter spezieller Berücksichtigung der Minussymptomatik. In: Möller HJ, Pelzer E (eds) Neuere Ansätze zur Diagnostik und Therapie schizophrener Minussymptomatik. Springer, Berlin Heidelberg New York, pp 223–230
Gibbons RD, Lewine RRJ, Davis JM, Schooler NR, Cole JO (1985) An empiricial test of a Kraepelinian vs a Bleulerian view of negative symptoms. Schizophr Bull 11:390–396
Goldberg SC (1985) Negative and deficit symptoms in schizophrenia do respond to neuroleptics. Schizophr Bull 11:453–456
Haag H, Greil W, Rüther E (1987) Zusammenhang zwischen Spätdyskinesie und verschiedenen Variablen der neuroleptischen Behandlung. In: Heinrich K, Klieser E (eds) Probleme der neuroleptischen Dosierung. Schattauer, Stuttgart, pp 237–249
Hansen LB, Larsen N-E (1985) Therapeutic advantages of monitoring plasma concentrations of perphenazine in clinical practice. Psychopharmacology 87:16–19
Heinrich K (1967) Zur Bedeutung des postremissiven Erschöpfungssyndroms für die Rehabilitation Schizophrener. Nervenarzt 38:487–491
Helmchen H (1988) Methodologische und strategische Erwägungen in der Schizophrenie-Forschung. Fortschr Neurol Psychiatr 56:379–389

Hoffman WF, Labs SM, Casey DE (1987) Neuroleptic-induced Parkinsonism in older schizophrenics. Biol Psychiatry 22:427–439
Huber G (1957) Pneumencephalographische und psychopathologische Bilder bei endogenen Psychosen. Springer, Berlin Göttingen Heidelberg
Johnstone EC, Crow TJ, Frith CD, Husband J, Kreel L (1976) Cerebral ventricular size and cognitive impairment in chronic schizophrenia: Lancet II:924–926
Kay SR, Opler LA (1987) The positive-negative dimension in schizophrenia: its validity and significance. Psychiatr Develop 5:79–103
Lehmann E, Quadbeck H, Tegeler J, Fararuni M, Heinrich K (1980) Wirkungsdifferenzen bei Hoch- und Standarddosierung von Fluphenazin-Decanoat in Abhängigkeit von Patienten-Merkmalen. Pharmakopsychiat Neuropsychopharmakol 13:117–129
Lewine RJ, Fogg L, Meltzer HY (1983) Assessment of negative and positive symptoms in schizophrenia. Schizophr Bull 9:368–376
Liddle PF (1987) The symptoms of chronic schizophrenia: a reexamination of the positive-negative dichotomy. Br J Psychiatry 151:145–151
Lindström LH (1985) Low HVA and normal 5-HIAA CSF levels in drug-free schizophrenic patients compared to healthy volunteers: correlations to symptomatology and family history. Psychiatry Res 14:265–273
Maier W, Schlegel S, Klinger T, Hillert A, Wetzel H (1990) Die Negativsymptomatik im Verhältnis zur Positivsymptomatik und zur depressiven Symptomatik der Schizophrenie: Eine psychometrische Untersuchung. In: Möller HJ, Pelzer E (eds) Neuere Ansätze zur Diagnostik und Therapie schizophrener Minussymptomatik. Springer, Berlin Heidelberg New York, pp 69–78
Mayer-Gross W (1920) Über die Stellungnahme zur abgelaufenen akuten Psychose. Z Ges Neurol Psychiatr 60:160–212
Meltzer HY, Zureick J (1989) Negative symptoms in schizophrenia: a target for new drug development – In: Dahl SG, Gram LF (eds) Clinical pharmacology in psychiatry. Springer, Berlin Heidelberg New York, pp 68–77
Möller HJ (1987a) Indikation und Differentialindikation der neuroleptischen Langzeitmedikation. In: Pichot P, Möller HJ (eds) Neuroleptika. Rückschau 1952–1986. Künftige Entwicklungen. Springer, Berlin Heidelberg New York, pp 63–79
Möller HJ (1987b) Konsequenzen aus der klinischen Psychopharmakologie für die nosologische und syndromatologische Klassifikation funktioneller psychischer Störungen. In: Simhandl C, Berner P, Luccioni H, Alf C (eds) Klassifikationsprobleme in der Psychiatrie. Med-pharmazeutische Verlagsgesellschaft, Purkersdorf, pp 163–188
Möller HJ, Kissling W (1987) Zur Frage der Beziehung zwischen Haloperidol-Serumspiegel und antipsychotischem Effekt. In: Heinrich K, Klieser E (eds) Probleme der neuroleptischen Dosierung. Schattauer, Stuttgart, pp 85–95
Möller HJ, Von Zerssen D (1981) Depressive Symptomatik im stationären Behandlungsverlauf von 280 schizophrenen Patienten. Pharmacopsychiatria 14:172–179
Möller HJ, Von Zerssen D (1982) Depressive states occurring during the neuroleptic treatment of schizophrenia. Schizophr Bull 8:109–117
Möller HJ, Von Zerssen D (1986) Depression in schizophrenia. In: Burrows GD, Norman TR, Rubinstein G (eds) Handbook of studies on schizophrenia, Part I. Elsevier, Amsterdam, pp 183–191
Möller HJ, Kissling W, Maurach R, Schmid W, Doerr P, Pirke K, Von Zerssen D (1981) Beziehungen zwischen Haloperidol-Serumspiegel, Prolactin-Serumspiegel, antipsychotischem Effekt und extrapyramidalen Begleitwirkungen. Pharmacopsychiatria 14:27–34
Möller HJ, Scharl W, Von Zerssen D (1985) Vorhersage des Therapieerfolges unter neuroleptischer Akutbehandlung: Ergebnisse einer empirischen Untersuchung an 243 stationär behandelten schizophrenen Patienten. Fortschr Neurol Psychiatr 53:370–383
Möller HJ, Kissling W, Dietzfelbinger T, Stoll K-D, Wendt G (1989) Efficacy and tolerability of a new antipsychotic compound (savoxepine): results of a pilot study. Pharmacopsychiatry 22:38–41

Müller WE (1987) Neurobiochemie der Neuroleptika. In: Pichot P, Möller HJ (eds) Neuroleptika. Rückschau 1952–1986. Künftige Entwicklungen. Springer, Berlin Heidelberg New York, pp 9–26
Nedopil N, Rüther E (1981) Initial improvement as predictor of outcome of neuroleptic treatment. Pharmacopsychiatry 14:205–207
Niemegeers C (1988) Pharmakologie und Biochemie niedrig dosierter Neuroleptika. In: Hippius H, Laakmann G (eds) Therapie mit Neuroleptika – Niedrigdosierung. Perimed, Erlangen, pp 10–18
Niemegeers C, Awouters F, Janssen PAJ (1990) Pharmakologie der Neuroleptika und relevante Mechanismen zur Behandlung von Minussymptomatik. In: Möller HJ, Pelzer E (eds) Neuere Ansätze zur Diagnostik und Therapie schizophrener Minussymptomatik. Springer, Berlin Heidelberg New York, pp 185–197
Nybäck H, Bergen BM, Hindmarsh T, Sedvall G, Wiesel F (1983) Cerebroventricular size and cerebrospinal fluid monoamine metabolites in schizophrenic patients and healthy volunteers. Psychiatry Res 9:301–308
Pinder RM, Brogden RN, Sawyer PR, Speight T, Spencer R, Avery GS (1976) Pimozide, a review of its pharmacological properties and therapeutic uses in psychiatry. Drugs 12:1–40
Prosser ES, Csernansky JG, Kaplan H, Thiemann S, Becker TJ, Hollister LE (1987) Depression, Parkinsonian symptoms, and negative symptoms in schizophrenics treated with neuroleptics. J Nerv Ment Dis 175:100–105
Richelson E (1984) Neuroleptic affinities for human brain receptors and their use in predicting adverse effects. J Clin Psychiatry 45:331–336
Rösler M, Hengesch G (1990) "Negative" Symptome im AMDP-System. In: Baum U, Fähndrich E, Stieglitz R-D, Woggon B (eds) Veränderungsmessung in Psychiatrie und Klinischer Psychologie. Profil, München, pp 329–339
Rüther E (1986) Wirkungsverlauf der neuroleptischen Therapie: Verlaufsuntersuchungen bei der antipsychotischen Therapie mit Haloperidol und Clozapin. Fischer, Stuttgart
Rüther E, Müller-Spahn F (1987) Neurobiochemische Untersuchungen bei Akut- und Langzeitbehandlung mit Neuroleptika. In: Pichot P, Möller HJ (eds) Neuroleptika. Rückschau 1952–1986. Künftige Entwicklungen. Springer, Berlin Heidelberg New York, pp 27–35
Sieberns S (1986) Darstellung der Depotneuroleptika. In: Heinrich K, Sieberns S (eds) Internationales Fluanxol-Depot-Kolloquium. Das ärztliche Gespräch, 40. Tropon, Cologne, pp 7–18
Sommers AA (1985) "Negative symptoms": conceptual and methodological problems. Schizophr Bull 11:364–379
Strauss JS, Carpenter WT jr, Bartko JJ (1974) The diagnosis and understanding of schizophrenia. III. Speculations on the processes that underlie schizophrenic symptoms and signs. Schizophr Bull 1:61–69
Tansella M, Balestrieri A (1976) The choice of neuroleptics in the treatment of schizophrenia. Arzneimittelforsch 26:943–945
Tegeler J (1981) Dosierung und Verträglichkeit der Depot- und Langzeitneuroleptika. In: Erfahrungsaustausch über die Anwendung von Depotneuroleptika – unter besonderer Berücksichtigung der Thioxanthen-Depotneuroleptika. Das ärztliche Gespräch, 35. Tropon, Cologne, pp 52–63
Van Kammen DP, Van Kammen WB, Mann LS, Seppala T, Linnoila M (1986) Dopamine metabolism in the cerebrospinal fluid of drug-free schizophrenic patients with and without cortical atrophy. Arch Gen Psychiatry 43:978–983
Van Kammen DP, Hommer DW, Malas KL (1987) Effect of pimozide on positive and negative symptoms in schizophrenic patients: are negative symptoms state dependent? Neuropsychobiology 18:113–117
Waddington JL, Youssef HA, Molloy AG, O'Boyle KM, Pugh MT (1985) Association of intellectual impairment, negative symptoms, and aging with tardive dyskinesia: clinical and animal studies. J Clin Psychiatry 46:29–33
Wiesel F-A, Farde L, Nordström A-L, Sedvall G (1990) Die Bedeutung der D_1 und D_2

Dopaminrezeptor-Blockade für die antipsychotische Wirkung von Neuroleptika. Eine PET-Studie an schizophrenen Patienten. In: Müller-Oerlinghausen B, Möller HJ, Rüther E (eds) Thioxanthene in der neuroleptischen Behandlung. Springer, Berlin Heidelberg New York, pp 13–20

Wilson LG, Roberts RW, Gerber CJ, Johnson MH (1982): Pimozide versus chlorpromazine in chronic schizophrenia: a 52 week double-blind study of maintenance therapy. J Clin Psychiatry 43:62–65

Wing JK (1978) Clinical concepts of schizophrenia. In: Wing JK (ed) Schizophrenia: toward a new synthesis. Academic, London, pp 1–30

Woggon B (1983) Prognose der Psychopharmakotherapie. Klinische Untersuchungen zur Voraussagbarkeit des Kurzzeittherapieerfolges von Neuroleptika und Antidepressiva. Enke, Stuttgart

Woggon B (1990) Wirkprofile klassischer Neuroleptika und die Beeinflussung von Minussymptomatik. In: Möller HJ, Pelzer E (eds) Neuere Ansätze zur Diagnostik und Therapie schizophrener Minussymtomatik. Springer, Berlin Heidelberg New York, pp 199–205

Woggon B, Beckmann H, Heinrich K, Linden M, Krebs E, Küfferle B, Pflug B, Rüther E, Schied HW (1986) Clinically relevant differences in the therapeutic profile of fluperlapine compared to haloperidol in the treatment of schizophrenic psychosis. Results of a multicentre double-blind study. Pharmacopsychiatria 19:204–205

Zinner HJ, Kraemer S, Möller HJ (1990) Empirische Untersuchungen zur Konkordanz verschiedener Minussymptomatik-Skalen sowie zur Korrelation mit testpsychologischen Befunden. In: Möller HJ, Pelzer E (eds) Neuere Ansätze zur Diagnostik und Therapie schizophrener Minussymptomatik. Springer, Berlin Heidelberg New York, pp 59–68

The Effect of Clozapine and Other Atypical Antipsychotic Drugs on Negative Symptoms

H. Y. MELTZER [1]

Introduction

The historical and theoretical basis for the division of the symptoms of schizophrenia into positive and negative has been reviewed by Berrios (1985) and Trimble (1986). There is general agreement that delusions and hallucinations are the cardinal positive symptoms of schizophrenia, but there is more controversy about the domain of negative symptoms. There is general agreement that flat affect, loss of volition, and loss of interest are negative symptoms. Motor retardation and poverty of thought content have also been included (Meltzer and Zureick 1989). There is less concurrence whether bizarre behavior and some types of thought disorder, e.g., marked incoherence, tangentiality, or illogicality, also should be considered positive symptoms (Andreasen and Olson 1982). In the absence of any definitive means of determining which symptoms are positive or negative, it seems appropriate at this time to take a conservative and operational viewpoint as to what constitutes each type.

Much of the recent interest in positive and negative symptoms has stemmed from consideration of the relative responsiveness of positive and negative symptoms to antipsychotic drug treatment. There is considerable evidence that the neuroleptic drugs such as haloperidol, chlorpromazine, molindone, thiothixene, and other members of the class of neuroleptic drugs are more effective in treating positive than negative symptoms (Meltzer et al. 1986). Some investigators have suggested that negative symptoms are unresponsive to neuroleptic drugs (Johnstone et al. 1978; Crow 1980). However, there is substantial support for the conclusion that typical neuroleptic drugs are effective, albeit in a limited way, against negative symptoms (see Meltzer 1985; 1987, 1989, 1990; Goldberg 1985; Meltzer et al. 1986). For example, using a negative symptom scale (Lewine et al. 1983) comprised of 11 items from the Schedule for Affective Disorders-Change scale (SADS-C; Endicott and Spitzer 1978) namely blunted affect, inappropriate affect, incoherence, loose associations, poverty of content, loss of interest, loss of sexual interest, slowed speech, slowed body movements, fatigue, and depressed appearance, Meltzer (1987) reported a 34.1 % decrease between admission and discharge in a group

[1] Department of Psychiatry, Case Western Reserve University, School of Medicine, Cleveland, OH 44106, USA

A. Marneros / N. C. Andreasen / M. T. Tsuang (Eds.)
Negative Versus Positive Schizophrenia

of 73 schizophrenic patients treated with typical neuroleptic drugs. This compared with a 69.4% decrease in positive symptoms (various hallucinations and delusions) in the same subjects.

Recently, finding more effective treatments for negative symptoms has become a major goal of new drug development for schizophrenia. As discussed elsewhere (Meltzer 1990), negative symptoms may be as much of a handicap to schizophrenic patients and their families and a burden to clinicians who work with schizophrenic patients as positive ones. The development of more effective treatment depends, in part, upon rating scales designed to assess symptoms accurately and comprehensively (Meltzer 1990). The most widely used means of assessing negative symptoms for psychopharmacologic purposes has been the Brief Psychiatric Rating Scale (BPRS, Overall and Gorham 1962), Anergia-Withdrawal subscale. This is comprised of blunted affect, emotional withdrawal and motor retardation, and disorientation items. More comprehensive negative symptom scales have been proposed (Meltzer 1990). The Scale for the Assessment of Negative Symptoms (SANS, Andreasen 1983) has achieved the widest acceptance, but its advantage for psychopharmacology has not been intensively explored.

We have suggested that changes in social function may, under some circumstances, be used as a measure of drug effects on negative symptoms (Meltzer 1990). While positive symptoms are a major determinant of social function, it is likely that improvement in volition, attention, motor activation, speech, and thought content will also have an influence.

Atypical Antipsychotic Drugs

There are numerous definitions of atypical antipsychotic drugs. It is an accepted requirement that they produce little or no extrapyramidal symptoms (EPS). These agents also do not lead to the marked increases in plasma prolactin (PRL) levels seen with typical neuroleptic drugs (Meltzer et al. 1989c). The prototype is clozapine, a dibenzodiazepine. Other drugs for which there is evidence of low EPS and an atypical plasma PRL response pattern in humans are fluperlapine, amperozide, melperone, RMI-81582, setoperone, and tiospirone (Meltzer et al. 1989d). There are other candidates, but there is much less clinical evidence to support the belief that they too are atypical antipsychotic drugs, e.g., zotepine, HP370, and pipamperone (Meltzer et al. 1989d).

Atypical Antipsychotic Drugs Other Than Clozapine

Fluperlapine, a dibenzazepine closely related to clozapine, was reported to decrease symptoms of apathy and retardation/depression in 46 chronic schizophrenic patients (Woggon et al. 1984). It had only a weak effect on anergia ratings in more acute patients (Dieterle et al. 1984). Zotepine, a dibenzothiepine, has been reported to be effective in treating some negative symptoms such as akinesia and anhedonia at low doses (Yamawaki 1987).

Setoperone, a thiazolpyrimidinone, was reported to decrease negative symptoms in schizophrenic patients with predominantly negative symptoms (Ceulemans et al. 1985).

Risperidone is a benzisoxazol derivative with an atypical preclinical profile (Janssen et al. 1988). It is currently undergoing extensive clinical testing, and there have been preliminary reports that it is effective in treating negative symptoms (Gelders et al. 1989).

Amperozide is a piperazine carboxamide compound with atypical antipsychotic properties (Haskins et al. 1987). It has been noted to have significant effects on negative symptoms in schizophrenic patients (Mertens et al. 1989).

Melperone is a butyrophenone with atypical antipsychotic properties (Christensson 1989). I have found that it produces significant decreases in negative symptoms in treatment-resistant schizophrenia (Meltzer et al. 1989a).

Some investigators refer to substituted benzamides as atypical antipsychotic agents, but they produce marked increases in plasma PRL levels. There have been a number of reports that sulpiride, a substituted benzamide, may be effective in decreasing apathy and withdrawal and increasing social participation in patients with marked negative symptoms (Toru et al. 1972; Cassari et al. 1975; Elizur et al. 1975; Mielke et al. 1977). These results could not be confirmed by Edwards et al. (1980) in a 6-week, double-blind trial comparing high dose sulpiride (1800 mg/day) and trifluoperazine (15–45 mg/day) in 38 chronic schizophrenic patients, using the BPRS negative symptoms subscale as the response measure. Alfredsson et al. (1985) compared the effect of moderate doses of sulpiride (800 mg/day) and chlorpromazine (400 mg/day) in 50 schizophrenic patients in a double-blind trial. Sulpiride significantly decreased the rating of negative symptoms using the Comprehensive Psychiatric Rating Scale (Asberg et al. 1978) and the nurses' observation scale for inpatient evaluation (NOSIE); Honigfeld and Klett (1965) during the first 2 weeks of treatment. Chlorpromazine was effective after 4 weeks of administration.

Remoxipride is a novel substituted benzamide which was reported to decrease the BPRS anergia scores in 10 schizophrenic patients (Lindstrom et al. 1985). Amisulpride is another substituted benzamide recently introduced in Europe. High-dose amisulpride (500–1200 mg/day) was found not to decrease BPRS anergia ratings in 14 schizophrenic patients (Mann et al. 1984). There is some evidence that at low doses it is effective in treating the negative symptoms of schizophrenia (Boyer 1989).

Clozapine

The strongest body of evidence which supports the ability of atypical antipsychotic drugs to improve negative symptoms is available from studies of clozapine. The early literature, including the pivotal study of Kane et al. (1988), has been reviewed elsewhere (Meltzer, in press) and only the highlights will be briefly discussed here.

Claghorn et al. (1987) reported that clozapine was significantly more effective than chlorpromazine in reducing BPRS Anergia-Withdrawal ratings in 150 schizophrenic patients with tardive dyskinesia or moderate-severe EPS who were randomly assigned to either treatment. Patients who had been chronically hospitalized were excluded. At both 8 weeks and with an end-point analysis, the improvement in this factor with clozapine compared with chlorpromazine treatment was greater than that for any other BPRS factor. This was true despite the fact that the two drugs were equivalent in improving motor retardation. Nurses' ratings supported the superiority of clozapine in improving social function. This study is of particular importance because it is the best one to date concerning the possible advantage of clozapine in treating non-neuroleptic-resistant schizophrenic patients. However, it is difficult to tell from a short-term study of this kind whethr the advantages are significant enough to warrant consideration of usage in the treatment of schizophrenic patients who are neither unresponsive to nor intolerant of neuroleptic drugs. Of course, factors other than improvement in negative symptoms would be relevant to such considerations.

The study of Kane et al. (1988) examined the effectiveness of clozapine in treatment-resistant schizophrenic patients. Some 305 schizophrenic patients with a history of failure to respond to at least three neuroleptic agents of two different classes were included. In the first phase, these patients were treated with high doses of haloperidol for 6 weeks, and less than 2% responded. The nonresponders plus a small group of haloperidol-intolerant patients were then randomly assigned to clozapine or chlorpromazine for 6 weeks. Clozapine was superior to chlorpromazine in decreasing BPRS positive symptoms from weeks 1 to 6; BPRS anergia-withdrawal scale showed greater improvement in the clozapine- than the chlorpromazine-treated group between weeks 2 and 6. Significantly greater improvement in social function in the clozapine-treated group was noted in the nurses' rating. This study established that clozapine was sufficiently superior to standard neuroleptic treatment to justify to the United States Food and Drug Administration that the benefit of clozapine in treatment-resistant or neuroleptic-intolerant schizophrenic patients outweighed its risks.

Long-Term Effects of Clozapine on Negative Symptoms

Meltzer et al. (1989b) reported preliminary results of an open, prospective study of the effect of clozapine with 51 treatment-resistant schizophrenic patients. These patients were similar in severity to those studied by Kane et al. (1988). The duration of treatment with clozapine was 1.5–35.2 months (mean $\pm$ SD 10.3 $\pm$ 8.1 months). Significant decreases were noted in the BPRS Withdrawal-Retardation scale, with an increasing improvement over time. An analysis of covariance demonstrated that the improvement in BPRS Withdrawal-Retardation ratings was independent of the improvement in positive symptoms.

Table 1. Effect of clozapine treatment on Brief Psychiatric Rating Scale (BPRS) total, positive, and negative symptoms

Time	*n*	Total	Positive	Negative
Baseline	70	54.4 ± 10.8	16.2 ± 5.5	10.1 ± 4.4
6 weeks	56	44.1 ± 11.8***	12.3 ± 5.1***	9.6 ± 4.0
3 months	50	39.5 ± 11.1***	11.6 ± 5.1***	8.8 ± 3.8*
6 months	45	40.2 ± 11.9***	11.9 ± 4.9***	8.4 ± 3.5*
9 months	40	40.2 ± 10.2***	11.6 ± 5.4***	8.8 ± 3.4**
12 months	39	37.1 ± 9.8***	10.3 ± 4.9***	8.2 ± 3.2**

* $P < 0.02$; ** $P < 0.01$; *** $P < 0.0001$.

Some subsequent results of this ongoing study in a larger sample of patients will be briefly reported here. Data are now available on 85 patients whose treatment with clozapine was begun 12 months prior to the point of data analysis. The methods used in this study have been described elsewhere (Meltzer et al. 1989 b). All were treatment-resistant by the criteria of Kane et al. (1988). The mean age was 34.6 ± 8.5 years. The mean age of onset was 20.7 ± 6.2 years. The number of previous hospitalizations was 8.7 ± 6.9. There were 60 males and 25 females. Negative symptoms were assessed with the BPRS (Overall and Gorham 1962), the SANS (Andreasen 1982) and the SADS-C (Endicott and Spitzer 1978).

Of the 85 patients, 70 (82.3%) had an admission total BPRS ≧ 36, one of the criteria used to select subjects for the study of Kane et al. (1988) to enter the double-blind phase of that study. This report will present data on these 70 patients. The initial total BPRS of those 70 patients was 54.4 ± 10.8. Of these 70 patients, 21 (30%) dropped out before the end of 12 months. The BPRS total, positive, and negative symptom scores at baseline, 3, 6, 9, and 12 months are given in Table 1. As there were some missing data and drop-outs at each time period, the number of subjects at each period decreases significantly. The baseline BPRS negative symptom score was 10.1 ± 4.4. There was no significant change in these ratings after 6 weeks despite a highly significant fall in BPRS total and positive symptoms ratings at this time. There was a significant improvement over baseline ratings in BPRS negative symptom scores for all subsequent time periods, but the extent of improvement did not greatly increase over time. The percentage of change in negative symptoms at 3 months was 5.4% and at 12 months 11.4% compared with 23.4% and 33.8%, respectively, for positive symptoms. The median BPRS negative symptom rating changed from 9 at baseline to 8 at 12 months in this sample whereas the median positive symptom score changed from 15 at baseline to 10 at 12 months. The median percentage improvement in BPRS negative and positive symptom scores at 12 months was 14% and 35.5%, respectively. Thus, there was a relatively slight overall improvement in BPRS negative symptom ratings in this group.

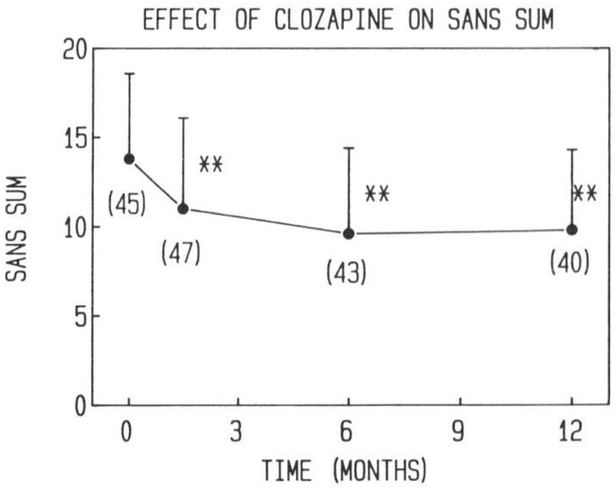

Fig. 1. Scale for the Assessment of Negative Symptoms (SANS) sum ratings in clozapine-treated, treatment-restistant schizophrenic patients ($p < 0.01$)

Table 2. Scale for the Assessment of Negative Symptoms (SANS) subscale global scores following clozapine treatment

Time	Alogia	Anhedonia	Attentional impairment	Affective flattening	Avolition
Baseline	2.5 ± 1.5	3.4 ± 1.0	2.1 ± 1.7	2.9 ± 1.0	3.3 ± 1.2
6 weeks	1.8 ± 1.4**	2.6 ± 1.3**	1.6 ± 1.5	2.5 ± 1.3	2.8 ± 1.2
6 months	1.4 ± 1.2***	2.2 ± 1.4**	1.1 ± 1.2***	2.2 ± 1.2•	2.9 ± 1.3
12 months	1.1 ± 1.3***	2.7 ± 1.2	1.3 ± 1.3*	2.4 ± 1.1•	2.9 ± 1.4

• $P < 0.10$; * $P < 0.05$; ** $P < 0.01$; *** $P < 0.001$ compared with baseline.

Analysis of the SANS ratings in a subgroup of the same subjects shows a greater but selective change in negative symptoms. As can be seen in Fig. 1, there was a significant improvement in the SANS sum score of all global items at 6 weeks, 6, and 12 months. Data in Table 2 indicate that the alogia global score also improved at all time points. Anhedonia global score improved at 6 weeks and 6 months only. Attentional impairment improved at 6 and 12 months only. There was a trend for improvement in affective flattening at 6 and 12 months. Avolition did not improve at any time point. The order of magnitude of the improvement was 28% at 12 months in the SANS sum and 56% for alogia. Thus, the SANS items (affective flattening and avolition) which parallel the BPRS negative symptom scale items (blunted affect and emotional withdrawal) also showed little or no change over a 12-month period.

These results must be viewed in the context of marked changes in the quality of life of these patients on clozapine. Data were available for 27 of the patients on the Quality of Life Scale (QLS; Heinrichs et al. 1984). The total QLS score increased from 28.7 ± 22.5 to 52.7 ± 31.7 ($P = 0.0001$). The Intrapsychic Function Score, which includes a number of negative symptom items, e.g., motivation, pleasure, and emotional interaction, increased from 5.2 ± 3.8 to 10.6 ± 3.1 ($P < 0.0001$). With the Interpersonal Relations Factor, which also includes negative symptom items, e.g., social participation and social initiative, absence of withdrawal improved from 11.6 ± 10.5 to 23.1 ± 10.4 ($P < 0.0001$).

Relationship of Change in Negative Symptoms to Change in Positive Symptoms

A critical issue in the consideration of the effect of typical and atypical antipsychotic drugs on negative symptoms is whether any effect is independent of the effect on positive symptoms. For example, improvement in withdrawal may be secondary to improvement in paranoid delusions; improvement in anhedonia or alogia may be secondary to decreased hallucinations, etc.

I have utilized several methods to examine this issue. Firstly, the correlations were examined between the change in positive and negative symptoms at 6 weeks, 6, and 12 months. None were significant in the clozapine-treated patient: $\varrho = -0.01$, $n = 48$; $\varrho = 0.25$, $P = 0.11$, $n = 43$; $\varrho = 0.00$, $n = 48$). Next, I used two multiple regression models. In the first, the final BPRS negative symptom scale rating was the dependent measure in a model which included BPRS negative and positive symptoms at baseline and the corresponding final BPRS positive symptom scale score. In the second model, the final BPRS negative symptom scale rating was the dependent measure in a model with included BPRS negative symptom ratings at baseline and the change in BPRS positive symptoms between baseline and either 6 weeks, 6, or 12 months. The results for both models were identical. Bothy types of models were significant at 6 weeks and 12 months but not at 6 months. However, only the baseline BPRS negative symptom score was significantly related to the 6-week or 12-month BPRS negative symptom score. The results for the 6-week change are given in Tables 3 and 4. It may be seen that they are virtually identical. Similar negative results were obtained when the SANS sum and the five global items were related to the BPRS positive symptom scale scores (data not presented). This indicates the improvement in negative symptoms during clozapine treatment are independent of the improvement in positive symptoms.

I have also examined the same effect in schizophrenic patients treated with typical neuroleptic drugs. Baseline and discharge data from my former Chicago site were utilized. Mean BPRS positive and negative symptom ratings at baseline and discharge and the change between these two periods are given in Table 5. Marked decreases in both positive and negative symptoms were

Table 3. Prediction of BPRS negative symptom score at 6 weeks in clozapine-treated schizophrenia: baseline and 6-week measures

Source	Regression coefficient	*F*	*P*
BPRS negative baseline	0.38	9.06	0.004
BPRS positive baseline	−0.09	0.59	0.45
BPRS positive 6 weeks	0.02	0.02	0.88

$F = 3.48$; df = 3.44; $P = 0.02$.
BPRS, Brief Psychiatric Rating Scale.

Table 4. Prediction of BPRS negative symptom score at 6 weeks in clozapine-treated schizophrenia: change between baseline and 6 weeks

Source	Regression coefficient	*F*	*P*
BPRS negative baseline	0.38	9.46	0.004
BPRS change in positive	0.04	0.15	0.70

$F = 4.80$; df = 2.45; $P = 0.01$.
BPRS, Brief Psychiatric Rating Scale.

Table 5. BPRS positive and negative symptom ratings in typical neuroleptic-treated schizophrenic patients

	Mean ± SD
Positive symptoms	
Baseline	14.6 ± 5.0 (182)
End point	8.8 ± 4.3 (177)***
Delta	6.0 ± 5.8 (173)
Negative symptoms	
Baseline	9.4 ± 4.5 (173)
End point	7.2 ± 3.0 (179)***
Delta	2.3 ± 4.2 (176)

*** $P < 0.0001$ compared with baseline.
BPRS, Brief Psychiatric Rating Scale.

Table 6. Prediction of BPRS negative symptom score at 6 weeks in typical neuroleptic-treated schizophrenic patients

Source	Regression coefficient	*F*	*P*
BPRS negative baseline	0.30	43.19	0.0001
BPRS positive baseline	−0.08	3.05	0.08
BPRS positive 6 weeks	0.11	5.38	0.02

$F = 5.54$; df = 3.169; $P = 0.0001$.
BPRS, Brief Psychiatric Rating Scale.

observed. There was a significant correlation between the change in positive and negative symptoms: $\varrho = 0.21$, $n = 173$, $P = 0.005$. However, there was no correlation between the baseline positive and negative symptom ratings. Multiple regression analysis also showed a relationship between positive and negative symptoms. As can be seen in Table 6, BPRS positive symptoms positively predicted BPRS negative symptoms at 6 weeks, after adjusting for

Table 7. Change in BPRS total, positive, and negative symptoms in type P and type N schizophrenic patients at 3 months

BPRS measure	Type P (35)	Type N (7)
Change in total	6.5 ± 12.5	4.4 ± 9.1
Change in positive	2.6 ± 3.9	− 0.86 ± 4.1 *
Change in negative	− 1.8 ± 4.1	6.0 ± 3.2 ****
% Change in total	12.1 ± 24.5	10.4 ± 22.3
% Change in positive	14.0 ± 28.3	−24.7 ± 65.0 ***
% Change in negative	−24.3 ± 48.3	39.4 ± 19.7 ***

* $P < 0.05$; *** $P < 0.001$; **** $P < 0.0001$.
BPRS, Brief Psychiatric Rating Scale.

BPRS negative and positive symptoms at baseline ($P = 0.02$). The results were identical using the change in BPRS positive symptoms in the model (data not shown). Thus, these data indicate that typical neuroleptic drugs in a group of schizophrenic patients not selected for treatment resistance produces improvement in negative symptoms but that this is not independent of the improvement in positive symptoms. Clozapine produces a smaller improvement in negative symptoms in treatment-resistant schizophrenia, but it is not related to the improvement in positive symptoms.

Effect of Clozapine in Patients with Mainly Negative Symptoms

Crow (1980) divided schizophrenia into two types: type I and type II. Among other differences, type I schizophrenia was identified as patients with predominantly positive symptoms and a good response to neuroleptic drugs. Type II was identified as patients with predominantly negative symptoms and a poor response to neuroleptic drugs. I have criticised this theory elsewhere (Meltzer 1985). Because of its widespread influence in current thinking, it was of interest to examine the effect of clozapine in type II schizophrenia. While nearly all of our patients meet the criteria for treatment resistance, they were, in fact, usually selected for the presence of positive symptoms. This alone suggests that the type I – type II distinction is only an abstraction. Nevertheless, I decided to identify the group of clozapine-treated patients with high positive and low negative symptoms using the BPRS. Patients with scores of moderate or worse on any one of BPRS items 4, 11, 12, and 15 and mild or less on all BPRS items 3, 13, 16, and 18 were considered high positive/low negative (type P) and patients with the reverse were considered high negative/low positive (type N). The BPRS negative symptom scores of the type P patients were 6.9 ± 4.4 versus 13.6 ± 4.3 for type N patients ($P < 0.001$). Of the 85 patients, there were 46 type P and 12 type N. The two groups did not differ in age, sex, or duration of illness, but the type P members had more often been previously hospitalized

(9.7 ± 8.4) than the type N ones (4.1 ± 4.3), $P < 0.01$. The change in BPRS total score was not significant in type P or type N patients after 3 months of treatment. However, the type P patients showed a greater improvement in positive symptoms whereas the reverse was true for type N patients (Table 7). Six of the 12 type N patients exhibited a decrease in BPRS negative symptom scores ≧ 50% within 12 months of treatment. These results further indicate that clozapine can improve negative symptoms independently of its effects on positive symptoms and that schizophrenic patients with predominantly negative symptoms are able to respond to antipsychotic drug treatment.

Conclusions

The results reported here demonstrate that atypical antipsychotic drugs can ameliorate negative symptoms, even in treatment-resistant schizophrenia. A variety of atypical antipsychotic drugs may be effective, but the evidence is strongest for clozapine. The SANS scale appears to be a useful means of identifying this improvement, perhaps more so than the BPRS negative symptom scale. There appears to be differences in the responses of specific types of negative symptoms to clozapine treatment. Alogia may be the most responsive and avolition, the least. The improvement in negative symptoms with clozapine appears to be independent of the improvement in positive symptoms. This is not so with typical antipsychotic drugs.

References

Alfredsson G, Härnryd C, Wiesel F-A (1985) Effects of sulpiride and chlorpromazine on autistic and positive psychotic symptoms in schizophrenic patients – relationship to drug concentrations. Psychopharmacology (Berlin) 85:8–13

Andreasen NC (1983) The scale for the assessment of negative symptoms (SANS). University of Iowa, Iowa City

Andreasen NC, Olsen S (1982) Negative vs. positive schizophrenia: definition and validation. Arch Gen Psychiatr9 39:789–794

Asberg M, Montgomery S, Perris, et al. (1978) CPRS - The psychopathological rating scale. Acta Psychiatr Scand 271:5–27

Berrios GE (1985) Positive and negative symptoms and Jackson: a conceptual history. Arch Gen Psychiatry 42:95–97

Boyer P (1989) Opposite therapeutic effects of amisulpride with different dosages. Excerpta Med Congr Ser 899:228

Cassario GB, Castrogiovanni P, Conti L (1975) Sulpiride versus haloperidol in schizophrenia: a double-blind comparative trial. Curr Ther Res 17:189–201

Ceulemans D, Gelders Y, Hoppenbrouwers M-L, Reyntjens A, Janssen P (1985) Effect of serotonin antagonism in schizophrenia: a pilot study with setoperone. Psychopharmacology (Berlin) 85:329–332

Christensson E (1989) Pharmacologic data of the atypical neuroleptic compound melperone (Burnont). Acta Psychiatr Scand [Suppl] 80:7–15

Claghorn J, Honigfeld G, Abuzzahab PS, Wang R, Steinbook R, Tuason V, Klerman G (1987) The risks and benefits of clozapine versus chlorpromazine. J Clin Psychopharmacol 7:377–384

Crow TJ (1980) Positive and negative schizophrenic symptoms and the role of dopamine. Br J psychiatry 139:379–386
Dieterle D, Eben E, Einhaupi K, Hippius H, Klein H, Rüther E, Schmauss M (1984) The effect of fluperlapine in acute psychotic patients. Pharmacopsychiatry 17:57–60
Edwards JG, Alexander JR, Alexander MS, et al. (1980) Controlled trial of sulpiride in chronic schizophrenic patients. Brit J Psychiatry 137:522–529
Elizur A, Davidson S, Psych FRC (1975) The evaluation of the anti-autistic activity of sulpiride. Curr Ther Res 18:578–584
Endicott J, Spitzer R (1978) A diagnostic interview. A schedule for affective disorders and schizophrenia. Arch Gen Psychiatry 35:837–844
Goldberg SC (1985) Negative and deficit symptoms in schizophrenia do respond to neuroleptics. Schizophr Bull 11:453–456
Haskins JT, Muth EA, Andree T (1987) Biochemical and electrophysiological studies of the psychotropic compound, amperozide. Brain Res Bull 19:465–471
Heinrichs DW, Hanlon TE, Carpenter WT Jr (1984) The quality of life scale: an instrument for rating the schizophrenic deficit syndrome. Schizophr Bull 10:388–396
Honigfeld G, Klett J (1965) The nurses' observation scale for inpatient evaluation (NOSIE): a new scale for measuring improvement in chronic schizophrenia. J Clin Psychol 21:65–71
Janssen PAJ, Niemeegeers CJE, Awouters F, Schellenkens KHL, Megens AAHP, Meert TF (1988) Pharmacology of risperidone (R64766), a new antipsychotic with serotonin-S_2 and dopamine-D_2 antagonistic properties. J Pharmacol Exp Ther 244:685–693
Johnstone EC, Frith CD, Crow TJ, Carney MWP, Price JS (1978) Mechanism of the antipsychotic effect in the treatment of acute schizophrenia. Lancet 1:848–851
Kane J, Honigfeld G, Singer J, Meltzer HY (1988) Clozapine for the treatment-resistant schizophrenic: a double-blind comparison versus chlorpromazine/benztropine. Arch Gen Psychiatry 48:789–796
Lewine RJ, Fogg L Meltzer HY (1983) Assessment of negative and positive symptoms in schizophrenia. Schizophr Bull 9:368–376
Lindström L, Besev G, Stening G, Widerlöv E (1985) An open study of remoxipride, a benzamide derivative, in schizophrenia. Psychopharmacology (Berlin) 86:241–245
Mann K, Bartels M, Bauer H, Gaertner HJ (1984) Amisulpride – an open clinical study of a new benzamide in schizophrenic patients. Pharmacopsychiatry 17:111–115
Meltzer HY (1985) Dopamine and negative symptoms in schizophrenia: critique of the type I–type II hypothesis. In: Alpert M (ed) Controversies in schizophrenia: changes and constancies. Guilford, New York, pp 110–136
Meltzer HY (1987) Effect of neuroleptics in the schizophrenia syndrome. In: Dahl SG, Gram LF, Paul SM, Potter WZ (eds) Clinical pharmacology in psychiatry. Selectivity in psychotropic drug action – promises or problems? Springer, Berlin Heidelberg New York, pp 255–265
Meltzer HY (1990) Pharmacological treatment of negative symptoms. In: Greden JF, Tandon R (eds) Negative schizophrenic syptoms: pathophysiology and clinical implications. American Psychiatric Press, Washington (in press)
Meltzer HY, Zureick J (1989) Negative syptoms in schizophrenia: a target for new drug development. In: Dahl SG, Gram LF (eds) Clinical pharmacology in psychiatry: from molecular studies to clinical reality. Springer, Berlin Heidelberg New York, pp 68–77
Meltzer HY, Sommers AA, Luchins DJ (1986) The effect of neuroleptics and other psychotropic drugs on negative symptoms in schizophrenia. J Clin Psychopharmacol 6:329–338
Meltzer HY, Alphs LD, Bastani B, Ramirez L (1989a) Effect of melperone in treatment-resistant schizophrenia. Excerpta Med Int Congr Ser 899:502
Meltzer HY, Bastani B, Kwon KY, Ramirez LF, Burnett S, Sharpe J (1989b) A prospective study of clozapine in treatment-resistant patients. I. Preliminary report. Psychopharmacology [Suppl] (Berlin) 99:S68–S72
Meltzer HY, Bastani B, Kwon KY, Ramirez LF, Matsubara S (1989c) Clozapine: new research on efficacy and mechanism of action. Eur Arch Psychiatry Neurol Sci 238:332–339

Meltzer HY, Matsubara T, Lee JC (1989d) Classification of typical and atypical antipsychotic drugs on the basis of dopamine D-1, D-2 and serotonin$_2$ pKi values. J Pharmacol Exp Ther 257:238–246
Mertens C, DeWilde J, Dierick M, Bergman I, Gustavsson G (1989) Clinical trials of amperozide in schizophrenia (Abstr. Excerpta Med Int Congr Ser 899:502
Mielke DH, Gallant DM, Roniger JJ, et al. (1977) Sulpiride: evaluation of antipsychotic activity in schizophrenic patients. Dis Nerv Syst 38:569–571
Overall JE, Gorham D (1962) The brief psychiatric rating scale. Psychol Rep 10:799–812
Toru M, Moriya H, Yamamoto K, Shimzono Y (1972) A double-blind comparison of sulpiride with chlorpromazine in chronic schizophrenia. J Clin Pharmacol 12:221–229
Trimble MR (1986) Positive and negative symptoms in schizophrenia. Br J Psychiatry 148:587–589
Woggon B, Heinrich K, Kuefferle B, Muller-Oerlinghausen B, Poldinger W, Ruther E, Schied HW (1984) Results of a multicenter AMDP study with fluperlapine in schizophrenic patients. Arzneimittelforschung 34:122–124
Yamawaki S (1987) Profiles of clinical efficacy and pharmacological action of zotepine. Pharmacopsychiatry 20:4–7

The Treatment of Positive and Negative Schizophrenic Symptoms with Dopamine Agonists

A. KLIMKE and E. KLIESER [1]

Dopamine Hypothesis and "Autoreceptor Concept"

The introduction of chlorpromazine in psychiatry (Delay and Deniker 1952) demonstrated that acute schizophrenic symptoms can successfully be treated with drugs, and this finding stimulated the search for the pathophysiological and pathobiochemical changes underlying schizophrenia. Steck (1954) and Haase (1955) first described extrapyramidal symptoms and drug-induced parkinsonism as possible side-effects occurring during treatment with neuroleptic agents. The investigation of dopamine as a neurotransmitter (Carlsson et al. 1958; Carlsson and Lindqvist 1963), the dopaminergic deficit in the basal ganglia of patients suffering from Parkinson's disease (Ehringer and Hornykiewicz 1960) as a result of the degeneration of nigral dopaminergic cells (Hornykiewicz 1973) and the efficacy of L-dopa in the treatment of parkinsonism, especially of akinesia (Birkmayer and Hornykiewicz 1962), led to the hypothesis that dopamine antagonism was responsible for both anti-psychotic and extrapyramidal effects of neuroleptics. The "dopamine hypothesis" of schizophrenia supposes that a functional overactivity of dopaminergic neurotransmission results in acute schizophrenic symptoms (van Rossum 1966; Meltzer and Stahl 1976). According to the positive symptoms appearing during an acute episode of schizophrenia, on the biochemical level an overstimulation of postsynaptic dopamine receptors in the mesolimbic and mesocortical projection areas is hypothesised. The efficacy of classic neuroleptic agents is explained by their ability to block post-synaptic dopamine receptors of the D2 type.

Although neuroleptic agents were introduced nearly 40 years ago it was not possible to prove the general validity of the dopamine hypothesis in schizophrenia.

According to clinical experience it seems questionable whether dopamine overactivity is present in all forms of acute schizophrenia. Extensive, controlled, double-blind studies of acute schizophrenia in our psychiatric hospital in Düsseldorf (performed from 1982–1986) demonstrated a sufficient response (markedly improved or improved) in 69% of 495 patients after 3 weeks of treatment with D2 antagonists like haloperidol, remoxipride or raclopride (Klieser et al. 1988, 1990). Additionally, it must be assumed that some of these

[1] Psychiatrische Klinik der Heinrich-Heine Universität, W-4000 Düsseldorf, FRG

A. Marneros / N. C. Andreasen / M. T. Tsuang (Eds.)
Negative Versus Positive Schizophrenia

responders would improve without neuroleptics on placebo (Klieser 1988). A remarkably large proportion of the patients who do not respond to low or high dosage of D2 antagonists improves markedly up to full remission of resistant positive symptoms during treatment with the atypical neuroleptic clozapine (Honigfeld et al. 1984; Kane et al. 1988) or after a series of electroconvulsive therapy (ECT) (Klimke and Klieser 1990). These clinical findings strongly support the view that in some cases the additional pharmacological manipulation of non-dopaminergic neurotransmitter systems by atypical neuroleptic agents or by ECT is necessary for sufficient symptom remission. As a possible pharmacotherapeutical principle for clozapine (Fink et al. 1984; Meltzer 1989) and some other new potential anti-psychotic drugs like risperidone (Janssen et al. 1988), serotonin antagonism has been discussed. More recently, for clozapine an influence on the glutamate system via the *N*-methyl-D-aspartate (NMDA) receptor was proposed as a possible explanation for efficacy in therapeutically resistant schizophrenia and phencyclidine (PCP)-induced refractory psychosis (Janowsky and Berger 1989).

Neuroanatomical mapping of dopaminergic pathways, physiological (extra- and intracellular single-cell recordings during electrical stimulation and after pharmacological and iontophoretical manipulation) and biochemical examinations (receptor binding studies in vitro, post-mortem, in vivo using positron emission tomography, PET) and animal behavioural studies have led to an abundance of new data. The two fundamental questions referring to the location of the primary disturbance in schizophrenia and to the functional meaning of D2 receptor antagonism (especially in mesolimbic and mesocortical projection areas) for the anti-psychotic efficacy of neuroleptic agents can, however, not definitively be answered.

A functional disturbance of the dopaminergic neuron itself, which results in increased synaptical dopamine release and dopamine turnover, is one possible explanation. The reasons for such a potential neuronal overactivity are not clear. Subsensitivity of presynaptical and somatodendritic autoreceptors (Carlsson 1975; Meltzer 1979) may result in a loss of autoregulatory inhibition. Alternatively, the dopaminergic overactivity may be secondary to pathological changes that are primary in other systems. According to the great number of different neurotransmitter systems which act on each other in part via feedback loops, a loss of usually inhibiting or an increase of excitatory afferents may lead to dopaminergic disinhibition (Reynolds 1989) or overstimulation. Examples for such inhibitory influences are serotonergic projections from raphe nuclei, γ-aminobutyrc acid (GABA) ergic striatomesencephalic projections (Nieuwenhuys et al. 1988) or enkephalinergic interneurons in the striatum ventrale and accumbens nucleus (Kuschinski and Hornykiewicz 1974; Biggio et al. 1978; Mulder et al. 1988).

A further hypothesis to explain postsynaptic overstimulation points at the dopamine receptors. It is suggested that there are at least two types of dopamine receptors, called according to Kebabian and Calne (1979) D1 and D2, which probably exist in different conformations. According to Seeman (1987) both D1 and D2 receptors have a low and a high affinity state with greatly different affinities to dopamine agonists and antagonists. A pathological increase of number and/or affinity for agonists of post-synaptic D2 receptors resulting in increased post-synaptic efficacy of dopamine was discussed as a possible disturbance underlying schizophrenia.

Nevertheless, we must draw conclusions cautiously if functional changes in the dopaminergic system in vivo or post-mortem are demonstrated. It has to be taken into consideration that the dopaminergic system is controlled by feed-back mechanisms and has a marked adaptivity under physiological conditions. As a possible explanation, it was hypothesized that the dopaminergic system may have the function of stabilizing central nervous functions (Friedhoff and Miller 1983; Friedhoff 1988). Changes of dopaminergic function found in schizophrenia may be the result of compensatory feed-back regulation as a reaction to pathological changes located primarily elsewhere or simply to neuroleptic agents.

In summary, only the assumption that D2 antagonism is the main factor for the anti-psychotic efficacy of classic neuroleptic agents seems to be certain.

All clinically effective anti-psychotic drugs including the atypical neuroleptic clozapine have dopamine D2 receptor antagonistic properties. Vice versa, all newly synthesised substances with D2 antagonistic properties which are able to permeate the blood/brain barrier have anti-psychotic efficacy in principally neuroleptic-responsive patients. Moreover, the dosages used clinically correlate well with the substance-specific D2 receptor affinity. PET examinations demonstrate a close relationship between customary dosage and central D2 receptor occupation in vivo (Farde et al. 1988).

The therapeutic principle D2 receptor antagonism is (with the exception of clozapine) regularly but in variable percentage (depending on drug-specific properties) coupled with extrapyramidal side-effects, as clinical investigations with pure D2 antagonists like remoxipride (Klieser et al. 1988) and raclopride (unpublished results) demonstrate. Such side-effects like acute dyskinesia and drug-induced parkinsonism, which are in some cases subjectively perceived as extremely uncomfortable, and the risk of possibly irreversible tardive dyskinesia (APA 1980; Wöller and Tegeler 1983) justify the search for new anti-psychotic drugs with low or no incidence of side-effects.

In this context Carlsson (1975, 1985, 1987, 1988) proposed the so-called autoreceptor concept as a possible pharmacological alternative for the treatment of schizophrenia. Autoreceptors (Roth 1979; Andén et al. 1983a; Clark et al. 1985) are dopamine receptors of the D2 type, which are located somatodendritically and presynaptically on the dopaminergic neuron itself. The stimulation of somatodendritic autoreceptors leads to the inhibition of firing, whereas stimulation of pre-synaptic receptors results in the inhibition of dopamine synthesis and release. As a consequence, the synaptical dopamine turnover is reduced. Under physiological conditions autoreceptors may be stimulated after the release of dopamine and so may have autoregulatory functions. The autoreceptor concept for the treatment of schizophrenia suggests that the selective pharmacological stimulation of autoreceptors without concomitant post-synaptic stimulation opens a new perspective for inhibiting (excessive) dopaminergic activity in the brain. In the case of dopaminergic hyperactivity as the main reason for acute positive symptoms, treatment with selective autoreceptor agonists should result in the reduction or remission of schizophrenic symptoms without extrapyramidal side-effects.

Classic Low-Dose Dopamine Agonists

Clinical Studies

The first clinical investigations to prove the autoreceptor concept in humans were performed using low-dose dopamine agonists (Table 1). This was substantiated with the observation of a biphasic action profile of the dopamine agonist apomorphine in animal studies. It has been postulated that apomorphine in low dosages stimulates dopaminergic autoreceptors. The resulting inhibition of firing rate and the reduction of dopamine release lead to motoric inhibition and sedation, whereas at higher dosages an additional post-synaptic stimulation results in increased activity and stereotyped behaviour. Results of

Table 1. Low-dosed apomorphine treatment in schizophrenia

Author(s)	Year	Diagnosis	Medic	*n*	*n/i*
Short-lasting antipsychotic effects after single-dose					
Smith et al. [a]	1977	chronic, NL-resistant	Yes	4	3
Tamminga et al.	1978	chronic, NL-resistant	Yes	18	9
Tamminga et al. [a]	1986	chronic	No	9	5
Corsini et al. [b,c]	1977a	chronic, NL-resistant	No	24	7
Corsini et al. [b,c]	1977b	acute symptoms	No	58	21
Cutler et al. [c]	1982	chronic, NL-resistant	Yes	5	2
No effect after single-dose administration					
Meltzer [b,c]	1980	schizophrenia	No	22	
Jeste et al.	1983	NL-resistant	8/12	12	
Ferrier et al.	1984	positive symptoms	No	15	
		mixed symptoms	No	15	
Levy et al.	1984	positive symptoms	No	15	
		only residual symptoms	No	10	
Syvälahti et al.	1986	chronic	Yes	12	
No effect after sub-chronic administration					
Hollister et al.	1980	schizophrenia (RDC-criteria)	Yes	11	
Tamminga et al.	1986	mixed symptoms	No	9	

NL, neuroleptic; Medic, concomitant neuroleptics: *n/i* number of patients who improved.
[a] Serious methodological objections.
[b] Open uncontrolled studies.
[c] Further details missing (methods, characteristics of patients).

first clinical studies in humans suggested a possible clinical importance of the autoreceptor concept.

Smith et al. (1977) reported casuistically a placebo-controlled study investigating four chronic schizophrenic patients with persisting positive symptoms, in three cases during continuing neuroleptic treatment. In three patients positive symptoms like hallucinations, delusions, thought disorder and paranoid ideas were markedly reduced 30–60 min after s.c. administration of 1.5–6 mg apomorphine.

Tamminga et al. (1978) found in 18 neuroleptic-resistant, chronic schizophrenic patients with prominent psychotic symptoms and during concomitant neuroleptic treatment a statistically significant reduction of positive symptoms after administration of 3 mg apomorphine s.c. as compared with placebo. The amelioration was observed 20 min after apomorphine administration and lasted maximally 60 min. Nine patients were improved, four revealed no difference to placebo, and five patients were slightly worsened. This bimodal distribution was interpreted as a possible hint for the existence of an apomorphine-sensitive sub-population of schizophrenic patients.

Corsini et al. (1977a) examined sedation and sleep induction after i.m. application of 1 mg apomorphine in 24 neuroleptic-free, chronic schizophrenic patients and reported as a by-product a sudden and marked reduction of psychotic symptoms in 7 schizoaffective patients which lasted, however, only 20–50 min. In a further, not placebo-controlled study Corsini et al. (1977b) and Di Chiara et al. (1978) described a rapid, short-lasting reduction of acute psychotic symptoms after i.m. administration of 1 mg apomorphine followed by a return to the previous psychotic condition. Altogether 21 of 58 unmedicated schizophrenic patients (7 of 12 hebephrenic type, 8 of 24 paranoid type, 6 of 18 schizoaffective type and none of 4 catatonic type) were beneficially influenced. The anti-psychotic action of 10 mg apomorphine was markedly reduced by haloperidol pretreatment (4–8 mg/day).

Cutler et al. (1982) examined in a placebo-controlled study the influence of low-dose apomorphine (0.005 mg/kg i.v.) during constant neuroleptic medication (1068 mg chlorpromazine equivalent/day) on serum homovanillic acid in five neuroleptic-resistant, chronic schizophrenic patients. As a secondary finding they reported in comparison with placebo significant improvement in the Brief Psychiatric Rating Scale (BPRS) score in two patients, whereas three remained psychopathologically unchanged.

Several investigators were not able to confirm these results. Meltzer (1980) did not find any marked change in psychosis in any of his subjects after administering a single dose of 0.75 mg apomorphine to 22 unmedicated schizophrenic patients, but as to methodology or characteristics of the patients no further information is given.

Jeste et al. (1983) found no significant effects after placebo-controlled administration of a single dose of apomorphine (0.01 mg/kg s.c.) in 12 neuroleptic-resistant schizophrenic patients (8 receiving concomitant neuroleptic agents, 4 unmedicated). Three patients improved (more than 25% reduction of BPRS score), 4 remained unchanged and 3 worsened. Two patients developed marked hypotension after apomorphine and could not be rated adequately. However, the explorative analysis revealed a statistically significant improvement in the anxiety/depression subscales. A significant difference was also found on the computed tomography (CT) scan. Patients with an abnormal CT scan result were improved or unchanged, whereas patients with a normal one tended to worsen after apomorphine administration.

Ferrier et al. (1984) examined in a placebo-controlled study the effects of 0.75 mg apomorphine s.c. in 30 unmedicated schizophrenic patients. Neither in 15 patients with mainly positive symptoms nor in 15 chronically ill patients with mixed positive and negative symptoms (rated according to a scale of Krawiecka et al. 1977 using interviews recorded on videotape) could a specific anti-psychotic efficacy be demonstrated. However, they reported a significant reduction of anxiety symptoms in acute schizophrenic patients.

Levy et al. (1984) carried out a placebo-controlled trial of the effects of a single dose of 0.75 mg apomorphine s.c. in 25 schizophrenic patients with differing courses of disease and symptomatology who were at least 2 weeks drug-free. Fifteen patients suffered mainly from positive symptoms, whereas 10 patients revealed only a residual symptomatology. Using the BPRS both placebo and apomorphine treatments tended to increase scores, but there was no difference between the treatment conditions and no hint of a better response in certain subgroups with different symptomatology. That apomorphine was centrally active was proved by concomitant measures of plasma prolactin, growth hormone (GH) and cerebrospinal fluid (CSF) homovanillic acid (HVA) levels.

Syvälahti et al. (1986) in a placebo-controlled study administered as single dose 0.005 mg/kg apomorphine s.c. (8 patients) and 5 months later 0.015 mg/kg over 90 min apomorphine i.v. (7 patients) to altogether 12 medicated, chronic schizophrenic patients with acute psychotic symptomatology. After s.c. application there was a slight, but statistically insignificant decrease of the mean BPRS score, and no difference was found after i.v. administration.

To examine the possible influence of adaptative phenomena in the dopaminergic system, Tamminga et al. (1986) administered under placebo-controlled conditions *N*-propyl-nor(NPN)apomorphine to 9 neuroleptic-free acute schizophrenic patients with mixed positive and negative symptoms in seven different dosages (2.5–40 mg orally) as a single dose and to a further 9 patients sub-chronically over 6 weeks (cross-over design, 3 weeks placebo and 3 weeks NPN-apomorphine). They reported a significant reduction of psychotic symptoms after NPN-apomorphine (2 h after administration) which became more obvious when the patients were separated according to their previous response to neuroleptic agents. Neuroleptic responders (with mainly positive symptoms like hallucinations and formal thought disorder) experienced a mean reduction of 20% in the BPRS score and revealed a significant anti-psychotic effect in comparison with placebo, whereas neuroleptic non-responders (with mainly deficit symptoms) remained unchanged or worsened slightly. With a sub-chronic dosage schedule there was no anti-psychotic efficacy, possibly as a result of adaptative changes and the development of tolerance to apomorphine.

Hollister et al. (1980) found no therapeutic effects during sub-chronic treatment of 11 carefully selected schizophrenic patients with 20 mg/day apomorphine (orally) as an additional medication to neuroleptic agents over 2 weeks. In one patient there was a marked exacerbation of psychosis after 8 days of treatment, and he was dropped from the study.

Investigations of low-dose ergot derivatives with dopamine agonistic properties revealed no clear results. It has to be stressed that these substances may agonistically influence serotoninergic and noradrenergic receptors (Burki et al. 1978).

Casuistically Colonna et al. (1978) reported marked and longer-lasting improvements of excited schizophrenic patients during combination therapy with 5–15 mg bromocriptine and benzodiazepine over several days.

Tamminga and Schaffer (1979) found no anti-psychotic effects after placebo-controlled treatment of neuroleptic-resistant, chronic schizophrenic patients. Three of seven neuroleptic-free patients developed marked deterioration (exacerbation of psychotic symptoms) after a 3-week treatment course with 10 mg bromocriptine per day. The treatment with the ergot derivative CF 25-397 did not change the psychopathology of 8 schizophrenic patients who were treated in part with concomitant neuroleptics.

Meltzer et al. (1983) treated in an open study nine chronic schizophrenic probands who were not taking neuroleptic agents with 0.5–6 mg/day bromocriptine over 3–4 weeks. One patient improved markedly and long-lasting, four improved partly but developed after 1 week of further treatment increased psychotic symptoms, two were unchanged, and two revealed a slight exacerbation of psychosis.

Gattaz et al. (1989) administered 2.5 mg/day bromocriptine in comparison with placebo to 30 neuroleptic-treated schizophrenic patients. After 24 h the verum group tended to have a more marked decrease in BPRS score, which lasted over 10 days. After 21 days of treatment there was no significant difference between the groups.

Critical Remarks

The studies cited above give no strong support for the clinical importance of the autoreceptor concept in the treatment of schizophrenia. According to the studies which investigated the possible effects of a single low dose of dopamine agonists a quite different experimental setting was chosen. The majority of investigations with negative results (no hint for anti-psychotic efficacy) were placebo-controlled and used a fixed dose, and the difference in psychopathological ratings before and after double-blind administration was taken for the statistical analysis.

In contrast, two studies supporting the efficacy of low-dose apomorphine used variable dosages and a questionable methodology. Smith et al. (1977)

paired post-treatment New Haven Schizophrenia Index (NHSI) scores of different treatment days, but they did not calculate the difference between the NHSI scores before and after application, so that fluctuations from day to day in psychopathology may have influenced the results.

Tamminga et al. (1986) used for statistical evaluation only 2 BPRS scores from 10 days of single-dose treatment, during which NPN-apomorphine in 7 variable dosages (2.5–40 mg) or placebo was randomly administered. Independent of the succession of treatment days, they took the day with maximal response to placebo and to verum, respectively, and the difference between the application-induced decrease of these scores was statistically significant. According to the authors this procedure was chosen because they found no clear dose-response correlation after looking into the randomisation list, and so they took the two days with maximal response. In our view this proceeding is not compatible with present statistical demands. The significance of the results presented is questionable if such an unusual statistic procedure is chosen after looking into the randomisation list and after the raw data were inspected.

Two further studies supporting the therapeutic implications of the autoreceptor concept are open, uncontrolled studies (Corsini et al. 1977a, b). Characteristics of the patients or details of psychopathology are lacking. Therefore, it cannot be excluded that the sedation and sleep induction described by Corsini et al. may have consecutively induced secondary reduction of psychotic symptoms similarly to results of Douglas (1900) and Feldman et al. (1945), who reported calming effects of low-dose apomorphine in excited schizophrenic and manic patients.

Corsini et al. (1977b) reported that acute sulpiride (100 mg i.m.) or subchronic haloperidol pre-treatment prevented apomorphine-induced sedation. This observation was interpreted as a clear argument for the involvement of dopamine autoreceptors. In fact, the efficacy of apomorphine at a *low* dosage suggests a stimulation of highly sensitive dopamine receptors, but it is not clear whether these receptors are autoreceptors or actually receptors in the brain. It has been shown that the pharmacological properties of the peripheral dopamine receptors (DA 1 and DA 2) correspond to those of the central D 1 and D 2 receptors. It is possible that the marked hypotension observed in several patients especially after an increase of dosage (Jeste et al. 1983) is mediated by peripheral dopaminergic stimulation, e.g. by inhibition of noradrenaline release from sympathic terminals via the DA 2 receptor (see Creese 1987).

The investigated population of schizophrenic patients was heterogeneous. In nearly all, positive symptoms predominated. However, depending on the study design patients with a different course of disease (acute, first episode vs. chronically ill), different response to classic neuroleptic agents (especially a high percentage of neuroleptic non-responders) and with or without concomitant neuroleptic medication were included. Today, it is believed generally that schizophrenia is a pathologically heterogeneous disease. It has to be supposed that only in a remarkable part but not all patients can the dopamine hypothesis be a valid explanation for positive symptoms and therefore that a clinical effect of autoreceptor stimulation can be expected. In contrast, it seems unlikely that patients who do not respond to strong post-synaptic receptor occupation by dopamine antagonists in high dosage will alternatively respond to autoreceptor stimulation. Furthermore, results from animal studies suggest that a stimulation of autoreceptors may antagonize the effects of concomitant neuroleptic treatment (i.e. reversal of depolarization inactivation of dopaminergic neurons, which is induced by sub-chronic neuroleptic treatment, see Bunney and Grace 1978). So far, the observation of reduced anti-psychotic efficacy of apomorphine after neuroleptic pretreatment (Corsini et al. 1977b) is in contrast to the findings of Smith et al. (1977), Tamminga et al. (1978) and Cutler et al. (1982).

In sub-chronic oral administration none of the apomorphine studies (Hollister et al. 1980; Tamminga et al. 1986) revealed anti-psychotic effects superior to placebo in medicated schizophrenic patients, and this was interpreted by Tamminga et al. as a possible result of pharmacological adaptation after repeated application.

Low-dose applications of ergot derivatives with dopamine agonistic properties give similarly contradictory results. Here, the additional stimulation of other receptor systems has to be taken in consideration.

After administration of the same dosage of low-dose dopamine agonists, totally different behavioural changes like sedation, sleep induction, hypotensive dysregulation, antipsychotic, anxiolytic, and antidepressant effects on the one hand, and, on the other hand, increase of activity and exacerbation of psychosis (Frye et al. 1982) have been described. This might be explained with the hypothesis of a dose-dependent action of dopamine agonists. However, the changes observed in open studies after apomorphine administration may be the result of other, for example, non-pharmalogical influences, which occurred during the test period. This should underline the necessity to confirm the results of open studies involving variable dosages with methodologically unobjectionable, placebo-controlled, double-blind studies.

Considering the methodological and theoretical objections stated above, in our view it is questionable whether a single dose of low-dose dopamine agonists of apomorphine type has really short-lasting, specific anti-psychotic effects. Moreover, and this is of great clinical relevance, there is no apomorphine study which found longer-lasting effects after a single dose or any effect after sub-chronic administration.

New Autoreceptor Specific Dopamine Agonists

The autoreceptor concept has stimulated the search for new drugs with selective agonistical affinity to dopamine autoreceptors without post-synaptic stimulation. In the past decade several new substances claimed to have this pharmacological profile, for example (−)-3-PPP (Carlsson 1985), (+)N-0437 (van der Weide et al. 1988), EMD 23448 (Seyfried et al. 1982, 1983) and EMD 49980 (Seyfried et al. 1989), B-HT 920 (Andén et al. 1982, 1983b) and (−)SND 919Y.

Table 2. Characteristics of the new putative autoreceptor-selective dopamine agonists B-HT 920 and EMD 49980

- Strong autoreceptor stimulation (inhibition of dopamine release, reduction of dopamine synthesis, inhibition of firing)
- Post-synaptic D2 stimulation after chronic denervation
- Significant lowering of plasma prolactin level

Additional properties

B-HT 920:
- Inhibition of acetylcholine release (pre-synaptically)
- α_2-adrenoreceptor stimulation (clonidine-like)

EMD 49980:
- Strong 5-hydroxytryptamine-1 A agonist and inhibition of serotonin uptake
- High first-pass effect (>95%)

Whereas some of these substances like (−)3-PPP were extensively pharmacologically characterised, there are first results of clinical studies using B-HT 920 (talipexole) and EMD 49980 (roxindol) (Table 2) in the treatment of acute schizophrenia with mainly positive symptoms.

B-HT 920 (Talipexole)

B-HT 920 is an azepin derivative (6-allyl-2-amino-5,6,7,8-tetrahydro-4*H*-thiazolo [4,5-D] azepin) and was originally regarded as a potential antihypertensive agent because of its clonidine-like action on adrenergic α_2 receptors (Pichler and Kobinger 1981). Andén et al. (1982) found additionally strong effects selectively on dopaminergic autoreceptors.

B-HT 920 inhibits γ-butyrolacton-induced dopa accumulation with an ED_{50} of 0.05 mg/kg as a result of a marked influence on the rate of dopamine synthesis, which is founded in an inhibition of striatal tyrosine hydroxylase activity (Jennewein et al. 1986). The inhibition of α-methyl-paratyrosine-induced disappearance of dopamine ($ED_{50} = 0.04$ mg/kg) reflects a marked reduction of dopamine release and turnover. These effects can be antagonized by haloperidol as a hint for the dopamine agonist activity of B-HT 920. The activity of nigral dopamine neurons in the substantia nigra is dose-dependently reduced ($ED_{50} = 2.3$ µg/kg).

In vitro, a marked inhibition of potassium-induced [^{3}H]acetylcholine release can be demonstrated, and recent results show that the striatal concentration of acetylcholine in vivo increases markedly (Seyfried et al. 1989) as a hint for an additional post-synaptic stimulation at the cholinergic preterminal (for review see Lehmann and Langer 1983).

The receptor binding profile reveals no marked affinity to α_1 adrenoreceptors and to 5-hydroxytryptamine (5-HT)-1, 5-HT-2 and muscarinergic acetylcholine receptors but a high affinity for α_2 adrenoreceptors.

In animal studies locomotor activity in mice and rats is inhibited as a result of autoreceptor stimulation. The motoric inactivation in mice caused by reserpine pretreatment is – in contrast to apomorphine – not antagonized, and this finding was interpreted as a lack of postsynaptic dopamine agonism. In dogs there is a marked emetic action (ED_{50} s.c. = 3.8 μg/kg). In rhesus monkeys sedation and sleepiness are observed with increasing dosage above 30 μg/kg. B-HT 920 antagonises haloperidol-induced acute dyskinesia in haloperidol-hypersensitive monkeys (after chronic treatment) at a dosage of 50–100 μg/kg B-HT 920. After the same dosage parkinsonian symptoms in *N*-methyl-4-phenyl-1,2,3,6-tetrahydropyridine (MTPT)-pretreated rhesus monkeys are totally reversed.

In summary B-HT 920 is a potent autoreceptor agonist with additional afficity to α_2 adrenoreceptors. Since Andén et al. (1982) reported first a selective action on dopamine autoreceptors, which is confirmed in some animal paradigms, more recent studies suggest agonistic effects on the cholinergic preterminal in the striatum. Furthermore, B-HT 920 has a marked postsynaptic action on supersensitive dopamine D 2 receptors after chronic denervation (Hinzen et al. 1986; Hjorth and Carlsson 1987; Pifl and Hornykiewicz 1988).

EMD 49980 (Roxindol)

EMD 49980 is a neurotrope dopamine agonist and belongs to the group of indolalkylamines. The chemical denotation is: 5-hydroxy-3(4-4-phenyl-1,2,3,4-tetrahydropyridol-(1)-)-butyl-(1)indol, methansulfonat.

It presents a high affinity for dopamine D 2 receptors and is highly active in displacing spiperone and domperidone in ligand binding assays (Seyfried et al. 1988). It is more than 1000-fold less effective in the SKF 38393 binding assay as a test for affinity to dopamine D 1 receptors.

In vivo EMD 49980 antagonises as effectively as apomorphine the γ-butyrolactone-induced inhibition of dopaminergic impulse flow as a result of stimulation of presynaptic and somatodendritic autoreceptors. In contrast to the biphasic profile of apomorphine, EMD 49980 presents in rats a dose-dependent decrease of locomotoric activity at dosages comparable with those of apomorphine when parenterally given. However, the dosage to cause the same behavioural effects is much higher when EMD 49980 is orally administered (more than 4 mg/kg body weight) as a result of a low bioavailability.

The inhibition of acetylcholine release in vitro is 10-fold lower for EMD 49980 as compared with apomorphine or pergolide. Therefore, a comparably low effect on normosensitive dopamine receptors is assumed. In vivo EMD 49980 increases the levels of striatal acetylcholine not more than 30% without reaching an ED_{50}, and only when parenterally given in a higher dosage of 3–30 mg/kg. Even at higher dosages, stereotyped behaviour is not evoked.

However, in the case of chronic denervation and consecutive development of post-synaptic receptor hypersensitivity (after unilateral lesioning of nigrostriatal dopamine fibres using 6-OH-dopamine), EMD 49980 also acts postsynaptically as a potent dopamine agonist. In contrast to haloperidol it produces no catalepsy in dosages up to 2 mg/kg s.c. (64 mg/kg orally).

EMD 49980 presents a high agonistic affinity to 5-HT-1A binding sites and leads, possibly by pre-synaptic inhibition of serotonin re-uptake, to an inhibition of reserpine-induced 5-hydroxytryptophan (5-HTP) accumulation in serotonergic neurons of the raphe nucleus (Seyfried et al. 1989).

When given to healthy volunteers, some developed after a single oral dose of 1 mg or more orthostatic dysregulation or gastrointestinal complaints which can be interpreted in general as dopaminergic side-effects. Repeated oral administration of 0.5 mg/day over a period of 1 week ($n = 12$) did not influence blood pressure, and this dosage was subjectively well tolerated.

Pharmacokinetic investigations in humans using the ^{14}C-labelled substance show a good resorption after oral administration and a marked first-pass metabolism with a bioavailability of less than 5%. The finding of unchanged substance in the faeces suggests in analogy to findings in animal studies a hydrolysis of conjugates which are secreted by the bile and supports the existence of an enterohepatic circle also in humans. The pharmaco-electroencephalogram (EEG) presented a typically neuroleptic profile after 0.5 mg with increased power in the slow frequency band and a decrease in the middle and fast beta bands, whereas a dose of 1 mg (no difference to placebo in the slow frequency band, increase of power in the beta band) produces changes similar to the effects of non-sedating anti-depressants. According to these findings it can be suggested that both dosages are effective in the central nervous system 1 h after application and over a period of at least 4 h.

In healthy volunteers no hints of extrapyramidal side-effects were found.

In summary, EMD 49980 acts in animal studies as an autoreceptor-specific dopamine agonist with only a low affinity to normosensitive postsynaptic receptors but a marked influence on hypersensitive receptors. Additionally, it has 5-HT-1A agonist and serotonin re-uptake inhibiting properties. Finally, a marked first-pass effect (> 95%) after oral administration in humans was observed.

Clinical Studies with B-HT 920 and EMD 49980

Lipka et al. (1988) and Wiedemann et al. (1989, 1990) treated under open conditions 12 patients suffering from acute paranoid schizophrenia (International Classification of Diseases, ICD no. 295.3 and 295.3 X according to the Diagnostic and Statistical Manual (DSM)-III classification), starting with 0.1 mg t.i.d. B-HT 920 orally as monotherapy. The dosage was increased over 3 weeks to 1.2 mg/day, and during the 4th week it was step-wise reduced to zero.

The statistical evaluation of 10 patients revealed no statistically significant anti-psychotic effect according to the difference in BPRS score between day 0 and day 21. Seven patients developed a marked, unexpected (from the preclinical data) increase of activity, which resulted in two drop-outs on day 1. Four patients were responders (more than 50% reduction in BPRS score), and 6 remained nearly unchanged. Only in the BPRS subscale anxiety/depression

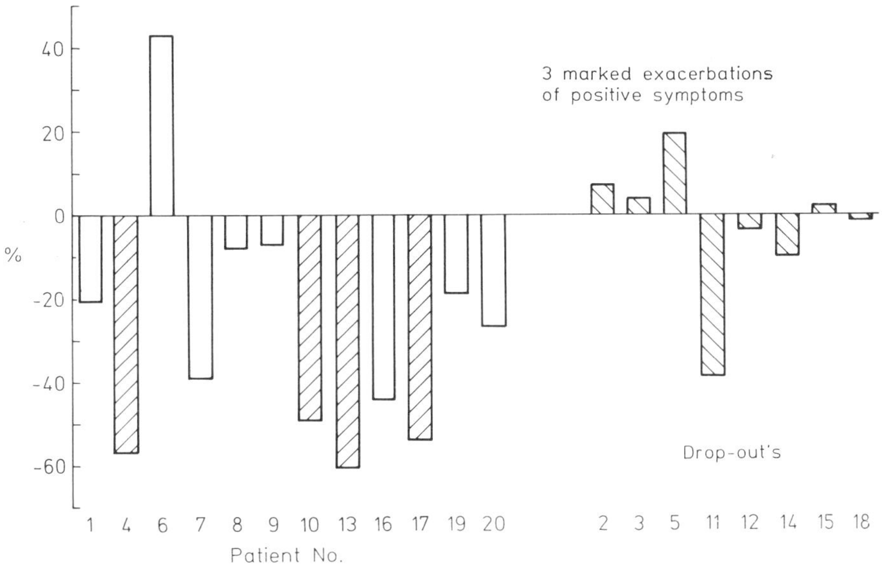

Fig. 1. Percentage reduction of Brief Psychiatric Rating Scale score during treatment with EMD 49980 over 4 weeks

was a statistically significant difference in favour of B-HT 920 found. There were not treatment-induced extrapyramidal syndromes. Examination of the plasma prolactin level revealed a significant reduction 2 h after application of the morning dose, indicating a central nervous system action on D2 receptors located in the tuberoinfundibular system, which are probably comparable with autoreceptors according to their receptor affinity (Carlsson 1985). All patients responded satisfactorily to subsequent treatment with classic neuroleptic agents.

Our working group examined in an open study the potential anti-psychotic efficacy of EMD 49980 in 20 carefully selected, acute schizophrenic patients (ICD no. 295.3) at an increasing dosage up to 3–9 mg over 4 weeks (Fig. 1). In all patients investigated positive symptoms predominated.

According to a priori defined criteria (50% reduction of BPRS score), 4 patients were clear responders; however, none of them achieved full remission. Ten patients were non-responders, and 3 of them were dropped because of marked exacerbation of psychotic symptoms. The explorative analysis of BPRS subscales revealed significant improvements of anxiety/depression and anergia but no effect for the subscales thought disturbance (THOT), hostility (HOST) and activation (ACTV), which are more specifical for acute psychosis. EMD 49980 was subjectively well tolerated, and in no case were extrapyramidal side-effects observed. Similar to the findings of Lipka et al. (1988) referring to B-HT 920, in our patients there was also a clear superiority of a consecutive treatment with classic neuroleptic agents. Seven of 10 EMD 49980 non-responders were fully remitted after 3 weeks of treatment with 15 mg/d haloperidol, and discharge from the hospital was possible within a further 6 weeks.

The Autoreceptor Concept: Discussion of the Discrepancy Between Pharmacology and Clinic

The therapeutic value of dopamine agonists in the treatment of positive schizophrenic symptoms could not be confirmed up to now, although from a theoretical point of view the autoreceptor concept developed by pharmacologists is a convincing new treatment principle. Neither the studies examining low-dose dopamine agonists nor trials with B-HT 920 and EMD 49980 have revealed convincing evidence for an anti-psychotic efficacy nearly comparable with that of classic neuroleptic agents. If the lack of anti-psychotic efficacy of autoreceptor agonists in a remarkable proportion of principally neuroleptic-responsive patients can be confirmed in further studies (our working group has started a placebo-controlled, double-blind investigation with SND 919 Y, which has structural similarity to B-HT 920 but with low α_2 adrenergic affinity), it has to be clarified how autoreceptor stimulation and classic neuroleptic treatment differ on the neuronal and receptor levels in schizophrenic patients. This question is of great heuristic interest and could possibly lead to a further development of the dopamine hypothesis.

It may simply be, as has been speculated in the past, that it is necessary for an effective anti-psychotic treatment to block mesocortical projections, which lack autoreceptors (Bannon et al. 1981). It is also possible that maximal stimulation of autoreceptors is not sufficient for inhibiting dopaminergic neurons (especially after chronic treatment) or that additionally a postsynaptic stimulation takes place. Several recent investigations suggest that probably not the anatomical location but the sensitivity of D2 receptors is crucial for stimulation by autoreceptor agonists. Several animal studies proved that the sensitivity and number of dopaminergic receptors (and the apomorphine response) can be substantially influenced by drug treatment or hormonal influences.

Chronic morphine administration leads to an increased inhibition of presynaptic dopamine turnover by apomorphine, possibly as a result of autoreceptor hypersensitivity (Kuschinski 1975). Chronic treatment with dopamine antagonists (neuroleptics) results similarly in pre-synaptical supersensitivity (Nowycky and Roth 1977), which is prevented by chronic lithium administration (Gallager et al. 1978). Furthermore, after subchronic administration of neuroleptics, an increase of number and a hypersensitivity of postsynaptic D2 receptors were reported (Christensen et al. 1976; Lee and Seeman 1978; Seeman 1987), and it was hypothesised whether the postsynaptic hypersensitivity could be responsible both for the development of tardive dyskinesia (Gerlach et al. 1974) and in certain cases for the re-exacerbation of schizophrenic psychosis after omitting neuroleptic treatment (Chouinard et al. 1978; David and Rosenberg 1979; Hunt et al. 1988). There is additional evidence for hormonal influences on the receptor sensitivity. Oestradiol and oestrogens have marked antidopaminergic properties similar to prolactin (Bédard et al. 1984) and lead to dopaminergic hypersensitivity and with long-term administration to an increase in number of D2 receptors (for review see Seeman 1980). ECT and repeated administration of anti-depressant drugs results in dopamine autoreceptor sub-sensitivity, which has been discussed as the reason for anti-depressive efficacy (Serra et al. 1979; Chiodo and Antelman 1980).

Several animal studies suggest a development of autoreceptor sub-sensitivity after administration of dopamine agonists (Baudray et al. 1977; Ljungberg 1979). Furthermore, recent findings suggest that dopamine D2 agonists can be ranked according to gradually increasing agonist efficacies rather than classified into autoreceptor-selective versus nonselective D2 agonists (Arnt and Hyttel 1990).

Animal studies suggest that the new autoreceptor agonists have a marked postsynaptic activity in the case of hypersensitive receptors, e.g. after chronic denervation (Carlsson 1985; Seyfried et al. 1989). This would lead in a subgroup of schizophrenic patients to dopaminergic behavioural effects; the psychomotoric activation with B-HT 920 and the exacerbation of symptoms with EMD 49980 may partly be explained by an additional post-synaptic influence.

Finally, in the past years there has been a renewed discussion about the possibility of reduced activity of corticostriatal and temporoamygdalar (Deakin et al. 1989) glutamatergic projections (Kim et al. 1980; Carlsson 1988), which are controlled by the dopaminergic system via inhibition at the glutamatergic pre-terminal (Schwarcz et al. 1978; Garau et al. 1978; Brown and Arbuthnott 1983). These receptors are of D2 type (Seeman 1980; Mitchell and Doggett 1980; Rowland and Roberts 1980; Nieoullon et al. 1982), which are estimated (from degeneration experiments) to constitute one-third of D2 receptors in the striatum and nucleus accumbens.

Up to now there have been no pharmacological studies referring to the important question of whether or not the new autoreceptor agonists act on these D2 receptors and inhibit glutamate release.

Negative Symptoms: Treatment with Autoreceptor Agonists?

Negative symptoms may develop at different times during the course of schizophrenia. In contrast to the dopamine hypothesis which explains acute schizophrenic symptoms by enhanced dopaminergic neurotransmission, there is no generally accepted pathophysiological theory for negative symptoms. There is no clear animal paradigm for negative symptoms, and different possible neurotransmitter systems are under discussion, e.g. a dysfunction of the noradrenergic reward system (Stein and Wise 1971; Strauss and Carpenter 1972) or of the serotonergic system (Bleich et al. 1988) or a (muscarinergic) cholinergic hyperactivity (Tandon and Greden 1989). The observation of the development or increase of negative symptoms during neuroleptic treatment led (in analogy to the dopamine hypothesis) to the speculation that a dysfunction, down-regulation (Friedhoff 1988) or degeneration of the dopaminergic system (Crow 1980) may partly account for negative symptoms. Negative symptoms occurring in Parkinson's disease and in encephalitis lethargica can be regarded as a result of a dopaminergic disturbance. Partly transient improvements of negative symptoms were reported after amphetamine (Angrist et al. 1980; Cesarec and Nyman 1985), but it remains unclear whether these were purely dopamine agonistic effects. Meltzer et al. (1986) reviewed six open and four controlled studies according to treatment of negative symptoms with L-dopa as monotherapy or concomitant with neuroleptic agents. The results of placebo-controlled studies in particular suggest that psychotic exacerbations during L-dopa therapy are rare and that additional medication with L-dopa in neuroleptic-treated patients may lead to an improvement, mainly in those with a duration of schizophrenia of 5 years or less. However, it is possible that these improvements are partially founded on an antagonism of L-dopa to neuroleptic side-effects (e.g. akinesia and drug-induced parkinsonism) and are not due to a specific effect on negative symptoms in type II schizophrenia in the sense of Crow (1980).

There is no specific reason to expect clinical efficacy of new autoreceptor agonists for negative symptoms. The reported psychomotoric activation (B-HT 920) and the significant improvement in the anxiety/depression (B-HT 920, EMD 49980) and anergia subscales (EMD 49980) of BPRS has led to first trials with negative schizophrenic symptomatology, but because of the small number of patients it is too early to draw conclusions. The totally different possible reasons for a high score in any negative symptom scale should be considered in further investigations.

Carpenter et al. (1985) differentiate between primary enduring negative or deficit symptoms, which are the basis for the type I/type II classification of Crow, and secondary negative symptoms. Secondary negative symptoms can be associated with an exacerbation of psychosis, and the improvement of negative symptoms after neuroleptic agents reported in literature (Davis 1980; Meltzer et al. 1986) supports this view. Studies in primates (McKinney et al. 1980) and in non-psychotic human controls (Baldessarini 1980) demonstrated that the side-effects of neuroleptic agents like sedation, drug-induced parkinsonism, akinesia and impairment of cognitive functioning may imitate negative symptoms. Here, an additional anti-cholinergic therapy or a reduction of neuroleptic medication may be indicated. Affective disturbances like depression during an acute episode or post-psychotic depression after remission of acute symptoms, psychotic anxiety or increase of dysphoria and/or anxiety as a result of neuroleptic side-effects can intensify preexisting negative symptoms. Finally, the custodial environment in hospital and active social withdrawal (e.g. to avoid emotional stimuli) are further possible contributing influences.

As a consequence, for investigations of new autoreceptor agonists in the treatment of negative symptoms the patients have to be carefully selected. It may be necessary to investigate separately different sub-populations, e.g.

patients suffering from post-psychotic depression, from schizodepressive psychosis, from type II schizophrenia or from side-effects of long-term neuroleptic agent administration. Only in a part of them will it be ethically possible and methodologically rich in meaning to stop additional neuroleptic medication, and so with negative symptoms new autoreceptor agonists should not only be tested as monotherapy but also as additional medication to neuroleptic agents.

References

American Psychiatric Association (1980) The Task Force on late neurological effects of antipsychotic drugs: tardive dyskinesia: saummary of a Task Force report of the American Psychiatric Association. Am J Psychiatry 137:1163–1172

Andén NE, Golembiowska-Nikitin K, Thornström U (1982) Selective stimulation of dopamine and noradrenaline autoreceptors by B-HT 920 and B-HT 933 respectively. Naunyn Schmiedebergs Arch Pharmacol 321:100–104

Andén NE, Grabowska-Andén M, Liljenberg B (1983a) Demonstration of autoreceptors on dopamine neurons in different brain regions of rats treated with gammabutyrolactone. J Neurol Transm 58:143–152

Andén NE, Nilsson H, Ros E, Thornström U (1983b) Effects of B-HT 920 and B-HT 933 on dopamine and noradrenaline autoreceptors in the rat brain. Acta Pharmacol Toxicol (Copenh) 52:52–56

Angrist B, Rotrosen J, Gershon S (1980) Responses to apomorphine, amphetamine, and neuroleptics in schizophrenic subjects. Psychopharmacology (Berlin) 67:31–38

Arnt J, Hyttel J (1990) Dopamine D-2 agonists with high and low efficacies: differentiation by behavioural techniques. J Neural Transm Gen Sect 80(1):33–50

Baldessarini RS (1980) Drugs and the treatment of psychiatric disorders. In: Gilman AG, Goodman LS, Gilman A (eds) The pharmacological basis of therapeutics. MacMillan, New York, pp 397–404

Bannon MJ, Michaud RL, Roth RH (1981) Mesocortical dopamine neurons: lack of autoreceptors modulating dopamine synthesis. Mol Pharmacol 19:270–275

Baudrey A, Costentin J, Marcais M, Martres MP, Protais P, Schwartz JD (1977) Decreased responsiveness to low doses of apomorphine after dopamine agonists and the possible involvement of hyposensitivity of dopamine autoreceptors. Neurosci Lett 4:203–207

Bédard P., Boucher R, DiPaolo T, Labrie F (1984) Interaction between estradiol, prolactin, and striatal dopaminergic mechanism. Adv Neurol 40:489–495

Biggio G, Casu M, Corda MG, DiBello C, Gessa GL (1978) Stimulation of dopamine synthesis in caudate nucleus by intrastriatal enkepahlins and antagonism by naloxone. Science 200:552–554

Birkmayer W, Hornykiewicz O (1962) Der 1-Dioxyphenylalanin (= L-DOPA)-Effekt beim Parkinson-Syndrom des Menschen: zur Behandlung und Pathogenese der Parkinson-Akinese. Arch Psychiatr Nervenkr 203:560

Bleich A, Brown SL, Kahn R, van Praag HM (1988) The role of serotonin in schizophrenia. Schizophr Bull 14(2):297–315

Brambilla F, Scarone S, Pugnetti L, Massironi R, Penati G, Nobile P (1983) Bromocriptine therapy in chronic schizophrenia: effects on symptomatology, sleep patterns, and prolactin response to stimulation. Psychiatry Res 8:159–169

Brown JR, Arbuthnott GW (1983) The electrophysiology of dopamine (D2) receptors: a study of the actions of dopamine on corticostriatal transmission. Neuroscience 10(2):349–355

Bunney BS, Grace AA (1978) Acute and chronic haloperidol treatment: comparison of effects on nigral dopaminergic cell activity. Life Sci 23:1715–1728

Burki HR, Asper H, Ruch W, Zuger PE (1978) Bromocriptine, dihydroergotoxine, methysergide, d-LSD, CF 25-397 and 29-712: effects on the metabolism of biogenic amines in the brain of the rat. Psychopharmacology (Berlin) 57:227–237

Carlsson A (1975) Receptor mediated control of dopamine metabolism. In: Usdin E, Bunney WE (eds) Pre- and postsynaptic receptors. Dekker, New York, pp 49–65

Carlsson A (1978) Does dopamine have a role in schizophrenia? Biol Psychiatry 13(1):3–21

Carlsson A (1985) Pharmacological properties of presynaptic dopamine receptor agonists. Psychopharmacology [Suppl] (Berlin) 2:31 38

Carlsson A (1987) Historical perspective of the chemistry and pharmacological treatment of schizophrenia. In: Henn FA, DeLisi LE (eds) Neurochemistry and neuropharmacology of schizophrenia. Elsevier, Amsterdam (Handbook of schizophrenia, vol 2)

Carlsson A (1988) Role of dopamine in the interaction between cortical and subcortical mechanisms. Psychopharmacology [Suppl] (Berlin) 96:49

Carlsson A, Lindqvist M (1963) Effect of chlorpromazine or haloperidol on formation of 3-methoxytyramine and normetanephrine in mouse brain. Acta Pharmacol (Copenh) 20:140–144

Carlsson A, Lindqvist M, Magnusson T, Waldeck B (1958) On the presence of 3-hydroxytyramin in brain. Science 127:471

Carpenter WT Jr, Heinrichs DW, Alphs LD (1985) Treatment of negative symptoms. Schizophr Bull 11(3):440–452

Cesarek Z, Nyman AK (1985) Differential response to amphetamine in schizophrenia. Acta Psychiatr Scand 71:523–528

Chiodo LA, Antelman SM (1980) Electroconvulsive shock: progressive dopamine autoreceptor subsensitivity independent of repeated treatment. Science 210:799–801

Chouinard G, Jones B, Annabel L (1978) Neuroleptic-induced supersensitivity psychosis. Am J Psychiatry 135:1409–1410

Christensen A, Fjalland B, Moller-Neilsen I (1976) On the supersensitivity of dopamine receptors induced by neuroleptics. Psychopharmacology (Berlin) 48:1–6

Clark D, Hjorth S, Carlsson A (1985) Dopamine-receptor agonists: mechanisms underlying autoreceptor selectivity. I. Review of the evidence. J Neural Transm 62:1–52

Colonna L, Petit M, Lepine JP (1978) Intérêt de la bromocriptine dans les schizophrénies dysthymiques. Encephale 4:115–117

Corsini GU, del Zompo M, Manconi S, Piccardi MP, Onali PL, Mangoni A (1977a) Evidence for dopamine receptors in the human brain mediating sedation and sleep. Life Sci 20:1613–1618

Corsini GU, del Zompo M, Manconi S, Cianchetti C, Mangoni A, Gessa GL (1977b) Sedative, hypnotic and antipsychotic effects of low doses of apomorphine in man. Adv Biochem Psychopharmacol 16:645–648

Creese I (1987) Biochemical properties of CNS dopamine receptors. In: meltzer HY (ed) Psychopharmacology: the third generation of progress. Raven, New York, pp 257–264

Crow TJ (1980) Molecular pathology of schizophrenia: more than one disease process? Br Med J 280:1–9

Cutler NR, Jeste DV, Karoum F, Wyatt RJ (1982) Low-dose apomorphine reduces serum homovanillic acid concentrations in schizophrenic patients. Life Sci 30:753–756

David K, Rosenberg G (1979) Is there a limbic system equivalent of tardive dyskinesia? Biol Psychiatry 14:699–703

Davis J (1980) Antipsychotic drugs. In: Kaplan HI, Freedman AM, Sadock BJ (eds) Comprehensive textbook of psychiatry/III, 3rd edn. Williams and Wilkins, Baltimore

Deakin JF, Slater P, Simpson MD, Gilchrist AC, Skan WJ, Royston MC, Reynolds GP, Cross AJ (1989) Frontal cortical and left temporal glutamatergic dysfunction in schizophrenia. J neurochem 52(6):1781–1786

Delay J, Deniker P (1952) 38 cas de psychoses traités par la cure prolongée continué de 4568 RP. Ann Med Psychol (Paris) 110:364

Di Chiara G, Corsini GU, Mereu GP, Tissari A, Gessa GL (1978) Self-inhibitory dopamine receptors: their role in the biochemical and behavioral effects of low doses of apomorphine. Adv Biochem Psychopharmacol 19:275–292

Douglas CJ (1900) Hypnotic action of apomorphine without nausea. Mercks Arch 11:212–213

Ehringer H, Hornykiewicz O (1960) Verteilung von Noradrenalin und Dopamin (3-Hydroxytyramin) im Gehirn des Menschen und ihr Verhalten bei Erkrankungen des extrapyramidalen Systems. Klin Wochenschr 38:1236

Eriksson E, Svensson K, Clark D (1985) The putative autoreceptor agonist B-HT 920 decreases nigral dopamine firing rate and prolactin release in rat. Life Sci 36:1819–1827

Farde L, Wiesel F-A, Halldin C, Sedvall G (1988) Central D2-dopamine receptor occupancy in schizophrenic patients treated with antipsychotic drugs. Arch Gen Psychiatry 45(1):71–76

Feldman F, Susselman S, Barrera SE (1945) A note on apomorphine as a sedative. Am J Psychiatry 102:403–405

Ferrier IN, Johnstone EC, Crow TJ (1984) Clinical effects of apomorphine in schizophrenia. Br J Psychiatry 144:341–348

Fing H, Morgenstern R, Oelssner W (1984) Clozapine – a serotonine antagonist? Pharmacol Biochem Behav 20:513–517

Friedhoff AJ (1988) Dopamine as a mediator of a central stabilizing system. Neuropsychopharmacology 3(1):189–191

Friedhoff AJ, Miller JC (1983) Clinical implications of receptor sensitivity modification. Annu Rev Neurosci 6:121–148

Frye PE, Pariser SF, Kim MH, O'Shaugnessy RW (1982) Bromocriptine associated with symptom exacerbation during neuroleptic treatment of schizoaffective schizphrenia. J Clin Psychiatry 43(6):252–253

Gallager DW, Pert A, Bunney WE Jr (1978) Haloperidol-induced presynaptic supersensitivity is blocked by chronic lithium. Nature 273:309–312

Garau L, Govoni S, Stefanini E, Trabucchi M, Spano PF (1978) Dopamine receptors: pharmacological and anatomical evidence indicate that two distinct dopamine receptor populations are present in the rat striatum. Life Sci 23:1745–1750

Gattaz WF, Rost W, Huebner CK, Bauer K (1989) Acute and subchronic effects of low-dose bromocriptine in haloperidol-treated schizophrenics. Biol Psychiatry 25(3):247–255

Gerlach J, Reisby N, Randrup A (1974) Dopaminergic hypersensitivity and cholinergic hypofunction in the pathophysiology of tardive dyskinesia. Psychopharmacologia 34:21

Haase HJ (1955) Psychiatrische Erfahrungen mit Megaphen (largactil) und dem Rauwolfiaalkaloid Serpasil unter dem Gesichtspunkt des psychomotirschen Parkinsonsyndroms. Nervenarzt 26(12):507–510

Hinzen D, Hornykiewicz O, Kobinger W, Pichler L, Pifl C, Schingnitz G (1986) The dopamine autoreceptor agonist B-HT 920 stimulates denervated postsynaptic brain dopamine receptors in rodent and primate models of Parkinson's disease: a novel approach to treatment. Eur J Pharmacol 131:75–86

Hjorth S, Carlsson A (1987) Postsynaptic dopamine (DA) receptor stimulator properties of the putative DA autoreceptor-selective agonist B-HT 920 uncovered by co-treatment with the D1-agonist SKF 38393. Psychopharmacology (Berlin) 93:534

Hollister LE, Kenneth LD, Berger PA (1980) Apomorphine in schizophrenia. Commun Psychopharmacol 4:277–281

Honigfeld G, Patin J, Singer J (1984) Clozapine: antipsychotic activity in treatment-resistant schizophrenics. Adv Ther 1:77–97

Hornykiewicz O (1973) Parkinson's disease: from brain homogenate to treatment. Fed Proc 32:183–190

Hunt JI, Singh H, Simpson GM (1988) Neuroleptic-induced supersensitivity psychosis: retrospective study of schizophrenic inpatients. J Clin Psychiatry 49:258–261

Janowsky A, Berger SP (1989) Clozapine inhibits [3H]MK-801 binding to the glutamate receptor-ion channel complex. Schizophr Res 2:179

Janssen PAJ, Niemegeers CJE, Awouters F, Schellekens KHL et al. (1988) Pharmacology of risperidone (R 644766), a new antipsychotic with serotonin-S2 and dopamine-D2 antagonistic properties. J Pharmacol Exp Ther 244:685–693

Jennewein HM, Bruckwick EA, Hanbauer I, Mierau J, Lovenberg W (1986) Evidence for a specific effect of B-HT 920, an azepine derivate, on tyrosine hydroxilase in the dopaminergic system of the rat. Eur J Pharmacol 123:363–369
Jeste DV, Zalcman S, Weinberger DR, Cutler NR, Bigelow LB, Kleinman JE, Rogol A, Wyatt RJ (1983) Apomorphine response and subtyping of schizophrenia. Prog Neuro-psychopharmacol Biol Psychiatry 7:83–88
Kane J, Honigfeld G, Singer J, Meltzer H (1988) Clozapine for the treatment-resistant schizophrenic. Arch Gen Psychiatry 45:789–796
Kebabian JW, Calne DB (1979) Multiple receptors for dopamine. Nature 277:93–96
Kim JS, Kornhuber HH, Schmidt-Burgk W, Holzmüller B (1980) Low cerebrospinal fluid glutamate in schizophrenics and a new hypothesis on schizophrenia. Neurosci Lett 20:379–382
Klieser E (1988) Experimental investigation to evaluate differential indications of neuroleptics and antidepressants. *Habilitationsschrift*, Heinrich-Heine University of Düsseldorf
Klimke A, Klieser E (1990) Zur Wirksamkeit der neuroelektrischen Therapie (NET) bei pharmakotherapeutisch resistenten endogenen Psychosen. Fortschr Neurol Psychiatr (in press)
Klieser E, Lehmann E, Tegeler J (1988) Experimental comparison of remoxipride, clozapine and haloperidol in the treatment of acute schizophrenia. Psychopharmacology [Suppl] (Berlin) 96:100
Klieser E, Klimke A, Lehmann E (1990) Zur prädiktorischen Bedeutung einer neuroleptischen Probetherapie mit Haloperidol. In: Heinrich K, Klieser E, Lehmann E (eds) 9. Düsseldorfer Psychiatrie-Symposion. Schattauer, Stuttgart (in press)
Klimke A, Klieser E, Strauss WH (1990) The new antipsychotic EMD 49980 – results of an open clinical trial in the treatment of acute schizophrenia (Abstr). Regional Congress of the World Federation of Societies of Biological Psychiatry (WFSBP), Marokko
Kornhuber J, Fischer EG (1982) Glutamate acid diethyl ester induces catalepsy in rats. A new model for schizophrenia? Neurosci Lett 34:325–329
Krawiecka M, Goldberg D, Vaughan M (1977) A standardized assessment scale for rating chronic psychotic patients. Acta Psychiatr Scand 55:299–308
Kuschinsky K (1975) Dopamine receptor sensitivity after repeated morphine administrations to rats. Life Sci 17:43–48
Kuschinsky K, Hornykiewicz O (1974) Effects of morphine on striatal dopamine metabolism: possible mechanism of its opposite effect on locomotor activity in rats and mice. Eur J Pharmacol 26:41–50
Lee T, Seeman P (1978) Enhanced 3H-neuroleptic binding in postmortem schizophrenic brains. Soc Neurosci Abstr 4:496
Lehmann J, Langer SZ (1983) The striatal cholinergic interneuron: synaptic target of dopaminergic terminals? Neuroscience 10(4):1105–1120
Levy MI, Davis EM, Mohs RC, Kendler KS, Mathé AA, Trigos G, Horvath TB, Davis KL (1984) Apomorphine and schizophrenia. Arch Gen Psychiatry 41:520–524
Lipka G, Wiedemann K, Benkert O, Holsboer F (1988) Presynaptic dopamine receptor agonist (B-HT 920) treatment of schizophrenia. Psychopharmacology [Suppl] (Berlin) 96:333
Ljungberg T (1979) Evidence that time-related changes in apomorphine stimulation determines the behaviour response. Neuropharmacology 18:327–334
McKinney WT, Moran EC, Kraemer GW, Prange AJ (1980) Long-term chlorpromazine in rhesus monkeys. Production of dyskinesias and changes in social behaviour. Psychopharmacology (Berlin) 72:35–39
Meltzer HY (1979) Clinical evidence for multiple dopamine receptors in man. Commun Psychopharmacol 3:457–470
Meltzer HY (1980) Relevance of dopamine autoreceptors for psychiatry. preclinical and clinical studies. Schizophr Bull 6:456–475
Meltzer HY (1989) Clinical studies on the mechanism of action of clozapine: the dopamine-serotonin hypothesis of schizophrenia. Psychopharmacology [Suppl] (Berlin) 99:S 18–27

Meltzer HY, Stahl M (1976) The dopamine hypothesis of schizophrenia: a review. Schizophr Bull 2:19

Meltzer HY, Kolakowska T, Robertson A, Tricou BJ (1983) Effect of low-dose bromocriptine in treatment of psychosis: the dopamine autoreceptor-stimulation strategy. Psychopharmacology (Berlin) 81:37–41

Meltzer HY, Sommers AA, Luchins DJ (1986) The effect of neuroleptics and other psychotropic drugs on negative symptoms in schizophrenia. J Clin Psychopharmacol 6(6):329–338

Mitchell PR, Doggett NS (1980) Modulation of striatal [3H]-glutamic acid release by dopaminergic drugs. Life Sci 26:2073–2081

Mulder AH, Frankhuyzen AL, Schoffelmeer ANM (1988) Kappa-opioid receptor agonists as potent and selective inhibitors of dopamine release in rat neostriatum. Psychopharmacology [Suppl] (Berlin) 96:148

Nieoullon A, Kerkerian L, Dusticier N (1982) Inhibitory effects of dopamine on high affinity uptake from rat striatum. Life Sci 30:1165–1172

Nieuwenhuys R, Voogd J, van Huijzen C (1988) The human central nervous system. A synopsis and atlas, 3rd edn. Springer, Berlin Heidelberg New York

Nowycky MC, Roth RH (1977) Presynaptic dopamine receptors. Development of supersensitivity following treatment with fluphenazine decanoate. Naunyn Schmiedebergs Arch Pharmacol 300:247–254

Pichler L, Kobinger W (1981) Centrally mediated cardiovascular effects of B-HT 920, a hypotensive agent of the "clonidin type". J Cardiovasc Pharmacol 3:269

Pifl C, Hornykiewicz O (1988) Postsynaptic dopamine agonist properties of B-HT 920 as revealed by concomitant D1-receptor stimulation. Eur J Pharmacol 146:189–191

Reynolds GP (1989) Beyond the dopamine hypothesis. The neurochemical pathology of schizophrenia. Br J Psychiatry 155:305–316

Roth RH (1979) Dopamine autoreceptors: pharmacology, function and comparison with post-synaptic dopamine receptors. Commun Psychopharmacol 3:429–445

Rowlands GJ, Roberts PJ (1980) Activation of dopamine receptors inhibits calcium-dependent glutamate release from cortico-striatal terminals in vitro. Eur J Pharmacol 62:241–242

Schmidt CJ, Lobur W, Lovenberg W (1986) Inhibition of K^+-stimulated [^{3}H]dopamine and [^{14}C]acetylcholine release by the putative dopamine autoreceptor agonist, B-HT 920. Naunyn Schmiedebergs Arch Pharmacol 334:377–382

Schwarcz R, Fuxe K, Agnati LF, Gustafson JA (1978) Effects of bromocriptine on ^{3}H-spiroperidol binding sites in rat striatum. Evidence for actions on dopamine receptors not linked to adenylate cyclase. Life Sci 23:465

Seeman P (1980) Brain dopamine receptors. Pharmacol Rev 32:229–313

Seeman P (1987) Dopamine receptors and the dopamine hypothesis of schizophrenia. Synapse 1:133–152

Serra G, Argiolas A, Klimek V, Fadda F, Gessa GL (1979) Chronic treatment with antidepressants prevents the inhibitory effect of small doses of apomorphine on dopamine synthesis and motor activity. Life Sci 25:415:424

Seyfried CA, Fuxe K, Wolf H-P, Agnati LF (1982) Demonstration of a new type of dopamine receptor agonist: an indolyl-3-butylamine. Actions at intact versus supersensitive dopamine receptors in the rat forebrain. Acta Physiol Scand 116:465

Seyfried CA, Fuxe K, Wolf HP, Agnati LF (1983) Neurochemical and functional studies with EMD 23448, a novel dopamine agonist. Acta Pharm Suec [Suppl] 2:243

Seyfried CA, Greiner HE, Haase AF, Böttcher H (1988) Ligand-binding profile of EMD 49980. A selectively presynaptic dopamine (D2) agonist with potent actions on 5-HT-systems. Psychopharmacology [Suppl] (Berlin) 96:336

Seyfried CA, Greiner HE, Haase AF (1989) Biochemical and functional studies on EMD 49980: a potent, selectively presynaptic D-2 dopamine agonist with actions on serotonin systems. Eur J Pharmacol 160:31–41

Smith RC, Tamminga C, Davis JM (1977) Effect of apomorphine on schizophrenic symptoms. J Neural Transm 40:171–176

Steck H (1954) Le syndrome extra-pyramidal et diencéphalique au cours des traitements au largactil et au serpasil. Ann Med Psychol (Paris) 112(2):737–743
Stein L, Wise CD (1971) Possible etiology of schizophrenia: progressive damage to the noradrenergic reward system by 6-hydroxydopamine. Science 171:1032–1036
Strauss JS, Carpenter WT Jr (1972) Six-hydroxy-dopamine, noradrenergic reward, and schizophrenia. Science 175:921–922
Syvälahti EKG, Säkö E, Scheinin M, Pihlajamäki P, Hietala J (1986) Effects of intravenous and subcutaneous administration of apomorphine on the clinical symptoms of chronic schizophrenics. Br J Psychiatry 148:204–208
Tamminga CA, Schaffer MH (1979) Treatment of schizophrenia with ergot derivatives. Psychopharmacology (Berlin) 66:239–242
Tamminga CA, Schaffer MH, Smith RC, Davis JM (1978) Schizophrenic symptoms improve with apomorphine. Science 200:567–568
Tamminga CA, Gotts MD, Thaker GK, Alphs LD, Foster NL (1986) Dopamine agonist treatment of schizophrenia with N-propylnorapomorphine. Arch Gen Psychiatry 43:398–402
Tandon R, Greden JF (1989) Cholinergic hyperactivity and negative schizophrenic symptoms. A model of cholinergic/dopaminergic interactions in schizophrenia. Arch Gen Psychiatry 46(8):745–753
Van der Weide J, Tendijck MEC, Tepper PG, DeVries JB, Dubocovich ML, Horn AS (1988) The enantiomers of the D-2 dopamine receptor agonist N-0437 discriminate between pre- and postsynaptic dopamine receptors. Eur J Pharmacol 146:319
Van Rossum JM (1966) The significance of dopamine-receptor blockade for the mechanism of action of neuroleptic drugs. Arch Int Pharmacodyn Ther 160:492–494
Wiedemann K, Benkert O, Holsboer F (1989) B-HT 920 – a novel dopamine autoreceptor agonist in the treatment of patients with schizophrenia. Pharmacopsychiatry 22:221
Wiedemann K, Benkert O, Holsboer F (1990) B-HT 920 – a novel dopamine autoreceptor agonist in the treatment of patients with schizophrenia. Pharmacopsychiatry 23:50–55
Wöller W, Tegeler J (1983) Späte extrapyramidale Hyperkinesen. Klinik – Prävalenz – Pathophysiologie. Fortschr Neurol Pschiat 51:131–157

Nonpharmacological Treatment Concepts of Negative Symptomatology

H. D. BRENNER, B. HODEL, and M. C. G. MERLO [1]

Introduction

In the past decade, while various rating scales such as the Scales for the Assessment of Negative Symptoms (SANS) (Andreasen 1982), the Positive and Negative Syndrome Scale (PANSS; Kay et al. 1987), the Psychological Impairments Rating Schedule (PIRS; Jablensky 1978), and its revised version the Behavioral Observation Schedule (BOS; Atakan and Cooper 1989) were being devised to assess negative symptoms in schizophrenia, intensive research was being conducted on negative symptoms in the fields of psychopharmacology, pathophysiology, and brain morphology (see surveys, Den Boer et al. 1987; Crow 1989). Thus, biological research began to focus its attention on a syndrome which until then had been within the domain of psychosocial treatment. In cases where integrating studies of pharmacological, psychological, and social therapies into long-term treatment of schizophrenia have been carried out, they, however, did not especially aim at negative symptoms (Carpenter 1987). It is interesting to note that the lines along which research developed led researchers to test and adopt new and older substances which were known to be partly antagonistic to neuroleptics (e.g., amphetamines). There has also been growing interest lately in the observed behavior of chronic schizophrenics who attempt to "cure themselves" with drugs and medications (Liberman and Bowers 1990). Another approach to research in this field is to experiment with medications such as risperidon which have the ability to block not only D_2 but also S_2 receptors. Analogous to Wing and Brown's approach in rehabilitating schizophrenic patients (1970), we find a twofold strategy on the biological level: on the one hand, it aims at decreasing the level of stress to be coped with, and on the other hand, at stimulating and reinforcing the patient. This also holds true for psychologically and socially oriented interventions. The negative and the positive syndromes are the target syndromes for these two approaches in order to avoid both overstimulation and understimulation.

Despite the concentration on biological approaches to therapy, eminent authors have repeatedly drawn attention to the possibility of influencing negative symptoms by means of psychological and social treatment programs,

[1] Department of Theoretical and Evaluative Psychiatry, Psychiatric University Hospital Bern, Bollingenstraße 111, 3072 Ostermundingen, Switzerland

A. Marneros / N. C. Andreasen / M. T. Tsuang (Eds.)
Negative Versus Positive Schizophrenia

and have formulated suggestions accordingly (e.g., Carpenter 1986; Zubin 1985; Selzer et al. 1989). Although such suggestions have evidently emanated from quite different views of the nature and etiology of negative symptoms, interpersonal skills and coping skills have been consistently emphasized. Thus, for example in the various vulnerability models, negative symptoms have either been regarded as a manifestation of a more pronounced predisposition to illness (e.g., the threshold model of Pogue-Geile and Harrow 1985) or as independent of the genetic liability to schizophrenia primarily present or arising secondary to psychosis (vulnerability-stress concept of Zubin 1985). Irrespective of these divergent views, psychological training techniques appear to be indicated in both cases, regardless of whether these serve to mediate stress management in order to reduce suprathreshold levels of anxiety which result in psychotic breakdown, or serve to diminish or compensate deficits in psychosocial functioning which increase the probability of occurrence of a schizophrenic episode characterized by positive symptoms in vulnerable individuals. However, even advocates of a disease model of negative symptoms who regard them as primary and as the direct manifestation of a cortical and/or subcortical lesion point out the possible benefit of psychological therapy techniques analogous, for example, to neuropsychological approaches after a frontal lobe trauma (cf. Carpenter 1986).

Selzer and colleagues (1989) recently distinguished between negative symptoms which are due to prefrontal cortex dysfunctions (above all marked impairments in cognitive functioning resulting in a decrease of instrumental role performance) and those which are expressions of psychological responses to core illness. They argue that the cortical dysfunction may explain a major proportion of the negative symptoms, but not such complex behaviors as social withdrawal, lack of motivation, lack of interest in treatment, etc. In their view, these phenomena indicate interactions of psychology and physiology. They may be adaptive when they reduce stress or anxiety, but become maladaptive when they lead to demoralization or ineffective coping. Specifically, the authors subdivide psychological responses to core illness into efforts to achieve safety and decrease stress (e.g., social withdrawal, cognitive avoidance) and into maladaptive dysfunctional patterns (e.g., emotional withdrawal, excessive self-reproach). However, in the presence of further negative symptoms, which they consider as being of uncertain or mixed etiology (e.g., amotivation, avolition, apathy, and anhedonia), they also impute a major effect of psychological factors in terms of adaptation to physiological and psychological events within the individual. Accordingly, they regard the negative symptoms as being responsive to interpersonal therapies and the patient's own coping efforts.

Psychological and Social Therapy Forms

The most important psychological and social therapy forms will shortly be presented here as they are mentioned in the few reviews on nonpharmacological therapies of negative symptoms (Carpenter et al. 1985; Wixted et al. 1988; Slade and Bentall 1989). These therapies were primarily devised for treating the chronically mentally ill in general. Then an attempt will be made to demonstrate the importance of conceiving therapeutic interventions, which, analogous to more specific pharmacological approaches, are meant to treat negative symptoms in a specific way.

Inpatient therapy programs were initially developed in the United States based on token economy within the tradition of behavior therapy. The respective studies conducted by Ayllon and Azrin (1968) and by Paul and Lentz (1977) are well-known. Wong et al. (1986) distinguished three different ways of operating a token economy: by suppressing the reaction by means of "stimulus interference," by punishing undesirable behavior, or by assigning positive contigencies to behavior that is not symptomatic. The first method cited attempts to "distract" the patient from psychotic behavior by keeping him busy or by conversing with him. The second method, punishment, elicits negative consequences so as to reduce maladjusted behavior. In other words, both of these methods are aimed at reducing behavioral excesses. The third method, on the other hand, attempts to promote skills and abilities the patient already possesses. It does not attempt to directly alter the negative symptoms. Although this kind of intervention is proven to be effective in reducing the chronic schizophrenic's symptoms during inpatient treatment, only very few patients managed to generalize behaviors acquired during these interventions to their everyday lives outside the confines of the hospital.

In the following years, training programs were devised to teach skills required to cope with everyday situations, especially those involved in coping with interpersonal interaction. Data obtained in various recently conducted longitudinal studies (e.g., WHO 1979; Schubart et al. 1986; Moeller and von Zerssen 1986) showed that many patients already manifest a premorbid history of social maladjustment and that this factor also contributes to the course of the illness and its prognosis. These findings confirmed the importance of social skills, life skills, and problem-solving skills training programs. Brown (1982), Bellack (1989), and Liberman (1988) in conjunction with their co-workers won a great deal of recognition for the detailed and carefully planned training programs they developed. The targeted skills are usually practiced in highly structured sessions, usually in small groups. Once the interaction to be practiced has been carefully assessed, the purpose of acquiring the targeted skills is explained, and the skills to be acquired are defined. Then the targeted skills are "modeled" by the therapists. After that, the patients rehearse these skills in role-playing situations. Subsequently, feedback sessions provide the patients with positive reinforcement to bolster their self-confidence. And last of all, the patients are assigned homework so that they can practice the skills learned in therapy in their daily lives (Wixted et al. 1988; Brenner et al. 1991a). Concomitantly with trends in modern cognitive psychology, teaching of "problem-solving" skills was developed with the aim of changing attitudes or cognitions which are thought to cause interpersonal and instrumental difficulties (Shepherd 1988). These strategies are supposed to provide a bridge for transferring behavior changes to real-life situations. Wallace and Boone (1984) and Hansen et al. (1985) report the effectiveness of problem-solving programs. Perris (1988, 1989) developed an intensive cognitive-behavioral psychotherapy program for schizophrenic patients based on Beck's approach to cognitive therapy. The objective of this program is to correct the patient's faulty appraisals and cognitive schemata. These therapy forms have, however, not succeeded in generating a specific concept to deal with the negative syndrome. Much in the same way the "face validity" method operates, they are believed to be particularly appropriate for patients with negative symptoms due to the deficits they manifest in their social behavior.

In summary, the procedures mentioned so far aim at global changes and tend to overlock specific techniques for treating negative symptoms. The question which continually arises in daily clinical practice – How can we motivate an apathetic-abulic patient to take part in the therapy being offered? – must be dealt with separately. Just as pharmacotherapy attempts to stimulate and activate the patient by directly manipulating physiological processes, methods need to be developed which will do the same on a psychological level.

More or less the same applies to therapies which aim at influencing the patient's social network. Family therapy and group therapy are the most differentiated approaches on a social level. However, only psychoeducational family therapy presents controlled studies with schizophrenic patients. This approach has been strongly influenced by the concept of "expressed emotion" (EE) (Leff and Vaughn 1985), the goal of therapy being to reduce high EE. Various studies indicate that reducing high EE results in rather effective relapse prevention (cf. Goldstein and Strachan 1987). However, data on families rated low on EE indicate that reducing the negative emotions of significant others does not in itself suffice to prevent relapse. Instead, the chance of non-relapse seems unrelated to an increased incidence of negative symptoms. The same phenomenon can be observed in patients on antipsychotic medication. This is one reason why Vaughn (1987) calls for research to study the ways low EE interacts with negative symptoms. But not only the social field of the family should be studied in relation to negative symptoms. The influence of group structures (for instance the group on a rehabilitation ward) should also be considered in order to intervene on apathy, amotivation, and other negative symptoms.

During the last few years, there has been a remarkably growing interest in what is fundamentally feasible for these nonpharmacological treatment approaches. Criticism has primarily been expressed by Hogarty et al. (1987), who pointed out that there is a discrepancy between very good short-term effects and unsatisfactory long-term effects. In the view of these authors, relapses are delayed rather than prevented in the long-term, and relapse frequently occurs when the patients are confronted with an independent life situation or increased work demands. In addition, G. E. Hogarty (personal communication) believes that once the variance in social adjustment associated with differential relapse in consequence of treatment has been accounted for, treatment programs show very little in the way of positive effects among nonrelapsed patients. Liberman et al. (1987) profess the opposite view. They regard the available results especially in the treatment of chronic schizophrenic patients as convincing, but also admit that generalizing the gains achieved in therapy to real-life conditions and maintaining the effects of therapy over a long period of time are still unresolved problems.

Today a growing number of researchers assume that the attentional, perceptual, and cognitive disorders in information processing shown by schizophrenic patients strongly contribute to these problems. In these terms, Hemsley already postulated in 1977 that persistent cognitive disorders are responsible for the limited effect of the training of social skills and for the exacerbations of the psychosis repeatedly observed during treatment. Spaulding et al. (1986) and Brenner (1987) have discussed in detail the possibility that elementary cognitive dysfunctions have pervasive interfering effects on the levels of microsocial and macrosocial behavior. The assumption of such interfering effects can be inferred both from the traditional Anglo-American concept of "core psychological deficit" (Lang and Buss 1965) and from the concept of "uncharacteristic basic disorders" in German psychopathology as defined by Suellwold and Huber (1986).

In the given context, the ways cognitive disorders interact with negative symptomatology are also a matter of prime importance. To date, research conducted on the interactions between these two factors has primarily focused on the aspect of symptom correlates rather than on the aspect of therapeutic interventions. Increasingly, attentional and other information-processing disorders are rightfully regarded as relevant mediating processes between neuroanatomical and neurochemical abnormalities on the one hand, and clinical symptoms and certain aspects of the course on the other. Basically, however, information processing can be treated if we work on the assumption that the neurobiological substratum can undergo modification.

Researchers used to maintain that cognitive disorders were related to negative symptomatology in rather general terms. Nowadays, they define this relationship in much more differentiated terms. For example, Opler et al. (1984) came to the conclusion that there is a particularly strong mutual relationship between cognitive impairment and negative symptomatology manifested. Their subjects had shown lower perceptual performance, lower vocabulary scores, and less mature responses in the Color-Form Preference and Representation Test. Numerous studies conducted in the following years seemed to yield contradicting findings. Cornblatt et al. (1985) discovered that although positive symptoms correlated with increased distractibility, negative symptoms correlated with a poor ability to recall irrelevant stimuli in auditory-visual tasks. Thus negative symptoms would indicate a weak ability to process irrelevant auditory stimuli. Results obtained by Nuechterlein and Dawson (1986) on forced choice span of apprehension tasks and continuous performance tasks showed negative correlations between the level of test performance and the Brief Psychiatric Rating Scale (BPRS) subscores, "motor retardation," "emotional withdrawal," and "disorientation." Negative correlations were, however, not observed between test performance and the subscores, "thought disorder" and "activation." The authors contend that signal discrimination deficits in situations demanding high levels of effective processing are linked to vulnerability to negative schizophrenic symptoms. Green and Walker (1985) found correlations between positive symptoms and lower scores in verbal short-term memory as well as between negative symptoms and visual-motor deficits. As in the other studies cited above, their data were based on typical attentional tasks. Other studies conducted during the past few years where also able to show more differentiated relationships (cf. Walker and Lewine 1988).

On the whole, research findings indicate that positive as well as negative symptoms correlate with disordered information processing. Nevertheless, negative symptoms seem to be related to overall information-processing abnormalities on multiple levels. Furthermore, there seem to be cognitive deficits related to states and others related to traits. State-linked cognitive deficits can also be observed in patients suffering from other psychoses. On the other hand, trait-linked ones tend to present a specific pattern of defective central inhibitory operations characteristic of schizophrenic spectrum disorders. They might correlate with tonic or episodic stress directly related to destabilizing monoaminergic systems which, in the long run, cause disturbed neurotransmission. Harascz (1985) adhered to this approach in his studies on the vital role that neural plasticity plays in the interaction between stress originating in the family and monoaminergic-linked vulnerability in the development of the schizophrenic disorder. Braff and Geyer (1990) draw an analogy between this sort of destabilization process and the increased systematic aminergic activity and the increased nucleus accumbens dopamine tone in animal model studies, and developed a tentative model of multiple information-processing disorders which could bridge the gap between information-processing intake deficits, negative symptoms, and organic brain impairment. In his studies he collected data on visual backward masking tasks. He discovered that patients with negative symptoms have significant inflation of stimulus recognition thresholds. These are similar to the deficits previously reported in patients with head injuries resulting in organic brain syndromes and deficits in time-dependent processing of information. This model not only relates information-processing disorders to state- and trait-linked disturbances but also to negative and positive symptoms. State-linked disorders mostly manifest within a span of several hundred milliseconds once the stimulus has been registered by the "activity path" of monoaminergic neurons. The multiple-level disorders of patients with negative symptoms tend to be trait-linked and correlate with additional and more global brain impairments.

Thus, underlying cognitive disorders might very well be the origin of both symptom dimensions. On the other hand, cognitive deficits might be secondary to positive and negative symptoms. Two findings do, however, speak against this assumption. First cognitive deficits can be observed prior to the manifestation of clinical symptoms, and secondly, they interact with positive and negative symptoms in a differentiated way. Future research should strive to develop more specific models to explain the role basic deficits in information processing play in schizophrenia. It should also aim at developing psychophysiological tests and experimental designs to selectively measure separate brain functions. The simultaneous application of brain imaging methods and extended neuropsychological test batteries could provide even more understanding of the correlates of the various disorders.

The postulated pervasive influence of elementary disorders in information processing on social behavior as well as the assumed relations between cognitive disorders and negative symptoms have up to now hardly had major effects on therapeutical practice. If they are assigned greater importance, then the scope of the traditional treatment approaches is enlarged by explicitly including cognitive preparation and working out treatment contents (cf. Liberman 1988), or by focusing on verbal self-instructions (cf. Meichenbaum and Cameron 1973). It has also been attempted to directly reduce cognitive disorders by quasi-experimental training procedures based on laboratory techniques (Spaulding et al. 1986; Lamberti et al. 1988; Mussgay et al. 1991). However, this approach is still in its very beginning.

Our own research concentrated on the development of a therapy program integrating cognitive and social interventions in the treatment of chronic schizophrenic patients (Roder et al. 1988; Brenner et al. 1991 b). This integrated psychological therapy (IPT) is a step-by-step program appropriate for small groups. It consists of five subprograms: Cognitive Differentiation, Social Perception, Verbal Communication, Social Skills, and Interpersonal Problem Solving (see Table 1). Even though each IPT subprogram contains discrete steps which prescribe therapeutic tasks for improving social and cognitive skills, there is a shift in the therapeutic work: At the beginning, basic cognitive skills are targeted, later they are shaped into verbal and social responses, as well as into general social competence. Additional, emotionally charged material or themes are introduced more and more, and group processes are intensified.

Patients first work on improving basic cognitive abilities in the Cognitive Differentiation subprogram. During the first step of this subprogram patients learn to discriminate stimulus categories by participating in a card-sorting task. Four attributes are printed on the card: number, geometric form, day of the week, and different colors. Patients are instructed to sort cards by one or more attributes. When competent at the simple stimulus task, training moves to word problems. Concept formation is trained through a series of tasks in which patients identify autonyms and synonyms, distinguish concepts with different definitions, and establish a hierarchy of related concepts. Finally, systematic search strategies are trained through a variation of the game, "twenty questions," thereby improving retrieval of verbal concepts.

In the Social Perception subprogram, patients are trained to accurately encode social stimuli. In part, this requires the patient to be able to discriminate relevant elements of social stimuli from environmental noise. To accomplish this task, patients view a series of slides in which actors interact in different social activities and display emotions of various intensity. As the subprogram progresses, the representation of the emotions as well as of the interactions increases in complexity and distress. In the last steps, slides are purposefully ambiguous, making interpretation of the emotions and the interactions

Table 1. The integrated psychological therapy (IPT)

Subprogram	Focus of interventions	Intervention techniques
Cognitive Differentiation	Attentional skills: Selective attention Shifting attention Sustaining focused attention Conceptualization abilities: Stimuli abstraction Concept formation Concept discrimination Concept modulation	Card sorting exercises Verbal concept exercises: Concept hierarchies Synonyms Autonyms Word definitions Word distinctions Words with different contextual meanings Search strategies
Social Perception	Analysis of social information: Discrimination of relevant social stimuli Reality-related interpretation of social stimuli	Description of the slide content Interpretation of the slide content Discussion of the individual interpretations Elaboration of headlines for the slide content
Verbal Communication	Conversation skills: Shifting attention to statements of others Use of associative-semantic processes Necessary for adequate answering	Verbatim repetition exercises Analogous repetition exercises Exercises with interrogatives: Asking with interrogatives Answering appropriately Conversation about one topic Free conversation

difficult. For each slide, one patient in the group is asked to list the observable qualities of the individual: "Describe the person to me." "What is he/she doing?" The therapist prompts and directs patients' attention to relevant aspects of the slide. From the initial description, members of the group are asked to interpret the intent of the actions and the emotion displayed by the actors. The group as a whole discusses individual interpretations regarding its reality adequacy. The aim of the discussion is not to achieve a group consensus by all means, but to obtain the patients' understanding of the reality-related interpretations. Individuals who possess extremely discrepant interpretations are thus gently confronted with inconsistent evidence.

The first two subprograms target the patient's cognitive abilities, especially focusing on the processing of social information. The first steps of the Verbal Communication subprogram extrapolate skills learned in previous subprograms to improve the patient's ability to pay attention to voiced statements of

Table 1 (Continued)

Subprogram	Focus of interventions	Intervention techniques
Social Skills	Competence in social skills: Reality-related succession of behavioral patterns Coping with interfering difficulties in the application of social skills Non- and paraverbal skills	Cognitive prestructuring: Definition of the aim Elaboration of the dialogue used in the subsequent role play Elaboration of the roleplay headlines Analysis of the anticipated difficulties in the role play Rating of difficulties in the subsequent role play Assigning the tasks for the subsequent role play (active role play, observers) Role play: Modeling by the cotherapist Analysis of the modeling Role play by a patient Feedback by the observers and by the therapist Transfer of the role play to real-life situations
Interpersonal Problem Solving	Application of (interpersonal) problem solving steps: Recognition of problem aspects Generation of alternative solutions Evaluation of success or failure of applied solutions	Identification and analysis of a given problem Cognitive prestructuring: Separation of facts from assumptions Transfer of complex problems into easily recognizable aspects Correction of idiosyncratic perspectives Elaboration of solutions Discussion of the solutions Focusing on one of the solutions Transfer of the focused solution to real-life situations Feedback on success or failure (in the subsequent therapy session)

others, to improve the patient's ability to accurately understand what is being said, and to facilitate the associative-semantic processes necessary for answering. During initial exercises, patients are rewarded for verbatim repetition of the statements of their partner. Literal repetition is quickly replaced with the paraphrasing of these statements. Reciprocal communication is improved with questions that foster mutuality in both listening and talking. Patients are taught the utility of basic question words (who? what? where? why? how?) and prompted to use them in conversation practice. Successful patients are instructed to continue free communication without immediate prompts. Therapist feedback fine-tunes patient performance throughout this subprogram.

The Social Skill and Interpersonal Problem Solving subprograms closely parallel more conventional behavioral skills training (Bellack et al. 1989; Liberman 198; Wallace 1984). Individual social skills are modeled by co-therapists, patients rehearse the skills in role playing and feedback is provided by the trainers. However, the IPT Social Skills subprogram is facilitated by focusing an cognitive components. Similarly, the acquisition of traditional problem-solving steps is enhanced through accentuation of the cognitive elements in the task. For example, selecting a solution involves cognitive analysis of the success and failure of similar solutions in other problem situations.

Various evaluation studies in different clinics have proven significant favorable overall treatment effects for different groups of schizophrenic patients, especially chronic ones. Table 2 gives an overview of the main IPT overall evaluation studies. The table shows the group design of each study as well as the patients' characteristics, the IPT interventions, the measures used and the kind of treatment effects. The design and the results of each study are described in more detail by Brenner et al. (1990).

Summarized, IPT intervention effects are visible primarily in cognitive and in psychopathological measures. In the study by Brenner et al. (1987, 1990), these effects are also shown after an 18-month follow-up (see Table 2). Later investigations also indicated effectiveness in treating cognitive disorders alone (e.g., Kraemer et al. 1987; Roder 1988). However, the findings obtained in these studies have partially been questioned (Mussgay and Olbrich 1988; Funke et al. 1989). Mussgay and Olbrich (1988) argued that social behavior functioning is primarily optimized and not disordered information processing. They base their assessment on studies with modified IPT interventions and their results are contradictory to our own analyses of the effects of cognitive IPT interventions alone (Roder 1988; Brenner et al. 1991 a). However, other critical aspects pointed out by Mussgay and Olbrich (1988) are taken into account in our actual research: the IPT aims at elementary cognitive disorders as well as at higher-order functioning. The measures used in the evaluation studies, however, often demand more than dealing with the assigned tasks on cognitive levels (e.g., fine motor skills are also necessary). Furthermore, the results of our earlier evaluation studies could not explain whether improved cognitive processes were a direct result of cognitive-treatment interventions, were due to some kind of compensatory mechanisms, or were due to improved overall social functioning.

The theoretical foundations of the IPT are based on the assumption that in schizophrenia the relationships between cognitive disorders and deviant social behavior – especially under social stressors – are maintained by two vicious circles (Brenner et al. 1991 a). A vicious circle is a positive feedback loop with

Table 2. The main overall evaluation studies of the IPT

Authors Diagnosis	Groups eg	Groups pag	Groups cg	Patients' characteristics (average)		IPT interventions	Treatment duration	Measures	IPT effects (pre- and post-treatment comparison)
Brenner et al. (1987, 1990) ICD-9: 295 (except 295.5, 295.7)	14	15	14	Age (years): IQ: Illness duration (years): Hospitalization (years):	33 98 6 1	All sub-programs	12 weeks with 4 sessions each (60–75 min)	Benton [a] D2 [a] FCO [a] MMPI [b] (only Schizophrenia Scale) BPRS [b] PSA [c]	Significant effects in cognitive and psychopathological measures. After an 18-month follow-up significant effects in cognitive, psycho-pathological, and social measures
Brenner et al. (1987) ICD-9: 295 (except 295.5, 295.7)	6		6	Age (years): IQ: Illness duration (years): Hospitalization (years):	44 102 22 15	All sub-programs	20 weeks with 3 sessions each (60 min)	Benton [a] D2 [a] SASKA [a] KVT [a] FCO [a] BPRS [b] AMDP [b] PSA [c]	Significant effects in one cognitive measure and trend-effects in psycho-pathological measures
Brenner et al. (1987) ICD-9: 295 (except 295.5, 295.7)	10		8	Age (years): IQ: Illness duration (years): Hospitalization (years):	30 103 7 2	All sub-programs	16 weeks with 4 sessions each (75 min)	Benton [a] D2 [a] SASKA [a] KVT [a] FCO [a] BPRS [b] PSA [c]	Significant effects in cognitive and psycho-pathological measures

Table 2. Continued

Authors Diagnosis	Groups eg	pag	cg	Patients' characteristics (average)		IPT interventions	Treatment duration	Measures	IPT effects (pre- and post-treatment comparison)
Kraemer et al. (1987) DSM-III schizophrenia	17		13	Age (years): IQ: Hospitalization (years):	6 93 14	Cognitive differentiation Social perception Cognitive coping strategies	12 weeks with 5 sessions	Number crossing [a] Word recognizing [a] FCO [a] BPRS [b] PD-S [b] Bf-S [b]	Significant effects in cognitive and psycho-pathological measures

eg: experimental group; cg: control group; pag: placebo-attention group;
[a] cognitve measures;
[b] psychopathological measures;
[c] social measures.

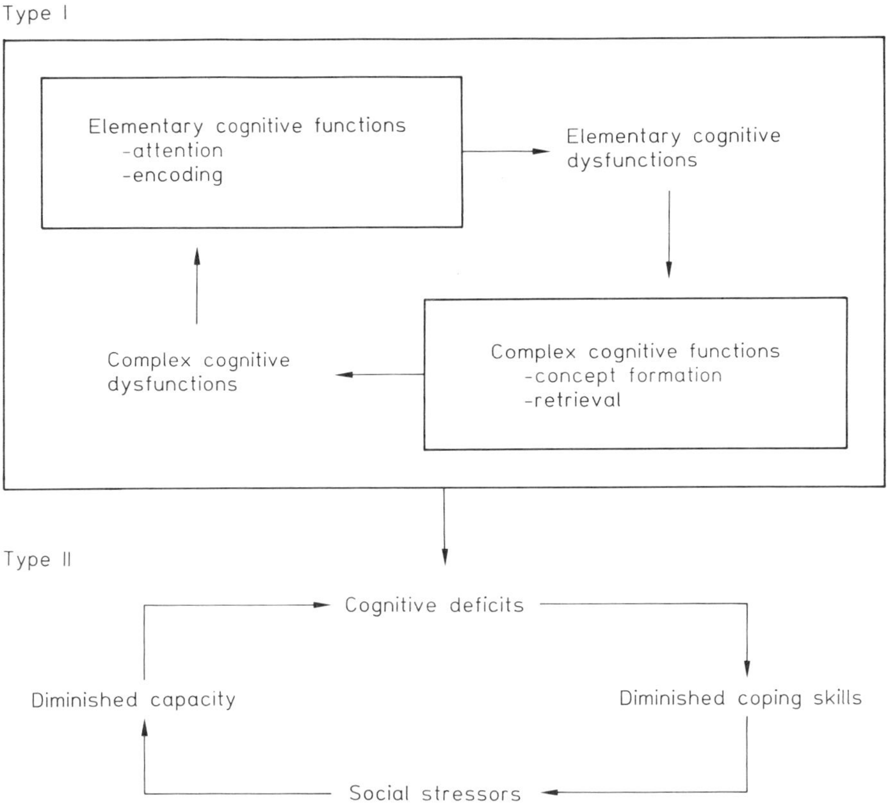

Fig. 1. Vicious circles in schizophrenia

elements exacerbating one another such that psychopathological symptoms may arise (see Ciompi 1982; Brenner 1989). The first vicious circle combines the top-down and bottom-up models of information processing in schizophrenia. Disorders in elementary cognitive processes diminish higher-order functioning which integrates incoming information. Diminution of the higher-order processes prevents coordination of elementary processes such that attention and basic perception are skewed. Like an overall spiral, this causes overall cognitive disorders (see Fig. 1).

Cognitive disorders are also one of the elements of the second vicious circle. They prevent sufficient acquisition of social skills such that the schizophrenic is unable to handle everyday social stressors. In the presence of such stressors, his level of arousal is heightened, symptoms recur, and cognitive processing decreases further (see Fig. 1). By combining cognitive and social interventions, the IPT is assumed to be a means of addressing the noxious continuing feedback loops of both vicious circles.

As both insufficient acquisition of social skills and deficits in cognitive processsing also seem to be linked to negative symptoms in schizophrenia, IPT

Table 3. Kendall's τ correlations between negative symptoms (high/low ratings in the BPRS subscore "anergia") and IPT interventions (pre- and post-treatment measurements)

Study 1 (Brenner et al. 1987, 1990)			
Negative symptoms, low ratings ($n = 5$) (BPRS anergia, $\bar{x} = 10.5$, SD = 1.9)		Negative symptoms, high ratings ($n = 5$) (BPRS anergia, $\bar{x} = 15.0$, SD = 1.9)	
Benton pre ($\bar{x} = 61.5$, SD = 5.9)	0.11	Benton pre ($\bar{x} = 77.2$, SD = 16.9)	−0.32
Benton post ($\bar{x} = 74.5$, SD = 15.8)	−0.67 [b]	Benton post ($\bar{x} = 94.8$. SD = 21.4)	−0.11
Saska pre ($\bar{x} = 93.0$, SD = 10.5)	−0.25	Saska pre ($\bar{x} = 102.8$, SD = 20.3)	−0.95 [a]
Saska post ($\bar{x} = 107.0$, SD = 14.2)	−0.11	Saska post ($\bar{x} = 121.4$, SD = 13.2)	−0.89 [a]
D2 pre ($\bar{x} = 86.7$, SD = 14.4)	0.11	D2 pre ($\bar{x} = 81.4$, SD = 13.1)	−0.89 [a]
D2 post ($\bar{x} = 88.5$, SD = 14.9)	−0.11	D2 post ($\bar{x} = 75.6$, SD = 33.1)	−0.95 [a]
KVT carefulness pre ($\bar{x} = 96.3$, SD = 8.7)	−0.44	KVT carefulness pre ($\bar{x} = 90.0$, SD = 15.6)	0.11
KVT carefulness post ($\bar{x} = 99.5$, SD = 4.7)	−0.88 [a]	KVT carefulness post ($\bar{x} = 98.2$, SD = 10.1)	−0.44
FCO pre ($\bar{x} = 25.8$, SD = 15.4)	0.74 [a]	FCO pre ($\bar{x} = 26.6$, SD = 17.6	0.11
FCO post ($\bar{x} = 24.2$, SD = 14.1)	0.44	FCO post ($\bar{x} = 25.0$, SD = 14.8)	−0.11
BPRS anxiety/depression pre ($\bar{x} = 18.7$, SD = 3.9)	−0.11	BPRS anxiety/depression pre ($\bar{x} = 17.8$, SD = 4.6)	0.53 [b]
BPRS anxiety/depression post ($\bar{x} = 13.8$, SD = 4.6)	0.53 [b]	BPRS anxiety/depression post ($\bar{x} = 12.6$, SD = 4.0)	0.53 [b]
BPRS thought disturbance pre ($\bar{x} = 9.7$, SD = 7.6)	0.00	BPRS thought disturbance pre ($\bar{x} = 8.2$, SD = 2.2)	−0.74 [a]
BPRS thought disturbance post ($\bar{x} = 10.7$, SD = 4.9)	−0.32	BPRS thought disturbance post ($\bar{x} = 9.0$, SD = 3.5)	0.11
BPRS activation pre ($\bar{x} = 7.7$, SD = 3.1)	0.00	BPRS activation pre ($\bar{x} = 8.8$, SD = 2.2)	−0.67 [b]
BPRS activation post ($\bar{x} = 10.0$, SD = 3.7)	−0.53 [b]	BPRS activation post ($\bar{x} = 5.8$, SD = 1.8)	−0.22
Study 2 (Hodel in preparation)			
Negative symptoms, low ratings ($n = 7$) (BPRS anergia, ($\bar{x} = 5.7$, SD = 1.9)		Negative symptoms, high ratings ($n = 9$) (BPRS anergia, ($\bar{x} = 8.7$, SD = 4.3)	
Self-Image-Scale (SIS) pre ($\bar{x} = 13.0$, SD = 22.5)	−0.75 [a]	Self-Image-Scale (SIS) pre ($\bar{x} = 15.3$, SD = 21.3)	−0.11
Self-Image-Scale (SIS) post ($\bar{x} = 14.5$, SD = 13.7)	−0.14	Self-Image-Scale (SIS) post ($\bar{x} = 15.1$, SD = 20.2)	−0.21

Table 3 (Continued)

Study 3 (Roder 1988)			
Negative symptoms, low ratings (n = 5) (BPRS anergia, $\bar{x}$ = 10.8, SD = 3.7)		Negative symptoms, high ratings (n = 6) (BPRS anergia, $\bar{x}$ = 12.3, SD = 2.1)	
Card Sorting Test pre ($\bar{x}$ = 1.0, SD = 1.7)	−0.73 [a]	Card Sorting Test pre ($\bar{x}$ = 2.0, SD = 1.6)	−0.44
Card Sorting Test post ($\bar{x}$ = 1.0, SD = 2.8)	−0.44	Card Sorting Test post ($\bar{x}$ = 1.0. SD = 1.4)	−0.49
Concept Formation Test pre ($\bar{x}$ = 8.5, SD = 12.1)	0.59 [b]	Concept Formation Test pre ($\bar{x}$ = 9.0, SD = 9.9)	0.41
Concept Formation test post ($\bar{x}$ = 8.3, SD = 6.2)	0.65 [b]	Concept Formation Test post ($\bar{x}$ = 6.3, SD = 7.1)	0.23
WAIS "picture completion" pre ($\bar{x}$ = 86.6, SD = 10.6)	0.80 [a]	WAIS "picture completion" pre ($\bar{x}$ = 90.0, SD = 15.7)	0.14
WAIS "picture completion" post ($\bar{x}$ = 100.0, SD = 20.0)	0.88 [a]	WAIS "picture completion" post ($\bar{x}$ = 88.3, SD = 3.7)	0.24

[a] strong correlation.
[b] moderate correlation.

should affect these symptoms, too. Therefore, we conducted sequential analyses of the data of three IPT studies to examine whether IPT intervention effects discriminate between patients who scored low and those who scored high on negative symptoms. The first was conducted for the IPT overall evaluation (Brenner et al. 1987, 1990), the second for the analysis of the influence of cognitive IPT interventions on the effects of subsequent social ones (B. Hodel, in preparation), and the third for the analysis of the influence of IPT cognitive interventions on social functioning (Roder 1988). All individuals who participated in the studies had an International Classification of Diseases (ICD-9) diagnosis of schizophrenia. In the first study the patients' average age was 29.7 years (SD 8.3) and their average IQ was 92.9 (SD 7.8). In the second study the patients' average age was 31.8 years (SD 6.7) and their average IQ was 95.7 (SD 7.6); and in the third study, the patients' average age was 29.3 years (SD 4.1) and their average IQ was 96.3 (SD 6.7).

In each study cognitive, social, and psychopathological measures were used for the pre- and post-treatment measurements. For the sequential analyses, only patients with high or low negative symptom ratings were considered. Negative symptoms were rated by the BPRS subscore "anergia." Extreme groups were created by splitting up the patient sample in each study along the median in the BPRS subscore "anergia" at the pre-treatment measurement. Only those patients were selected whose rating value deviated more than 25% from the sample median. From 44 patients, 37 patients (17 patients with low, 20 patients with high negative symptoms) were choosen. In Table 3, the extreme groups of each study are briefly described together with the results of the sequential analyses.

In each study the extreme groups showed comparable performances in the pre-treatment measurements (as assessed by the Kruskall-Wallis test). Furthermore, there was no significant difference between both extreme groups at treatment end. Additional Kruskall-Wallis tests showed that in all three studies the differences (i.e., the improvements) between the pre- and post-study measurements did not vary significantly between the two extreme groups either. Results of Kendall's τ correlations were mixed: In the first study (five patients with low and five with high negative symptom ratings), one strong correlation corresponded to our expectations (for the definition of strong, median, and weak correlation, see Friedrich and Hennig 1980): after treatment, "low negative symptoms" correlates negatively with the subscore "carefulness" of the concentration test (*Konzentrationsverlaufs-Test*, KVT). The strong correlations of "thought disorders" (assessed by the Frankfurt Complaints Questionnaire, FCQ, and by the BPRS subscore "thought disturbance") in the pre-treatment measurement do not discriminate between the extent of negative symptoms. "Low negative symptoms" correlates with FCQ, "high negative symptoms" with the BPRS subscore "thought disturbance." The correlations of the attention encumbrance test, D2, and of the verbal intelligence test, Saska, with "high negative symptoms" are also less valid because they hold before and after treatment. Valid median correlations, however, were found after treatment between "low negative symptoms" and the Benton as well as the BPRS subscores "anxiety/depression" and "activation." For "high negative symptoms," median correlations exist with the BPRS subscore, "anxiety/depression," before and after treatment. In the second study seven patients had low and nine, high negative symptom ratings. There is a strong negative correlation before treatment between the Self-Image Scale (SIS) and "low negative symptoms." In the third study of five patients with low and six patients with high negative symptom ratings, median correlations were found between the cognitive test of Concept Formation, and "low negative symptoms" before and after treatment. Though the subscore of the Wechsler Adult Intelligence Scale (WAIS) intelligence test, "picture completion," shows strong correlations with "low negative symptoms," it also does this before and after treatment. Only the Card Sorting Test has a valid, strong correlation with "low negative symptoms" before treatment.

The results of the three sequential analyses allow us to draw the conclusion that the effectiveness of the IPT is not affected by the extent of the patients' negative symptoms. Thus, the patients whose ratings showed high negative symptom values gain in the same degree from the IPT interventions as patients whose ratings showed low negative symptom values. However, this should not lead to the assumption that negative symptoms have no effects on treatment results. As Mussgay and Olbrich (1988) have assumed, the measures of the IPT studies seem to call for global rather than for specific cognitive performances. On the other hand, the BPRS subscore "anergia" may assess impairments which are of slighter significance for the acquisition of cognitive and social skills than, for example, specific attentional/perceptive and cognitive processes related to the manifestation of negative symptoms.

Another question still open with regard to the treatment of negative symptoms is whether training of very elementary cognitive processes either with laboratory methods developed in accordance with experimental investigations on disorders of information processing, or with computer-assisted neuropsychological techniques, constitutes an advance in treatment effectiveness. Spaulding et al. (1986), Lamberti et al. (1988) and Mussgay et al. (1991) have reported first experiences with this in schizophrenic patients. Contrary to earlier opinions (see Brenner 1987) but in view of such results and of the fact that our earlier global assumptions on the effects of the pervasiveness of cognitive disorders on social behavior could not be confirmed in our own investigation (Brenner et al. 1990, 1991a; Hodel et al. in preparation), the more definitive training of specific dysfunctions might prove to be useful. Our own therapeutic experiences as well as our own empirical data point in another direction. Accordingly, emotional factors should substantially weaken the effects of IPT interventions (Brenner et al. 1991a; Hodel et al. 1990). This seems to be caused by effects which emotions have on both vicious circles. At present, attempts are being made to evaluate the extent to which steps toward perceiving and appraising one's emotions could be included in the various subprograms of the IPT. In addition, efforts are also being made not only to make patients aware of what they feel, but also to help them to realize what caused them to feel the way they do, and to appraise the consequences. In addition, on the social level, so-called independent living skills (cf. Liberman et al. 1987) are also being incorporated into the IPT.

If more effective treatment techniques within the therapy approaches mentioned so for are to be developed, then further clarification is most likely needed of the reciprocal relationship between, on the one hand, disorders in information processing and social functioning, and, on the other, positive and negative schizophrenic symptoms. Today, too little emphasis has been laid on research which strives to apply the systems approach and to relate these different fields with one another, and thus, the information we have collected on this matter is correspondingly scanty.

However, as mentioned above, the treatment of negative symptoms should also be studied on the level of social interactions. Besides rules performances and other socially defined factors such as institutionalism, stigma, and the influence of the social benefit system (Strauss et al. 1989), the influence of the social field structure of a psychiatric ward has hitherto not been studied in relation to negative symptoms. In order to investigate the connection between negative symptoms and the ways patients relate on a ward, we conducted a 6-month study on a rehabilitation ward for young schizophrenic patients (Merlo et al., in preparation).

We used the Systematic Multiple Level Observation of Groups (SYMLOG) method as a measure of the group dynamics, and SANS as well as BPRS for the psychopathological ratings. This method has been developed by Bales and his colleagues (1979) as a new field theory for small group research. It includes instruments for measuring values and interpersonal behavior. In many years of direct interaction process analysis, Bales (1970) found three fundamental dimensions for characterizing the style of relating to one another. These three dimensions are: (1) U–D, upward, dominant–downward, submissive; (2) P–N, positive, friendly–negative, unfriendly; (3) F–B, forward, goal oriented–backward, not goal oriented. As shown in Figs. 3 and 5, these dimensions can be depicted as a field diagram with the U–D dimension represented by the size of the image circles. The upper right quadrant is the space where those members of the group are situated that connect in a functional way to each other. The three dimensions are obtained by 26 items which describe the behavior of a person in the group, for instance: appears friendly, reacts impulsively, or seems afraid and under tension.

Two single cases from the above-mentioned study are presented, each representative of different developments within the group. Patient A was a 29-year-old man with DSM-III-R (American Psychiatric Association 1987) schizophrenia first diagnosed at the age of 18. He did not finish school and had been living at home completely cut off from the outside world. He suffered from chronic hallucinations and delusions, as well as marked negative symptoms. As shown in Figs. 2 and 3, there was no meaningful improvement in his psychopathology as measured with SANS or BPRS sum scores within the 6-month study. His position in the social field of the rehabilitation ward also did not change. He remained in a nonfunctional position. Patient B, aged 27, was a theology student when she was admitted to our hospital for the second time with acute psychotic symptoms corresponding to DSM-III-R schizophrenic disorder, paranoid form. Two years beforehand, she had recovered from a similar psychotic episode. Since her symptomatology did not improve even after 3 months of treatment on an acute ward, she was transferred to the rehabilitation ward where she displayed marked positive and negative symptoms at the beginning of the therapy (see Figs. 4 and 5). In contrast to patient A, her psychopathological disturbances improved during 4 months of inpatient treatment. Concomitantly, she became an accepted member of the patient group. This change in her position within the group is depicted in the SYMLOG field diagram where her image circle moves from the left lower quadrant to the right upper quadrant.

Coping Behavior

Finally, a further possible treatment approach should be mentioned. It seems to be important to point out that repeated demands for special attention to be paid to coping processes in the treatment of negative symptoms have barely been acknowledged in practice. The systematic investigation of the coping behavior of schizophrenic patients in situations experienced as stressful or threatening has only just begun. In the last few years, however, some empirical investigations have been published, both in German (Lange 1982; Böker et al. 1984, 1989; Brenner et al. 1987; Thurm and Häfner 1987; Wiedl and

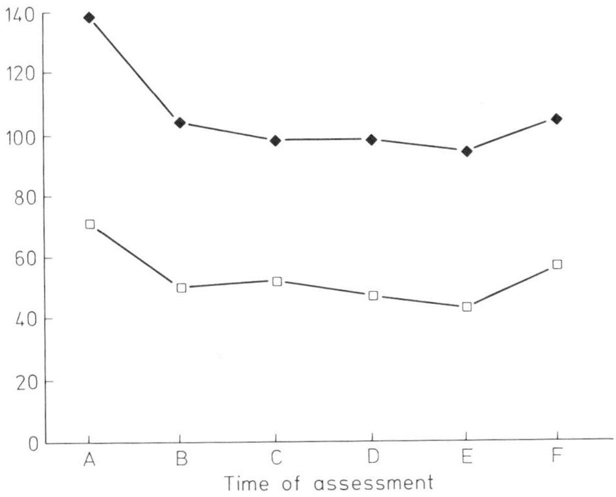

Fig. 2. BPRS (□) and SANS (◆) sum scores: patient A

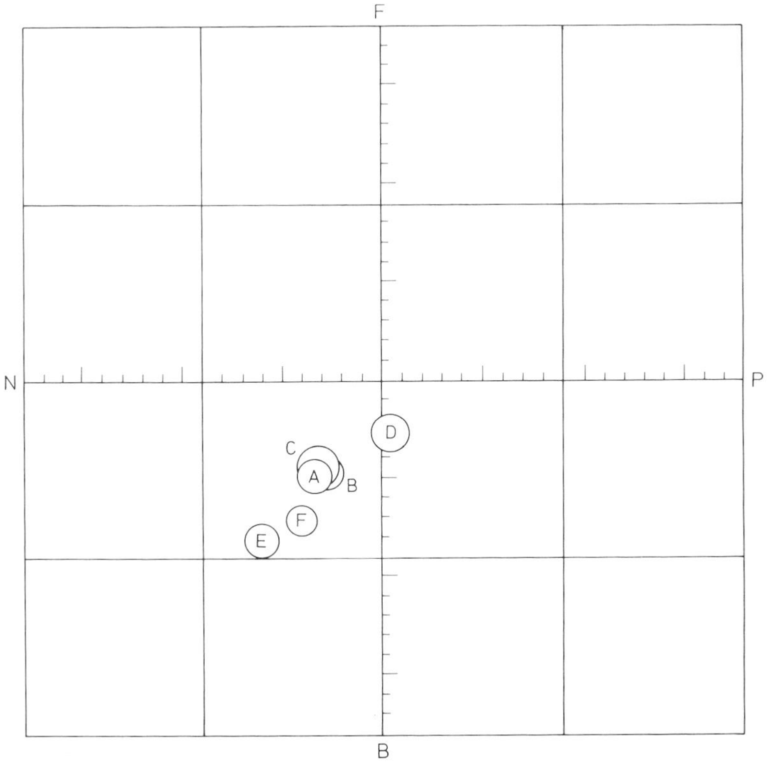

Fig. 3. SYMLOG field diagram: patient A

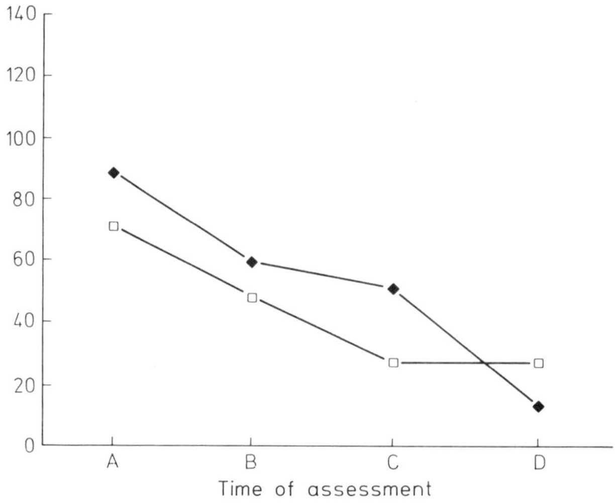

Fig. 4. BPRS (□) and SANS (◆) sum scores: patient B

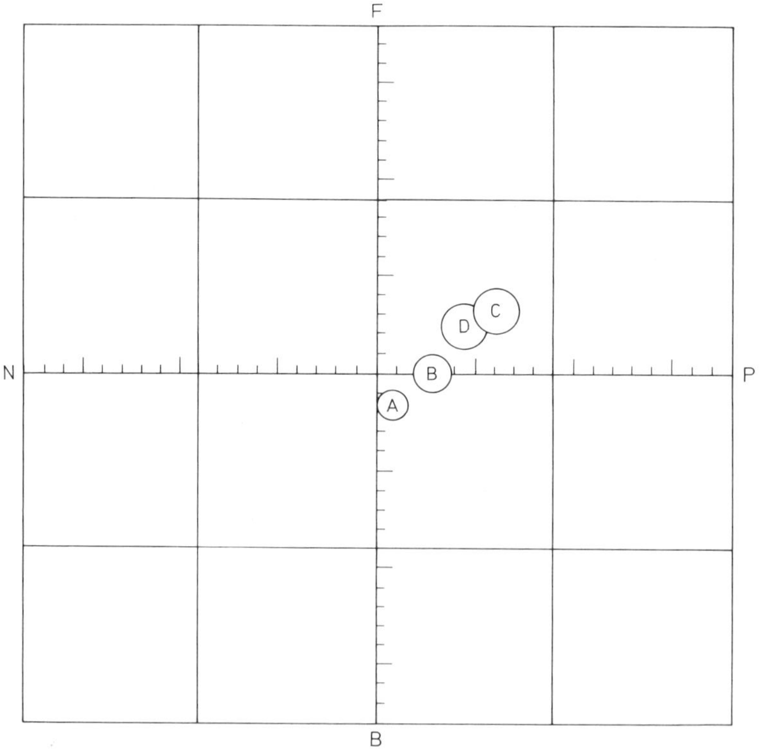

Fig. 5. SYMLOG field diagram: patient B

Schöttner 1989) and in English (Breier and Strauss 1983; Cohen and Berg 1985; Harding and Strauss 1985; Strauss et al. 1985; Godschalk 1987; Strauss 1989). This slowly increasing interest in the coping behavior of schizophrenic patients is connected with a paradigmatic reorientation in the understanding of psychopathology, especially with the development of the vulnerability-stress model (Zubin and Spring 1977) and its different modifications (e.g., Nuechterlein and Dawson 1984; Liberman et al. 1987). There are also connections with the process-oriented view of psychopathological phenomena in the sense of "performance theory" (Patterson 1982). This focuses on the interaction between the person and his environment, and thus differs from the traditional static understanding of psychological states; instead, these are investigated with regard to specific patterns of interaction with the environment, especially those factors causing stress. The evidence which is now available shows that schizophrenic patients consciously perceive with great regularity both threatening, stressful situations and prodromal and intermediate stages in the process of decompensation and attempt to cope with them. Surprisingly, the coping behavior used is active and problem centered, rather than passive and avoiding, and is furthermore, highly differentiated. It is also interesting that connections between the course of the illness and coping become apparent. However, all previous investigations have been exclusively retrospective and do not come to terms with coping behavior as a process. The methods of treatment thus lag considerably behind psychological research into coping. There, the interaction between stress, coping behavior, and mental illness – especially its microstructure – is almost always conceptualized as a variant of the model developed by Lazarus and Folkman (1984), which is centered on the transaction between person and situation. It postulates a continuum from the stressful event, to its appraisal, to an attempt at adaptation and reappraisal, and presupposes a mutual and progressive influencing of person and situation along the time axis. Coping is seen as a multifactorial process of problem solving and adaptation as well as of self-regulation of negative emotional conditions. Thus, further research into the role played by coping behavior in schizophrenia implies the necessity of developing models which diagnostically classify and describe the different forms of coping behavior, and then of applying these to the question of symptomatology, course, and outcome.

Using Hempel's (1965) analysis of the logical structure of causally based versus rational predictions of behavior and also the research of Perrez and Reicherts (1987) as a basis, we are presently investigating whether the coping attempts of schizophrenic patients follow certain rules formulated in accordance with theoretical and empirical evidence, and, if so, which and to what extent. This research is in its earliest stages and our results are so far purely descriptive. Nevertheless, we will outline it here in some detail in order to show its underlying philosophy and to encourage its further development as well as criticism. We proceed from a situational, operational theory of stress and coping that connects perceived situational characteristics as antecedents with behavior properties as consequents. In line with the transactional model of coping, the subjective cognitions are regarded as relevant characteristics in the subjects' perception of situations and their representations of controllability, changeability, and valence. Controllability is defined as the degree of probability that the situation can be influenced in its outcome, by the person's reactions: changeability as the degree of probability that the situation will change through its own dynamics; and valence as the degree of infringement or hindrance. Coping operations are distinguished according to whether they are problem oriented or not, and whether they occur on the level of action, cognition, or emotion.

The central question, then, is whether it would be possible to formulate intersubjectively valid rules or criteria for appropriate or inappropriate coping in the sense of criterion-oriented diagnosis. The formulation of such rules is based on empirical results from Becker (1984), Perrez and Reicherts (1987), and Wiedl et al. (in preparation) that in stressful situations healthy persons act according to particular rules, whereas disturbed persons do not, as well as on their "face validity" from clinical experience. This approach also seems to be of special interest insofar as it is exactly the regular linking of characteristics of a situation with behavior which is often disturbed in the case of schizophrenics (cf. Suellwold and Huber 1986). According to a contingency table, we initially formulated every conceivable rule concerning the relationship between cognitive representations and coping operations. From this complete list of rules, "functional" and "dysfunctional" rules of coping behavior were extracted, in accordance with the theoretical and empirical criteria mentioned above.

Our preliminary results from 25 chronic schizophrenic patients according to DSM-III-R point to the assumption that patients with pronounced negative symptoms as measured by the BPRS subscore "anergia" follow more dysfunctional rules than patients with fewer negative symptoms, and that rules are followed less consistently (Brenner et al., in preparation). In addition, they regularly seem to judge the controllability of stressful situations as lower and the changeability and valence as higher. Here we find interesting connections with the results of Reicherts (Reicherts 1988; Reicherts and Perrez 1989), who found increased signs of mental impairment where modes of coping were inconsistent. The results of Falloon and Talbot (1981) should also be mentioned, who found that a mode of coping with manifest positive symptoms was more useful if always carried out in the same way. Furthermore, while the dysfunctional coping behavior of patients with low ratings of negative symptoms is more on the action level, that of patients with high ratings of negative symptoms is more on the emotional level.

In addition to the preliminary character of these results, the observation of particular patterns of stress processing displayed by patients with negative symptoms does not of course allow conclusions to be drawn on possible causal relationships. It also would be desirable if the rules investigated concerning coping with stress could be oriented on empirically gained criteria of effectiveness (in the sense of leading to goal attainment) and appropriateness (which regardless of effectiveness in individual cases should correspond to several further criteria of rationality, e.g., the cost-benefit relation). Results of such research could provide valuable indications for methods of treatment of patients with prevailing negative symptoms concerned with coping with environmental challenges. It seems to us that one of the aims must lie in perceiving the stressful situation in a more differentiated and discriminating way, in learning to distinguish functional from dysfunctional coping, and in encouraging the regular use of particular coping strategies.

Summarizing, contrary to psychopathological, biological, or epidemiological research, the area of nonpharmacological approaches to the treatment of schizophrenic patients with negative symptoms has been neglected up until now. In our opinion, in addition to the more differentiated evaluation of existing cognitive and social therapy methods, investigations in coping with stressful situations could provide the basis for more effective therapeutic approaches and deserve our increased attention.

References

American Psychiatric Association (1987) Diagnostic and statistical manual of mental disorders, 3rd rev edn. American Psychiatric Association, Washington DC

Andreasen NC (1982) Negative symptoms in schizophrenia. Definition and reliability. Arch Gen Psychiatry 39:784–788

Atakan Z, Cooper GE (1989) Behavioural observation schedule (BOS), PIRS. Br J Psychiatry 155 [Suppl 7]:78–80

Ayllon T, Azrin NJ (1968) The token economy: a motivational system for therapy and rehabilitation. Appleton-Century-Crofts, New York

Bales RF (1970) Personality and interpersonal behavior. Holt, Rinehart and Winston, New York

Bales RF, Cohen SP, Williamson SA (1979) SYMLOG: a system for the multiple level observation of groups. Free Press, New York

Becker P (1984) Bewältigungsverhalten und Psychische Gesundheit. Universität Trier, Fachbereich I Psychologie, Trier (Trierer Psychologische Berichte, vol 11 (5))

Bellack AS (1989) A clinical guide for the treatment of schizophrenia. Plenum, New York

Bellack AS, Morrison RL, Mueser K (1989) Social problem solving in schizophrenia. Schizophr Bull 15:101–116

Boeker W, Brenner HD, Gerstner G, Keller F, Müller J, Spichtig L (1984) Self-healing strategies among schizophrenics: attempts at compensation for basic disorders. Acta Psychiatr Scand 69:373–378

Boeker W, Brenner HD, Würgler S (1989) Vulnerability-linked deficiencies, psychopathology and coping behavior in schizophrenics and their relatives. Br J Psychiatry 155 [Suppl 5]:128–135

Braff DL, Geyer MA (1990) Sensorimotor gating and schizophrenia. Human and animal model studies. Arch Gen Psychiatry 47:181–188

Breier A, Strauss JS (1983) Self-control in psychotic disorders. Arch Gen Psychiatry 40:1141–1145

Brenner HD (1989) The treatment of basic psychological dysfunctions from a systemic point of view. Br J Psychiatry 155 [Suppl 5]:74–83

Brenner HD (1987) On the importance of cognitive disorders in treatment and rehabilitation. In: Boeker W, Brenner HD (eds) Psychosocial treatment of schizophrenia. Huber, Toronto

Brenner HD, Hodel B, Kube G, Roder V (1987) Kognitive Therapie bei Schizophrenen: Problemanalyse und empirische Ergebnisse. Nervenarzt 58:72–83

Brenner HD, Kraemer S, Hermanutz G, Hodel B (1990) Cognitive treatment in schizophrenia. In: Straube ER, Hahlweg K (eds) Schizophrenia. Concepts, vulnerability and intervention. Springer, Berlin Heidelberg New York
Brenner HD, Hodel B, Roder V, Corrigan P (1991 a) Treatment of cognitive dysfunctions and behavioral deficits in schizophrenia. Integrated psychological therapy. Schizophr Bull (in press)
Brenner HD, Roder V, Kienzle N, Hodel B (1991 b) Treatment and rehabilitation of schizophrenic patients: an integrated psychological therapy program. Huber/Hogrefe, Toronto (in press)
Brown M (1982) Maintenance and generalization issues in skills training with chronic schizophrenics. In: Curran JP, Monti PM (eds) Social skills training: a practical handbook for assessment and treatment. Guilford, New York
Carpenter WT Jr (1986) Thoughts on the treatment of schizophrenia. Schizophr Bull 12:527–535
Carpenter WT Jr (1987) The phenomenology and course of schizophrenia: treatment implications. In: Meltzer HY (ed) Psychopharmacology: the third generation of progress. Raven, New York
Carpenter WT Jr, Heinrichs DW, Alphs LD (1985) Treatment of negative symptoms. Schizophr Bull 11:440–452
Ciompi L (1982) Affektlogik: Über die Struktur der Psyche und ihre Entwicklung. Klett-Cotta, Stuttgart
Cohen CI, Berg LA (1985) Personal coping styles of schizophrenic outpatients. Hosp Community Psychiatry 36:407–410
Cornblatt BA, Lenzenweger F, Dworkin RH, Erlenmeyer-Kimling L (1985) Positive and negative schizophrenic symptoms, attention and information processing. Schizophr Bull 11:397–407
Crow TY (1989) A current view of the type II syndrome: age of onset, intellectual impairment and the meaning of structural changes in the brain. Br J Psychiatry 155 [Suppl 7]: 15–20
Den Boer JA, Westemberg HGM, Verhoeven WMA (1987) Negative symptoms in schizophrenia; a review of diagnostic, pathophysiological and therapeutic aspects. New Trends. Exp Clin Psychiatry 3 (2): 109–145
Fallon IRH, Talbot RE (1981) Persistent auditory hallucinations: coping mechanisms and implications for management. Psychol Med 11:329–339
Friedrich W, Hennig W (1980) Der sozialwissenschaftliche Forschungsprozess. VEB, Berlin
Funke B, Reinecker H, Commichau A (1989) Grenzen kognitiver Trainingsmethoden bei schizophrenen Langzeitpatienten. Nervenarzt 60:750–756
Godschalk SM (1987) Experiences and coping strategies of people with schizophrenia. Diss Abst Int [B] 2:387
Goldstein MJ, Strachan AM (1987) The family and schizophrenia. In: Jacob T (ed) Family interaction and psychopathology: theories, methods and findings. Plenum, New York
Green M, Walker E (1985) Neuropsychological performance and positive and negative symptoms in schizophrenia. J Abnorm Psychol 94:460–470
Hansen DJ, Lawrence JSS, Christoff KA (1985) Effects of interpersonal problem-solving-training with chronic aftercare patients on problem-solving component skills and effectiveness of solutions. J Consult Clin Psychol 53:167–174
Harascz JL (1985) Neural plasticity in schizophrenia. Schizophr Bull 11:191–229
Harding CM, Strauss JS (1985) The course of schizophrenia: an evolving concept. In: Alpert M (ed) Controversies in schizophrenia, changes and constancies. Guilford, New York
Hempel CG (1965) Aspects of scientific explanations and othersays in the philosophy of science. Free Press, New York
Hemsley DR (1977) What have cognitive deficits to do with schizophrenic symptoms? Br J Psychiatry 130:167–173
Hodel B, Brenner HD, Merlo M (1990) Cognitive and social training for chronic schizophrenic patients: a comparison between two types of therapeutic interventions. In: Stefanis CN (ed) Psychiatry, vol 3. Elsevier, Amsterdam (International Congress Series 900-3)

Hogarty GE, Anderson CM, Reiss DJ (1987) Family psychoeducation, social skills training and medication in schizophrenia: the long and short of it. Psychopharmacol Bull 23(1)
Jablensky A (1978) Psychological impairments rating schedule. WHO, Geneva
Kay SR, Opler LA, Fissbein A (1987) The positive and negative syndrome scale (PANSS) for schizophrenia. Schizophr Bull 13:261–276
Kraemer S, Sulz KHD, Schmid R, Laessle R (1987) Kognitive Therapie bei standardversorgten schizophrenen Patienten. Nervenarzt 58:84–90
Lamberti G, Wieneke KH, Brauke N (1988) Der Computer als Hilfe beim Aufmerksamkeitstraining – Eine klinisch-experimentelle Studie. Rehabilitation 27:190–198
Lang PJ, Buss AH (1965) Psychological deficit in schizophrenia: interference and activation. J Abnorm Psychol 70:77–106
Lange HU (1982) Anpassungsstrategien, Bewältigungsreaktionen und Selbstheilungsversuche bei Schizophrenen. Fortschr Neurol Psychiatr 49:275–285
Lazarus RS, Folkman S (1984) Coping and adaption. In: Gentry WD (ed) Handbook of behavioral medicine. Guilford, New York
Leff JP, Vaughn C (1985) Expressed emotion in families. Guilford, New York
Liberman RP (ed) (1988) Psychiatric rehabilitation of chronic mental patients. American Psychiatric Press, Washington DC
Liberman RP, Bowers MB Jr (eds) (1990) Issue theme: substance abuse comorbidity in schizophrenia. Schizophr Bull 16(1)
Libermann RP, Jacobs HE, Boone SE, Foy DW, Donahoe CP, Fallon IRH, Blackwell G, Wallace CJ (1987) Skills training for the community adaption of schizophrenics. In: Boeker W, Brenner HD (eds) Psychosocial treatment of schizophrenia. Huber, Toronto
Meichenbaum D, Cameron R (1973) Training schizophrenics to talk to themselves: a means of developing attentional controls. Behav Ther 4:515–534
Moeller HJ, von Zerssen D (1986) Der Verlauf schizophrener Psychosen unter den gegenwärtigen Behandlungsbedingungen. Springer, Berlin Heidelberg New York
Mussgay L, Olbrich R (1988) Trainingsprogramme in der Behandlung kognitiver Defizite Schizophrener. Z Klin Psychol 17:341–353
Mussgay L, Olbrich R, Ihle W, Handtmann T (1991) Das Training kognitiver Fertigkeiten bei schizophrenen Patienten und seine Effekte auf elementare Informationsverarbeitungsmasse. Z Klin Psychol 20:103–114
Nuechterlein KH, Dawson ME (1984) Information processing and attentional functioning in the developmental course of schizophrenic disorders. Schizophr Bull 10:160–203
Nuechterlein KH, Dawson ME (1986) Attentional vulnerability indicators, thought disorder and negative symptoms. Schizophr Bull 12:408–426
Opler L, Kay S, Rosado V, Lindemeyer JP (1984) Positive and negative syndromes in chronic schizophrenic inpatients. J Nerv Ment Dis 172:317–325
Patterson GR (1982) Coercive family process: a social learning approach. Castalia, Oregon
Paul GL, Lentz RJ (1977) Psychosocial treatment of chronic mental patients: milieu versus social-learning programs. Harvard University Press, Cambridge
Perrez M, Reicherts M (1987) Behavior and cognition analysis of coping with stress by depressed persons. In: Huber W (ed) Progress in psychotherapy research. Presses Universitaires de Lauvain, Lauvain-La Neuve
Perris C (1988) Intensive cognitive-behavioral psychotherapy with patients suffering from schizophrenic psychotic or postpsychotic syndroms. Theoretical and practical aspects. In: Perris C, Blackburn IM, Perris H (eds) Cognitive psychotherapy, theory and practice. Springer, Berlin Heidelberg New York
Perris C (1989) Cognitive therapy with schizophrenic patients. Cassell, London
Pogue-Geile MF, Harrow M (1985) Negative symptoms in schizophrenia: their longitudinal course and prognostic importance. Schizophr Bull 11:427–439
Reicherts M (1988) Diagnostik der Belastungsverarbeitung. Huber, Bern
Reicherts M, Perrez M (1989) Prediction of behavior in the natural setting. In: Keats JA, Taft R, Heath RA, Lovibond SH (eds) Mathematical and theoretical systems. Elsevier, Amsterdam

Roder V (1988) Untersuchungen zur Effektivität kognitiver Therapie mit schizophrenen Patienten. Dissertation, University of Bern, Department of Psychology

Roder V, Brenner HD, Kienzle N, Hodel B (1988) Intergriertes Psychologisches Therapieprogramm für schizophrene Patienten (IPT). Psychologie Verlags Union, Munich

Schubart C, Schwarz R, Krumm B, Biehl H (1986) Schizophrenie und soziale Anpassung – eine prospektive Längsschnittuntersuchung. Springer, Berlin Heidelberg New York

Selzer MA, Sullivan TO, Carsky M, Terkelsen KG (1989) Working with the person with schizophrenia. The treatment alliance. New York University Press, New York

Shepherd G (1988) The contribution of psychological interventions to the treatment and management of schizophrenia. In: Bebbington P, McGuffin P (eds) Schizophrenia. The major issues. Heinemann, Oxford

Slade P, Bentall R (1989) Psychological treatment for negative symptoms. Br J Psychiatry 155 [Suppl 7]:133–135

Spaulding W, Storms L, Goodrich V, Sullivan M (1986) Applications of experimental psychopathology in psychiatric rehabilitation. Schizophr Bull 12:560–577

Strauss JS (1989) Mediating processes in schizophrenia towards a new dynamic psychiatry. Br J Psychiatry 155 [Suppl 5]:22–28

Strauss JS, Hafez H, Lieberman P, Harding CM (1985) The course of psychiatric disorders. III. Longitudinal principles. Am J Psychiatry 142:289–296

Strauss JS, Rakfeldt J, Harding CM, Liberman P (1989) Psychological and social aspects of negative symptoms. Br J Psychiatry 155 [Suppl 7]:128–132

Suellwold L, Huber G (1986) Schizophrene Basisstörungen. Springer, Berlin Heidelberg New York

Thurm I, Häfner H (1987) Perceived vulnerability, relapse risk and coping in schizophrenia – an explorative study. Eur Arch Psychiatry Neurol Sci:46–53

Vaughn CE (1987) Patterns of emotional response in the families of schizophrenic patients. In: Goldstein MJ, Hand J, Hallweg K (eds) Treatment of schizophrenia. Family assessment and intervention. Springer, Berlin Heidelberg New York

Walker E, Lewine RJ (1988) The positive/negative symptom distinction in schizophrenia. Validity and etiological relevance. Schizophr Res 1:315–328

Wallace CJ (1984) Community and interpersonal functioning in the course of schizophrenic disorders. Schizophr Bull 10:233–257

Wallace CJ, Boone SE (1984) Cognitive factors in the social skills of schizophrenic patients: implications for treatment. Nebraska Symposion on Motivation. University of Nebraska Press, Lincoln

WHO (1979) Schizophrenia: an international follow-up study. Wiley, Chichester

Wiedl KH, Schöttner B (1989) Die Bewältigung von Schizophrenie (I): theoretische Perspektiven und empirische Befunde. Z Klin Psychol Psychopathol Psychother 37:176–194

Wing JK, Brown GW (1970) Institutionalism and schizophrenia. Cambridge University Press, London

Wixted JT, Morrison RL, Bellack AS (1988) Social skills training in the treatment of negative symptoms. Int J Ment Health 17:3–21

Wong SE, Massel HK, Mosh MD, Liberman RP (1986) Behavioral approaches to the treatment of schizophrenia. In: Burrows GD et al. (eds) Handbook of studies on schizophrenia. Elsevier, Amsterdam

Zubin J (1985) Negative symptoms: are they indigenous to schizophrenia? Schizophr Bull 11:461–469

Zubin J, Spring B (1977) Vulnerability: a new view of schizophrenia. J Abnorm Psychol 86:103–126

The Demise of the Kraepelinian Binary Concept and the Aetiological Unity of the Psychoses *

T. J. Crow [1]

Emil Kraepelin's key contribution was to establish that there is a relationship between the form of a psychotic illness and its outcome. Illnesses in which affective change is a prominent component have a better outcome than those in which affective features are less prominent and in which the psychotic phenomena cannot be understood as secondary to affective change. The success of the Kraepelinian system, even its survival, owes everything to the reality of this relationship. Yet the independence of the two Kraepelinian entities has never been satisfactorily established (and Kraepelin himself had doubts). Notwithstanding this, the influence of the Kraepelinian concept is pervasive: every textbook has separate chapters on schizophrenia and affective disorder. A major objective of operational diagnostic criteria such as the Research Diagnostic Criteria (RDC) and Diagnostic and Statistical Manual (DSM) III is to separate these two entities with maximum reliability.

The assumption underlying such endeavours – that affective disorder and schizophrenia have different underlying pathogeneses and aetiology – has been paralytic to our thinking and stultifying to research. It obscures important general relationships that encompass both affective and schizophrenic psychoses and may provide a clue to aetiology. Such relationships include that both types of psychosis have an onset within the reproductive epoch and an incidence that is worldwide and without established relation to environmental or cultural variables.

If, as seems increasingly likely, the psychoses are genetic in origin, our most urgent task is to identify the locus. The Kraepelinian binary concept generates the expectation that there are at least two loci; the concept of a continuum leads to the prediction that there is but a single locus. Here it will be argued that one particular site in the genome is compatible with established observations on familial clustering and can explain some other enigmas.

---

* This paper will also appear as a chapter entitled "The Failure of the Kraepelinian Binary Concept and the Search for the Psychosis Gene". In: Kerr A, McClelland H (eds) (1991) Concepts of mental disorder. Gaskell, Royal College of Psychiatrists, London.

[1] Division of Psychiatry, Clinical Research Centre, Northwick Park Hospital, Harrow, HA1 3UJ, United Kingdom

A. Marneros / N. C. Andreasen / M. T. Tsuang (Eds.)
Negative Versus Positive Schizophrenia

Do Family Studies Support the Kraepelinian Separation?

Until recently the challenge to the Kraepelinian system has come from a small band of workers with interests in fields other than genetics. Thus, Kendell (1987) has approached the problem through phenomenology and nosology, Menninger et al. (1958) and Beck (1972) have been interested in therapeutic strategies and Flor-Henry (1983), in neuropsychology. Almost without exception, those who have relied upon family studies (e.g. Winokur 1984; Gershon and Rieder 1980; Cloninger et al. 1985; Kendler and Hays 1983) have followed Kraepelin in adopting a binary view. Only Angst et al. (1979) with an early interest in schizoaffective psychoses, and Karlsson (1974), who applied a global concept of psychosis to the historical records in Iceland, have adopted positions of relative agnosticism. An order of battle (Fig. 1) illustrates the predilection of geneticists for the Kraepelinian viewpoint and the diversity of interests of the protagonists of the continuum viewpoint.

At first sight it appears ominous for the continuum concept that those who have been most concerned with the genetic basis, who might therefore be expected to be the most hard-headed and quantitative, have been the strongest advocates of the Kraepelinian position. Thus, Gershon and Rieder (1980) wrote that "evidence from twin and family studies suggests that bipolar manic-depressive illness and chronic schizophrenia are distinct entities". According to Reich et al. (1982), "The genetic diathesis for affective disorders is independent of that for other psychiatric disorders", and Loranger (1981) on the basis of a family study using DSM III criteria concluded that "manic-depression and schizophrenia are genetically unrelated diseases".

Part at least of the confidence that genetic researchers have had in the Kraepelinian concept is based upon the fallacy of the excluded middle. Such studies are almost invariably conducted upon samples which are "purified" (as in Loranger's study) so that they include only probands who meet standard criteria for either classic Kraepelinian affective disorder or schizophrenia. Schizoaffective or atypical cases are excluded, and the conclusion drawn is that there is relatively little overlap in family studies between the psychoses. Such a

Binary Theorists		*Continuum Theorists*
Kraepelin		
		Menninger
Winokur		
		Kendell
		Beck
		Karlsson
	Angst	
Gershon		
Kendler		
		Flor-Henry
Cloninger		
		Crow

Fig. 1. Protogonists of the binary and continuum theories as judged from published contributions up to 1986, excluding Kraepelin (1920)

strategy is clearly inadequate to demonstrate the bimodality that is assumed in the Kraepelinian two-entities principle.

As we shall see, some workers have come to realise that the intermediate psychoses raise real problems for the binary system; others have yet to appreciate the difficulties presented by recent studies even in some cases where these are their own. Kraepelin himself was aware of the problem. In one of his last contributions (Kraepelin 1920) he wrote

> Perhaps it is also possible to tackle the difficulties which prevent us from distinguishing reliably between manic-depressive insanity and dementia praecox. No experienced psychiatrist will deny that there is an alarmingly large number of cases in which it seems impossible, in spite of the most careful observation, to make a firm diagnosis... Nevertheless it is becoming increasingly clear that we cannot distinguish satisfactorily between these two illnesses and this brings home the suspicion that our formulation of the problem may be incorrect.

In family studies what is required to test the two-entities principle is a sample of probands that includes a representative selection of both typical states and intermediate psychoses. The question to be asked is whether the distribution of illness in relatives is or is not bimodal along the axis that separates the typical syndromes. Bimodality supports the two-entities principle, failure to find it in a suitably selected sample favours the continuum concept.

Ødegaard (1972) was perhaps the first to mount such an investigation. In a series of consecutive admissions with a diagnosis of psychosis to the Oslo mental hospitals he included schizophrenic psychoses with three grades of defect, reactive, atypical affective and typical manic-depressive psychoses, in his classification of probands. In this typology it is likely that those illnesses which in other systems would be described as schizoaffective will be included in one of the categories of schizophrenia without defect, "reactive" and "atypical affective" psychoses. Illnesses in first and second degree relatives are classified into the three categories of "schizophrenia" and "reactive" and "affective" psychoses. When illness in the proband is arranged along a continuum, the percentage of ill relatives in each of these categories can be examined (Fig. 2).

The percentage suffering from schizophrenia is highest amongst the relatives of probands with schizophrenia with severe defect and declines progressively across the continuum, as the percentage of relatives with affective disorder rises. The percentage with reactive psychosis is highest in the relatives of probands with that diagnosis and declines in either direction from this point to minima at the pure defect and manic-depressive extremes.

The findings are more readily assimilated to a continuum than to a binary concept. At each point on the proband diagnostic scale there is overlap with adjacent categories. The intermediate classes of psychosis do not form discrete and separate entities; rather they appear to have clear and quantitatively varying relationships with the prototypical symptom patterns. Of particular interest is the fact that within the three categories of schizophrenic illness the proportion of illnesses amongst the relatives that are schizophrenic declines while that of those that are affective increases as the severity of defect in the proband changes from severe to slight to absent. Similar relationships between

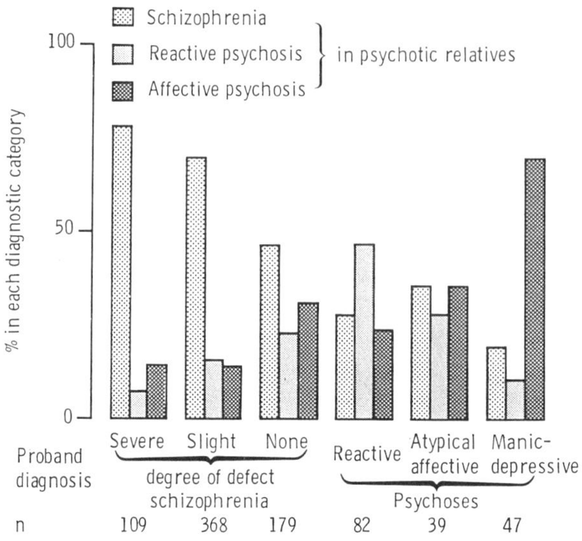

Fig. 2. Relative risks of psychiatric disorder, classified from case histories, in the first and second degree relatives of a consecutive series of admissions of patients with psychosis (data taken from Ødegaard 1972)

form of illness in the proband and the presence of affective disorder in the relatives were reported by Kant (1942) in a study of recovered and deteriorated (e.g. with defect states) schizophrenic patients. Affective illness was more commonly seen in the former class of patients. It is unclear why this should be the case if schizophrenia and affective illness are genetically unrelated.

Similar findings on the spectrum of psychotic illness are reported by Angst et al. (1979) from Zurich. These workers started with the question whether schizoaffective disorders are related to affective or to schizophrenic illness and later extended the scope of their inquiries to include the prototypical syndromes. In a recent analysis (Table 1) their findings are presented with probands classified as unipolar (UP) and bipolar (BP) affective disorder, schizoaffective illness of a predominantly affective (ASA) and predominantly schizophrenic (SSA) type and schizophrenia (S). Relatives were classified into the categories of schizophrenia and affective disorder. As in Ødegaard's study (1972) the proportion of schizophrenic to affective relatives increases across the spectrum from unipolar illness to typical schizophrenia.

In an earlier report Angst et al. (1983) had written

The obtained results are certainly puzzling in certain aspects. The underlying hypothesis of a continuum of psychosis is not disproved by our results. They show that on a descriptive level of symptoms and syndromes, taking into account the whole course of a psychosis, the dichotomy into schizophrenia and affective disorders is highly questionable. We do not only find transitional groups but also marked affective symptomatology underlying or superimposed to schizophrenia... Based on our findings, we do not conclude that a unitary psychosis exists but we think of a continuum of psychopathological subgroups with a lot of overlap which may also differ to a certain extent in other respects such as course, genetics and response to treatment.

Table 1. Morbid risk in first-degree relatives

	UP	BP	ASA	SSA	S
Probands	58	31	34	35	105
No. of affected relatives:					
schizophrenia (S)	10	4	19	18	31
affective psychoses (A)	24	6	14	4	5
S:A ratio (age-corrected)	0.30	0.47	0.92	2.99	5.05

From Angst and Scharfetter (1990).
UP, unipolar; BP, bipolar affective disorder; ASA, schizoaffective illness predominantly affective; SSA, predominantly schizophrenic; S, schizophrenia.

In their later discussions these authors write that "our analyses reveal no clear breeding true of either affective disorders or schizophrenia" (Stassen et al. 1988) and "The group of schizobipolar patients survives despite all attempts to break them down and to allocate them to schizophrenia and to affective disorder" (Angst and Scharfetter 1990).

A further indicator of a sea change in the literature comes from the studies of Gershon and colleagues at the National Institute of Mental Health. Whereas in 1980 Gershon and Rieder concluded that mania and schizophrenia could be considered as distinct genetic entities, subsequent work significantly modified this view. Thus, in a family study of affective and schizoaffective probands Gershon et al. (1982) concluded the data were compatible with the different affective disorders representing thresholds on a continuum that extends from unipolar through bipolar I and bipolar II to schizoaffective illness "representing greatest vulnerability"; and in a study (Gershon et al. 1988) of the relatives of patients with chronic psychosis (schizophrenia or schizoaffective disorder), this group found that there was no tendency for schizoaffective diagnosis or acute psychoses to aggregate separately from schizophrenia. Increased incidence of affective disorder (bipolar plus unipolar) was found in the relatives of patients with both schizoaffective disorder and schizophrenia. Gershon et al. (1988) considered a number of possible interpretations and concluded that

> There is much evidence suggesting that there must be at least gradations of affectivity and schizophrenicity. Presence of schizoaffective disorder in relatives, for example, is more associated with schizophrenic probands than with probands with chronic schizoaffective disorder... Patients with schizoaffective disorder have more relatives with bipolar disorder than do schizophrenic patients. Studied by the same methods, patients with affective disorders have a lower incidence of psychosis... in their relatives than do the patients with schizophrenia or chronic schizoaffective disorder.

The most recent contribution is that of Maier et al. (1989) who studied 450 probands with affective, schizoaffective and schizophrenic psychoses. Some 1250 first-degree relatives were interviewed with the Schedule for Affective Disorders and Schizophrenia–Lifetime Assessment (SADS–LA) supplemented by interviews for polydiagnostic classification and personality disorders. In

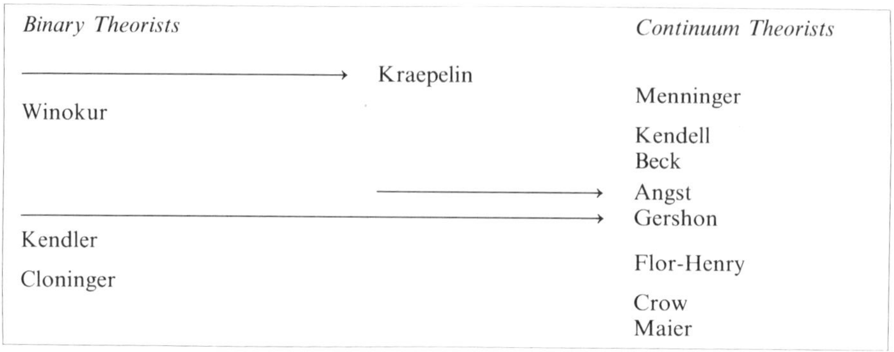

Fig. 3. Status of adherence to the binary and continuum theories in 1990, including Kraepelin (1920)

general agreement with a continuum concept these authors found (in a preliminary report) that "the familial pattern of disorders found is characterised by an unspecificity of diagnostic entities". Further analyses of this large and systematic investigation will be of considerable interest.

Thus, support for the Kraepelinian position is somewhat less than that represented in Fig. 1. Kraepelin's adherence to the two-entities principle was conditioned by reservations. Angst has moved from a position of agnosticism toward the continuum viewpoint and Gershon, on the basis of the studies that he and his colleagues have carried out at NIMH, has switched from adherence to the classic two-entities principle to the view that no clear lines can be drawn, i.e. to a version of the continuum concept (Fig. 3).

The Case of the Palaeo-Kraepelinians

Three strong protagonists of the binary concept remain: Cloninger, Kendler and Winokur. Their views and the evidence that they use to support them deserve careful consideration.

Cloninger et al. (1985) at St. Louis conducted the only study so far to challenge the conclusion of Kendell and Brockington (1980) that no bimodal separation of the prototypical psychoses can be achieved on the basis of phenomenology or outcome. These authors derived a discriminant function to distinguish schizophrenic from other psychiatric patients and normal individuals, that relied upon a constellation of four features (persecutory delusions, delusions of control, firmly fixed, mood-incongruent delusions, and auditory hallucinations) occurring together through a 6- to 12-year follow-up. Scale scores for the total of the four symptoms (minus one for the presence of a history of spending sprees plus elation) were used to demonstrate a bimodal separation of schizophrenic patients, defined by the Feighner criteria, from other subjects. The authors claim that not only did their scale identify 68% of schizophrenics and achieve separation from other subjects but that it was also useful for predicting outcome and the presence of a similar syndrome in relatives. A number of points are relevant:

1. The strategy adopted identifies a concept of schizophrenia that is notably restricted. The Feighner criteria require a history of 6 months' continuous illness and exclude a large number of patients who by other criteria (e.g. the RDC and Catego system) will be classified as schizophrenic. Yet by the Cloninger rule 32% even of the Feighner-positive schizophrenic patients will be excluded. Therefore, if as the authors claim these patients form a separate category of psychotic illnesses (possibly "true Kraepelinian schizophrenia"), it is not one that corresponds to several other concepts of the extent and frequency of occurrence of the disease. Many non-affective, non-schizophrenic psychoses remain to be accounted for.
2. The family history part of the study is not a critical test of bimodality. The fact that schizophrenic illnesses are found more commonly amongst the relatives of probands with typical schizophrenic illnesses than amongst those of affective and other psychoses and normal individuals is the generally accepted finding. The question to be addressed is whether accepting the Cloninger et al. definition of schizophrenia allows one to identify families that include an excess of individuals with schizophrenia but no excess of schizoaffective or atypical psychoses. The findings of Gershon et al. (1988) and Angst and Scharfetter (1990) suggest that this will not be the case.
3. An index of absence of affective disorder (history of spending sprees with marked elation) is used to identify the group of "true" schizophrenic probands. It would be interesting to know how much the findings depend upon this. Perhaps it is another indication of the way in which the propensity for affective change diminishes as the severity of schizophrenia increases along the psychotic continuum.

For each of these reasons the Cloninger study remains indecisive. If bimodality has been established, the region of rarity is located far to the right (i.e. the schizophrenic extreme) on the line along which affective disorder and schizophrenia are separated. If this definition of schizophrenia is substantiated many psychoses hitherto labelled schizophrenic will require a new name.

A notable illustration of the relevance of atypical psychoses and of the bias introduced by sampling as probands only those patients who suffer from classic affective and schizophrenic psychoses is provided by Kendler et al. (1986). Whereas previously they had applied DSM III criteria for affective disorder and schizophrenia to the Iowa 500 series of patients and controls and their relatives and had concluded that the Kraepelinian separation was generally supported by the findings in the relatives, in this study they examined a series of probands with a chart diagnosis of schizophrenia who did not meet the Feighner criteria. These individuals were allocated to the DSM III diagnostic categories of schizophreniform disorder, schizoaffective disorder and psychotic affective illness. Kendler et al.'s conclusions deserve full quotation:

The pattern of psychopathology in relatives of schizophreniform probands closely resembled that found previously in relatives of schizophrenic probands. Relatives of schizoaffective probands had an excess risk for schizophrenia, other psychoses, and bipolar illness. The pattern of illness found in relatives of probands meeting Research Diagnostic Criteria for mainly schizophrenic schizoaffective disorder appeared indistinguishable from that of relatives of schizophrenic probands. Relatives of probands with psychotic affective disorder had an excess risk for schizophrenia and for unipolar and bipolar affective disorder.

It is instructive to examine these conclusions in an attempt to determine where the dividing line between schizophrenia and affective disorder might be drawn. Firstly, since the spectrum of symptoms in the schizophreniform disorders is the same as in schizophrenia while their duration is less, a similarity in genetic relationships is to be expected. However, as some of these schizophreniform ilnesses (and also the DSM III schizophrenia cases) are unlikely to meet the Cloninger criterion of true schizophrenia, the overlap here is an embarassment for Cloninger et al.'s definition. Secondly, the finding that the relatives of patients with schizoaffective psychoses have an excess risk for both schizophrenia and affective illness is problematic for the Kraepelinian viewpoint unless these psychoses can be subdivided into schizophrenic and affective subtypes. But this is just what the studies of Angst and co-workers have failed to establish – no such distinction can be justified. Lastly, the findings in the relatives of patients with psychotic affective disorder in this series suggest a greater overlap between the prototypical psychoses than was apparent in the earlier DSM III-based studies with the Iowa series.

Overall, the findings give no comfort to the Kraepelinian concept. The impact on Kendler's own thinking is interesting to follow. Previously, in collaboration with Hays (Kendler and Hays 1983), he had studied patients with schizophrenia defined by DSM III criteria and had identified a group of 28 with a first-degree relative with affective disorder. These were compared with a group of 98 with no history of affective disorder in a first-degree relative. Patients with a family history of affective disorder were more likely to have suffered from affective symptoms on follow-up. The conclusion was that "even when DSM III criteria are met hesitation is indicated in diagnosing schizophrenia in patients with a first degree relative with bipolar illness".

In the later paper, however, Kendler et al. (1986) conclude that

The familial link between schizophrenia and at least a subgroup of schizoaffective disorders argues that the presence of prominent affective features, both depressive and manic, during the course of a chronic "schizophrenic-like" illness need not indicate a familial predisposition to affective illness.

Thus in 1983 it was argued that affective illness in a relative cast doubt on the diagnosis of schizophrenia in the proband, but by 1986 it was conceded that prominent affective features even in the proband were consistent with a diagnosis of schizophrenia.

The question must be asked of the defenders of the Kraepelinian concept, where is the line to be drawn? Is it to be drawn so as to define schizophrenia restrictively as Cloninger et al. (1985) instruct us to do and as it seems that Kendler and Hays in 1983 would have accepted, or is it to be drawn to include a substantial fraction of schizoaffective disorders, as Kendler et al. in 1986 recommend? In this case we are faced with the problem of distinguishing the "affective" types of schizoaffective disorder from the "schizophrenic" types, but this is just what the investigations of Angst et al. (1983; Angst and Scharfetter 1990) and Gershon et al. (1982, 1988) suggest cannot be achieved. The very existence of these illnesses is a challenge to the two-entities principle, as Kraepelin himself appreciated. Their genetic relationships as demonstrated by the recent studies deal a death-blow to the Kraepelinian system.

Winokur (1984) has wrestled long and hard with these problems and has been one of the stoutest defenders of the dichotomy. Even he, in collaboration with the Zurich group, has recognised the problems that the Kraepelinian system now faces. As a co-author (Stassen et al. 1988) reporting a study of 350 affected first-degree relatives of 269 hospitalized patients with functional psychoses, he writes that "typical syndrome patterns clearly appeared in both populations... Nevertheless our analyses revealed no clear breeding true of either affective disorders or schizophrenia."

Thus, it is difficult to identify a coherent defence in the literature of the classic Kraepelinian position. It must be assumed that that position has given way to some form of the continuum hypothesis – either that there are a large number of different genetic entities, each with its own locus, which show a substantial overlap in their phenotypic manifestations (Kendell 1987), or that there are a number of different alleles at a single genetic locus (Crow 1986a, 1987a). The first view has difficulty in explaining the extent and source of variation within families. The second faces the problem of the nature of the variation at the hypothetical locus. What sort of genes are these that show an apparently continuous variation? What sort of change in the gene could take place between different members of the same family?

Inter-generational Change in the Form of Psychosis

One manifestation of within-family variation noted by a number of authors is an apparent increase in the severity and change in the form of psychosis between generations. One of the first to draw attention to this phenomenon was Rosenthal (1970). In a survey of risk of other psychiatric illness in first-degree relatives of patients with affective disorder he noted an excess of schizophrenia in children (a mean of 2.3% in 5 studies), while the risk in parents and siblings remained within the 0.8% lifetime prevalence for the general population. Rosenthal asked, "From a genetic viewpoint why should schizophrenia have occurred at all in these families?"

Pollock and Malzberg (1940) collected family histories of psychosis over three generations and classified the probands as suffering from affective disorder or schizophrenia. In siblings the ratio of schizophrenia to affective disorder was as predicted from the proband diagnosis (8:2 for schizophrenic probands, and 3:11 for affective), but for preceding generations the ratio was similar for the two groups of probands, 11:15 for schizophrenic and 3:7 for affective probands. Thus, it appears that in preceding generations but not in

Table 2. Psychotic offspring of psychotic parents classified by diagnosis

Parents	Offspring	
	Affective disorder	Schizophrenia
Penrose (1968):		
Affective	232	205
Schizophrenic	34	150
	Manic-depressive psychosis	Schizophrenia
Powell et al. (1973):		
Manic-depressive psychosis	10	15
Schizophrenia	0	9

siblings the rate of affective disorder is higher than would be predicted in relatives of patients with schizophrenia on a conventional view.

Slater (1953) reported similar findings. In his study of twins he recorded psychiatric illness in other relatives and found the ratio of affective disorder to schizophrenia (4:3) to be particularly high in the parents of patients with schizophrenia. No excess of schizophrenia was found in the parents or siblings of patients with affective disorder. In an earlier study (Slater 1936) of manic-depressive illness:

A surprising feature had been the number of schizophrenics among the children ... In 10 of the 15 cases where manic-depressive subjects had been found by Dr Slater to have schizophrenic children he had been unable to find schizophrenia in other members of the patient's family or that of the husband or wife.

Two studies have examined parent-child pairs in which both members suffered from psychosis (Table 2). Penrose (1968) identified 621 such pairs in a series of 5456 pairs of relatives with psychiatric disease admitted over a period of 18 years to the Ontario mental hospitals. Among the ill children of schizophrenic parents, a diagnosis of schizophrenia preponderated over affective disorder in a ratio of almost 5:1. Among the hospitalised children of affectively ill parents the ratio was only a little less than 1; schizophrenia was almost as common as affective disorder. In a similar study in the Aberdeen case register, Powell et al. (1973) found schizophrenia in the children of schizophrenic parents and affective illness among the children of parents with affective disorder as expected. However, among the latter they found that for 10 cases of affective disorder, 15 cases of schizophrenia were also present.

The latest contribution to this literature is a study by Decina et al. (1989) of a series of 24 parent-child pairs both admitted over a period of about 60 years to the same institution with diagnoses meeting DSM III criteria for schizophrenia or affective disorder. While no case of affective disorder was found in the children of schizophrenic parents, 50% of children with psychotic affective disorders presented with schizophrenia. The authors concluded that:

The findings are consistent with the view that, in affected families, the severity of psychopathology increases from one generation to the next... psychotic affective disorder in the parents may predispose to schizophrenia in the children.

Again the question must be asked – what sort of genes are these that change their phenotype so readily? What happens between generations in these cases? Do the genes reassort, recombine or even jump, or does their mode of expression change?

Table 3. Risk of illness in different categories of first-degree relative of probands with affective disorder and schizophrenia

	Bipolar affective disorder (Price et al. 1985)	Schizophrenia (Zerbin-Rudin 1972)
Parents	4.8	6.3
Siblings	6.0	10.4
Children	9.5	13.7

From Crow (1986b).

A related phenomenon is the relative risk of psychosis in the different categories of first-degree relative with both affective disorder and schizophrenia (Table 3). The risk is different in the different categories of first-degree relative, being greater in children than siblings, and greater in siblings than in parents. This is true of both affective disorder and schizophrenia. The phenomenon may be relevant to recent reports (for example from the NIMH Epidemiological Catchment Area Study; Klerman et al. 1985) of an apparent secular increase in affective disorder. These reports are generally based upon studies of affective disorder within families; again, it may be that what we see is an increase in frequency or severity of illness between generations.

Here we approach the central paradox of psychosis – why, if these diseases are genetic in origin, do they persist? Why are they so prevalent? Book (1953) first suggested that schizophrenia was associated with a high rate of mutation and was followed in this view by Lewis (1958) in his paper on fertility and mental illness. The suggestion may be relevant to affective disorders as well as to schizophrenia and might relate also to inter-generational change. Perhaps what we see is a high rate of change at a particular locus that has the evolutionary advantage of generating new variants.

Where Is the Gene?

In October, 1987, the Lancet (Leader 1987) discussed the alternative to Kraepelin's binary viewpoint – the continuum concept – emphasising what I accept as its corollary, that there should be a single genetic locus. Yet quite apart from the various claims for an established linkage for one or more of the psychoses, we have reasonable evidence that the affective disorders at least are sometimes sex-linked and sometimes not (Risch et al. 1986). Does this not indicate that heterogeneity is already established?

There remained one way[2] in which homogeneity could yet be maintained – the locus for psychosis should be within the pseudoautosomal or exchange region of the sex chromosomes (Crow 1987b, 1988), that small region of the short arms within which there is exchange of genetic material between X and Y chromosomes in male meiosis (Ferguson-Smith 1965; Burgoyne 1986). At such a locus there is the possibility of apparent sex linkage in a condition that generally follows an autosomal mode of inheritance.

There are other reasons for taking a sex chromosomal locus for psychosis seriously. In a discussion of the excess of cases of sex chromosome aneuploidy (particularly XXY and XXX) that have consistently been observed in populations of patients with psychosis, Forssman (1970) wrote:

> Myself I am convinced that study of aberrations of the sex chromosomes will prove to have a radical effect on large sections of psychiatric thinking... That several different types of gonosomal aberration are associated with an increased risk of functional psychosis is an observation which should make us stop and think.

A gene for psychosis on the sex chromosomes is widely discounted on the grounds of the autosomal pattern of transmission. A locus in the pseudoautosomal region circumvents this problem.

The defining characteristic of pseudoautosomal transmission is same-sex concordance: within families there is an above chance expectation that individuals carrying a gene in this region will be of the same sex. When such a gene is inherited from a father it will be preferentially passed either on the X chromosome to daughters or on the Y chromosome to sons. By contrast when the disease is inherited on an X chromosome from the mother it is equally likely to be passed to a daughter or a son. Thus, assuming a dominant mode of transmission, concordance by sex is associated with a paternal origin of the gene.

Same-sex concordance in schizophrenia was first noted by Mott (1910) and was discussed in some detail by Penrose (1942) and Rosenthal (1962). The prediction that concordance by sex for psychosis will apply particularly to those cases in which inheritance is through the father has been tested in a series of 120 sibships that include at least two psychotic members (Crow et al. 1989). With paternal inheritance pairs of siblings with schizophrenia were more likely to be of the same sex. Neither same-sex concordance itself nor its association with paternal transmission are dependent upon the excess of males that is present in this and some previous series (Crow et al. 1990).

The prediction of same-sex concordance in affective disorder can be tested in the existing literature for bipolar disorder (Table 4). There is an excess of same-sex over opposite-sex pairs, and this cannot be accounted for by the excess of females that is also present.

The findings of the NIMH Collaborative Program on the Psychobiology of Depression with respect to familial transmission of bipolar illness (Rice et al. 1987) are also relevant. In this study of 187 families of bipolar patients the risk

[2] A second possibility is that an X – Y homologous gene is involved – Crow TJ, DeLisi LE X and Y linkage in schizophrenia. Psychiatric Genetics 2:102–103, 1991

Table 4. Distribution by sex in sibling pairs with bipolar affective illness

	Winokur et al. (1969)	Goetzl et al. (1974)	Mendlewicz and Rainer (1974)	Gershon et al. (1982)	Totals
MM	3	0	19	7	29
MF	4	0	19	15	38
FF	5	3	21	9	38
Same sex	67	Sign test (against 50:50 expectation)			
Opposite sex	38	$z = 2.83$, $P < 0.0025$			

The data from Winokur et al. (1969) are as summarised by van Eerdewegh et al. (1980). The data from Mendlewicz and Rainer (1974) and Gershon et al. (1982) are as abstracted by Risch et al. (1986).
M, male; F, female.

to relatives was found to be unrelated to the sex of the proband or relative. However, there was sex-specific sibling heterogeneity in that brother-sister correlations (0.36 for interview, and 0.23 for history data) were significantly ($P < 0.05$ and $P < 0.005$, respectively) less than brother-brother (0.63 and 0.53) and sister-sister (0.53 and 0.54) correlations. The authors conclude that "the exact source of this heterogeneity is unclear... the mode of transmission appears to be complex and may suggest that the environmental similarity for siblings is sex specific". It could be that the correlation is genetic and that it reflects a locus in the pseudoautosomal region.

Evidence from a sibling pair study suggesting linkage to the pseudoautosomal telomere has recently been presented (Collinge et al., 1989, 1991).

Conclusions

Contrary to established opinion one is forced to conclude that little support for the Kraepelinian binary concept is to be found in genetic studies. Unquestionably, there is a relationship between the form of psychotic illness in a proband and form of illness in the first-degree relatives, but there is also a lot of variation, and, crucially, no lines of separation between the prototypical syndromes can be drawn on genetic grounds. Those studies that have included an unselected series of patients with psychotic illness as probands have failed to identify any natural line of cleavage that could serve to separate disorders that are predominantly affective from those that are primarily schizophrenic. Workers who claim that such a line can be drawn are not in agreement with each other, or on occasion with themselves, as to where it should be drawn. It has to be concluded that there is a continuum of psychotic illness including variations within the affective (to include unipolar, bipolar and schizoaffective) and schizophrenic (to include variations in severity of defect symptoms) realms as well as between the major Kraepelinian prototypes.

Since this variation rests upon a genetic base, it must be assumed that the psychosis gene either exists in different forms or is expressed in different ways. Further evidence for such genetic variation comes from studies indicating that the risk of a schizophrenic type of psychosis is increased in children of parents with affective illness. Already (to account for a persistently high prevalence in the face of a fertility disadvantage) it has been proposed that the genes related to psychosis are subject to a high rate of mutation. Variation in the form of illness within families and between generations further emphasises the possible role of mutation, epimutation (Holliday 1987) or variations in mode of expression of the psychosis gene.

A locus for psychosis has been suggested in the pseudoautosomal (exchange) region of the sex chromosomes. This could explain (a) how apparent X-linkage in some families with affective disorder could co-exist with autosomal transmission in others without the necessity to invoke heterogeneity, (b) the association between sex chromosomal aneuploidies and psychosis and (c) the phenomenon of concordance by sex for psychosis within families. Such concordance is found in family studies involving both schizophrenic and affective illnesses.

References

Angst J, Scharfetter C (1990) Schizoaffective Psychosen. Ein nosologisches Ärgernis. In: Lungershausen E, Kaschka WP, Witkowski RJ (eds) Affektive Psychosen. Schattauer, Stuttgart

Angst J, Felder W, Lohmeyer B (1979) Schizoaffective disorders. I. Results of a genetic investigation. J Affective Disord 1:139–153

Angst J, Scharfetter C, Stassen HH (1983) Classification of schizo-affective patients by multidimensional scaling and cluster analysis. Psychiatr Clin (Basel) 16:254–264

Beck AT (1972) Depression: causes and treatment. University of Pennsylvania, Philadelphia

Book JA (1953) Schizophrenia as a gene mutation. Acta Genet Stat Med 4:133–139

Burgoyne PS (1986) Mammalian X and Y crossover. Nature 319:258–259

Cloninger CR, Martin RL, Guze SB, Clayton PJ (1985) Diagnosis and prognosis in schizophrenia. Arch Gen Psychiatry 42:15–25

Collinge J, Boccio A, DeLisi LE, Johnstone EC, Lofthouse R, Owen F, Poulter M, Risby D, Shah T, Crow TJ (1989) Evidence for a pseudoautosomal locus for schizophrenia: a sibling pair analysis. Cytogenet Cell Genet 51:978

Collinge J, DeLisi LE, Boccio A, Johnstone EC, Lane A, Larkin C, Leach M, Lofthouse R, Owen F, Poulter M, Shah T, Walsh C, Crow TJ (1991) Evidence for a pseudoautosomal locus for schizophrenia using the method of affected sibling pairs. Br J Psychiatry 158:624–629

Crow TJ (1986a) The continuum of psychosis and its implication for the structure of the gene. Br J Psychiatry 149:419–429

Crow TJ (1986b) Secular changes in affective disorder and variations in the psychosis gene. Arch Gen Psychiatry 43:1013–1014

Crow TJ (1987a) Psychosis as a continuum and the virogene concept. Br Med Bull 43:754–767

Crow TJ (1987b) Pseudoautosomal locus for psychosis? Lancet 2:1532

Crow TJ (1988) Sex chromosomes and psychosis: the case for a pseudoautosomal locus. Br J Psychiatry 153:675–683

Crow TJ, DeLisi LE, Johnstone EC (1989) Concordance by sex in sibling pairs with schizophrenia is paternally inherited: evidence for a pseudoautosomal locus. Br J Psychiatry 155:92–97

Crow TJ, DeLisi LE, Johnstone EC (1990) Reply... a locus closer to the telomere? Br J Psychiatry 156:416–420
Decina P, Luscas LR, Linder JR, Horwath E (1989) Parent-child pairs with major psychiatric diseases (Abstr 105). 142nd Meeting of the American Psychiatric Association, Washington
Ferguson-Smith MA (1965) Karyotype-phenotype correlations in gonadal dysgenesis and their bearing on the pathogenesis of malformations. J Med Genet 2:142–155
Flor-Henry P (1983) Cerebral basis of psychopathology. Wright, Bristol
Forssman H (1970) The mental implications of sex chromosome aberrations. Br J Psychiatry 117:353–363
Gershon ES, Rieder RO (1980) Are mania and schizophrenia genetically distinct? In: Belmaker RH, van Praag HM (eds) Mania, an evolving concept. Spectrum, New York, pp 97–109
Gershon ES, Hamovit J, Guroff JJ, Dibble E, Leckmann JF, Sceery W, Targum SD, Nurnberger JI, Goldin LR, Bunney WE (1982) A family study of schizo-affective, bipolar I, bipolar II, unipolar and normal control patients. Arch Gen Psychiatry 39:1157–1167
Gershon ES, DeLisi LE, Hamovit J, Nurnberger JI, Maxwell ME, Schreiber J, Dauphinais D, Dingman CW, Guroff JJ (1988) A controlled family study of chronic psychoses: schizophrenia and schizo-affective disorder. Arch Gen Psychiatry 45:328–336
Goetzl U, Green R, Whybrow P, Jackson R (1974) X linkage revisited; a further study of manic-depressive illness. Arch Gen Psychiatry 31:665–672
Holliday R (1987) The inheritance of epigenetic defects. Science 238:163–170
Kant O (1942) The incidence of psychoses and other mental abnormalities in the families of recovered and deteriorated schizophrenic patients. Psychiatr Q 16:176–186
Karlsson JL (1974) Inheritance of schizophrenia. Acta Psychiatr Scand [Suppl] 274:1–116
Kendell RE (1987) Other functional psychoses. In: Kendell RE, Zealley AK (eds) Companion to psychiatric studies, 4th edn. Livingstone, Edinburgh, pp 363–377
Kendell RE, Gourlay J (1970) The clinical distinction between the affective psychoses and schizophrenia. Br J Psychiatry 117:261–266
Kendell RE, Brockington IF (1980) The identification of disease entities and the relationship between affective and schizophrenic psychoses. Br J Psychiatry 137:324–331
Kendler KS, Hays P (1983) Schizophrenia subdivided by the family history of affective disorder. Arch Gen Psychiatry 40:951–955
Kendler KS, Gruenberg AM, Tsuang MT (1986) A DSM-III family study of the non-schizophrenic psychotic disorders. Am J Psychiatry 143:1098–1105
Klerman GL, Lavori PW, Rice J, Reich T, Endicott J, Andreasen NC, Keller MB, Hirschfield RMA (1985) Birth-cohort trends in rates of major depressive disorder among relatives of patients with affective disorder. Arch Gen Psychiatry 42:689–693
Koller PC, Darlington CD (1934) The genetical and mechanical properties of the sex chromosomes I rattus norvegicus. J Genet 29:159–173
Kraepelin E (1920) Die Erscheinungsformen des Irreseins. Z Gesamte Neurol Psychiatr 62:1–29 (In English 1974: Patterns of mental disorder. In: Hirsch SR, Shepherd M (eds) Themes and variations in European psychiatry. Wright, Bristol, pp 7–30)
Leader (1987) A continuum of psychosis? Lancet 2:889–890
Lewis AJ (1958) Fertility and mental illness. Eugen Rev 50:91–106
Loranger AW (1981) Genetic independence of manic-depression and schizophrenia. Acta Psychiatr Scand 63:444–452
Maier W, Hallmayer J, Heun R (1989) A controlled family study in affective and schizophrenic disorders: support for continuum models and spectrum concepts. Abstracts of the 1st World Congress of Psychiatric Genetics, vol 1, p 35
Mendlewicz J, Rainer JD (1974) Morbidity risk and genetic transmission in manic depressive illness. Am J Hum Genet 26:692–701
Menninger K, Ellenberger H, Pruyser P et al. (1958) The unitary concept of mental illness. Bull Menninger Clin 22:4–12
Mott FW (1910) Hereditary aspects of nervous and mental disease. Br Med J 2:1013–1020

Ødegaard O (1972) The multifactorial inheritance of predisposition to schizophrenia. In: Kaplan AR (ed) Genetic factors in "schizophrenia". Thomas, Springfield, pp 256–275
Penrose LS (1942) Auxiliary genes for determining sex as contributory causes of mental illness. J Ment Sci 88:308–316
Penrose LS (1968) Critical survey of schizophrenia genetics. In: Howells JG (ed) Modern perspectives in world psychiatry. Oliver and Boyd, Edinburgh, pp 3–19
Pollock HM, Malzberg B (1940) Hereditary and environmental factors in the causation of manic-depressive psychosis and dementia praecox. Am J Psychiatry 96:1227–1247
Powell A, Thomson N, Hall DJ, Wilson L (1973) Parent-child concordance with respect to sex and diagnosis in schizophrenia and manic-depressive psychosis. Br J Psychiatry 123:653 658
Price RA, Kidd KK, Pauls DL, Gershon ES, Prusoff BA, Weissman MM, Goldin LR (1985) Multiple threshold models for affective disorders: the Yale-NIMH collaborative family study. J Psychiatr Res 19:533–546
Reich T, Cloninger CR, Suarez B, Rice J (1982) Genetics of the affective psychoses. In: Wing L, Wing JK (eds) Psychoses of uncertain aetiology. Cambridge University Press, Cambridge, pp 147–159 (Handbook of psychiatry, vol 3)
Rice J, Reich T, Andreasen N, Endicott J, van Eerdewegh M, Fishman R, Hirschfeld RMA, Klerman GL (1987) The familial transmission of bipolar illness. Arch Gen Psychiatry 44:441–447
Risch N, Baron M, Mendlewicz J (1986) Assessing the role of X-linked inheritance in bipolar-related major affective illness. J Psychiatr Res 20:275–288
Rosenthal D (1962) Familial concordance by sex with respect to schizophrenia. Psychol Bull 59:401–421
Rosenthal D (1970) Genetic theory and abnormal behavior. McGraw-Hill, New York
Slater ETO (1936) Inheritance of manic-depressive insanity. Lancet 1:429–431
Slater ETO (1953) Psychotic and neurotic illness in twins. HMSO, London
Stassen HH, Scarfetter C, Winokur G, Angst J (1988) Familial syndrome patterns in schizophrenia, schizoaffective disorder, mania, and depression. Eur Arch Psychiatry Neurol Sci 237:115–123
Van Eerdewegh MM, Gershon ES, van Eerdewegh PM (1980) X-chromosome threshold models of bipolar manic-depressive illness. J Psychiatr Res 15:215–238
Winokur G (1984) Psychosis in bipolar and unipolar affective illness with special reference to schizo-affective disorder. Br J Psychiatry 145:236–242
Winokur G, Clayton PJ, Reich T (1969) Manic-depressive illness. Mosby, St. Louis
Zerbin-Rudin E (1972) Genetic research and the theory of schizophrenia. Int J Ment Health 1:42–62

Positive and Negative Symptomatology: The State of Affairs

A. MARNEROS [1] and N. C. ANDREASEN [2]

Introduction

Distinctions and dichotomies within the groups of schizophrenic disorders are as old as the concept of schizophrenia itself. Some of the distinctions were made according to the phenomenology, like the classical distinction of paranoid-hallucinatory, hebephrenic, catatonic, and simplex forms. Other distinctions are based on the prognosis (benign/non-benign, process/non-process, deficit/non-deficit, good prognosis/poor prognosis, etc.). Others are based on an assumed etiology, such as reactive (psychogenic)/process schizophrenia, or organic/endogenous schizophrenia (Marneros and Tsuang, 1991).

The importance of Bleuler's "fundamental symptoms" (E. Bleuler 1911, 1950) for the identification of schizophrenic syndromes was unfortunately covered mainly in the 1970s and the beginning of 1980s, as a result of the increasing use of Schneider's first rank symptoms. However, in the last decade "a return to an interest in negative symptoms brought the study of clinical psychopathology back to a more central and balanced position. Now, most clinicians and investigators recognise that in order to comprehensively evaluate and describe their patients, they must include a discussion of negative symptoms as well as positive symptoms" (Andreasen 1990 a). Crow's delineatio of the type I versus type II dichotomy and Andreasen's distinction of positive and negative schizophrenic syndromes (Andreasen 1982, 1985 a, b, c, 1989; Andreasen and Olsen 1982; Crow 1980, 1985) mark the beginning of ongoing research. The positive/negative dichotomy originated research in phenomenology, etiopathogenesis, course and outcome, treatment, biology and genetics, and social and psychological coping strategies. The fruitful work of many researchers and teams all over the world is, however, often marked by controversial findings. In the last decade the positive/negative distinction was able to answer some of the questions in schizophrenia research. However, some essential questions still remain unanswered. The aim of the European-American Workshop on Positive and Negative Schizophrenia in Bonn, on which this book is based, was to discuss arguments for and against the positive/negative distinction. In the following chapter we will try to summarize

[1] Psychiatrische Universitätsklinik, Sigmund-Freud-Straße 25, W-5300 Bonn, FRG
[2] University of Iowa, Department of Psychiatry, 500 Newton Road, Iowa City, 10 52242, USA

A. Marneros / N. C. Andreasen / M. T. Tsuang (Eds.)
Negative Versus Positive Schizophrenia

the most important conclusions of the contributions in this book and hope we can do this in an unbiased way.

The Historical Point

In his contribution in this volume, as well as in an earlier work (Berrios 1985), Berrios gives a fundamental view of the creation and meaning of the terms "positive" and "negative" in psychiatry. He shows that the terms coined by Reynolds in the 1850s as independent forms of physical sign (Reynolds 1858) were first brought together by Jackson (1887) who asserted that they depended upon one another. DeClérambault (1927, cited in Berrios 1991) spoke about positive, negative, and mixed phenomena, whereby negative phenomena were considered to be the result of "deficits" and "inhibitions." Berrios pointed out that Henri Ey emphasized a "dialectic interaction" between positive and negative symptoms and, according to whether the disorganization occurred in a cross-sectional or a longitudinal frame, he classified negative symptoms into synchronic and diachronic. Ey, deeply influenced by Jackson, considered negative symptoms as organic and the real manifestations of the disease, while positive symptoms were restitutive, a healthy reaction of the "psychological frame," and hence not a manifestation of disease. As Berrios pointed out, the Jacksonian usage of the positive/negative symptoms distinction was highly theoretical, and the question with respect to current usage is whether these terms can be divested of all their theoretical underpinnings.

The usage of the positive/negative concept in modern clinical and theoretical relevance with respect to schizophrenia is based mainly on the work of Kraepelin, E. Bleuler, and Kurt Schneider, although none of them used the term "positive" or "negative." All of them focused on the relevant point in a very different way. Although Kraepelin assumed that disturbances of some processes (which in current terms could be described as negative, such as volitional, cognitive, and affective) are the central symptoms of schizophrenia (Andreasen 1990b), he divided schizophrenia into various subtypes, some of them characterized mainly by negative symptoms, i.e., hebephrenia; and others by positive symptoms, like the paranoid-hallucinatory subtype. E. Bleuler's concept (1911, 1950) of fundamental schizophrenic symptoms concerning loss of the continuity of associations, loss of attention and volition, ambivalence and autism (most of them can be defined as negative symptoms) became for a long time predominant in diagnosing schizophrenia (Andreasen 1990b).

In the 1960s and 1970s, however, the interest of clinicians and researchers focused on the so-called first rank schizophrenic symptoms which can be assumed to be the core of positive symptoms. Schneiderian first rank symptoms are reliable enough, easy to detect – in spite of partial difficulties (Mellor 1991) – and clearly pathological (Andreasen 1990b; Marneros 1984a, b, 1985, 1988; Mellor 1970; Mellor 1991).

This was one of the most important reasons for their incorporation in the well-established diagnostic schedules and systems. However, very soon "clinicians with an interest in phenomenology and direct clinical experience in diagnosing and treating patients suffering from schizophrenia recognised that delusions and hallucinations, although relatively easy to be defined reliably, were not necessarily the most characteristic symptoms of schizophrenia" (Andreasen 1990b). It became clear that negative symptoms, either referred to by that name or by other terms (such as "basic symptoms," "deficit symptoms," "apathy syndrome," "minus symptoms," etc.) are clinically and theoretically the most important (Andreasen 1990c; Andreasen et al. 1991; Huber 1983; Gross 1989; Gross and Huber 1985; Gross et al. 1986; Süllwold and Huber 1987).

Definition and Assessment

Following the Jacksonian opinion, positive symptoms can be defined as the presence of a behavior or function that is otherwise normally not present in an individual. Negative symptoms are defined as the absence of behavior or function that is usually present in the normal individual. Negative symptoms seem to have in common the loss of an important cognitive or behavioral function, while positive symptoms represent an exaggeration or distortion of a normal function. Thus, positive and negative symptoms have to represent general cognitive and behavioral dominance. Symptoms representing negative and positive domains were already identified at the very beginning of schizophrenia research, but under various other names (Berrios 1985, 1991; E. Bleuler 1911; Janzarik 1968; Kraepelin 1919).

Following mainly the work of Andreasen and co-workers, a set of rating scales has been formed in order to assess both positive and negative symptoms. The Scale for the Assessment of Negative Symptoms (SANS; Andreasen 1983, 1990c) evaluates five major negative symptoms: alogia, affective blunting, anhedonia-asociality, avolition-apathy, and attentional impairment are assumed to be representative of the negative domain. The Scale for the Assessment of Positive Symptoms (SAPS; Andreasen 1984) evaluates four major positive symptoms assumed to be representative of a positive domain of psychopathology; delusions, hallucinations, positive thought disorder (i.e., derailment, tangentiality, incoherence, illogicality, circumstantiality, etc.), and bizarre behavior (Andreasen 1983, 1984, 1990b, c; Andreasen et al. 1991). The reliability of SANS and SAPS was investigated in different centres in the United States, Europe, and Japan, and was found to be consistently high (Andreasen 1990b, c; Andreasen et al. 1991).

A result of the increasing interest in the central role of negative symptoms is the plethora of scales assessing negative symptoms phenomena like negative symptoms. Stieglitz (1991) quoted 14 such scales and instruments, apart from other general psychopathological scales involving subscales which are connected to negative symptomatology, such as IMPS, BPRS, and AMDP. The application of different assessment instruments is certainly one of the reasons for the partly discrepant results regarding the positive/negative dichotomy reported in the literature. Moreover, the resulting limited comparability makes an aggregation of data and results difficult for the purposes of meta-analyses (Stieglitz 1991).

In assessing negative symptoms, one has to be aware of following points (Stieglitz 1991):

- Clarification of the question, which measurement models and test-theoretical approaches are appropriate for assessing negative symptoms, particularly when probabilistic test models are also included.
- Mathematical-statistical clarification of the question of the multidimensionality of negative symptomatology.
- Meta-analyses of previous studies with the same instruments.
- Multimodal analyses with regard to construct validity when experimental techniques and elementary characteristics of negative symptoms are included.

Carpenter and co-workers (1991) illustrated three main problems in the study of negative symptoms. The *first* is the inclusion of secondary negative symptoms when the aims of the study relate only to primary negative symptoms (i. e., negative symptoms which are primary to the disease process versus those which are secondary to associated conditions, e. g., neuroleptic-induced akinesia or anhedonia induced by depression). The *second* is the definition of a negative symptom subtyp in the presence or absence of criteria other than negative symptoms. According to the opinion of Carpenter and coworkers, in the most commonly used approaches, categorization of a patient relative to a putative negative symptom subtype is influenced by the presence or absence of positive symptoms. The *third* is, in many studies, that the differences in a validating variable between the negative symptom subtype and a comparative cohort cannot be traced directly to the negative symptoms as such comparison groups may systematically differ in age of onset, duration of illness, drug responsiveness, severity of psychosis, or other associated features.

In a somewhat similar way, Mundt assumed (1985, 1991) that either negative or positive symptoms of schizophrenia are a kind of epiphenomenon of a qualitative core phenomenon of the psychopathology of schizophrenia, which is the disturbed ability to constitue reality (Mundt 1991).

According to Lieberman and co-workers (1991) primary negative symptoms appear to have prognostic importance regarding treatment response. Patients in whom they occur have a poor response in terms of their positive symptoms. The interaction between positive and negative symptoms and different pharmacology was demonstrated by the patients' response to Methyl after remission. In the absence of positive symptom activation, negative symptoms actually declined with Methyl. This effect is similar to previously reported effects with psychostimulants (Angrist et al. 1980, 1982; Lieberman et al. 1985). It has been interpreted as negative or deficit symptomatology reflecting a condition of refused dopaminergic activity. The authors assume that the neurochemical process mediating primary negative symptoms is different from that mediating positive symptoms and is likely located in a different anatomic region. Since brain morphology has been found to be preferentially associated with male gender (Andreasen et al. 1990; Bogerts et al. 1990; Lieberman et al., 1991), and a relationship was found between enduring negative symptoms and abnormal brain morphology, Lieberman and co-workers assumed a connection between male gender and a more unfavorable course, treatment response, and outcome in schizophrenia.

According to Lieberman and co-workers (1991), positive and negative symptoms are highly correlated during the acute phase of schizophrenia and periods of symptom exacerbation. At these times when positive symptom levels are high it is difficult or impossible to identify primary negative symptoms accurately, and therefore it may be necessary to assess negative symptoms following remission of positive symptoms or during the residual phase of the illness.

One has to be aware of the problems associated with the primary versus secondary distinction of negative symptoms and the interference with other psychodynamically or sociodynamically determined variables (Brenner et al. 1991, Carpenter et al. 1991, Lewine 1991, Mundt 1991). The data of Andreasen (1990b, c; Andreasen et al. 1991), however, suggest that negative symptoms within the context of a schizophrenic syndrome can be distinguished from depressive symptoms within the context of a depressive syndrome. However the issue of phenomenological overlap between negative symptoms and depressive symptoms remains; that is, specific symptoms of depression and the negative symptoms of schizophrenia may be similar descriptions and definitions. As symptoms of schizophrenia, alogia and avolition overlap closely with psychomotor retardation. The anhedonia and asociality of schizophrenia could be similar to the anhedonia of depression.

Lewine (1991) pointed out that a distinction between anhedonia as a state and as a trait condition must be made, and that the relationship between physical and social anhedonia has to be clarified. Physical anhedonia was found to be more discriminating for schizophrenia and much more stable than social anhedonia (Lewine 1991). Nevertheless, the above-mentioned overlaps can make it quite difficult to determine whether negative symptoms are secondary to depression or whether they represent primary or core negative symptoms (Andreasen et al. 1991). The results of a variety of studies regarding this problem are controversial. Nevertheless, the consistent theme that emerges from the bulk of these studies is that affective blunting is consistently distinguishable from depressed mood, suggesting that the presence of this symptom may be particularly powerful in investigations that attempt to separate core negative symptoms from negative symptoms that may be secondary to depression (Andreasen et al. 1991).

The group of Huber in Germany paid a lot of attention to and pointed out the importance of the distinction between subjective and objective assessment (Huber 1983; Gross 1989; Gross and Huber 1985; Gross et al. 1986).

However, the correlation between subjective and objective signs reported in the literature is very poor, perhaps as a reflection of the relatively poor insight that patients have about their deficits (Andreasen 1990b). The exploration of the interrelationship between subjective and objective measures remains an important field of research in psychopathology (Gross and Huber 1985).

Symptoms Versus Syndromes Versus Diseases

Based on the phenomenological distinction of positive and negative symptoms, Crow (1980) proposed a linkage between phenomenology and external validators. He suggested that positive symptoms were associated with good premorbid functioning, relatively favorable outcome, acute onset, good response to treatment, hyperdopaminergic activity in a structurally normal brain, while negative symptoms correlated with poor premorbid functioning, impaired cognition, poor response to treatment, and also structural brain abnormality. The two-syndrome hypothesis, namely type I or "positive schizophrenia" and type II or "negative schizophrenia," became a very creative but also very controversial construct. In order to facilitate testing of the two-syndrome hypothesis, Andreasen and Olsen (1982) proposed a set of criteria based on clinical symptoms alone. Because it was clear that many patients had a combination of both positive and negative symptoms, they proposed a definition for three subtypes: positive, negative, and mixed. Criteria for the positive and negative subtypes are shown in Tables 1 and 2. The category of mixed schizophrenia includes those patients who do not meet the criteria for either positive or negative schizophrenia, or who meet criteria for both.

In their own work with these criteria, Andreasen and Olsen (1982) found that approximately one-third of patients fell into each of these three subtypes, although in a second replication the proportion of patients who were "predominantly positive" or "predominantly negative" was considerably smaller (Andreasen et al. 1990). Marneros and co-workers (Marneros and Tsuang, Marneros et al. 1991, Deister et al. 1991, Rohde et al. 1991), found that 32% of the *initial* episodes fell into the negative category, 44% into the positive category, and 24% into the mixed category. Andreasen observed that the negative patients had many correlates that confirmed the original Crow hypothesis (Andreasen 1990b; Andreasen et al. 1991).

Carpenter and co-workers (Carpenter and Buchanan 1988; Carpenter et al. 1988; Carpenter et al. 1991; Kirkpatrick et al. 1989; Wagman et al. 1987) modified these concepts by stressing the importance of the "deficit syndrome" and by ruling out a variety of contaminating variables (Table 3).

However, one of the main questions is: how stable are these and similar syndromes during the long-term course (Carpenter et al. 1991, Marneros et al. 1991, Häfner and Maurer 1991, Maurer and Häfner 1991)? Long-term investigations on the course of schizophrenia covering more than 20 years (M. Bleuler 1972; Ciompi and Müller 1976; Huber et al. 1979; Janzarik 1968; Marneros et al. 1991) have found a kind of "side-finding" that positive episodes usually change into negative episodes – although under different names – and vice versa. The groups of Häfner and of Marneros (Häfner and Maurer 1991, Maurer and Häfner 1991, Marneros et al. 1991, Rohde et al.

Table 1. Positive schizophrenia

1. At least one of the following is a prominent part of the illness:
   a. Severe hallucinations that dominate the clinical picture (auditory, haptic, or olfactory). (The judgement of severity should be based on various factors such as persistence, frequency, and effect on life-style)
   b. Severe delusions (may be persecutory, jealous, somatic, religious, grandiose, or fantastic)
   c. Marked positive formal thought disorder (manifested by marked incoherence, derailment, tangentiality, or illogicality)
   d. Repeated instances of bizzare or disorganized behavior

2. None of the following is present to a marked degree:
   a. Alogia
   b. Affective flattening
   c. Avolition-apathy
   d. Anhedonia-asociality
   e. Attentional impairment

Table 2. Negative schizophrenia

1. At least two of the following are present to a marked degree:
   a. Alogia (e.g., marked poverty of speech, poverty of content of speech)
   b. Affective flattening
   c. Anhedonia-asociality (e.g., inability to experience pleasure or feel intimacy, few social contacts)
   d. Avolition-apathy (e.g., anergia, lack of impersistence at work or school)
   e. Attentional impairment

2. None of the following dominates the clinical picture or is present to a marked degree:
   a. Hallucinations
   b. Delusions
   c. Positive formal thought disorder
   d. Bizarre behavior

1991, Deister et al. 1991) have investigated schizophrenia particularly from the viewpoint of change from one type of episode into another during the long-term course and the longitudinal dependence of positive and negative symptoms.

It is interesting that both the above-mentioned German groups, although using different designs, different samples, and testing different hypotheses, came to the same conclusion: negative and positive phenomena are longitudinally not independent, and a pure negative or a pure positive long-term course of schizophrenic illness is extremely rare.

With the aim of analyzing dichotomy models of schizophrenia from the developmental or longitudinal viewpoint, Häfner and Maurer formulated six different models and possible testing hypotheses and related them to the early development of schizophrenia *from first real onset* of symptoms *until the first hospitalization*. Marneros and co-workers tried to identify the type of episodes

Table 3. Criteria for schizophrenia with deficit syndrome according to Carpenter

1. The patient meets DSm-III criteria for schizophrenia.
2. At least two of the following negative symptoms must be present:
   a. Flattened or restricted affect
   b. Anhedonia
   c. Poverty of speech with curbing of ideational field and decrease of curiosity
   d. Lack of sense of purpose
   e. Lack of social drive
3. The negative symptoms are not fully accounted for by one or more of the following:
   a. Depression or anxiety
   b. Drug effect
   c. Environmental deprivation
4. Some combination of two or more of the negative symptoms listed above have been present for the preceding 12 months and were always present during periods of clinical stability (including chronic psychotic states) or during recovery from psychotic exacerbation. These symptoms may not be detectable during transient episodes of acute psychotic disorganisation or decompensation.

Patients meeting only criterion 1 can be designated as "schizophrenic without negative symptoms." Patients meeting criteria 1 and 2 and possibly 4, but not 3, can be designated as "schizophrenic with deficit syndrome." Patients meeting all four criteria can be designated "schizophrenic with deficit syndrome." Patients meeting criteria 1, 2, and 3, but not 4 could either be cases of "schizophrenia with primary, nonenduring negative symptoms" or instances that with time will meet the full criteria for "schizophrenia with deficit syndrome." Clearly, the former designation can be made with confidence only after negative symptoms have remitted. However, since there may be considerable research interest in this group, it is desirable to have criteria that exclude most cases that will progress to schizophrenia with deficit syndrome without waiting to see if current negative symptoms remit. Hence, the following criteria were proposed for schizophrenia with primary, nonenduring negative symptoms:

1. The patient meets criteria 1, 2, and 3 for "schizophrenia with deficit syndrome"
2. The patient does not meet criterion 4 for schizophrenia with deficit syndrome
3. The patient has had two or more prior periods of primary negative symptoms (criteria 1, 2, and 3 for schizophrenia with deficit syndrome), followed by at least 3 months of remission of negative symptoms
4. The current period of primary negative symptoms is not more than of 4 months duration

This would leave a residual, ambiguous category of patients meeting criteria 1, 2, and 3 for schizophrenia with deficit syndrome, but not meeting full criteria for schizophrenia with primary nonenduring negative symptoms. Such cases would require further observation to determine if they subsequently meet criteria for schizophrenia with deficit syndrome.

from first episode (excluding "prodromal symptoms") *until the last episode of the illness* (excluding the so-called "residual symptoms") after a long-term course (on average more than 23 years).

Häfner and Maurer (1991) concluded that in their representative sample of first hospitalized schizophrenics the found significant correlation of the sum values of positive and negative symptoms from the time of true onset until first admission contradicts the hypothesis of Crow and Andreasen, postulating an independence of positive and negative syptomatology. Although Andreasen's original report (1982) appears to suggest the independence of positive and negative symptoms, since factor analysis elicited a bipolar factor, subsequent work disconfirmed independence of positive and negative symptoms. Subsequent factor analyses have consistently yielded three factors – psychotic, disorganized, and negative – and in a series of overview articles Andreasen and her co-workers have consistently stressed the overlap of positive and negative symptoms in individual patients, suggesting the importance of a mixed clinical picture (Andreasen 1985a; Andreasen and Grove 1986; Arndt et al. 1991). A stability of Andreasen's subtypes during the phase of early development of schizophrenia was found by the Mannheim group quite good only within two years after onset. However, in the last 2-year segment before admission, the pure subtypes become less stable. It seems that the categorical change of symptomatology is also a function of the duration of the illness. The opinion regarding the duration of the illness was also confirmed by Marneros and co-workers, investigating the opposite point in time, namely *after* first hospitalization. Furthermore, the results of Häfner and Maurer support the hypothesis of preceding negative symptoms.

According to Huber and co-workers (Huber 1983; Gross 1989), the basic symptoms are so termed because they represent the basis of productive-psychotic symptomatology. Basic symptoms occur not only initially, but also in later stages and especially in so-called uncharacteristic residual states. According to Huber, it is not possible to separate between positive and negative symptoms, acute and chronic schizophrenia, and a type I and a type II syndrome because all of these distinctions are stages of the same disease, and the negative symptoms can progress into positive symptoms and vice versa (Huber 1983). Basic symptoms can change from uncharacteristic symptoms to other characteristic symptoms, and into productive-psychotic symptoms and vice versa. These three developmental levels can be, according to Huber (1983), conceptualized as existing on a psychopathological continuum.

However, Kraepelins's model of negative symptoms occurring only as a consequence of positive symptoms could not be upheld by the Mannheim team. By testing further models the authors found that negative and positive symptoms are obviously not independent phenomena. Negative symptoms as the direct expression of the disease process seem to announce the occurrence of positive symptoms. Furthermore, they rise steeply and concomitantly with the positive sumptoms and clearly recede again after the acute state, though not always to the initial level before the "true" onset of the disease.

The similarity of the findings and therefore the conclusions in the work of the groups of Häfner and of Marneros are clearly demonstrated in the contribution of Maurer and Häfner in this volume. Using the data of a 5-year follow-up study, Maurer and Häfner found that is was impossible to identify convincing proportions of pure positive and negative subtypes. Moreover, these subtypes did not prove to be stable during the course of the disease. Marneros and co-workers (1991) came to the same conclusion using the data of a long-term (23-year), partly retrospective, partly prospective study. They found that only six patients remained purely negative from the beginning to the end of the observation time, and only 18 patients remained purely positive, even after exclusion of "prodromal" and "residual" states. They concluded that schizophrenia is bimorphous in the long-term course. A higher stability of negative symptoms in comparison to positive symptoms has been repeatedly reported in the literature (Barnes and Liddle 1990; Johnstone et al. 1987; Pogue-Geile and Harrow 1984; Biehl et al. 1989). Some studies have suggested that the stability of negative symptoms depends on the chronicity of the illness; acute forms of the illness having more unstable negative symptoms (Lindenmayer et al. 1986; Kay and Opler 1987). However, the question regarding the dichotomy of the two types of schizophrenia does not concern the stability of symptoms per se, but the monomorphism (that is, one and the same type of episode, positive or negative) or bimorphism (that is, either the change of negative episodes into positive or vice versa, or mixed positive and negative symptomatology) of the long-term course of the illness (Marneros et al. 1991).

The group of Marneros tried to find some premorbid or prognostic correlations between the type of *initial* episode and premorbid features or outcome factors. They found that patients with a negative initial episode had, in comparison to patients with a positive onset, a significantly lower age at onset, significantly fewer social contacts before onset, a stable heterosexual relationship significantly less frequently, and therefore significantly fewer patients with a negative onset were married at the time of the initial episode (Rohde et al. 1991). Regarding the long-term outcome (on average after 23 years), it was found that 80% of the patients who had no persistent alterations at the end of the observation time had had a positive onset. On the other hand, it was found that about one-third of the patients with a negative onset had to be permanently hospitalized. It was concluded that the type of initial symptomatology might have a predictive value with regard to long-term outcome, however, probably not as an isolated factor but in combination and interaction with other premorbid and sociodemographic features (Deister et al. 1991).

The positive/negative dichotomy and other dichotomies close to this distinction – such as Crow's dichotomy (1980) in type I and type II, or the dichotomy of Farmer et al. (1983, 1984) in H-type and P-type, or the dichotomy of Carpenter and co-workers (Carpenter et al. 1988) in deficit/non-deficit schizophrenia – aim, among other things, to identify correlations between phenomenology and severity of the illness. However, the results regarding the relationship between phenomenology and long-term outcome are still contradictory. Some studies have found correlations between negative symptomatology and unfavorable outcome (Astrup et al. 1962; Carpenter et al. 1988; Pogue-Geile and Harrow 1985), while other studies have not (Bland et al. 1978; Gift et al. 1980; Knight and Roff 1985; Lindenmayer et al. 1986; Johnstone et al. 1979).

There are many potential reasons for the contradictory results. One of them could be the bimorphous long-term course (Marneros et al. 1991). A second possible reason has been pointed out by Barnes and Liddle (1990): Some scales for rating negative symptoms include items which are related to social functioning, such as the impersistence at work or school in the SANS (Andreasen 1983), work impairment and social withdrawal in the High Royds Evaluation of Negativity (HEN; Mortimer et al. 1989), passive-apathetic social withdrawal which takes into account the neglect of activities of daily living in the Positive and Negative Syndrome Scale (PANSS; Kay et al. 1989), or patients' ability to plan and carry out work, school, or self-care tasks (Iager et al. 1985).

Thus, according to Barnes and Liddle (1990), the apparent ability of negative syndrome scores to predict poor social functioning may in some cases partly reflect some overlap between some rating scales for negative symptoms and those used to rate impairment of social functioning and role performance, as well as the relative stability and chronic nature of these features. Another reason could be the correlation of negative symptoms with some unfavorable premorbid, sociodemographic, and social parameters (Marneros et al. 1989a, b; Steinmeyer et al. 1989; Deister et al. 1991; Marneros et al. 1991; Rohde et al. 1991).

Genetics

Genetic data currently available allow fairly limited conclusions regarding the negative/positive symptom dichotomy in schizophrenia. According to the conclusion of McGuffin and co-workers (1991), the twin data, based on a reworking of previously published studies, do not allow a clear separation into two distinct subtypes of schizophrenia. According to the authors, there is fairly consistent evidence from the published twin results and from their own family data that probands who have experienced negative symptoms tend to have more affected relatives than probands who have had only positive symptoms. The authors tested a liability/threshold model in which negative or mixed schizophrenia was postulated to be a more severe disorder lying beyond a more extreme threshold on a liability continuum than positive symptom schizophrenia, which was postulated to be a less severe condition lying beyond a less extreme threshold. The simple model where negative and positive symptom schizophrenia differ only quantitatively in terms of their positions on the same continuum of liability cannot be rejected and, on grounds of parsimony, can even be favored over a model where the two clinical forms are constructed as two separate conditions (McGuffin et al. 1991).

The findings of Tsuang and co-workers (1991) from the Brockton-Harvard family project, while preliminary in nature, suggested that negative symptomatology appears to serve as a more powerful descriptor of the relatives of schizophrenics than positive symptomatology. In particular, affective flattening and apathy/avolition appear to be relevant dimensions in this description. First-degree relatives of DSM-III-R schizophrenic and depressed control probands were interviewed and rated utilizing Andreasen's SANS and SAPS. A statistical model, including the negative symptom scales, successfully differentiated the two sets of relatives, with the first-degree relatives of schizophrenics scoring higher on an overall level of negative symptoms. A model including positive symptom scales failed to discriminate among family members (Tsuang et al. 1991).

Biology

Crows conceptualization of the type I and type II schizophrenia, together with the operationalization of negative symptoms, mainly using Andreasen's SANS, became a model for studying subtypes in particularly negative schizophrenic symptoms. Findings, discussion, and conclusions are still controversial. While Crow assumed that type II schizophrenia was a non-dopaminergic form, other authors challenged this concept and hypothesised that type II was a hypodopaminergic form of schizophrenia. As van Kammen and co-workers (1991) pointed out, the type I/type II division has led investigators to define negative symptoms as a component of an irreversible deficit syndrome with large ventricles or lesions in the prefrontal cortex. However, these findings are not shared by all studies (references in van Kammen et al. 1991; Andreasen 1990b; Andreasen et al. 1991; Marks and Luchins 1990; Bogerts et al. 1991). Referring to the literature, van Kammen and coworkers summarized that decreased dopaminergic turnover and activity are associated with severe, stable, chronic, and poor prognosis forms of schizophrenia. They concluded that decreased dopamine turnover is related to the presence of negative symptoms during residual states, whereas increases in noradrenaline turnover are associated with increased schizophrenic symptomatology.

As Pickar and co-workers (1990) pointed out, it is difficult to review pharmacological and metabolite studies without concluding that dopaminergic mechanisms play a significant role in mediating both negative and positive symptoms. Nevertheless, the characteristics of dopaminergic involvement are unclear. Whereas compelling evidence continues to link the mechanism of action of neuroleptic drugs, including therapeutic effects on positive and negative symptoms, to the blockade of D2 receptors, neuroleptic-induced alterations in dopaminergic functions are time dependent and may include reductions in variability as well as in net dopamine activity (Pickar et al. 1990). The authors close their large review of the literature with the conclusion that the separation of positive from negative symptoms of schizophrenia in terms of biological substrates has yet to be fully realized. Van Kammen and co-workers (1991) suggested that negative symptomatology has to be better differentiated, for example, into primary/non-primary, drug responsive/drug non-responsive, and residual or non-residual symptoms.

Summarizing the most recent neuropathological, CT, PET, SPECT, and MRI studies, Bogerts et al. (1991) conclude that positive schizophrenic symptoms is caused by left limbic temporal lobe diseases, while negative symptoms might be related to a more diffuse cortical pathology, including bilateral temporal lobe dysfunction and prefrontal cortical hypoactivity. However, a review of the literature given by the authors shows that most of these findings are still controversial. Nevertheless, the positive/negative distinction focused the interest of research not on a global correlation of the schizophrenic disease with morphological changes but with single symptoms or groups of symptoms having some consistency, such as a positive or negative cluster.

Marks and Luchins (1990) reviewed 28 articles on brain imaging in schizophrenia. Eighteen of them provide some support for the view that structural brain abnormalities detected by imaging technics, such as large ventricles or sulci, are associated with fewer positive and/or more negative symptoms, five studies cannot support this view, and three of them provide evidence for the opposite correlation. Marks and Luchins conclude that the next task seems to be to pay more attention to the development of hypotheses linking particular brain regions to specific symptoms.

Treatment

The positive/negative dichotomy became a very interesting domain for pharmacological research (Barnes and Liddle 1990; Boyer et al. 1990; Pickar et al. 1990; Meltzer 1991; Möller 1991). As Meltzer (1991) pointed out, much of the recent interest in positive and negative symptoms has stemmed from consideration of the relative responsiveness of positive and negative symptoms to antipsychotic drug treatment (see also Möller, 1991). Although negative symptoms were initially characterized as being unresponsive to drug treatment (Crow 1980), some studies showed a beneficial effect with some antipsychotic drugs, particularly pimozide, sulpiride, and clozapine (Barnes and Liddle 1990; Meltzer 1991, Möller 1991). There is considerable evidence that the so-called typical neuroleptics, like butyrophenone or phenothiazine, are more effective in treating positive than negative symptoms. In discussing the literature, Möller (1991) came to the conclusion that there is some evidence that typical neuroleptics are also able to reduce negative symptoms. However, because most of these trials were performed during acute exacerbations of schizophrenic psychoses, the question arises as to whether only negative symptoms secondary to productive symptoms might be involved (Möller 1991, Pickar et al. 1990).

The results reported by Meltzer (1991) demonstrate that atypical antipsychotic drugs can ameliorate negative symptoms, even in treatment-resistant schizophrenia. Clozapine may be the most effective of these atypical antipsychotic drugs (Meltzer 1991, Pickar et al. 1990). There appear to be diffferences in the responses of specific types of negative symptoms to clozapine treatment: alogia may be the most responsive and avolition the least. The improvement in negative symptoms with clozapine appears to be independent of the improvement in positive symptoms. According to the opinion of Meltzer (1991) this is not so with typical antipsychotic drugs.

The treatment of negative schizophrenic symptoms with dopamine agonists is unclear. The findings are only preliminary in nature (Klimke and Klieser 1991) although some studies have reported improvement in positive as well as in negative symptoms (Klimke and Klieser 1991, Lieberman et al. 1985; Pickar et al. 1990). Other studies found a lack of correlation between the improvement of negative and positive symptoms and concluded that they represent distinct components of psychosis (Barnes and Liddle 1990).

Negative symptoms could be primary – related to the illness – or secondary as a consequence of the illness (Brenner et al. 1991; Carpenter et al. 1991; Lewine et al. 1991; Mundt 1991). Drug treatment alone is, in these cases, not sufficient; additional psychosocial treatment is necessary (McGlashan et al. 1990). However, as Brenner et al. (1991) pointed out, the area of non-pharmacological approaches to the treatment of schizophrenic patients with negative symptoms has been neglected up to now. Strategies and methods of coping with stressful situations, suggested by Brenner and co-workers (1991), could provide the basis for more effective therapeutic approaches.

Negative and Positive Symptomatology in Childhood Schizophrenia

Only a few studies have applied the concept of positive and negative schizophrenia to childhood schizophrenia (Betts and Walker 1987; Eggers 1991, Remschmidt et al. 1991). Betts and Walker found a correlation between age at onset of childhood schizophrenia and manifestation of positive and negative symptoms. Negative symptoms were most frequent in early childhood, while positive symptoms increased with increasing age. Remschmidt and co-workers investigated 113 adolescents diagnosed as having a schizophrenic disorder according to a multiaxial classification scheme (according to ICD-9). Most of them were found to have a mixed type of schizophrenia (approximately 42%); approximately 30% were diagnosed as having a negative type of schizophrenia, and fewer than 30% as having a positive type of schizophrenia. A syndrome shift occurred up to the end of the episode, mostly in only one direction: positive to negative (Remschmidt et al. 1991). The findings of Remschmidt and co-workers are not contradictory to the finding of Marneros and co-workers (1991) because Marneros and co-workers investigated the shift from one type of episode to another during course of the illness, while Remschmidt and co-workers investigated the interaepisodic shift. Remschmidt and co-workers conclude that the concept of positive and negative schizophrenia is also a useful one in differentiating schizophrenic psychoses in late childhood and adolescence; however, positive and negative symptomatoloy cannot be looked upon as stable traits of schizophrenic psychoses. There are other dynamic symptoms that change remarkably during treatment and during the course of the schizophrenic disorder (Remschmidt et al. 1991).

Eggers (1991) investigated the long-term prognostic value of negative symptoms in 57 patients with childhood schizophrenia on average 16 years later. He found that negative symptoms occurred in patients in good remission whose psychosis followed an acutely recurring course as well as in patients with chronically deteriorating psychoses. However, the way the negative symptoms manifested themselves depended largely on the course of the disease.

In childhood schizophrenia which became chronic the negative symptoms were found to be present from the beginning of the illness. There was also found to be an overrepresentation of premorbidly maladjusted children in the group of patients with negative schizophrenia. Some of the negative symptoms, especially if they were present in acutely recurring productive episodes with positive symptoms, prooved to be reactions to the psychotic experiences.

The findings of the reported studies show that the concept of positive and negative symptoms of schizophrenia can be applied in childhood psychiatry and that much more research is needed.

Epilogue

The contributions in this book underline the relevance of negative symptomatology in schizophrenia. In the words of Andreasen (1990b), they show that:

> A relative balance has been restored to descriptive psychopathology, giving more equal emphasis on florid colourful symptoms such as delusions and hallucinations as well as the more debilitating negative symptoms. An emphasis on considering the neural mechanisms that may underlie both positive and negative symptoms has led to a more focused approach to asking questions about psychopathology, particularly emphasising the importance of longitudinal perspectives and the possible interaction between treatment effects and psychopathology.

They also show an interaction between negative and positive symptomatology, especially on the long-term perspective (Häfner and Maurer 1991, Maurer and Häfner 1991, Marneros et al 1991). Perhaps the study of interaction between distinct symptoms and syndromes can contribute to answer some aspects of the question of psychotic continuum and "etiological unity of the psychoses" (Crow 1991). Several contributions in this book do not support a clear-cut distinction of schizophrenias into a positive and a negative syndrome. There are several factors that confound a simple dichotomy, in accordance with other studies (see contributions in Andreasen 1990a). However, the modus of linkage and interaction between positive and negative symptomatology can certainly be another field of fruitful research.

References

Andreasen NC (1982) Negative syndromes in schizophrenia: definition and reliability. Arch Gen Psychiatry 39:784–788

Andreasen NC (1983) The scale for assessment of negative symptoms. University of Iowa, Iowa City

Andreasen NC (1984) The scale for assessment of positive symptoms. University of Iowa, Iowa City

Andreasen NC (1985a) Positive versus negative schizophrenia. A critical evaluation. Schizophr Bull 11:380–389

Andreasen NC (1985b) Negative syndromes in schizophrenia: strategies for longterm management. Adv Biochem Psychopharmacol 40:1–7

Andreasen NC (1985c) Positive versus negative schizophenia: criteria and validation. In: Pichot P, Berner P, Wolf R, Thau K (eds) Psychiatry. The state of the art, vol. 1: clinical psychopathology, nomenclature and classification. Plenum, New York

Andreasen NC (1989) Neural mechanisms of negative symptoms. Br J Psychiatry 155 (Suppl 7): 93–98

Andreasen NC (1990a) Schizophrenia: positive and negative symptoms and syndroms. Karger, Basel
Andreasen NC (1990b) Positive and negative symptoms: historical and conceptual aspects. In: Andreasen NC (ed) Schizophrenia: positive and negative symptoms and syndromes. Karger, Basel
Andreasen NC (1990c) Methods for assessing positive and negative symptoms. In: Andreasen NC (ed) Schizophrenia: positive and negative symptoms and syndromes. Karger, Basel
Andreasen NC, Grove WM (1986) Evaluation of positive and negative symptoms in schizophrenia: definition and prevalence. Psychiatr Psychobiol 12:108–121
Andreasen NC, Olsen S (1982) Negative versus positive schizophrenia. Arch Gen Psychiatry 39:789–794
Andreasen NC, Flaum M, Swayze VW, Tyrell G, Arndt S (1990) Positive and negative symptoms in schizophrenia. Arch Gen Psychiatry 47:615–621
Andreasen NC, Flaum M, Arndt S, Alliger R, Swayze VW (1991) Positive and negative symptomes: assessment and validity. In: Marneros A, Andreasen NC, Tsuang MT (eds) Negative vs. positive schizophrenia. Springer, Berlin Heidelberg New York
Angrist B, Rotrosen J, Gershon S (1980) Differential effects of amphetamine and neuroleptics on negative vs. positive symptoms in schizophrenia. Psychopharmacology 72:17–19
Angrist B, Peselow E, Rubinstein M, Corwin J, Rotrosen J (1982) Partial improvement in negative schizophrenic symptoms after amphetamine. Psychopharmacology 78:128–130
Arndt S, Alliger RJ, Andreasen NC (1991) The positive and negative distinction: failure of the two dimensional model. Br J Psychiatry (in press)
Astrup C, Fossum A, Holmboe R (1962) Prognosis in functional psychoses. Thomas, Springfield
Barnes TRE, Liddle PF (1990) Evidence for the validity of negative symptoms. In: Andreasen NC (ed) Schizophrenia: positive and negative symptoms and syndromes. Karger, Basel
Berrios GE (1985) Positive and negative symptoms and Jackson. Arch Gen Psychiatry 42:95–97
Berrios GE (1991) Positive and Negative Signals: A conceptual history. In: Marneros A, Andreasen NC, Tsuang MT (eds) Negative vs. positive schizophrenia. Springer, Berlin Heidelberg New York
Betts BA, Walker E (1987) Positive and negative symptoms in psychotic and other psychiatrically disturbed children. J Child Psychol Psychiatry 28:555–568
Biehl H, Maurer K, Jablensky A, Cooper JE, Tomov T (1989) The WHO Psychological Impairments Rating Schedule (WHO/PIRS). I. Introducing a new instrument for rating observed behaviour and the rationale of the psychological impairment concept. Br J Psychiatry 155 (Suppl 7):68–70
Bland RC, Parker JH, Orn H (1978) Prognosis in schizophrenia: prognostic predictors and outcome. Arch Gen Psychiatry 35:72–77
Bleuler E (1911) Dementia praecox oder Gruppe der Schizophrenien. In: Aschaffenburg G (ed) Handbuch der Psychiatrie. Spezieller Teil, vol 4. Deuticke, Leipzig
Bleuler E (1950) Dementia praecox or the group of schizophrenias. International University Press, New York
Bleuler M (1972) Die schizophrenen Geistesstörungen im Lichte langjähriger Kranken- und Familiengeschichten. Springer, Berlin Heidelberg New York
Bogerts B, Ashtari M, Degreef G, Alvir JM, Bilder RM, Lieberman JA (1990) Reduced temporal limbic structure volumes on magnetic resonance images in first episode schizophrenia. Psychiatry Res 35:1–13
Bogerts B, Falkai P, Degreef G, Lieberman J (1991) Neuropathological and brain imaging studies in positive and negative schizophrenia. In: Marneros A, Andreasen NC, Tsuang MT (eds) Negative vs. positive schizophrenia. Springer, Berlin Heidelberg New York

Boyer P, Lecrubier V, Puech AJ (1990) Treatment of positive and negative symptoms: pharmacologic approaches. In: Andreasen NC (ed) Schizophrenia: Positive and negative symptoms and syndromes. Karger, Basel

Brenner HD, Hodel B, Merlo MCG (1991) Nonpharmacological treatment concepts of negative symptomatology. In: Marneros A, Andreasen NC, Tsuang MT (eds) Negative vs. positive schizophrenia. Springer, Berlin Heidelberg New York

Carpenter WT, Buchanan RW (1988) Domains of psychopathology relevant to the study of etiology and treatment in schizophrenia. Schizophrenia: scientific progress. Oxford University Press, New York

Carpenter WT, Heinrichs DW, Wagman AMI (1988) Deficit and nondeficit forms of schizophrenia: the concept. Am J Psychiatry 145:578–583

Carpenter WT, Buchanan RW, Kirkpatrick B, Thaker G, Tamminga C (1991) Negative symptoms: a critique of current approaches. In: Marneros A, Andreasen NC, Tsuang MT (eds) Negative vs. positive schizophrenia. Springer, Berlin Heidelberg New York

Ciompi L, Müller C (1976) Lebensweg und Alter der Schizophrenen. Eine katamnestische Langzeitstudie bis ins Senium. Springer, Berlin Heidelberg New York

Crow TJ (1980) Positive and negative schizophrenic symptoms and the role of dopamine. Br J Psychiatry 137:383–386

Crow TJ (1985) The two syndrome concept: origins and current status. Schizophr Bull 11:471–186

Crow TJ (1991) The demise of the Kraepelinian binary concept and the etiological unity of the psychoses. In: Marneros A, Andreasen NC, Tsuang MT (eds) Negative vs. positive schizophrenia. Springer, Berlin Heidelberg New York

Deister A, Marneros A, Rohde A (1991) Long-term outcome of patients with a positive initial episode versus patients with a negative initial episode. In: Marneros A, Andreasen NC, Tsuang NC (eds) Negative versus positive schizophrenia. Springer, Berlin Heidelberg New York

Eggers C (1991) Negative symptoms in the long-term course of childhood schizophrenia. In: Marneros A, Andreasen NC, Tsuang MT (eds) Negative vs. positive schizophrenia. Springer, Berlin Heidelberg New York

Farmer AE, McGuffin P, Spitznagel E (1983) Heterogeneity in schizophrenia. A cluster analytic approach. Psychiatry Res 8:1–12

Farmer AE, McGuffin P, Gottesman II (1984) Searching for the split in schizophrenia: a twin study perspective. Psychiatry Res 13:109–118

Gift TE, Strauss JS, Kokes RF et al. (1980) Schizophrenia: affect and outcome. Am J Psychiatry 137:580–585

Gross G (1989) The 'basic' syptoms of schizophrenia. Br J Psychiatry 155 (Suppl 7): 21–25

Gross G, Huber G (1985) Psychopathology of basic stages of schizophrenia in view of formal thought disturbances. Psychopathology 18:115–125

Gross G, Huber G, Schüttler R (1986) Long-term course of Schneiderian schizophrenia. In: Marneros A, Tsuang MT (eds) Schizoaffective psychoses. Springer, Berlin Heidelberg New York

Häfner H, Maurer K (1991) Are there two types of schizophrenia? True onset and sequence of positive and negative syndromes prior to first admission. In: Marneros A, Andreasen NC, Tsuang MT (eds) Negative vs. positive schizophrenia. Springer, Berlin Heidelberg New York

Huber G (1983) Das Konzept substratnaher Basissymptome und seine Bedeutung für Theorie und Therapie schizophrener Erkrankungen. Nervenarzt 54:23–32

Huber G, Gross G, Schüttler R (1979) Schizophrenie. Eine verlaufs- und sozialpsychiatrische Langzeitstudie. Springer, Berlin Heidelberg New York

Iager AC, Kirch DG, Wyatt RJ (1985) A negative symptom rating scale. Psychiatry Res 16:27–36

Jackson JH (1887) Remarks on evolution and dissolution of the nervous system. J Ment Sci 33:25–48

Janzarik W (1968) Schizophrene Verläufe. Eine strukturdynamische Interpretation. Springer, Berlin Heidelberg New York

Johnstone EC, Frith CD, Gold A, Stevens M (1979) The outcome of severe acute schizophrenic illnesses after one year. Br J Psychiatry 134:28–33

Johnstone EC, Owens DGC, Frith CD, Crow TJ (1987) The relative stability of positive and negative features in chronic schizophrenia. Br J Psychiatry 150:65–71

Kay SR, Opler LA (1987) The positive-negative dimension in schizophrenia: its validity and significance. Psychiatr Dev 2:79–103

Kay SR, Opler LA, Fiszbein A (1989) PANSS rating criteria: Negative Scale (N). Br J Psychiatry 155 (Suppl 7):66–67

Kirkpatrick B, Buchanan RW, McKenney PD, Alphs LD, Carpenter WT (1989) The Schedule for the Deficit Syndrome: an instrument for research in schizophrenia. Psychiatr Res 30:119–124

Klimke A, Klieser E (1991) The treatment of positive and negative schizophrenic symptoms with dopamine agonists. In: Marneros A, Andreasen NR, Tsuang MT (eds) Negative vs. positive schizophrenia. Springer, Berlin Heidelberg New York

Knight RA, Roff JD (1985) Affectivity in schizophrenia. In: Alpert M (ed) Controversies in Schizophrenia. Guilford Press, New York London

Kraepelin E (1919) Dementia praecox and paraphrenia. Livingstone, Edinburgh

Lewine RJ (1991) Anhedonia and the amotivational state of schizophrenia. In: Marneros A, Andreasen NC, Tsuang MT (eds) Negative vs. positive schizophrenia. Springer, Berlin Heidelberg New York

Lieberman JA, Kane JM, Gadalletta D, Ramos-Lorenz J, Bergmann K, Wegner J, Novacenko H (1985) Methylphenidate challenge tests and course of schizophrenia. Psychopharmacol Bull 21:123–129

Lieberman JA, Jody D, Alvir JMJ, Borenstein M, Mayerhoff DI (1991) Negative symptoms in schizophrenia: relationship to positive symptoms and outcome. In: Marneros A, Andreasen NC, Tsuang MT (eds) Negative vs. positive schizophrenia. Springer, Berlin Heidelberg New York

Lindenmayer JP, Kay SR, Friedman C (1986) Negative and positive schizophrenic syndromes after the acute phase: a prospective follow-up. Compr Psychiatry 27:276–286

McGuffin P, Harvey I, Williams M (1991) The negative/positive dichotomy: does it makes sense from the perspective of the genetic researcher? In: Marneros A, Andreasen NC, Tsuang MT (eds) Negative vs. positive schizophrenia. Springer, Berlin Heidelberg New York

Marks RC, Luchins DJ (1990) Relationship between brain imaging findings in schizophrenia and psychopathology. In: Andreasen NC (ed) Schizophrenia: Positive and negative symptoms and syndromes. Karger, Basel

Marneros A (1984a) The pathognomonic value of K Schneider's first rank symptoms in schizophrenia. Psychiatr Fenn 15:99–105

Marneros A (1984b) Frequency of occurrence of Schneider's first rank symptoms in schizophrenia. Eur Arch Psychiatry Neurol Sci 234:78–82

Marneros A (1985) Schneiderian first rank symptoms in organic psychoses. In: Pichot P, Berner P, Wolf R, Thau K (eds) Psychiatry. The state of the art, vol 1. Plenum, New York

Marneros A (1988) Schizophrenic first-rank symptoms in organic mental disorders. Br J Psychiatry 152:625–628

Marneros A, Tsuang MT (1991) Dichotomies and other distinctions in schizophrenia. In: Marneros A, Andreasen NC, Tsuang NC (eds) Negative versus positive schizophrenia. Springer, Berlin Heidelberg New York

Marneros A, Deister A, Rohde A, Steinmeyer EM, Jünemann H (1989a) Long-term outcome of schizoaffective and schizophrenic disorders: a comparative study. Part I: definitions, methods, psychopathological and social outcome. Eur Arch Psychiatry Neurol Sci 238:118–125

Marneros A, Steinmeyer EM, Deister A, Rohde A, Jünemann H (1989b) Long-term outcome of schizoaffective and schizophrenic disorders: a comparative study. Part III: social consequences. Eur Arch Psychiatry Neurol Sci 238:135–139

Marneros A, Deister A, Rohde A (199) Long-term investigations in stability of negative/positive distinction. In: Marneros A, Andreasen NC, Tsuang NC (eds) Negative versus positive schizophrenia. Springer, Berlin Heidelberg New York

Maurer K, Häfner H (1991) Dependence, independence or interdependence of positive and negative symptoms. In: Marneros A, Andreasen NC, Tsuang MT (eds) Negative vs. Positive Schizophrenia. Springer: Berlin Heidelberg New York

McGlashan TH, Heinssen RK, Fenton WS (1990) Psychosocial treatment of negative symptoms in schizophrenia. In: Andreasen NC (ed) Schizophrenia: Positive and negative symptoms and syndromes. Karger, Basel

Mellor CS (1970) First rank symptoms of schizophrenia. Br J Psychiatry 140:423–424

Mellor CS (1991) Methodological problems in identifying and measuring first-rank symptoms of schizophrenia. In: Marneros A, Andreasen NC, Tsuang NC (eds) Negative versus positive schizophrenia. Springer, Berlin Heidelberg New York

Meltzer HY (1991) The effect of clozapine and other atypical antipsychotic drugs on negative symptoms. In: Marneros A, Andreasen NC, Tsuang MT (eds) Negative vs. positive schizophrenia. Springer, Berlin Heidelberg New York

Möller HJ (1991) Typical neuroleptics in the treatment of positive and negative symptoms. In: Marneros A, Andreasen NC, Tsuang NC (eds) Negative versus positive schizophrenia. Springer, Berlin Heidelberg New York

Mortimer AM, McKenna PJ, Lund CE, Mannuzza S (1989) Rating of negative symptoms using the High Royds Evaluation of Negativity (HEN) Scale. Br J Psychiatry 155 (Suppl 7):89–91

Mundt C (1985) Das Apathiesyndrom der Schizophrenen. Eine psychopathologische und computertomographische Untersuchung. Springer, Berlin Heidelberg New York

Mundt C (1991) Constituting reality – Its decline and repair in the long-term course of schizophrenic psychoses. In: Marneros A, Andreasen NC, Tsuang MT (eds) Negative vs. positive schizophrenia. Springer, Berlin Heidelberg New York

Pickar D, Litman RE, Konicki PE, Wolkowitz OM, Breier A (1990) Neurochemical and neural mechanisms of positive and negative symptoms in schizophrenia. In: Andreasen NC (ed) Schizophrenia: Positive and negative symptoms and syndromes. Karger, Basel

Pogue-Geile MF, Harrow M (1984) Negative and positive symptoms in schizophrenia and depression. Schizophr Bull 10:371–387

Remschmidt H, Martin M, Schulz E, Gutenbrunner C, Fleischhaker C (1991) The concept of "positive and negative schizophrenia" in child and adolscent psychiatry. In: Marneros A, Andreasen NC, Tsuang MT (eds) Negative vs. positive schizophrenia. Springer, Berlin Heidelberg New York

Reynolds JR (1858) On the pathology of convulsions, with special reference to those of children. Liverpool Med Chir J:1–14

Rohde A, Marneros A, Deister A (1991) Premorbid and sociodemographic features of initially positive and initially negative schizophrenia. In: Marneros A, Andreasen NC, Tsuang NC (eds) Negative versus positive schizophrenia. Springer, Berlin Heidelberg New York

Steinmeyer EM, Marneros A, Deister A, Rohde A (1989) Long-term outcome of schizoaffective and schizophrenic disorders: a comparative study. Part II: causal-analytic investigations. Eur Arch Psychiatry Neurol Sci 238:126–134

Stieglitz RD (1991) Assessment of negative symptoms: instruments and evaluation criteria. In: Marneros A, Andreasen NC, Tsuang MT (eds) Negative vs. positive schizophrenia. Springer, Berlin Heidelberg New York

Süllwold L, Huber G (1987) Schizophrene Basisstörungen. Springer, Berlin Heidelberg New York

Tsuang MT, Gilbertson MW, Faraone SV (1991) Genetic transmission of negative and positive symptoms in the biological relatives of schizophrenics. In: Marneros A, Andreasen NC, Tsuang MT (eds) Negative vs. positive schizophrenia. Springer, Berlin Heidelberg New York

van Kammen DP, Peters JL, Yao J, van Kammen WB, Neylan T, Shaw D (1991) Noradrenergic mechanisms, state dependency, and negative symptoms in schizophrenia. In: Greden JF, Tandon R (eds) Negative schizophrenic symptoms: pathophysiology and clinical implications. American Psychiatric Press, Washington DC
Wagman AMI, Heinrichs DW, Carpenter WT (1987) The deficit and non-deficit forms of schizophrenia: neuropsychological evaluation. Psychiatry Res 22:319–330

Subject Index